McGraw-Hill
SPECIALTY BOARD REVIEW

Dermatology

A Pictorial Review

NOTICE

Medicine is an ever-changing science. As new research and clinical experience broaden our knowledge, changes in treatment and drug therapy are required. The authors and the publisher of this work have checked with sources believed to be reliable in their efforts to provide information that is complete and generally in accord with the standards accepted at the time of publication. However, in view of the possibility of human error or changes in medical science, neither the editors nor the publisher nor any other party who has been involved in the preparation or publication of this work warrants that the information contained herein is in every respect accurate or complete, and they disclaim all responsibility for any errors or omissions or for the results obtained from use of the information contained in this work. Readers are encouraged to confirm the information contained herein with other sources. For example and in particular, readers are advised to check the product information sheet included in the package of each drug they plan to administer to be certain that the information contained in this work is accurate and that changes have not been made in the recommended dose or in the contraindications for administration. This recommendation is of particular importance in connection with new or infrequently used drugs.

McGraw-Hill
SPECIALTY BOARD REVIEW

Dermatology

A Pictorial Review

Asra Ali, MD
Assistant Professor
Department of Dermatology
University of Texas at Houston Medical School
Houston, Texas

McGraw-Hill
Medical Publishing Division

New York   Chicago   San Francisco   Lisbon   London   Madrid   Mexico City
Milan   New Delhi   San Juan   Seoul   Singapore   Sydney   Toronto

The McGraw·Hill Companies

Dermatology: A Pictorial Review

Copyright © 2007 by The McGraw-Hill Companies, Inc. All rights reserved.
Printed in China. Except as permitted under the United States Copyright
Act of 1976, no part of this publication may be reproduced or distributed
in any form or by any means, or stored in a data base or retrieval system,
without the prior written permission of the publisher.

1 2 3 4 5 6 7 8 9 0 CTP 0 9 8 7 6

ISBN: 0-07-142293-5

This book was set in Slimbach by TechBooks, Inc.
The editors were Anne M. Sydor, Karen G. Edmonson, and Peter J. Boyle.
The production supervisor was Sherri Souffrance.
The indexer was Kathrin Unger.
China Translation and Printing Services was printer and binder.

This book is printed on acid-free paper.

Cataloging-in-Publication data is on file with the Library of Congress.

International ISBN: 0-07-110547-6
Copyright © 2007. Exclusive right by The McGraw-Hill Companies, Inc. for
manufacture and export. This book cannot be re-exported from the coun-
try to which it is consigned by McGraw-Hill. The International Edition is
not available in North America.

CONTENTS

CONTRIBUTORS

A. Sohail Ahmed, MD
Assistant Professor of Medicine
Division of Rheumatology
Department of Medicine
Boston University School of Medicine
Boston, Massachusetts

Asra Ali, MD
Assistant Professor
Department of Dermatology
University of Texas at Houston Medical School
Houston, Texas

Nishath Ali, MD
Chief Resident, Obstetrics and Gynecology
Department of Obstetrics and Gynecology
Baylor College of Medicine
Houston, Texas

Vaseem Ali, MD
Associate Professor
Department of Obstetrics and Gynecology
University of Texas at Houston Medical School
Houston, Texas

Syed Azhar, MD
Associate Professor
Department of Family Medicine
University of Texas, Medical Branch
Galveston, Texas

Rajesh Balkrishnan, PhD
Merrell Dow Professor
Ohio State University School of Public Health and College
    of Pharmacy
Columbus, Ohio

Holly Bartell, BS
Medical Student-IV
Department of Dermatology
University of Texas at Houston Medical School
Houston, Texas

Melissa A. Bogle, MD
Clinical Assistant Professor
Department of Dermatology
University of Texas, M.D. Anderson Cancer Center
Houston, Texas

Jennifer Clay Cather, MD
Professor
Department of Dermatology
Co-Director, CTCL and GVHD Clinic
Baylor University Medical Center
Dallas, Texas

Nor Chiao, MD
Resident in Dermatology
Department of Dermatology
University of Texas, M.D. Anderson Cancer Center
Houston, Texas

Fran E. Cook-Bolden
Assistant Professor
Department of Dermatology
Columbia University
New York, New York

Manuel Davila, MD
Clinical Dermatologist
Southeast Harris County Dermatology Associates, PA
Pasadena, Texas

A. Hafeez Diwan, MD, PhD
Assistant Professor of Dermatology
Division of Pathology and Laboratory Medicine
Department of Anatomic Pathology
University of Texas, M.D. Anderson Cancer Center
Houston, Texas

Madeleine Duvic, MD
Professor and Deputy Chair
Division of Internal Medicine
Department of Dermatology
University of Texas, M.D. Anderson Cancer Center
Houston, Texas

Adrienne M. Feasel, MD
Ladera Park Dermatology
Austin, Texas

Adelaide A. Hebert, MD
Professor of Dermatology and Pediatrics
Department of Dermatology
University of Texas at Houston Medical School
Houston, Texas

Kelly L. Herne, MD
Advanced Dermatology
Houston, Texas

Sylvia Hsu, MD
Professor
Department of Dermatology
Baylor College of Medicine
Houston, Texas

Jennifer L. Jones, MD
Instructor in Dermatology
Department of Dermatology
Harvard Medical School
Boston, Massachusetts

Robert E. Jordon, MD
Professor
Department of Dermatology
University of Texas at Houston Medical School
Houston, Texas

Rajani Katta, MD
Assistant Professor
Department of Dermatology
Baylor College of Medicine
Houston, Texas

Mark LaRocco, PhD
Adjunct Associate Professor
Department of Pathology and Laboratory Medicine
University of Texas at Houston Medical School
Houston, Texas

Victor R. Lavis, MD
Professor
Division of Endocrinology
Department of Internal Medicine
University of Texas at Houston Medical School
Houston, Texas

Steven Marcet, MD
Dermatologist
Newnan Dermatology
Newnan, Georgia

Ramsey Markus, MD
Assistant Professor of Dermatology
Department of Dermatology
Baylor College of Medicine
Houston, Texas

Denise W. Metry, MD
Associate Professor
Departments of Dermatology and Pediatrics
Baylor College of Medicine
Houston, Texas

Mark Naylor, MD
Adjunct Assistant Member
Clinical Pharmacology Program
Oklahoma Medical Research Foundation
Oklahoma City, Oklahoma

Tri H. Nguyen, MD
Associate Professor, Dermatology and Otophinolaryngology
Division of Medicine
Department of Dermatology
University of Texas, M.D. Anderson Cancer Center
Houston, Texas

Ida Orengo, MD
Professor
Department of Dermatology
Baylor College of Medicine
Houston, Texas

Victoria G. Ortiz, MD
Resident
Department of Dermatology
University of Texas at Houston Health Science Center
Houston, Texas

Danette M. Persyn, MD
Private Practice
Houston, Texas

Clare Pipkin, MD
Instructor
Department of Dermatology
Beth Israel Deaconess Medical Center
Boston, Massachusetts

Victor G. Prieto, MD, PhD
Professor
Division of Pathology and Laboratory Medicine
Department of Anatomic Pathology
University of Texas, M.D. Anderson Cancer Center
Houston, Texas

Bryan Selkin, MD
Instructor of Dermatology
Department of Dermatology
Beth Israel Deaconess Medical Center
Boston, Massachusetts

Benjamin Solky, MD
Winchester, Massachusetts

Tahniat S. Syed, MD, MPH
Assistant Professor of Pediatrics
Division of Adolescent Medicine
Department of Pediatrics
St. Christopher's Hospital for Children
Philadelphia, Pennsylvania

Marziah Thurber, MD
Resident
Mount Sinai Medical Center
Miami, Florida

Stephen K. Tyring, MD, PhD, MBA
Professor
Department of Dermatology
University of Texas at Houston Health Science Center
Houston, Texas

Genevieve Wallace, MD
Dermatology Resident, PGY2
Department of Dermatology
University of Texas at Houston Health Science Center
Houston, Texas

Stephen E. Wolverton, MD
Professor of Clinical Dermatology
Department of Dermatology
Indiana University School of Medicine
Indianapolis, Indiana

CHAPTER 1

HAIR FINDINGS

MELISSA A. BOGLE
ASRA ALI

- Development
  - Follicles formed during 3rd month of gestation; form first on head
  - Lining of follicle = ectodermal origin
  - Dermal papilla = mesodermal origin
  - Epidermal invaginations occur at an angle to the surface and over sites of mesenchymal cell collections
  - Eventually these epidermal cells form a column that surrounds the mesenchymal dermal papilla to form the bulb
  - The dermal papilla (along with "stem" cells in the bulge) induce hair follicle formation by the overlying epithelium
  - Additionally, two or three other collections of cells form along the follicle
    - Upper collection becomes the mantle from which the sebaceous gland will develop
    - Lower swelling becomes the attachment for the arrector pili muscle and where follicle germinal cells reside in telogen phase
    - If a third collection of cells exists, it is found opposite and superior to the sebaceous gland and develops into the apocrine gland
- Structure (Fig. 1-1)
  - Longitudinal structure: seven regions of the hair follicle (superior to inferior)
    - Permanent portion of the hair follicle
      - ▲ Hair canal region: distinct only during fetal development; from skin surface to the dermal-epidermal junction
      - ▲ Infundibulum
      - ▲ Area of the sebaceous gland
      - ▲ Isthmus: begins at sebaceous gland and ends at the bulge (site of insertion of arrector pili muscle)
      - ▲ Area of the bulge: site of insertion of the arrector pili muscle
    - Transient portion of the hair follicle (also called matrix): contains melanocytes
      - ▲ Lower hair follicle
      - ▲ Hair bulb: envelopes the dermal papilla; contains the critical line of Auber at the widest diameter; below the critical line of Auber is the bulk of mitotic activity
  - Microscopic structure (Fig. 1-2)
    - The hair follicle is arranged in concentric circles (from outer to inner)
      - ▲ Basement membrane (glassy membrane): PAS-positive, acellular; thin during anagen and thickens during catagen
      - ▲ Outer root sheath (ORS): present the length of the follicle; never keratinizes; stays fixed in place
      - ▲ Inner root sheath (IRS): grows toward cell surface
        - △ Henle's layer: one cell thick and first to cornify
        - △ Huxley's layer: two cells thick; eosinophilic-staining trichohyalin granules
        - △ Cuticle
    - Hair shaft: grows toward cell surface; cornifies without trichohyalin or keratohyalin granules
      - ▲ Cuticle: shingle-like hair cells that interlock with cuticle cells of IRS
      - ▲ Cortex: arises from cells in center of hair bulb; disulfide bonds in this region give hair its tensile strength; keratinizes to form shaft; contains pigment of hair
      - ▲ Medulla: contains melanosomes; found only in terminal hairs
  - Hair cycle: Follicles cycle in a mosaic pattern (adjacent hairs in different stages) (Fig. 1-3)
    - Anagen: growth phase, stages I–VI
      - ▲ 84 percent of hair follicles at any one time; last a few months to 7 years
      - ▲ Cells in the hair bulb are actively dividing

1

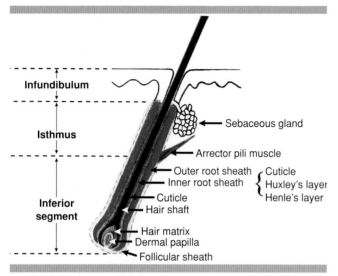

FIGURE 1-1 Diagram of a normal anagen hair follicle. *(From Freedberg IM et al: Fitzpatrick's Dermatology in General Medicine, 6th ed. New York: McGraw-Hill, 2003, p. 633.)*

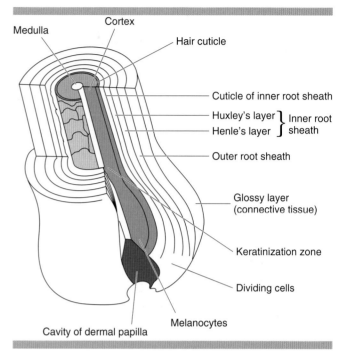

FIGURE 1-2 Diagrammatic representation of the cross section of a hair shaft. *(From Freedberg IM et al: Fitzpatrick's Dermatology in General Medicine, 6th ed. New York: McGraw-Hill, 2003, p. 150.)*

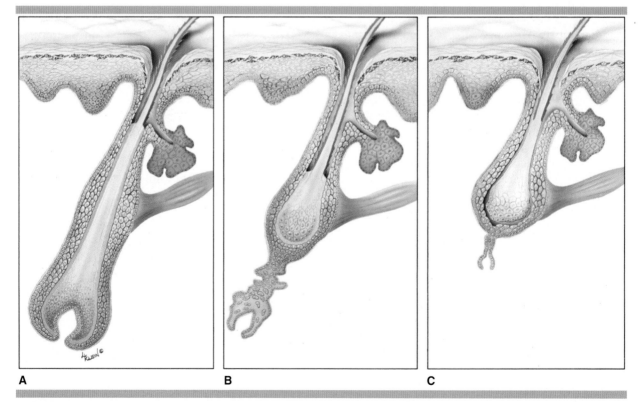

A   B   C

FIGURE 1-3 Changes during hair growth. **A.** Anagen (growth stage). **B.** Catagen (degenerative stage). **C.** Telogen (resting stage). *(From Freedberg IM et al: Fitzpatrick's Dermatology in General Medicine, 6th ed. New York: McGraw-Hill, 2003, p. 151.)*

TABLE 1-1 Effects of Medications/Hormones on Hair

Substance	Effect on Hair Growth
Androgens	Shortens duration of anagen in androgen-sensitive areas of scalp; enlarges follicles in androgen-dependent areas
Estrogen	Prolongs anagen; postpartum decrease in estrogen can cause telogen effluvium
Growth hormone	Synergistic with androgens
Prolactin	Hirsutism
Thyroxine	High or low level can cause telogen effluvium
Oral contraceptives	Telogen effluvium when stopped
Finasteride	Prolongs anagen phase for scalp hairs; may convert vellus to terminal
Minoxidil	Induces and prolongs anagen phase
Cyclosporine	Hypertrichosis
Retinoids	Telogen effluvium due to early onset of catagen

– Catagen: transitional or degenerative stage
- ▲ 2 percent of hair follicles at any one time
- ▲ Last a few days to weeks
- ▲ Matrix cells have stopped dividing
- ▲ Incomplete keratinization
- ▲ Thickened basement membrane (glassy layer)
- ▲ Transient, lower portion of follicle is broken down

– Telogen: resting phase
- ▲ 14 percent of hair follicles at any one time
- ▲ Last about 3 months
- ▲ "Club hair"; no inner root sheath
- ▲ Dermal papilla retracted to higher position in dermis

• Hair pigmentation
- – Pigment comes from melanocytes located in the matrix, above the dermal papilla
- – Eumelanin: pigment of brown-black hair
- – Pheomelanin: pigment of blonde-red hair
- – Loss of melanocytes causes graying of hair—poliosis (can be seen in regrowth of hair after alopecia areata)

• Hair growth
- – Hair grows approximately 0.35–0.37 mm/day
- – Longer anagen phase = longer hair
- – Medications can affect hair growth (see Table 1-1)

HAIR DISORDERS

Alopecia, Nonscarring

1. Alopecia areata (Fig. 1-4)
   - Abrupt onset ± exclamation-point hairs
   - Follicular damage in anagen; then rapid transformation into telogen
   - Patchy hair loss
   - Alopecia totalis: total scalp hair loss
   - Alopecia universalis: total scalp and body hair loss
   - Ophiasis: localized hair loss along the periphery of the scalp
   - Nails: pitting, mottled lunula, trachyonychia, or onychomadesis
   - Histology: peribulbar infiltrate of T cells and macrophages ("swarm of bees")
   - Associations: vitiligo, diabetes mellitus, pernicious anemia, systemic lupus erythematosus (other autoimmune conditions)
   - Treatment: intralesional steroids, topical steroids, prednisone, topical immunotherapy [squaric acid dibutylester (SADBE) and diphencyprone (DPCP)], anthralin, psoralen plus ultraviolet A (UV-A), cyclosporine, tacrolimus

2. Androgenetic alopecia
   - Hereditary thinning in genetically susceptible men and women

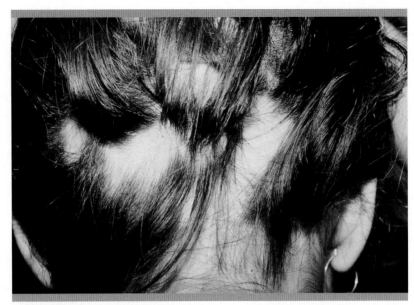

FIGURE 1-4 Alopecia areata. *(Courtesy of Dr. Ali Asra.)*

- Anagen shortens, follicles become smaller, miniaturized hairs, number of follicles remains the same
- Linked to conversion of testosterone to dihydrotestosterone (DHT) by 5α-reductase (type II, outer root sheath and dermal papillae of hair follicles) at hair follicles
- Male pattern: frontotemporal recession and vertex balding (Hamilton-Norwood stages) (Fig. 1-5)
- Female pattern: diffuse thinning over the vertex and parietal scalp (Fig. 1-6)
- Histology: miniaturization, increased vellus-to-terminal-hair ratio
- Treatment: 5α-reductase inhibited by finasteride
- Minoxidil: peripheral vasodilator, increases the number of follicles in anagen, converts vellus hairs to terminal hairs
- Surgical treatment: hair transplantation with minigrafts and micrografts

3. Triangular (temporal) alopecia (Fig. 1-7)
   - Triangular patch of vellus hairs or complete hair loss
   - Frontal-temporal region
   - Histology: vellus hairs
   - No treatment, usually persistent

4. Loose anagen syndrome
   - Fair-haired children with easily dislodgable hair
   - Examination reveals sparse growth of thin, fine hair and diffuse or patchy alopecia
   - Anagen hairs are easily and painlessly pulled from scalp
   - Diagnosis: Epilated hairs are predominantly in anagen phase; trichograms (forcible hair plucks) reveal an abnormally large percentage of anagen hairs lacking inner and outer sheaths
   - Histology: ruffled cuticle, distorted anagen bulb; premature and abnormal keratinization of the inner root sheath
   - Improves with age

5. Telogen effluvium
   - Hair shedding, often with an acute onset
   - Reactive process caused by a reaction to physical or mental stressors; any drug can potentially cause it
   - A large number of hairs shift from anagen to telogen at one time
   - Telogen hairs move back to anagen in 3–4 months following the inciting event; hair density may take 6–12 months to return to baseline
   - The percentage of hairs in telogen rarely goes beyond 50 percent
   - Forced extraction of 10–20 hairs; diagnosis is made if greater than 25 percent of extracted hairs are in telogen
   - Histology: increased number of telogen hairs
   - Prognosis: Recovery is spontaneous and occurs within 6 months

6. Anagen effluvium
   - Always abnormal to shed anagen hairs
   - Hair usually broken off and not shed
   - Radiation therapy and chemotherapy agents
   - Hair shafts are abruptly thinned (Pohl-Pinkus constructions) and break off at skin surface
   - Other causes: mercury intoxication, boric acid intoxication, thallium poisoning, colchicine, severe protein deficiency
   - Histology: normal follicles

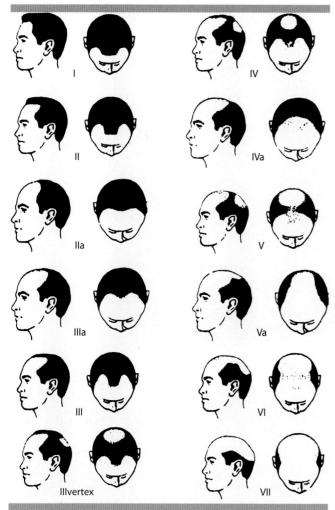

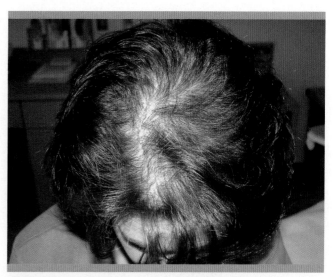

FIGURE 1-6 Androgenetic alopecia, typical female pattern. *(Courtesy of Dr. Adelaide Hebert.)*

FIGURE 1-5 Androgenetic alopecia in men. Hamilton-Norwood classification. *(From Olsen EA et al: Female pattern hair loss. J Am Acad Dermatol 45:S70, 2001.)*

- Scarring alopecia can result
- Treatment: keratolytics, improves with age
9. Traction alopecia (Fig. 1-9)
   - Prolonged traction on the scalp by physical pressure: tight braids, foam rollers, tight pony tail
   - Hair loss may be persistent if the traction is unrelenting
10. Endocrine related
    - Hypothyroidism: sparse, coarse, dry, brittle hair
    - Hyperthyroidism: sparse, fine hair
    - Androgen-dominant oral contraceptives: androgenetic alopecia

7. Trichotillomania
   - Impulse-control disorder
   - Repeated plucking or pulling of hairs
   - Confluence of short sparse hairs within an otherwise normal area of the scalp
   - Varying lengths of regrowth
   - Microscopic examination: tapered tips of newly regrowing anagen hairs or bluntly cut hairs
   - Histology: pigment casts, increased catagen hairs, trichomalacia
   - Treatment: psychological intervention and/or medication to modify behavior; clomipramine
8. Pityriasis amiantacea (Fig. 1-8)
   - Thick scale, matted hair
   - May mimic severe seborrheic dermatitis or psoriasis; however, hair that is involved is dislodged on attempts to physically remove the scale

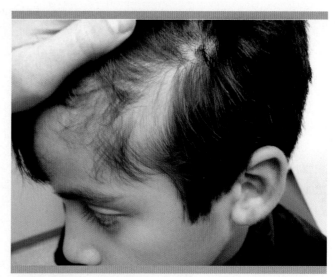

FIGURE 1-7 Triangular alopecia. *(Courtesy of Dr. Adelaide Hebert.)*

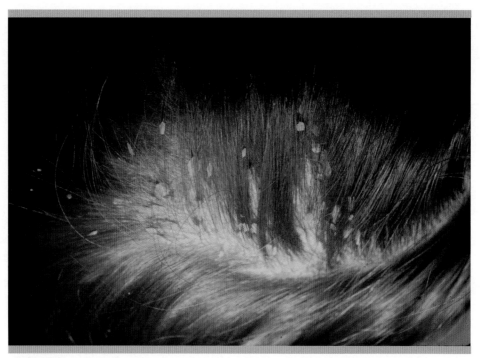

FIGURE 1-8 Pityriasis amiantacea. *(Courtesy of Dr. Adelaide Hebert.)*

Alopecia, Scarring

1. Pseudopelade (of Brocq)
   - End-stage scarring alopecia
   - Oval or irregularly shaped atrophic patches with area of hair growth ("footprints in the snow")
   - Histology: atrophy, perifollicular inflammation at the level of the infundibulum, loss of sebaceous epithelium, fibrotic streams into the subcutis

2. Lichen planopilaris
   - Perifollicular erythema and/or a violaceous discoloration of the scalp
   - > 50 percent associated with cutaneous or oral lichen planus
   - Involves scalp alone or scalp and other hair-bearing areas (Graham Little syndrome)
   - Frontal fibrosing alopecia: frontotemporal hairline recession and eyebrow loss in postmenopausal

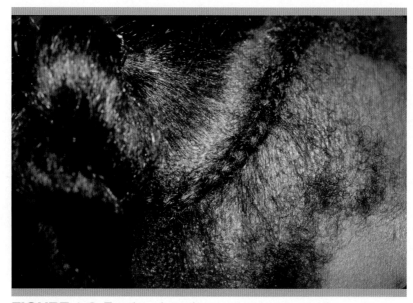

FIGURE 1-9 Traction alopecia.

women that is associated with perifollicular erythema, especially along the hairline
- Histology: lichenoid interface dermatitis of the superficial follicular epithelium

3. Aplasia cutis congenita
   - Congenital absence of skin and subcutaneous tissue; may involve cranium
   - Coin-sized defect or larger
   - Often midline scalp vertex
   - Hair collar sign: ring of dark hair encircling aplasia lesion; suggests neural tube defect
   - Adams-Oliver syndrome: severe aplasia cutis congenita, cutis marmorata telangiectatica congenita, limb defects, and atrial septal defect

4. Lupus erythematosus
   - Chronic cutaneous (discoid) lupus erythematosus: erythema, scarring alopecia; dilated follicles ± keratin plugs
   - Systemic lupus erythematosus: diffuse, nonscarring alopecia; broken hairs in frontal region ("lupus hairs")
   - Diagnostic biopsy and direct immunofluorescence
   - Treatment: topical, intralesional, or oral steroids; systemic retinoids; antimalarials

5. Central centrifugal cicatricial alopecia (CCCA)
   - Follicular degeneration syndrome; hot-comb alopecia
   - Follicular loss mainly on the crown of the scalp
   - Possibly secondary to tight braids, ponytails, hair straighteners, or curlers

- Histology: premature desquamation of the inner root sheath, mononuclear infiltrate at the isthmus, loss of the follicular epithelium with fibrosis

6. Alopecia mucinosa (follicular mucinosis)
   - Erythmatous plaques or flat patches without hair
   - Children: head and neck, benign, self-resolving
   - Adults: more widespread distribution; may be associated with cutaneous T-cell lymphoma
   - Histology: mucin in the outer root sheath and sebaceous glands, perifollicular lymphohistiocytic infiltrate

7. Acne keloidalis (Fig. 1-10)
   - Follicular pustules and papules that progress to firm, keloidal papules
   - Commonly on occiput of African-Americans
   - Foreign-body reaction to trapped hair shaft fragments
   - Often bacterial superinfection
   - Histology: follicular dilatation and mixed peri-infundibular infiltrate with follicular rupture and foreign-body granulomas
   - Treatment: systemic antibiotics, topical and/or intralesional steroids

8. Dissecting folliculitis
   - Perifolliculitis capitis abscedens et suffodiens of Hoffman
   - Suppurative folliculitis
   - Fluctuant nodules on vertex, occiput
   - Histology: sinus tracts, sterile abscesses
   - Treatment: systemic steroids, systemic antibodies, dapsone, retinoids, surgical excision

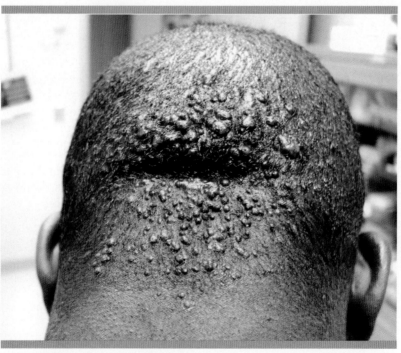

FIGURE 1-10 Acne keloidalis.

9. Folliculitis decalvans
   - Bogginess of scalp with pustules and erosions
   - *Staphylococcus aureus* cultured
   - Histology: acute suppurative folliculits with neutrophils and eosinophils; later mixed with lymphocytes and histiocytes
   - Loss of sebaceous epithelium and perifollicular fibrosis
   - Treatment: systemic antibiotics with or without rifampin, systemic and/or topical steroids, systemic retinoids

10. Morphea
    - En coup de sabre: linear morphea on frontal scalp and forehead
    - Parry-Romberg syndrome: linear morphea with alopecia, facial hemiatrophy, epilepsy, and exophthalmos

Genetic Syndromes (Table 1-2)

1. Anhidrotic ectodermal dysplasia (Christ-Siemens-Touraine syndrome)
   - X-linked recessive form associated with defect in Ectodysplasin, pegged teeth

TABLE 1-2 Hair Shaft Disorders

Hair Finding	Microscopic Description	Associations
Trichorrhexis nodosa	Frayed nodes spaced along hair (brooms stuck end to end)	Most common hair shaft dystrophy Congenital or acquired Arginosuccinic aciduria, Menkes' kinky hair syndrome, citrullinemia, trichothiodystrophy Acquired disease: Proximal: common in black female hair after chemical or hot comb straightening Distal: excessive brushing
Pili trianguli et cannaliculi	Hair has triangular cross section with longitudinal groove on electron microscopy	Uncombable hair syndrome
Flag sign	Intermittent reddish discoloration of hair	Kwashiorkor, anorexia nervosa
Trichorrhexis invaginata	"Bamboo hair" with intussusception of the hair shaft (ball and socket)	Netherton's syndrome; abnormal keratinization of hair shaft in the keratogenous zone
Pili torti	Twisted flattened from 90–360 degrees, multiple irregular intervals	Björnstad syndrome, citrullinemia, Menkes' kinky hair syndrome, Crandall's syndrome, Bazex's syndrome, Salamon's syndrome, Beare's syndrome, trichothiodystrophy, isotretinoin therapy
Monilithrix	Elliptical nodes with a regular periodicity of 0.7–1 mm between nodes, hair shaft is constricted (fractures common)	Autosomal dominant variable expressivity; short, brittle hairs emerging from keratotic follicular papules
Pili annulati	"Zebra-striped hair" with alternating segments of light and dark color due to air cavities	Pili annulati
Trichoschisis	Clean transverse break along hair shaft where a local absence of cuticle is present	Trichothiodystrophy

- Rare autosomal dominant, autosomal recessive forms associated with defect in NEMO gene, immunodeficiency disorders
- Thin, sparse hair
- Absent pilosebaceous units in Blaschko's lines
- Hypohidrosis, atopic dermatitis, nail dystrophy
- Abnormal facies: saddle nose, frontal bossing, thick lips, and peg teeth
- Hair has longitudinal groove on electron microscopy
- Female carriers must be watched for hyperpyrexia

2. Argininosuccinic aciduria
- Autosomal recessive decrease in argininosuccinase
- Most common urea cycle defect
- Hyperammonemia, failure to thrive, hepatomegaly, seizures, ataxia, mental retardation
- Trichorrhexis nodosa
- Low-protein diet and arginine supplementation may reverse hair anomalies

3. Björnstad syndrome
- Pili torti (spares eyelashes)
- Bilateral sensorineural deafness correlates with the severity of hair defects
- Crandall syndrome is pili torti and deafness with hypogonadism

4. Hidrotic ectodermal dysplasia (Clouston's syndrome)
- Autosomal dominant defect in gap junction protein (connexin 30)
- Thin, sparse hair after puberty
- Palmoplantar keratoderma, nail dystrophy, bulbous fingertips, tufted terminal phalanges
- Normal sweating, facies, and dentition

5. KID syndrome
- Autosomal dominant mutation in gap junction protein GJP2 (connexin 26)
- Keratitis ($\pm$ blindness), ichthyosis, and deafness
- Scarring alopecia, dystrophic nails

6. Menkes kinky hair syndrome
- XLR defect in MKHD gene (copper transport ATPase 7A)
- Decreased serum copper and ceruloplasmin with increased copper in all organs *except* the liver
- Sparse, light-colored, "steel wool" hair; pili torti (most common), trichorrhexis nodosa
- Skin is pale with laxity and a "doughy" consistency
- Progressive cerebral degeneration

- Radiologic findings: wormian bones in cranial sutures, metaphyseal widening, spurs in long bones
- Tortuous arteries, genitourinary anomalies

7. Monilothrix
- Autosomal dominant defect in keratins 1 and 6
- See Table 1-2

8. Netherton's syndrome
- Autosomal recessive defect in *SPINK5*
- Ichthyosis linearis circumflexa, atopic dermatitis
- Trichorrhexis invaginata (bamboo hair) is the most common hair abnormality, but trichorrhexis invaginata is the most characteristic

9. Piebaldism
- Autosomal dominant defect in *C-KIT*
- White forelock, depigmented patches on ventral midline

10. Trichothiodystropy
- Autosomal recessive defect in *XPB/ERCC3* DNA repair transcription gene (analogous to xeroderma pigmentosum group D)
- Ataxia but no freckling or UV-induced skin cancers
- Trichoschisis, banding with polarized microscopy ("tiger tail")
- Hairs have 50 percent reduction in sulfur (cysteine) content
- PIBIDS: photosensitivity, intellectual impairment, brittle hair, ichthyosis, decreased fertility and short stature

11. Uncombable hair syndrome
- Autosomal dominant or sporadic
- Defect: an abnormal configuration of inner root sheath that keratinizes before the hair shaft
- Blonde, shiny, "spun glass" hair
- Electron microscopy: pili trianguli et canaliculi, longitudinal groove, triangular shape on cross section
- Lashes and brows are not affected
- Biotin may help symptoms

12. Wooly hair
- Autosomal dominant
- Negroid hair on the scalp of person of non-Negroid background
- Involves only scalp hair
- Microscopy: hair shaft tightly coiled
- Improves with age

13. Cronkhite-Canada syndrome
- Sporadic
- Extensive alopecia
- Melanotic macules on the fingers, gastrointestinal polyposis, generalized hyperpigmentation, onychodystrophy, malabsorption/diarrhea

TABLE 1-3 Presentations of Tinea Capitis

Tinea	Fungus	Treatment
"Black dot" tinea: alopecia with pinpoint black dots (infected hairs that have broken off) (see Fig. 1-9)	*Trichophyton tonsurans*, endothrix	Griseofulvin 20–25 mg/kg per day; terbinafine, itraconazole
Kerion: boggy lesions with crust, severe inflammatory reaction (see Fig. 1-10)	*T. mentagrophytes, T. verrucosum*	Griseofulvin 20–25 mg/kg per day; terbinafine, itraconazole
Favus: large crust of matted hyphae (scutula)	*T. schoenleinii*	Griseofulvin 20–25 mg/kg per day; terbinafine, itraconazole

Infectious

1. Tinea capitis (Table 1-3; Fig. 1-11 and 1-12)
2. Piedra
   - Gritty nodules on the hair in temperate climates
   - White piedra is caused by *Trichosporon beigelii*
   - Black piedra is caused by *Piedraia hortai*
3. Syphilis (Fig. 1-13)
   - Moth-eaten alopecia
4. Trichomycosis nodosa
   - Granular sheath around hair shaft
   - Axilla or pubic area
   - *Corynebacterium tenuis,* poor hygiene

Miscellaneous

1. Pseudofolliculitis (Fig. 1-14)
   - Occurs at any site where hair is shaved, most common in beard
   - Curved hair follicle
   - Ingrown hairs, foreign-body reaction
2. Green hair
   - Reaction to copper in pools
   - Treat with chelating agents
3. Bubble hair
   - Brittle, fragile hair from excessive heat
   - Hairdryers, straightening irons

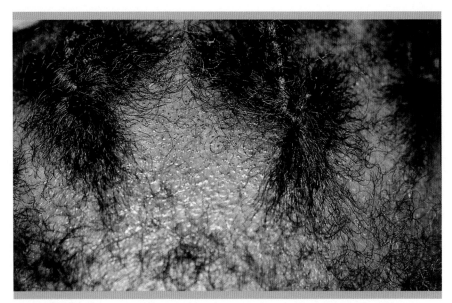

FIGURE 1-11 Tinea capitis: black dot variant. *(From Wolff K et al. Fitzpatrick's Color Atlas & Synposis of Clinical Dermatology, 5th ed. New York: McGraw-Hill, 2005, p. 709.)*

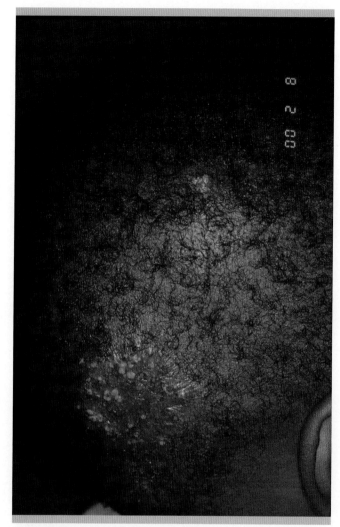

FIGURE 1-12 Kerion on scalp.

4. Acquired progressive kinking
- Kinking and twisting of hair shaft at irregular intervals
- Most common in young men in frontotemporal or vertex scalp as a precursor of androgenetic alopecia
- Rarely occurs in women or prepubertal men without progression to alopecia
- Widespread kinking of the hair: AIDS, drugs (retinoids)

Hypertrichosis

- Overgrowth of hair not localized to androgen-dependent areas
- Local congenital or acquired hypertrichosis: melanocytic nevi, Becker's nevus (smooth muscle hamartoma), meningioma, porphyria, spinal dysraphism
- Generalized congenital hypertrichosis: X-linked dominant congenital hypertrichosis lanuginosa, fetal hydantoin syndrome, fetal alcohol syndrome

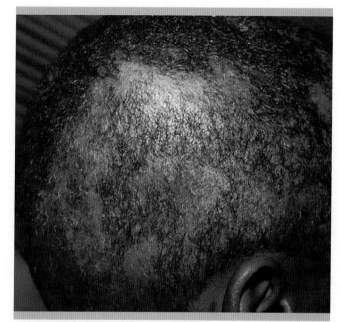

FIGURE 1-13 Syphilis. *(Courtesy of Dr. Robert Jordan.)*

- Generalized acquired hypertrichosis: acquired hypertrichosis lanuginosa, internal malignancy, Rubenstein-Taybi, Cornelia de Lange, minoxidil, cyclosporine, phenytoin, anorexia nervosa

Hirsuitism

- Excessive terminal hair growth in androgen-dependent areas
- Usually related to hyperandrogenism
- Polycystic ovarian syndrome: hirsuitism, acne, abnormal periods, obesity
- Ovarian, adrenal, pituitary tumors
- Medications (Table 1-1): androgens, high-progesterone oral contraceptives, minoxidil

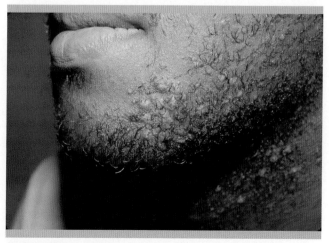

FIGURE 1-14 Pseudofolliculitis. *(Courtesy of Dr. Robert Jordan.)*

REFERENCES

Birnbaum PS, Baden HP: Heritable disorders of hair. *Dermatol Clin* 1987;5:137–153.

Dawber RP: An update of hair shaft disorders. *Dermatol Clin* 1996;14:753–772.

Freedberg IM et al. *Fitzpatrick's Dermatology in General Medicine,* 6th Ed. New York: McGraw-Hill; 2003.

McKee PH. *Pathology of the Skin: With Clinical Correlations.* London: Mosby-Wolfe; 1996.

Mulinari-Brenner F, Bergfeld WF: Hair loss: diagnosis and management. *Cleve Clin J Med* 2003;70:705–712.

Pomeranz AJ, Sabnis SS: Tinea capitis: epidemiology, diagnosis and management strategies. *Paediatr Drugs* 2002;4: 779–783.

Sperling LC, Mezebish DS: Hair diseases. *Med Clin North Am* 1998;82:1155–1169.

Stratigos AJ, Baden HP: Unraveling the molecular mechanisms of hair and nail genodermatoses. *Arch Dermatol* 2001;137: 1465–1471.

Sullivan JR, Kossard S: Acquired scalp alopecia. *Australas J Dermatol* 1998;39:207–219.

CHAPTER 2

EYE FINDINGS

MELISSA A. BOGLE
SYED AZHAR

EYELID ANATOMY (FIG. 2-1)

Upper Eyelid

- Extends superiorly to the eyebrow
- Upper eyelid skin crease (usually 8–12 mm superior to eyelid margin where muscle fibers of pretarsal orbicularis, levator aponeurosis, and skin insert onto the superior edge of the tarsus)
- Upper lid retractor: levator palpebrae superioris (LPS) and Müller's muscle
- Lid margin has horizontal row of eye lashes anteriorly and approximately 25 openings of Meibomian glands posteriorly

Lower Lid

- Extends below the inferior orbital rim to join the cheek
- Inferior eyelid fold (usually 3–5 mm inferior to eyelid margin where muscle fibers of orbicularis and capsulopalpebral fascia attach to inverior edge of tarsus)
- Lower eyelid retractors
  - Fascial extension (capsulopalpebral fascia) from the terminal muscle fibers and tendon of the inferior rectus and inferior oblique muscles
  - Lid margin is similar to upper eye lid, with eye lashes in front and openings of Meibomian glands posteriorly
- Nasojugal fold
  - Runs inferiorly and laterally from the inner canthal region, forming the tear trough
- Malar fold
  - Runs inferiorly and medially from the outer canthus toward the inferior aspect of the nasojugal fold
- Interpalpebral fissure
  - Fusiform space between the eyelid margins (usually 10–11 mm in youth; decreases with age to 8–10 mm)

- Tarsal plates
  - Composed of dense fibrous tissue and are responsible for the structural integrity of the lids
- Sensory innervation of the eyelids
- Terminal branches of the ophthalmic [cranial nerve (CN) V1] and maxillary (CN V2) divisions of the trigeminal nerve (CN V)

Glands of the Eyelid

- Zeis glands
  - Small, modified sebaceous glands
  - Open into the hair follicles at the base of the eyelashes
- Meibomian glands
  - Sebaceous glands, present within the tarsus secrete lipid layer of tear film
- Glands of Moll
  - Apocrine glands
  - Located anterior to the meibomian glands within the distal eyelid margin

CONGENITAL ABNORMALITIES

Albinism

- Oculocutaneous albinism
  - Involves both the skin and eyes
  - Divided into approximately 10 different types
  - Mostly autosomal recessive
  - Type I due to tyrosinase defect: results in a decrease in the amount of melanin present in each of the melanosomes chromosome 11
  - Type II: defect in P polypeptide chromosome 15
- Ocular albinism:
  - Mainly affects the eyes with minimal to no skin involvement
  - Four different forms noted near birth with poor vision and nystagmus

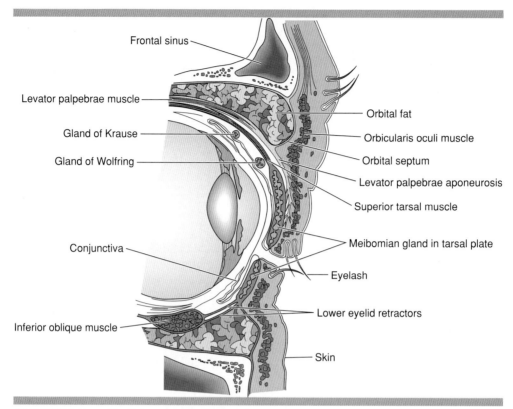

FIGURE 2-1 Eyelid anatomy. *(From Riordan-Eva P, Richter JP: Vaughan & Ashbury's General Ophthalmology, 16th ed. New York: McGraw-Hill, 2004, Fig. 1-22.)*

- Sex-linked or autosomal recessive disease: reduction in the number of melanosomes
- Ocular anomalies
  - Photophobia, refractive errors, strabismus, pendular nystagmus, iris transillumination defects, hypopigmented fundus, foveal hypoplasia, and abnormal decussation of the temporal optic nerve fibers (monocular vision and poor stereopsis and strabissmus)
  - Color of the iris usually is blue (can vary from blue to brown)

- Visual acuity, pupillary reflex responses, and fundi are normal

Juvenile Xanthogranuloma

- Non-Langerhans' histiocytosis with Touton giant cells (under age 2 years)
- Ocular anomalies
  - Ocular involvement is the most common extracutaneous site

ATAXIA-TELANGIECTASIA (LOUIS-BAR SYNDROME) (FIG. 2-2)

- Autosomal recessive
- Defect in *ATM* gene on 11q22-23
- Ocular anomalies
  - Telangiectasia of the bulbar conjunctiva (first appears at 3–5 years)
  - Accelerated aging of skin and vessel changes on eyelids (rare)
  - Strabismus and nystagmus
  - Poor ability to initiate saccades

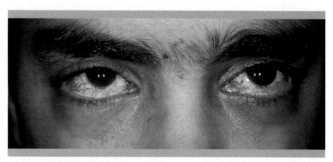

FIGURE 2-2 Ataxia-telangiectasia. *(From Paller AS: Hereditary immunodeficiency disorders, in Alper JC (ed): Genetic Disorders of the Skin. Chicago: Mosby Year Book, 1991, p. 105.)*

- Orbital masses, unilateral glaucoma, yellowish brown iris lesions resulting in iris heterochromia and spontaneous hyphema, uveitis

Nevus of Ota (Ocular Melanocytosis or Melanosis Oculi)

- (See Chap.8, Fig. 8-2.)
- Unilateral congenital pigmentary lesion of sclera (bluish or slate gray)
- May involve eyelid or adjacent skin with dermal hyperplasia (Asians)
- Higher incidence of glaucoma and possibly malignant melanoma

Cockayne's Syndrome (CS)

- CS type 1 is caused by a defect in the Cockayne syndrome type A gene (CSA or ERCC8) located on chromosome 5
- Mutations in the DNA excision repair gene ERCC6 located on band 10q11 cause CS type 2
- AR defect in xeroderma pigmentosum complementation group G (DNA helicase)
- Autosomal recessive disorders
- Ocular anomalies
  - Retinitis pigmentosa ("salt and pepper retina")
  - Cataracts in children younger than 3 years
  - Optic atrophy or optic disk pallor

Gardner Syndrome

- Autosomal dominant
- Mutations in the tumor suppressor adenomatous polyposis coli gene (APC)
- Mutations on the APC gene that correlate with congenital hypertrophy of the retinal pigment epithelium (CHRPE) are between codon 311 on exon 9 and codon 1444 on exon 15
- Bilateral CHRPE
  - Benign hyperpigmented lesion of the retinal pigment epithelium
  - Typically smaller, multiple, and bilateral in Gardner syndrome (50–80 percent)

Hypomelanosis of Ito (Incontinentia Pigmenti Achromians)

- Mosaicism of the X chromosome
- Ocular anomalies
  - Retinal pigment abnormalities: radial hypopigmented streaks, unilateral heterochromic iris, hypopigmentation of the cornea, strabismus, and hypertelorism
  - Cataracts and retinal detachment

Incontinentia Pigmenti (Bloch-Sulzberger Syndrome)

- X-linked dominant defect in NEMO
- Ocular anomalies

- Occurs in one-third of patients, lethal to hemizygous male
- Retina with mottled, diffuse hypopigmentation (nearly pathognomonic)
- Abnormal peripheral retinal vessels with areas of nonperfusion (very common), retrolental membrane formation (pseudoglioma), cataracts, glaucoma, microphthalmos, nystagmus, and strabismus
- Optic atrophy or foveal hypoplasia

Leopard Syndrome (Moynahan Syndrome)

- Lentigines (spares the mucous membranes), electrocardiographic (ECG) conduction defects, ocular hypertelorism, pulmonic stenosis, abnormal genetalia, retardation of growth, deafness

Nail Patella Syndrome

- Also known as hereditary osteoonychodysplasia (HOOD)
- Autosomal dominant
- Defect in gene LMX1B
- Ocular anomalies
  - Lester iris: hyperpigmentation of the pupillary margin of the iris (45 percent of patients)
  - Heterochromia of the iris with cloverleaf deformity, cataracts, microcornea, and glaucoma

CONNECTIVE TISSUE DISORDERS

Ehlers-Danlos Syndrome

- Abnormalities in the synthesis and metabolism of collagen
- Most ocular abnormalities occur in the kyphoscoliosis type (previously known as type VI)
  - Autosomal recessive
  - Defect in lysyl hydroxylase
  - Mutations in the PLOD gene
- Ocular anomalies
  - Retinal detachments, microcornea, myopia, blue sclera, angioid streaks, keratoconus, myopia, lens subluxation, and ocular fragility can lead to a ruptured globe/blindness

Marfan's Syndrome

- Autosomal dominant
- Defect mutations in the fibrillin-1 (FBN1) gene located on chromosome 15q21.1
- Fibrillin needed to form microfibrils
  - Structural component of the suspensory ligament of the lens
- Ocular anomalies
  - Lens subluxation (50–80 percent)
    - Lense tends to displace superotemporally

- – Typically present at birth and is nonprogressive
- – Can result in hyperopic or myopic shift, astigmatism
- Slit-lamp exam
  - – Displaced crystalline lens
  - – Appears as a black crescent at the edge of the lens against a red reflux from the fundus
- Other ocular anomalies
  - – Flat cornea
  - – Increased axial length of the globe resulting in myopia (nearsightedness) and retinal detachment
  - – Glaucoma and cataracts in patients younger than 50 years
  - – Hypoplastic iris or hypoplastic ciliary muscle causing decreased miosis

Osteogenesis Imperfecta

- Autosomal dominant defect of type I collagen synthesis
- Ocular anomalies
  - Type I: Premature arcus senilis, blue sclera
  - Type II: Dark-blue sclera may be present
  - Type III: Sclera of variable hue
  - Type IV: Normal sclera
  - Blue sclera is caused by thinness and transparency of the collagen fibers of the sclera allowing visualization of underlying uvea
  - Also may present with keratoconus, megalocornea, anterior embryotoxon, congenital glaucoma, zonular cataract, dislocated lens, choroidal sclerosis, retinal hemorrhage

Pseudoxanthoma Elasticum (PXE)

- Autosomal recessive
- Defect in *ABCC6* gene
- Cutaneous and ocular findings of PXE are referred to as Grönblad-Strandberg syndrome
- Increased amounts of elastic tissue that become calcified

- Ocular anomalies
  - Angiod streaks:
    - – Dark-red to brown bands that are breaks in the thickened and calcified Bruch membrane
    - – Radiate from the optic nerve
    - – Bruch's membrane is a collagen- and elastin-containing membrane between the retina and the choroid
  - Macular degeneration, retinal hemorrhage, choroidal ruptures

Waardenburg Syndrome (Table 2-1)

- Autosomal dominant defect of neural crest cell migration and differentiation
- Ocular anomalies
  - Dystopia canthorum (most common)
  - Distance between the inner angles of the eyelids is accompanied by increased distance between the inferior lacrimal points
  - Heterochromic irides, bilateral isohypochromia iridis (pale-blue eyes)
  - Strabismus
  - Albinotic fundi: generalized decrease in retinal pigment

Werner Syndrome (Progeria Adultorum)

- Autosomal recessive defect in the *WRN* gene (DNA helicase)
- Ocular anomalies
  - Posterior subcapsular cataracts (20–40 years)

Focal Dermal Hypoplasia of Goltz

- X-linked dominant, Xp22
- Ocular anomalies
  - Heterochromia, irregularity of the pupils, aniridia, lens subluxation
  - Colobomas of the iris, choroid, retina, or optic disc
  - Corneal defects, cloudiness of the vitreous, widely spaced eyes

TABLE 2-1 Waardenburg Syndrome: Defects and Associations

Type	Defect	Associations
I	*PAX3*	Dystopia canthorum, convergent strabismus (blepharophimosis), and reduced visibility of the medial sclera
II	*MITF*	Heterochromia iridium, no dystopia canthorum
III	*PAX3*	Dystopia canthorum
IV	*SOX10*	Hirschsprung's disease

- Microphthalmia, anophthalmia, optic nerve hypoplasia
- Ectropion, ptosis, nystagmus, photophobia, strabismus
- Naegeli syndrome
- Rare autosomal dominant form of ectodermal dysplasia
- Ocular anomalies
  - Dermatoocular syndrome (starting at age 2)
  - Spotlike pigmentation may be present around the mouth and eyes

KERATOTIC DISEASES

Ichthyosis

X-LINKED ICHTHYOSIS
- X-linked recessive
- Abnormal steroid sulfatase
- Ocular anomalies
  - Comma-shaped corneal deposits

LAMELLAR ICHTHYOSIS
- Autosomal recessive
- Abnormal transglutaminase
- Ocular anomalies
  - Ectropion, unilateral megalocornea

Refsum Syndrome
- Phytanic acid oxidase deficiency
- Ocular anomalies
  - Pigmentary retinopathy ("salt and pepper retina"), cataracts, nystagmus, night blindness

Sjögren-Larsson Syndrome
- Fatty alcohol oxidoreductase deficiency
- Ocular anomalies
  - Atypical retinal pigment with "glistening dots," pigmentary retinopathy

Conradi-Hunermann Syndrome
- *PEX7/EBP*
- Ocular anomalies
  - Asymmetric focal cataracts, optic nerve hypoplasia

KID (Keratitis, Ichthyosis, and Deafness) Syndrome
- Gene defect *GJP2/Connexin26*
- Ocular anomalies
  - Keratitis, blindness, photophobia

CHIME Syndrome
- Colobomas of the eye, heart defects, ichthyosiform dermatosis, mental retardation, and ear defects

Vogt-Koyanagi-Harada Syndrome
- (HLA-DR4) Granulomatous uveitis/iridocyclitis, swollen optic disc, chorioditis, vitreous opacities, and serous retinal detachments

VASCULAR DISORDERS

Osler-Weber-Rendu (Hereditary Hemorrhagic Telengiectasia) Syndrome
- Autosomal dominant
- Defects in endoglin and activin receptor-like kinase type I (*ALK-1*) genes
- Ocular anomalies
  - Conjunctival telangiectasias

Capillary Hemangiomas
- One of the most common benign orbital tumors of infancy (females 2:1)
- Benign endothelial cell and vascular channel neoplasms that are typically absent at birth and characteristically have rapid growth in infancy
- Ocular anomalies
  - Morbidity related to space-occupying effects
  - Amblyopia (43–60 percent), astigmatism, strabissmus with eyelid involvement
  - Presentation: unilateral, superonasal, eyelid, or brow lesion

Sturge-Weber Syndrome
- Disease characterized by facial capillary malformation with underlying soft tissue and skeletal hypertrophy, ipsilateral arteriovenous (AV) malformation, cerebral calcification, hemiparesis, hemianopia, contralateral seizures, and some mental deficiency
- Ocular anomalies
  - Glaucomas: 60 percent at birth or early infancy and 30 percent presenting during childhood, almost always unilateral and ipsilateral to the port-wine stain
  - "Tomato catsup" fundus with a bright-red or red-orange color
  - Tortuous conjunctival and episcleral vascular plexuses
  - Choroidal angiomas (indirect binocular ophthalmoscopy)
  - Anisometropic amblyopia

TUMORS

Basal Cell Carcinoma (BCC) (Fig. 2-3)
- Most common epithelial tumor of the eyelid
- Most common location is the lower eyelid (48.9–72.1 percent)

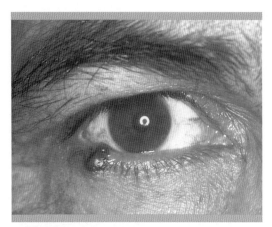

FIGURE 2-3 Basal cell carcinoma. *(From Lowenstein J, Lee S: Ophthalmology: Just the Facts. New York: McGraw-Hill, 2004, p. 75.)*

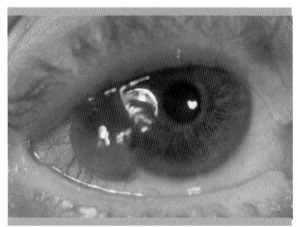

FIGURE 2-5 Melanoma. *(From Lowenstein J, Lee S: Ophthalmology: Just the Facts. New York: McGraw-Hill, 2004, p. 96.)*

- Highest recurrence in lesions arising from the medial canthus (60 percent)
- Nodular BCC most common type

Squamous Cell Carcinoma (SCC) (Fig. 2-4)

- Approximately 5 percent of malignant eyelid tumors
- Incidence of metastasis is 0.23–2.4 percent of cases
- Location of lesion (upper/lower eyelid, medial/lateral/central eyelid); SCC more common on lower eyelid

Sebaceous Cell Carcinoma

- May mimic either a chalazion or chronic blepharitis
- Invades locally and can spread to regional lymph nodes
- Predilection for the upper lid

- Yellowish, firm, painless, indurated papule or ulceration
- May arise from meibomian glands, Zeis glands, or glands associated with the caruncle
- Large anaplastic cells with open vesicular nuclei and prominent nuclei set in foamy or frothy cytoplasm

Melanoma (Fig. 2-5)

- Rare pigmented eyelid tumor
- Must be differentiated from nevi and BCC
- Change in the appearance of a pigmented lesion warrants excisional biopsy of the lesion

Chalazion (Fig. 2-6)

- Granuloma of a meibomian gland

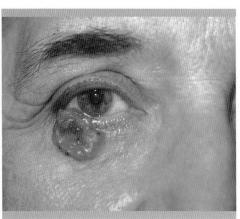

FIGURE 2-4 Squamous cell carcinoma. *(From Lowenstein J, Lee S: Ophthalmology: Just the Facts. New York: McGraw-Hill, 2004, p. 76.)*

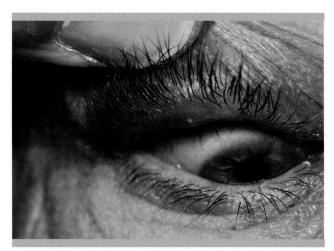

FIGURE 2-6 Chalazion. *(From Knoop K: Atlas of Emergency Medicine. New York: McGraw-Hill, 2002, p. 39.)*

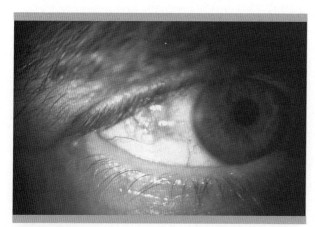

FIGURE 2-7 Nevus. *(From Lowenstein J, Lee S: Ophthalmology: Just the Facts. New York: McGraw-Hill, 2004, p. 92.)*

- Mass of granulation tissue and inflammation owing to lipid breakdown products from retained glandular secretions
- Nontender, firm nodule located deeply within the tarsal plate about 5 mm from the lid margins
- Eversion of the lid may reveal the inflamed meibomian gland

Hydrocystoma

- Translucent cyst located near the lid margin
- Resulting from blockage of the sweat glands of the eyelid

Nevus (Fig. 2-7)

- Nevi are well-demarcated, flat or elevated, pigmented or nonpigmented lesions
- May become more pigmented, more elevated, or cystic during adolescence or young adulthood
- Pigmented lesions that have changed in appearance should be excised

Seborrheic Keratosis

- Benign greasy hyperkeratotic lesions that appear to be stuck on the skin
- Commonly occurring in the elderly, may become irritated occasionally

SYSTEMIC HAMARATOMA SYNDROMES

Tuberous Sclerosis

- Autosomal dominant and spontaneous mutations
- Hamartin and tuberin found on chromosomes 9 and 16, respectively

- Ocular anomalies
  - Hypopigmented macule in the iris, seizures
  - Retinal hamaratomas (phakomas): whitish gray nodular lumps with a mulberriy appearance, glial cell in origin and may calcify, some lesions are flat and smooth
  - Nystagmus and angioid streaks

Neurofibromatosis I

- Autosomal dominant, nearly half are sporadic
- Neurofibromin gene found on 17q11.2
- Ocular anomalies
  - Lisch nodules (iris hamaratomas) (Fig. 2-8)
  - Hamartomas of the iris (tan nodules develop in childhood)
  - Asymptomatic dome-shaped nodules
  - Found on slit-lamp examination
    - Plexiform neurofibroma of the orbit or eyelid leading to glaucoma and ptosis, choroidal lesions (nevi), optic nerve gliomas, ectropion uveae, retinal hamartoma, prominent corneal nerves, sphenoid wing dysplasia

Neurofibromatosis II

- Autosomal dominant, rare melanocytic and cutaneous lesions
- Schwannomin gene codes for Merlin on chromosome 22
- Bilateral acoustic neuromas, meningiomas, schwannomas, and ependymomas
- Juvenile posterior subcapsular cataract

Von-Hippel–Lindau Syndrome

- Autosomal dominant inheritance with variable penetrance

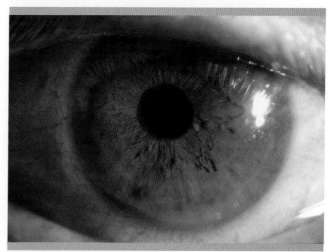

FIGURE 2-8 Lisch nodules. *(From Freedberg IM et al: Fitzpatrick's Dermatology in General Medicine, 6th ed. New York: McGraw-Hill, 2003, p. 1828.)*

- Gene on chromosome 3
- Ocular anomalies
  - Congenital capillary angiomatous hamartomas of the retina (50 percent of patients)
  - Serum leakage from these vessels
  - In patients with retinal angiomas, 25 percent have associated cerebellar hemangioblastomas
  - Congenital capillary angiomatous hamartomas of the optic nerve
  - Visual complications of retinal angiomas include macular exudation, retinal detachment, vitreous hemorrhage, cataract, glaucoma, and nerve damage
- Treatment: argon laser photocoagulation, cryotherapy, or irradiation, fluid drainage, scleral buckling, penetrating diathermy, vitreous surgery
- Angiomas have a poor prognosis unless they are treated

COLLAGEN-VASCULAR DISEASES

Sjögren's Syndrome

- Autoimmune condition (SSA and SSB antigens)
- Human leukocyte antigen B8 (HLA-B8) and DR3 antigens
- Ocular anomalies
  - Xerophthalmia, keratoconjunctivitis sicca, punctate keratopathy, uveitis, optic neuritis, scleritis

Relapsing Polychondritis (RP)

- Episodic inflammatory condition involving cartilaginous structures
- Ocular anomalies
  - Decreased visual acuity, conjunctivitis, episcleritis, scleritis, uveitis, retinopathy, diplopia, and eyelid swelling

Polyarteritis Nodosa (PAN)

- Disease with necrotizing inflammation of medium- or small-sized arteries
- Ocular anomalies
  - Hypertensive and ischemic retinopathy, central nervous system (CNS) lesions resulting in visual loss, CN palsies, scleritis, marginal corneal ulceration, interstitial keratitis

Dermatomyositis (DM)

- Heliotrope rash, violaceous to dusky erythematous rash
- With or without edema in a symmetric distribution involving the periorbital skin
- Rare ophthalmoplegia owing to myositis of extraocular muscles

Wegener Granulomatosis (WG)

- Autoimmune inflammatory process with necrotizing granulomas
- Antineutrophil cytoplasmic antibodies (c-ANCA) directed at neutrophil proteinase 3 (PR-3), ocular involvement (29–58 percent)
- Nodular scleritis, peripheral keratitis, orbital pseudotumor, and retinal vasculitis

Sarcoidosis (Fig. 2-9)

- Multisystem granulomatous disease of unknown etiology
- Lacrimal gland and conjunctival granulomatous nodules, interstitial keratitis
- Cataract and glaucoma: complication of uveitis and/or the corticosteroid treatment
- Anterior uveitis: most common ocular manifestation of sarcoidosis with mutton fat keratic precipitates, iris nodules (Busacca and Koeppe), iris synechae
- Glaucoma: both open-angle and angle-closure
- Retinal neovascularization, periphlebitis, perivascular cuffing and exudates
- Vitreous cavity inflammation (pars planitis), choriodal lesions
- Rarely neurosarcoid: granulomas of the optic nerve (CN II) along with oculomotor nerves (CNs III, IV, and VI)
  - May cause diplopia, ptosis, or paresis of extraocular muscles
- Heerfordt syndrome (uveoparotid fever)
  - Fever, uveitis, which may precede the parotid enlargement, and facial nerve palsy

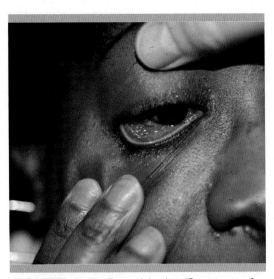

FIGURE 2-9 Sarcoidosis. *(Courtesy of Dr. Steven Mays.)*

- Löfgren syndrome
  - Fever, erythema nodosum, bilateral hilar adenopathy, and arthralgias
  - Associated with anterior uveitis in 6 percent of patients

BULLOUS DERMATOSES

Ocular Cicatricial Pemphigoid (OCP)

- Autoantibodies directed against
  - β_4 subunit of α_6,β_4-integrin (205-kDa protein, also known as CD104)
  - Epiligrin (laminin 5), ligand for α_6,β_4-integrin
  - α_6-Integrin subunit
- Ocular anomalies in older individuals (70 years mean age)
  - Chronic conjunctivitis, irritation, dry eye, discharge, subepithelial fibrosis
  - Cicatrization with conjunctival shrinkage, symblepharon, fibrotic bands

Stevens-Johnson Syndrome

- Delayed hypersensitivity reaction to drugs, usually acute (HLA-B12, -Bw44)
- Other causes: infection, vaccination, systemic diseases, physical agents, food
- Ocular anomalies
  - Conjunctivitis, chemosis, vesicles, bullae, membranes, ulceration
  - Swollen and ulcerated eyelids leading to entropion, dry eyes, trichiasis
  - Subepithelial fibrosis, lagophthamos, corneal ulceration, vascularization, opacification, and rarely, perforation
  - Conjunctival shrinkage, foreshortening of fornices resulting in symblepharon ankyloblepharon

METABOLIC DISORDERS

Alkaptonuria

- Autosomal recessive
- Deficiency of homogentisic acid oxidase
- Causes ochronosis
- Bluish black discoloration of certain tissues
- Osler sign: blue-black pigment in sclera near insertion of rectus muscles, oil-droplet opacities in cornea, pigmented pingucela, granules in episclera

Fabry's Disease

- X-linked recessive
- Defect in α-galactosidase

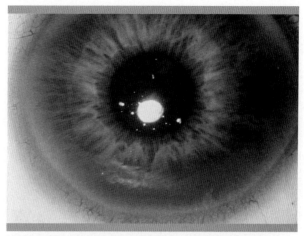

FIGURE 2-10 Hepatolenticular degeneration. *(From Lowenstein J, Lee S: Ophthalmology: Just the Facts. New York: McGraw-Hill, 2004, p. 123.)*

- Cornea verticillata (whorled corneal deposits), spokelike lens deposits, conjunctival and retinal tortuosity, oculomotor abnormalities

Hepatolenticular Degeneration (Wilson's Disease) (Fig. 2-10)

- Autosomal recessive
- Disorder of copper metabolism
- Keyser-Fleiser ring: greenish brown ring of copper in periphery of cornea

Homocystinuria

- Autosomal dominant
- Deficiency of cystathionine synthetase
- Downward lens dislocation

Primary Amyloidosis (Myeloma-Associated)

- Amyoid protein (AL) derived from immunoglobulin light chains
- Periorbital purpuric plaques ("pinch purpura"), amyloid deposition in the corneal stroma, conjunctiva and eyelid nodules, lattice corneal dystrophy

Richner-Hanhart Syndrome (Tyrosinemia II)

- Autosomal recessive
- Deficiency of hepatic tyrosine aminotransferase
- Severe keratitis and corneal ulcerations (blindness, photophobia, red eye

Xanthelasma Palpebrarum (Fig. 2-11)

- Asymptomatic bilateral and symmetric, yellow, flat, polygonal papules around the eyelids
- Most common in the upper eyelid near the inner canthus

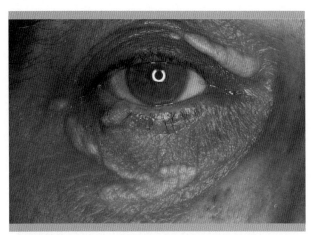

FIGURE 2-11 Xanthelasma palpebrarum. *(From Lowenstein J, Lee S: Ophthalmology: Just the Facts. New York: McGraw-Hill, 2004, p. 71.)*

- May be associated with hyperlipidemia
- Lesions characterized by accumulations of lipid-laden macrophages

Thyroid-Associated Ophthalmopathy (TSO)
- Also known as Graves' ophthalmopathy
- Autoimmune-mediated inflammation of the extraocular muscle and periorbital connective tissue

- Dalrymple sign: upper lid retraction
- Eyelid retraction, proptosis, chemosis, periorbital edema, and altered ocular motility (restrictive myopathy, usually of inferior rectus and medial rectus, resulting in hypotropia and esotropia and defective elevation and abduction), diplopia, congestion of orbit
- Exposure keratopathy is common and should be prevented
- Optic nerve damage with visual field loss can be gauged by relative afferent pupillary defects

ACNEIFORM CONDITIONS

Acne Rosacea
- Eyelid telangiectasias, blepharitis, recurrent chalazia, conjunctivitis, corneal scarring

VIRAL INFECTIONS

Varicella and Herpes Zoster Ophthlmicus
- Varicella-zoster virus (VZV) (Fig. 2-12)
- Herpes virus that causes both varicella (chicken pox) and herpes zoster (shingles)
- Herpes zoster ophthalmicus occurs in later life and causes ocular complications and severe neuralgic pain

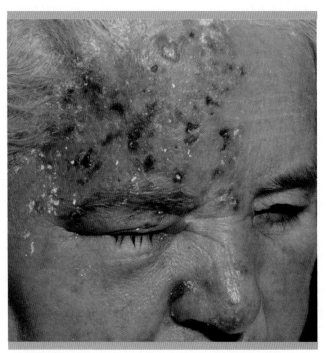

FIGURE 2-12 Varicella-zoster virus: ophthalmic herpes zoster. *(From Wolff K et al. Fitzpatrick's Color Atlas & Synopsis of Clinical Dermatology, 5th ed. New York: McGraw-Hill, 2005, p. 825.)*

- Ophthlmic branch of the trigeminal nerve is commonly involved
- More common in immunosuppressed individuals
- Prodrome of lancinating pain over the dermatome
- Eruption is maculopapular to vesiculopapular to ulcerative, and finally crust formation and scarring occurs
- Ocular complications such as keratitis and uveitis occur in 50 percent of patients with cutaneus eruption
- Most dreaded complication is postherpetic neuralgia

Herpes Keratoconjunctivitis

- Herpes zoster ophthalmicus (HZO)
- Tissues innervated by the ophthalmic division of the trigeminal nerve
- Acute orbital and globe lesions develop within 3 weeks of the rash
- Grouped vesicles usually involving one, but occasionally up to three adjacent dermatomes
- Vesicles become pustular and occasionally hemorrhagic with evolution to crusts in 7–10 days
- Punctate keratitis, corneal ulcers

Herpes Simplex Keratitis

- Antibodies present in 90 percent of the adult population in Western world
- Primary ocular herpes occurs as a follicular conjunctivitis, regional lymphadenitis, and ulcerative blepharitis
- Recurrent episodes of keratitis are common
- Dendritic corneal ulcers are pathognomonic
- Recurrent stromal keratitis causes structural damage to cornea resulting in corneal opacities often requiring corneal transplant
- Most common cause of corneal blindness in the United States

Molluscum Contagiosum

- Small, waxy nodules have a central umbilication
- If present on the eyelids, they may produce a follicular conjunctivitis

BACTERIAL DISEASES

Oculoglandular Sydrome of Parinaud

- Cat-scratch disease (Bartonella henselae)
- Unilateral granulomatous conjunctivitis

Syphilis

- Caused by the spirochete Treponema pallidum
- Secondary syphilis
- Ocular abnormalities
- Anterior uveitis

- Neurosyphilis
- Argyll Robertson pupil: small, irregular pupil that reacts normally to accommodation but not to light

Miliary Tuberculosis

- Caused by Mycobacterium tuberculosis
- Occurs when caseous material reaches the bloodstream from a primary focus
- Can cause choroidal tubercles in the retina

Lyme Disease

- Caused by Borrelia burgdorferi
- Transmitted by the bite of an infected Ixodes tick
- Stage 1: conjunctivitis and photophobia
- Stage 2: CN VII palsy (Bell palsy), blurred vision due to papilledema, optic atrophy, optic or retrobulbar neuritis, or pseudotumor cerebri
- Stage 2 or stage 3: episcleritis, symblepharon, keratitis, iritis, pars planitis, vitreitis, chorioretinitis, exudative retinal detachment, retinal pigment epithelial detachment, cystoid macular edema, and branch artery occlusion

Actinomyces

- Actinomyces israelii is a gram-positive anaerobic bacillus
- Actinomyces keratitis (keratoactinomycosis)
  - Dry ulceration with central necrosis surrounded by a gutter of demarcation
- Conjunctivitis, blepharitis
- Primary chronic canaliculitis of tear drainage apparatus

Hordeolum

- Painful, erythematous, and localized
- External hordeolum (stye)
  - Arises from a blockage and infection of Zeiss or Moll sebaceous glands
  - Abscess points at the lid margin.
- Internal hordeolum
  - Secondary infection of meibomian glands in the tarsal plate
  - Staphylococcus aureus is the infectious agent in 90–95 percent of cases
- Both types can arise as a secondary complication of blepharitis

INFESTATIONS AND BITES

Onchocerciasis (River Blindness)

- Onchocerca volvulus
- Simulium black fly vector
- Microfilariae in the anterior chamber
- Sclerosing keratitis, chorioretinitis, glaucoma, blindness

Loiais

- Filarial nematode: *Loa loa*
- Bite from *Chrysops*
- Calabar swellings: localized areas of angioedema
- Migration of adult worm across conjunctiva

Pediculosis Pubis

- Occasionally, infestation may be present in the eyebrows and eyelashes

DERMATOUVEITIDES

Behçet's Disease

- HLA-B5, -B51
- Major criteria
  - Recurrent oral aphthous ulcers (at least 3 in a 12-month period)
- Minor criteria (2/4)
  - Pathergy
  - Ocular findings: anterior uveitis, posterior uveitis, retinal vasculitis
  - Genital ulcers
  - Skin findings: pustules, erythema nodosum
- Ocular anomalies
  - Decreased visual acuity from severe uveitis, pain, redness, photophobia
  - Neovascular glaucoma, cataracts, vitreous hemorrhage, iritis, retinal vessel occlusions, and optic disc edema
  - Anterior uveitis (hypopyon uveitis): most common eye abnormality overall (a third of cases)
  - Posterior uveitis with retinal vasculitis is the most common cause of blindness.
- Treatment
  - Immunosuppressants for eye involvement
  - Azathioprine
  - Cyclosporin A

Reiter's Syndrome

- HLA-B27
- Conjunctivitis, acute iridocyclitis, keratitis, episcleritis

VITAMIN-RELATED DISORDERS

Vitamin A Deficiency

- Night blindness, dryness, corneal ulceration/keratomalacia, HSV infection
- Bitot's spots: foamy areas on conjunctiva from accumulation of keratin or bacteria

Scurvy

- Caused by a prolonged deficiency of vitamin C
- Ocular features include those of Sjögren syndrome, as well as subconjunctival hemorrhage and hemorrhage within the optic nerve sheath

MECHANICAL EYELID DISORDERS

Entropion

- Inward turning of the eyelid margin from infection, scarring, mechanical
- Causes irritation, redness, and stringy white mucoid discharge

Ectropion

- Outward turning of the eyelid margin from lower eyelid laxity, mechanical
- Causes tearing, corneal irritation and conjunctival redness, dry eyes
- Lower eyelid is involved most commonly

Trichiasis

- Misdirected eyelashes that rub on the cornea
- Ocular pain, tearing, and redness
- Commonly caused by chronic blepharitis, trauma, or chemical injuries to eyes

Dermatochalasis

- Redundant eyelid skin and fat
- May result in functional loss of superior vision if the tissue hangs over the eyelid margin

Blepharoptosis

- Drooping of the margin of the eyelid, may cause functional vision loss
- Etiology includes age-related dehiscence of the levator muscle, Horner's syndrome, third cranial nerve palsy, myasthenia gravis, and trauma

REFERENCES

Kanski JJ. *Clinical Ophthalmology. A Systematic Approach*, 4th Ed. Burlington, Massachusetts: Butterworth-Heinemann, 1999. Chapters 1.12 and 1.30.

Liesegang TJ. Herpes simplex virus epidemiology and ocular importance. *Cornea* 2001;20(1)1–13.

Liesegang TJ. Herpes zoster virus infection. *Curr Opin Ophthalmol* 2004;15(6):531–536.

Neoplastic and inflammatory tumors of the eye lids, in Tasman W, Jaeger E., ed. *Duane's Clinical Ophthalmology*, 2005 Ed. Philadelphia: Lippincott Williams & Wilkins, 2005.

CHAPTER 3

NAIL FINDINGS

MELISSA A. BOGLE
IDA ORENGO

NAIL ANATOMY (FIG. 3-1)

- Nail plate
  - Made up of dead, keratinized cells of the nail matrix epithelium firmly attached to the nail bed
  - Pink color owing to nail bed blood vessels
  - Lunula: visible portion of the nail matrix
  - Nail thickness depends on the length of the nail matrix and nail bed
  - Onychocorneal band: most distal portion of firm attachment of the nail plate to the nail bed
  - Onychodermal band: pink band that lies between the onychocorneal band and the nail plate white free edge
- Proximal nail fold
  - Dorsal portion: thinner than skin of the digit, devoid of pilosebaceous units
  - Ventral portion: in continuity with the matrix, adheres to the nail plate surface, and keratinizes with a granular layer
  - Horny layer forms the cuticle and prevents the separation of the plate from the nail fold
  - Dermis contains numerous capillaries that run parallel to the surface of the skin; morphology can be altered in connective tissue diseases
- Nail matrix
  - Lies above the midportion of the distal phalanx
  - Keratinization of the proximal nail matrix cells produces the dorsal nail plate
  - Keratinization of the distal nail matrix cells produces the intermediate nail plate
  - Lunula: where the distal matrix is not completely covered by the proximal nail fold but is visible through the nail plate as a white half-moon-shaped area
  - Cells are able to synthesize both "soft," or skin-type, and "hard," or hair-type, keratins
- Nail bed
  - Extends from the distal margin of the lunula to the onychodermal band
  - Completely visible through the nail plate
  - Epithelium is adherent to the nail plate, two to five cell layers
  - Nail bed keratinization produces a thin horny layer that forms the vental nail plate
  - No granular layer is present
- Hyponychium
  - Anatomic area between the nail bed and the distal groove, where the nail plate detaches from the dorsal digit
- Dermis
  - No subcutaneous tissue, no pilosebaceous units
  - Condensed connective tissue that forms a tendon-like structure connecting the matrix to the periosteum of the phalangeal bone
- Blood and nerve supply
  - Blood supply provided by the lateral digital arteries, arches supply the matrix and nail bed
  - Sensory nerves: originate from the dorsal branches of the paired digital nerves, run parallel to the digital vessels
- Nail growth
  - Fingernails: 3 mm/month
  - Toenails: 1 mm/month
  - After nail plate is avulsed, it takes 40 days before new fingernail will first emerge

NAIL DISORDERS

Chromonychia

- Abnormality in color of the substance and/or the surface of the nail plate and/or subungual tissue
- Systemic cause: All digits are usually involved
- Endogenous cause: Color corresponds to shape of lunula (concave)
- External contact: Color follows the shape of the proximal nail fold (convex)
1. Blue lunula
   - Wilson's disease

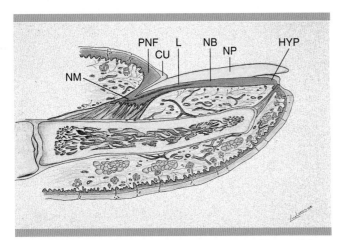

FIGURE 3-1 Drawing of a normal nail. CU, cuticle; HYP, hyponychium; L, lunula region; NB, nail bed; NM, nail matrix; NP, nail plate; PNF, proximal nail fold. *(From Freedberg IM et al: Fitzpatrick's Dermatology in General Medicine, 6th ed. New York: McGraw-Hill, 2003, p. 159.)*

- Argyria, silver nitrate
- Drugs: azidothymidine (AZT), quinicrine, busulfan, phenopthalein
2. Red lunula (Fig. 3-2)
   - Cardiac failure

- Heumatoid arthritis
- Alopecia areata
- Diabetes
- Polycythemia vera
- Carbon monoxide poisoning
3. Leukonychia
   - White color of nail in five patterns: total leukonychia (inherited usually), distal portion still appears pink, transverse leukonychia (systemic disorder), punctuate (from minor trauma), longitudinal (associated with Darier's disease)
   - Hereditary or acquired
   - Hereditary form is autosomal dominant and may be associated with epithelial cysts and renal stones
4. Melanonychia striata (Fig. 3-3)
   - Presence of a pigmented stripe, usually brown or black, along the length of the nail bed
   - Deposition of melanin in the nail plate from a variety of causes
   - Bands of nevocellular nevi
   - Idiopathic in dark-skinned individuals
   - Drugs: azidothymidine (AZT), antimalarials
   - Systemic diseases: AIDS, Addison's disease, Cushing's syndrome, hyperthyroidism, folic acid or vitamin B_{12} deficiency
5. Subungual melanoma
   - 0.7–3.5 percent of cutaneous melanomas
   - Longitudinal black or brown bands with different hues

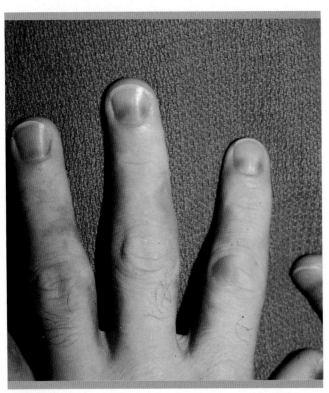

FIGURE 3-2 Red lunula. *(Courtesy of Adelaide Hebert.)*

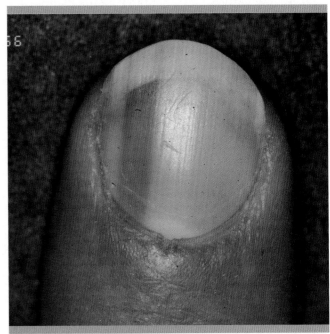

FIGURE 3-3 Melanonychia. *(Courtesy of Adelaide Hebert.)*

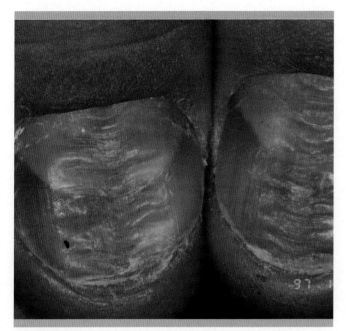

FIGURE 3-4 Habit tick. *(Courtesy of Adelaide Hebert.)*

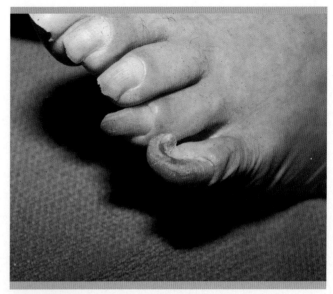

FIGURE 3-5 Onychogryphosis. *(Courtesy of Richard Krathen.)*

- Hutchinson's sign: spread of pigmentation into the nail folds
- Pigmentation in a single digit
- Occurs at age 50 or older

External Influences

1. Habit-tick deformity (Fig. 3-4)
   - Multiple transverse grooves (Christmas-tree pattern)
   - Thumbnails
   - Chronic mechanical injury to the cuticle
2. Onychogryphosis (Fig. 3-5)
   - Curved, thickened nail plate without attachment to the nail bed
   - Nail keratin is produced by the nail matrix at uneven rates, with the faster-growing side determining the direction of the deformity
   - Ill-fitting footwear, self-neglect, trauma, occasionally inherited as an autosomal dominant trait
   - Hemionychogryphosis with lateral deviation of the nail plate results from congenital malalignment of the big toenail
3. Onycholysis
   - Separation of the nail plate from the bed
   - Trauma, contact irritants
   - Dermatologic and systemic conditions: onychomycosis, diabetes mellitus, thyroid disorders, pregnancy, porphyria, pellagra, scurvy, psoriasis, scleroderma, lupus, hidrotic ectodermal dysplasia
   - Photo-induced onycholysis: tetracyclines, psoralens, 8-MOP, fluoroquinolones, chloramphenicol
   - Congenital

4. Onychoschezia
   - Distal horizontal nail splitting
   - External factors: water, chemicals
5. Splinter hemorrhages
   - Disruption of blood vessels in the nail bed can cause fine, splinter-like vertical lines to appear under the nail plate
   - Caused by injury to the nail or by certain drugs and diseases
   - Trauma is the most common cause
   - Resolve spontaneously
6. Ingrown nails
   - Great toenails are particularly vulnerable
   - Improper nail trimming, tight shoes, or poor posture can cause a corner of the nail to curve downward into the skin
   - Can lead to infection
7. Transverse overcurvature
   - Nail may be tile-shaped or may display an increase in curvature along the nail bed (pincer or trumpet nail)
   - Overcurvature may extend to the point of encompassing a cone of nail bed soft tissue
8. Chronic paronychia
   - Occurs in patients whose hands are subjected to moist local environments
   - Often due to contact dermatitis
   - Red, semicircular, indurated cushion around the base of the nail
   - Nail detaches from the distal portion of the proximal nail fold, which has lost its cuticle
   - May result in *Candida* invasion with discolored nail plate and cross-ridged lateral edges

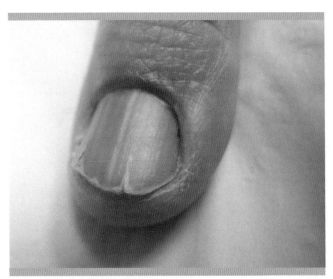

FIGURE 3-6 Darier nail. *(Courtesy of Adelaide Hebert.)*

9. Onychomadesis (nail shedding)
   • Spontaneous separation of the nail from the matrix
   • Usually latent
   • Nail plate shows a transverse split but continues growing for some time because there is no disruption in its attachment to the nail bed
   • Growth ceases when the nail is cast off after losing the connection

Genetic Syndromes

1. Keratosis follicularis (Darier's disease) (Fig. 3-6)
   • Defect in ATPase 2A2
   • Nails: red and white longitudinal streaks, wedge-shaped nicking, subungual hyperkeratosis
   • Follicular dyskeratosis, acrokeratosis verruciformis of Hopf
2. Nail-patella syndrome
   • Autosomal dominant
   • Defect in *LMX1B* gene
   • Nails: triangular lunula
   • Hypoplastic or absent patella, bilateral posterior iliac horns, radial head subluxation, scoliosis, palmoplantar hyperhidrosis
   • Glomerulonephritis ± renal failure
   • Eyes: heterochromic irides, lester iris, cataract
3. Congenital malalignment
   • Lateral deviation of the long axis of nail growth relative to the distal phlanx
   • Acquired traumatic malposition may follow acute trauma
4. Hook nail
   • Bowing of the nail bed owing to a lack of support from the short bony phlanx

5. Hereditary ectodermal dysplasia
   • Primary epidermal disorders in which one of the following signs occur: hypotrichosis, hypodontia, onychodysplasia, and anhidrosis
6. Epidermolysis bullosa (EB)
   • Junctional and dystrophic forms
   • Abnormalities of the nail matrix and nail bed associated with the pathogenetic alterations of the dermal-epidermal junction
   • Secondary trauma to the nail
7. Pachyonychia congenita
   • Autosomal dominant
   • Nails: thick subungual hyperkeratosis, pincer nails
   • Type I: Jadassohn-Lewandowsky
     – Keratins 6a and 17
     – Palmoplantar and follicular hyperkeratosis, benign oral leukoplakia
   • Type II: Jackson-Lawler
     – Keratins 6b and 17
     – Type I plus bullae on palms and soles, early dentition/natal teeth, steatocystoma multiplex
   • Type III: Shafer-Branauer
     – Type I plus corneal dystrophy, cataracts
   • Type IV: pachyonychia congenita tarda
     – Late onset, hyperpigmentation around the neck, waist, and flexures

Infection

1. Onychomycosis (Fig. 3-7)
   • *Trichophyton rubrum*
     – Distal subungual onychomycosis (DSO)

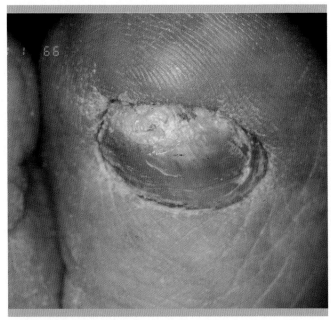

FIGURE 3-7 Onychomycosis. *(Courtesy of Adelaide Hebert.)*

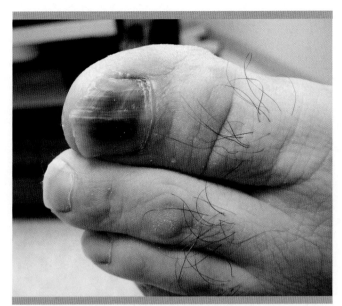

FIGURE 3-8 *Pseudomonas* nail. *(Courtesy of Richard Krathen.)*

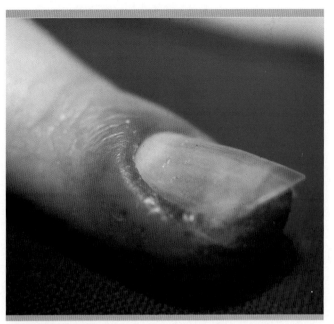

FIGURE 3-9 Acute paryonichia. *(Courtesy of Robert Jordon.)*

- Proximal subungual onychomycosis (PSO), associated with AIDS
- Superficial white onychomycosis (SWO) in children and HIV-positive individuals
- *Trichophyton mentagrophytes*
  - Superficial white onychomycosis (SWO)
2. *Pseudomonas* nails (Fig. 3-8)
   - *Pseudomonas* infection
   - Green (pyocyanin) or yellow (fluorescein)
3. Acute paryonichia (Fig. 3-9)
   - Follows any break in the skin
   - Starts in the paronychium at the side of the nail with local redness, swelling, and pain
   - Treat with antibiotics and possible partial avulsion, if necessary

Manifestations of Internal Disease

1. Alopecia areata (Fig. 3-10)
   - Geometric nail pitting (most common)
   - Twenty-nail dystrophy (generalized nail roughness)
2. Koilonychia
   - Naile is concave with raised edges (spoon nails)
   - Iron-deficiency anemia associated with Plummer-Vinson's syndrome
   - Normal finding in childhood
   - Mal de Maleda (keratoderma palmoplantaris transgrediens): painful glove-and-stocking keratoderma, psoriasiform hyperkeratotic plaques, koilonychia, onychogryphosis, scrotal tongue

3. Lichen planus
   - Dorsal pterygium (angel-wing deformity), longitudinal ridging/splitting, rarely yellow nails
4. Lindsey's nail (half-and-half nail)
   - Distal brown to pink nail bed with proximal pallor
   - Azotemia, chronic renal failure with uremia
5. Mees lines
   - Transverse white bands

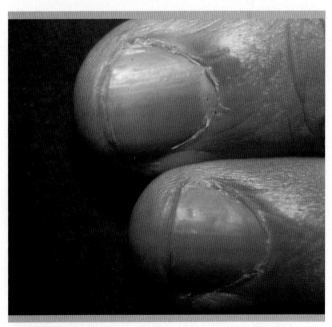

FIGURE 3-10 Nail pitting. *(Courtesy of Robert Jordan.)*

- Grow out with nail
- Arsenic poisoning
6. Meurke's lines
   - Paired white bands parallel the lunula
   - Do *not* grow out with nail
   - Hypoalbuminuria, nephrotic syndrome
   - Chemotherapy
7. Nail fold telangiectasias
   - Dermatomyositis
   - Scleroderma, systemic lupus erythematosus
8. Terry's nail
   - 1- to 2-mm distal pink band
   - Liver cirrhosis, hypoalbuminemia
   - Congestive heart failure
   - Diabetes mellitus
9. Twenty-nail dystrophy (trachyonychia)
   - Rough, sandpapered appearance
   - Autosomal dominant inherited form: present at birth and gets worse with age
   - Alopecia areata
   - Psoriasis
   - Lichen planus
10. Yellow-nail syndrome
    - Yellow nails with slow growth
    - Lymphedema
    - Pulmonary disorders, bronchiectasis
11. Psoriasis
    - 10–55 percent of adults with psoriasis
    - Salmon patches, "oil drop" defect in nailbed
    - Onycholysis
    - Irregular pitting—involvement of proximal nail fold
    - Subungual hyperkeratosis
12. Beau's lines (Fig. 3-11)
    - Recurrent disease will produce transverse grooves separated by normal nail.
    - Chronic paronychia
    - Chemotherapy, retinoids
    - Fever, illness
13. Median canaliform dystrophy of Heller
    - Midline split with backward-angled ridges ("fir tree")
    - Habit tick deformity-thumbs
    - Enlarged lunula resulting from pressure on the base of the nail
14. Pterygium
    - "Angel-wing" deformity
    - Dorsal: gradual shortening of the proximal nail groove, leading to progressive thinning of the nail plate and secondary fissuring caused by the fusion of the proximal nail fold to the matrix and then to the nail bed
    - Portions of the divided nail plate progressively decrease in size as the pterygium widens
    - Total loss of the nail with permanent atrophy

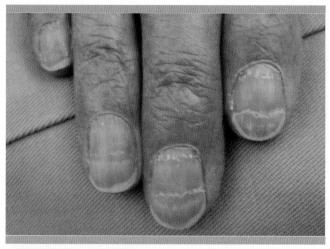

FIGURE 3-11 Beau's lines. *(Courtesy of Sharon Hymes.)*

- Lichen planus, bullous disorders, radiotherapy, digital ischemia, trauma, congenital
- Ventral: distal extension of the hyponychial tissue that is anchored to the undersurface of the nail, thereby obliterating the distal groove
- Scleroderma, Raynaud's disease, median nerve causalgia, formaldehyde/nail polish, trauma, congenital
15. Brachyonychia/racquet nail
    - Width of nail is greater than length
    - Thumb involvement autosomal dominant trait owing to obliteration of the epiphyseal line
    - Acroosteolysis
    - Down syndrome
    - Rubenstein-Taybi syndrome
16. Onychorrhexis
    - Nail longitundinal ridging (aged nails)
    - Brittle nail syndrome
    - Lichen planus, alopecia areata
    - Rheumatoid arthritis, graft-versus-host disease
    - Drug: isotretinoin, thallium poisoning
17. Clubbing (Fig. 3-12)
    - Increased transverse and longitudinal nail curvature
    - Hypertrophy of the soft tissue components of the digit's pulp
    - Hyperplasia of the fibrovascular tissue at the base of the nail
    - Early clubbing obliterates the normal diamond-shaped window formed at the base of the nail beds when there is opposition of the dorsum of two fingers from opposite hands
    - Causes of clubbing
18. Anonychia
    - Absence of all or part of one or several nails

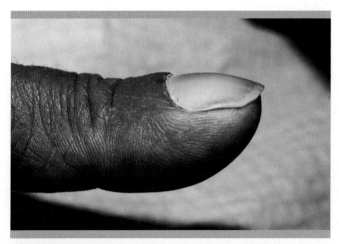

FIGURE 3-12 Clubbing. *(Courtesy of Robert Jordan.)*

- May be congenital (with underlying bone abnormalities) or acquired (through lichen planus)
19. Pitting
    - Depressions in the nail
    - Characteristic of psoriasis, alopecia areata, and eczema
    - Easily detachable parakeratotic cells in the superficial layers of the nail plate
    - Indicates a disturbance in the maturation and keratinization of the proximal nail matrix
20. Acrokeratosis paraneoplastica of Bazex
    - Psoriasiform changes
    - Associated with malignant epitheliomata of the upper respiratory tract or digestive tract and may precede the diagnosis of the tumor

Tumors of the Nail Area

1. Warts
    - Benign tumors caused by human papiloma virus, most frequently types 1, 2, and 4
2. Keratin implantation cysts
    - Lined with epidermis and filled with keratin
    - Occasionally observed under the nail
    - Most commonly due to trauma
    - May appear as a subungual tumor raising the nail plate or causing a bulbous enlartement of the terminal phlanx
    - X-ray will show a sharply dermarcated, round defect
3. Onychomatricoma
    - Tumor of the nail matrix
    - Longitudinal band of yellow thickening of the nail plate
    - Increased transverse curvature of the nail, splinter hemorrhages of the proximal nail

4. Keratoacanthomas
    - Rapidly growing, locally aggressive tumors
    - Most frequently on the hyponychium
5. Acquired periungual fibrokeratoma
    - Asymptomatic nodule with a hyperkeratotic tip, narrow base
    - Emerges from beneath the proximal nail fold, grows on the nail and causes sharp longitudinal depressions
6. Koenen's tumor
    - Periungual fibromas in tuberous sclerosis
    - Small, round, smooth, flesh-colored, asymptomatic
7. Infantile digital fibromatosis
    - Round, smooth, dome-shaped, shiny, firm red dermal nodules
    - Dorsal and axial surfaces of the fingers and toes
    - May present at birth or develop during infancy
8. Bowen's disease
    - Also known as *epidermoid carcinoma*
    - Etiology linked to HPV-16, -34, and -35; arsenic also may play a role (also think about association with genital warts)
    - Presents as a circumscribed plaque with a warty surface extending from the nail groove both under and around the nail
    - Nail dystrophy develops when the matrix is affected
    - Carcinoma cuniculatum: rare variant of squamous cell carcinoma with low biologic malignancy
9. Myxoid cysts
    - Asymptomatic, smooth swelling enlarges slowly
    - Usually located on one side of the midline
    - Transillumination reveals the cystic nature of the tumor
10. Exostosis and osteochondroma
    - Commonly on toes
    - Trauma is the main cause
    - Painful, elevates the nail plate
    - Bone-hard tumor, confirmed by x-ray

Vascular Tumors

1. Pyogenic granuloma
    - Eruptive hemangioma usually seen following trauma
    - Small, bluish red nodule develops rapidly on the periungual skin
    - Lesion becomes necrotic and forms a collarette of macerated white epithelium
2. Glomus tumor
    - Triad: pain, tenderness, temperature sensitivity
    - Reddish spot in the nail bed, distal fissured nail plate

REFERENCES

Daniel CR: Nail pigmentation abnormalities. *Dermatol Clin* 1985;3:431–443.

Faergemann J, Baran R: Epidemiology, clinical presentation and diagnosis of onychomycosis. *Br J Dermatol* 2003;149:1–4.

Fistarol SK, Itin PH: Nail changes in genodermatoses. *Eur J Dermatol* 2002;12:119–128.

Freedberg IM et al. *Fitzpatrick's Dermatology in General Medicine,* 6th Ed. New York: McGraw-Hill; 2003.

Herzberg AJ: Nail manifestations of systemic diseases. *Clin Podiatr Med Surg* 1995;12:309–318.

McKee PH. *Pathology of the Skin: With Clinical Correlations.* London: Mosby-Wolfe; 1996.

McLean WH: Genetic disorders of palm skin and nail. *J Anat* 2003;202:133–141.

Pappert AS, Scher RK, Cohen JL: Nail disorders in children. *Pediatr Clin North Am* 1991;38:921–940.

Rich P: Nail disorders. Diagnosis and treatment of infectious, inflammatory, and neoplastic nail conditions. *Med Clin North Am* 1998;82:1171–1183.

Telfer NR: Congenital and hereditary nail disorders. *Semin Dermatol* 1991;10:2–6.

CHAPTER 4

FUNGAL DISEASE

MELISSA A. BOGLE
MARK LAROCCO

SUPERFICIAL MYCOSES

Tinea Versicolor (Fig. 4-1)

- *Malassesezia furfur (Pityrosporum ovale)*
- Clinical
  - Hypo- or hyperpigmented macules on trunk, extremities
- Histology
  - Round to oval yeast with septate hyphae in stratum corneum
- Potassium hydroxide (KOH): "spaghetti and meatballs" (hyphae and spores)
- Culture: Saboroud dextrose agar (SDA) with olive oils (fatty acids essential for growth)
- Treatment: Selenium sulfide (2.5 percent), oral/topical ketoconazole cream, ketoconazole 400 mg

Tinea Nigra

- *Phaeoannellomyces (Exophiala) werneckii*
- Clinical
  - Brown-black nonscaly macules on the palms/soles
  - Transmitted by traumatic implantation
- Histology: brown hyphae in stratum corneum, no tissue response
- Microscopic: large, dematiacious hyphae
- Culture: SDA, brown-black colonies
- Treatment: topical keratolytics and antifungals; griseofulvin ineffective

Piedra

- *Piedraia hortae* (black piedra); *Trichosporon beigelii* (white piedra)
- Black piedra (BP): hard nodules on scalp hair; metallic sound when combing
- White piedra (WP): less adherent, light-brown to white nodules in beard, mustache, or pubic hair
- Histology
  - BP: well-organized stroma; hyphae aligned in periphery
  - WP: less organized; hyphae perpendicular to shaft

- Culture
  - *T. beigelii* requires cyclohexamide-free media; wrinkled, creamy white colonies
  - *P. hortae* grows slowly; dark-brown to black colonies with reddish brown pigment on reverse
- Treatment: shaving, improved hygiene

CUTANEOUS MYCOSES

- Filamentous fungi (molds)
- Possess keratinolytic enzymes that allow parasitization of all fully keratinized tissues of the body (hair, skin, and nails)
- Organisms do not usually penetrate beneath epidermal layer of skin
- Consist of three genera (Tables 4-1 and 4-2)
  - *Trichophyton*: affects hair, nails, skin (Table 4-3)
  - *Epidermophyton*: affects nails, skins
  - *Microsporum*: affects hair, skin
- Different species may show marked host preferences
  - Humans (anthropophilic species)
  - Animals (zoophilic species; Table 4-4)
  - Soil (geophilic species)

Tinea Capitis

- Endothrix infection (growth and sporulation within hair shaft) (Fig. 4-2 and Table 4-5)
  - *Trichophyton tonsurans*
    - Common isolate in the U.S. causes "black dot" presentation (weak hair shaft breaks at the skin surface)
  - *T. violaceum*: more common in Europe, North Africa, and Middle East
  - *T. schoenleinii*: cause of *favus*; see scutula (crusting) with permanent loss of hair, scarring
- Ectothrix infection (growth and sporulation around hair shaft); tend to fluoresce (see Table 4-6)
  - *Microsporum audouinii*: anthropophilic, causes epidemic tinea capitis, preveiously most common cause of tinea capitis

33

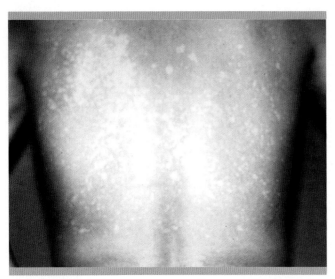

FIGURE 4-1 Tinea vesicolor. *(Courtesy of Adelaide Hebert.)*

- *M. canis:* zoophilic, can cause localized outbreaks, may be acquired from dogs and cats
- *T. mentagrophytes:* zoophilic

Tinea Favosa (Favus)

- *T. schoenleinii;* less commonly *T. violaceum* and *M. gypseum*
- Scutula (collections of hyphae and keratinous debris) on scalp; cicatricial alopecia
- Microscopic: linear arrangement of hyphae along longitudinal axis of hair shaft
- Kerion
- Suppurative folliculitis
- Deep boggy red areas characterized by a severe acute inflammatory infiltrate
- *Trichophyton* spp

Tinea Barbae

- Inflammatory or kerion-like: animal workers
- *T. verrucosum*
  - Zoophilic, ectothrix
  - Contracted from cattle
  - Superficial or sycosiform type: resembles bacterial folliculitis
- *T. mentagrophytes*
  - Contracted from dogs and cattle
- *M. canis, T. schoenleinii,* and *T megninii*
  - Circinate, spreading type: active, vesiculopustular border with central scaling

Tinea Corporis

- *T. rubrum, M. canis* (children), and *T. mentagrophytes*
  - Scaly erythematous patches with raised borders and central clearing
- Zoophilic fungi
  - *T. verrucosum* or *T. mentagrophytes*
  - Cause inflammatory reactions
- Variants
  - Tinea imbricata or Tokelau
    - *T. concentricum,* South Pacific
    - Concentric circles and polycyclic or serpiginous scaly plaques
  - Bullous tinea corporis
    - *T. rubrum*
  - Majocchi's granuloma (Fig. 4-3)
    - Deeper involvement of hair follicles with foreign-body granulomas
    - Erythematous patch with pustules
    - *T. rubrum, T. violaceum, T. tonsurans*
- Histology
  - "Sandwich sign": hyphae between orthokeratosis and compact hyperkeratosis or parakeratosis
- Potassium hydroxide (KOH) (Fig. 4-4)
  - Skin scrapings reveals numerous septate branching hyphae

TABLE 4-1 Key Morphologic Criteria for Identifying the Dermatophytes

Microscopic Morphology of:	*Epidermophyton*	*Microsporum*	*Trichophyton*
Macroconidia	Abundant, club-shaped, thick-walled, smooth, arranged in groups	Usually abundant, spindle-shaped, thick-walled, rough	Usually scarce, club-shaped, smooth, thin-walled
Microconidia	Absent	Usually scarce, elongate	Abundant, spherical, elongate, or pear-shaped

TABLE 4-2 Differentiating Characteristics of Dermatophytes

Dermatophyte	Colony	Microscopic	Characteristics
T. rubrum	Fluffy white; red on reverse (no diffusion) (see Fig. 4-6)	Smooth, pencil-shaped microconidia; "birds on a wire"	Urease (−) Hair perforation (−)
T. mentagrophyte var. mentagrophytes (zoophilic)	Tan granular, brown-red color on reverse	Grapelike clusters of microconidia and spiral hyphae (see Fig. 4-7)	Urease (+) Hair perforation (+) (+) Hair invasion: large spore ectothrix
T. mentagrophyte var. interdigitale	Cream fluffy; reverse yellow/brown	Few pyriform microconidia	(+) Hair invasion, large spore ectothrix; (+) hair penetration, urease positive
M. gypseum (geophilic)	Cinnamon, flat powdery with brown reverse color	Thin walled rough macroconidia, cucumber-z shaped	(+) Hair invasion: large spore ectothrix, hair fluorescence: none or dull green
M. canis	White fluffy, reverse yellow	Rough, canoe-shaped macroconidia; pointed tip ("snout") Note: *Epidermophyton* are smooth-walled	Grows on polished rice (+) hair invasion" small spore ectothrix; green fluorescence
M. audoinii	Downy beige; salmon pink on reverse	Micro- and macroconidia rarely present	Does not grow on polished rice (+) Hair invasion: small spore ectothrix (yellow/green)
T. tonsurans	Brown, yellow, white suedelike; reddish brown on reverse	Smooth balloon-shaped macroconidia (rare); teardrop-shaped microconidia with varying sizes and arrangement	(+) Hair invasion, requires thiamin
T. schoenleinii	Cream-colored, cerebriform, (glaborous), heaped	Antler-shaped hyphae (favic chandeliers)	(+) Hair invasion: fluorescence green causes scutula
T. verrucosum	Cream wrinkled, heaped, cream color on reverse	Smooth-walled macroconidia (rare) with "tails"	(+) Hair invasion: large spore ectothrix, requires thiamin and/or inositol
T. violaceum	Glaborous, wrinkled, reverse violet red	Micro- and macroconidia not present	(+) Hair invasion: endothrix, requires thiamine
T. concentricum	White glaborous, white color reverse	Micro- and macroconidia not present; narrow branching hyphae	Causes tinea imbricate: "tokelau"
E. floccosum	Flat, granular, khaki color front and reverse	Large, thin club-shaped macroconidia	Produces chlamydoconidia
M. nanum	Tan granular; beige color reverse	Rough-walled two-celled macroconidia ("pig snout")	(+) Hair invasion, large spore ectothrix, no fluorescence

TABLE 4-3 Nutritional Requirements of *Tricophyton* Species

Nutritional Requirement	Species
Thiamine	*T. tonsurans, T. violaceum, T. verrucosum,* some *T. concentricum*
Histidine	*T. megninii*
Niacin	*T. equinum*
Inositol and thiamine	*T. verrucosum*

TABLE 4-4 Zoophilic Dermatophytes

Dermatophyte	Natural hosts
M. gallinae	Chickens/other birds
M. nanum	Pigs (snouts)
M. canis	Cats, dogs, horses
T. verrucosum	Cattle, sheep, horses
T. equinum	Horses
T. simii	Monkeys, chickens
T. mentagrophytes var. *mentagrophytes*	Cats, dogs, rabbits

Tinea Cruris

- *Epidermophyton floccosum* (Fig. 4-5)
  - Groin, perineal, and perianal areas
- *T. rubrum* (Fig. 4-6)
  - May extend over buttocks and waist
  - Scrotum typically spared (versus candidiasis)

Tinea Pedis/Manuum

- Interdigital type
  - Maceration between the fourth and fifth toes
  - *T. rubrum, T. mentagrophytes* var. *interdigitale,* and *E. floccosum*
- Moccasin type
  - Erythema with slight scaling may extend to side of feet

- *T. rubrum*
- Vesicular type
  - Pruritic vesicles or bullae
  - *T. mentagrophytes* var. *mentagrophytes* (Fig. 4-7)

Tinea Unguium (Onychomycosis)

- Distal subungual onychomycosis (DSO)
  - Occurs at free nail edge
  - Thickened and yellow nail plate, subungual debris, and onycholysis
  - *T. rubrum*
- Proximal subungual onychomycosis (PSO)
  - Affects proximal nail plate
  - *T. rubrum,* associated with HIV

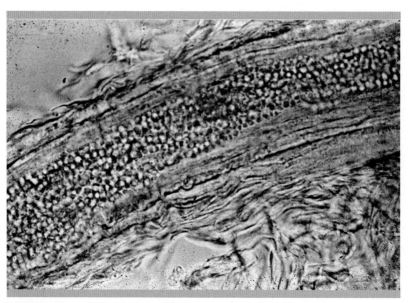

FIGURE 4-2 Endothrix. *(Courtesy of Mark LaRocco.)*

TABLE 4-5   Endothrix Fungi

T. tonsurans
T. schoenleinii
T. soudanese
T. gourvilli
T. yaoundie
T. violaceum

TABLE 4-6   Small Spore Ectothrix that Fluoresce

Name	Color
M. distortum	Yellow/green
M. audouinii	Yellow/green
M. canis	Yellow/green
M. ferrugineum	Yellow/green

Note: *T. schoenleinii* (favic type); causes blue/green fluorescence

- White superficial onychomycosis (WSO)
  - Occurs on the nail surface
  - *T. mentagrophytes* (adults), *T. rubrum* (children)
- Endonyx OM (EO)
  - White discoloration of the nail plate, no subungual debris

Id Reaction

- Host's immune response to dermatophytosis
- Occurs at a distant site from the fungal infection
- Lesions are devoid of organisms
- May be triggered by antifungal treatment
- Acute vesicular dermatitis of the hands and feet and evolves into a scaly eczematoid reaction
- Commonly due to *T. mentagrophyte*

SUBCUTANEOUS MYCOSES

- Three clinically distinct types of fungal infections
  - Sporotrichosis
  - Chromomycosis
  - Mycetoma

Sporotrichosis

- *Sporothrix schenckii:* zoonosis of cats, dimorphic fungus
- Lymphocutaneous form: (Fig. 4-8)
  - Acquired by traumatic implantation of soil fungus, often due to a rose thorn
  - Nodules with sporotrichoid spread (follows lymphatics) on extremities
- Fixed cutaneous form
  - Localized ulcers or granulomas on face, neck, and trunk
- Pulmonary or disseminated disease:
  - Occurs after inhalation; disseminated lesions in joints, lungs, mucous membranes
  - Seen in immunosuppressed individuals
- Histology:
  - Tissue phase (37°C) (Fig. 4-9)
    - Consists of elongated, cigar-shaped yeasts; rarely seen in histologic sections of tissue
  - Mold phase (25°C) (Fig. 4-10)
    - Consists of septate hyphae
    - Turn white to black with age
    - Delicate conidiophores bearing pyriform (pear-shaped) conidia in rosette clusters
  - Asteroid bodies
    - Yeast forms surrounded by eosinophilic halo
    - Histologic examination of tissue
    - Represent deposition of antigen-antibody complexes
- Culture (25°C): fast growing; no growth at greater than 39°C; inhibited by cycloheximide

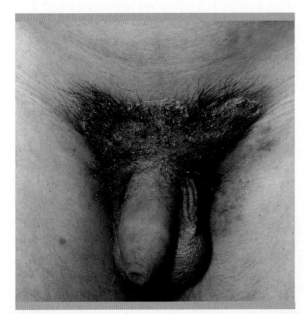

FIGURE 4-3 Majocchi's granuloma. *(From Wolff K et al: Fitzpatrick's Color Atlas & Synopsis of Clinical Dermatology, 5th ed. New York: McGraw-Hill, 2005, p. 715.)*

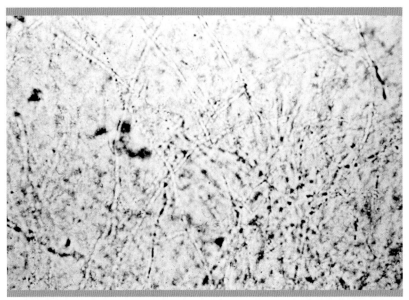

FIGURE 4-4 Potassium hydroxide (KOH). *(Courtesy of Mark LaRocco.)*

- Treatment
  - Lymphocutaneous disease: itraconazole, saturated solution of potassium iodide (SSKI)
  - Disseminated disease: amphotericin B

Chromoblastomycosis

- Localized, chronic infection
- Acquired by implantation of soil organisms

- Lesions are usually painless and "cauliflower-like," verucous plaques
- Etiologic agents
  - Slowly growing dematiaceous (pigmented) fungi
  - Most common agents include *Fonsecaea pedrosii, F. compactum, Cladophialophora carrionii, Rhinocladiella aquaspersa, Phialophora verrucosa,* and *Wangiella dermatitidis*

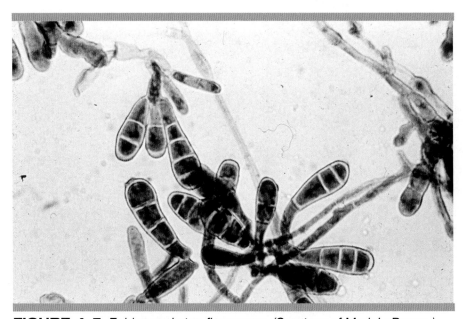

FIGURE 4-5 *Epidermophyton floccosum. (Courtesy of Mark LaRocco.)*

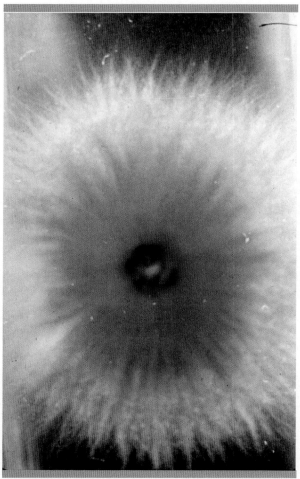

FIGURE 4-6 *T. rubrum. (Courtesy of Mark LaRocco.)*

- Histology
  - "Sclerotic bodies" (also called *Medlar bodies, copper penny bodies*) (Fig. 4-11)
  - Brown segmented hyphal forms seen in infected tissue
- Culture
  - Folded gray-green to black colonies
- Treatment
  - Itraconazole, surgical excision

Subcutaneous Phaeohyphomycosis

- Dematiaceous fungi
- *Exophala jeanselmei, Wangiella dermatitidis, Alternaria* spp., *Bipolaris* spp., *Curvularia* spp., *Phialophora* spp
- Clinical
- Solitary subcutaneous abcess; may drain
- Microscopic: branched, spetate dematiacious hyphae
- Histology: hyphae seen, no medlar bodies
- Culture: dark leathery or wooly colonies; microscopic evaluation varies with each species
- Example: Alternariosis: *Alternaria* spp.; conidia resemble "hand grenades" in chains
- Treatment: surgery, itraconazole

Mycetoma (Madura Foot, Maduramycosis)

- Includes both actinomycetoma (caused by bacteria) and eumycetoma (caused by fungi)
- Acquired from soil implantation

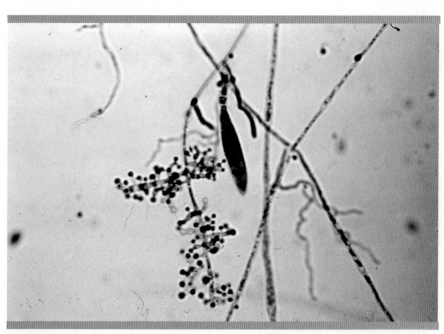

FIGURE 4-7 *T. mentagrophytes* var. *mentagrophytes. (Courtesy of Mark LaRocco.)*

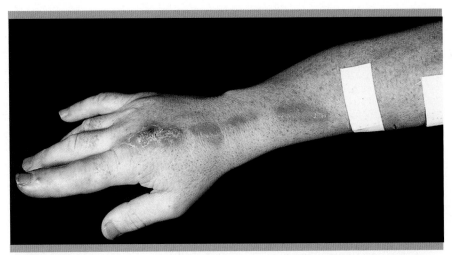

FIGURE 4-8 Sporotrichosis clinical. *(From Wolff K et al: Fitzpatrick's Color Atlas & Synopsis of Clinical Dermatology, 5th ed. New York: McGraw-Hill, 2005, p. 739.)*

- Lesions involve skin, subcutaneous tissue, fascia, and bone
- Painless subcutaneous nodule
- Formation of granulomas and abscesses that eventually drain by formation of sinus tracts
- May see "grains" in sinus tract drainage
  - Represent compact microcolonies of the pathogen(s) (useful for diagnosis)

- Etiologic agents
  - Eumycotic (fungal) mycetoma
    - *Pseudallescheria boydii* (most common in United States)
    - *Madurella mycetomatis*
    - *Acremonium* spp
    - *Curvularia* spp.
    - *Exophiala jeanselmei*

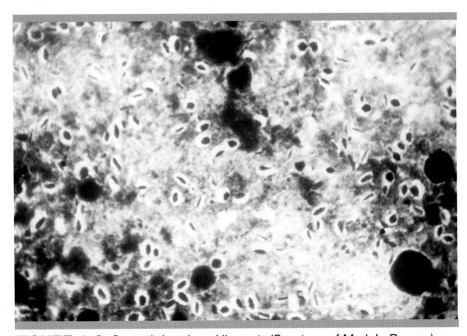

FIGURE 4-9 *Sporothrix schenckii* yeast. *(Courtesy of Mark LaRocco.)*

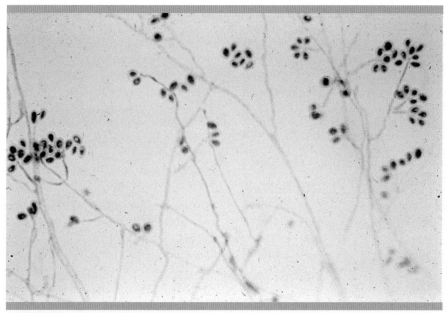

FIGURE 4-10 *S. schenckii* mold. *(Courtesy of Mark LaRocco.)*

- Actinomycotic (bacterial) mycetoma:
  actinomycetes
  - Gram-positive branching rods once thought to
    be primitive fungi but now recognized as true
    bacteria
  - Clinical: tumefaction, sinus tracts, and sulfur
    grains; muscle and bone invasion

  - *Nocardia asteroides, N. brasiliensis,
    Streptomyces somaliensis*
- Histology:
  - Eumycotic mycetoma: grains and fungal elements
    for (see Table 4-7)
  - Actinomycotic mycetoma: sulfur grains with fine
    threadlike filaments; stain gram positive (Fig. 4-12)

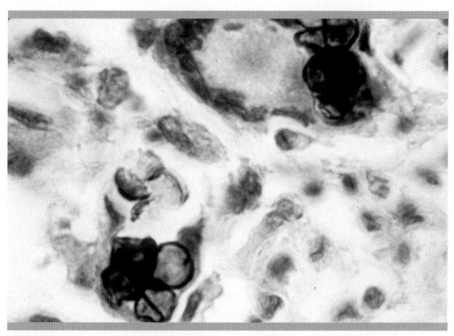

FIGURE 4-11 Chromoblastomycosis. *(Courtesy of Mark LaRocco.)*

TABLE 4-7　Identification of *Mycetoma* Microcolonies

Grain Color	Organism
White	Fungi or actinomycetes; *Acremonium* sp. *Pseudallescheria boydii*
Black	*Exophiala jeanselmei, Madurella mycetomatis, Curvularia* sp.
Red	*Actinomadura pelletieri*
Yellow	*Streptomyces, Nocardia*

- Need culture for confirmation
- Treatment
  - Eumycotic mycetoma: antifungals seldom effective, surgical excision
  - Actinomycotic mycetoma: antimicrobial therapy

Rhinosporidiosis

- *Rhinosporidium seeberi*
  - Caused by an aquatic protozoan (Mesomycetozoa)
  - Previously thought to be a fungus
  - Endemic in India and Sri Lanka
  - Chronic granulomatous infection
- Clinical
  - Typically limited to the mucosal epithelium
- Pink to deep-red polyps of the nasopharynx (70 percent)
- Can obstruct breathing, sensation of an intranasal foreign body
- Polyps in the lacrimal sac (15 percent) also can occur: photophobia, redness, and secondary infection
- Histology: thick-walled sporangium of 150–350 micrometers containing tens of thousands of endospores
- Treatment: local surgical excision

Lobomycosis (Keloidal Blastomycosis or Lobo's Disease)

- *Lacazia loboi* (previously *Loboa loboi)*
- Zoonosis of freshwater dolphins
- Clinical
  - Develops at sites of minor trauma
  - Lesions develop slowly over time
  - Keloidal nodules, verrucoid to nodular lesions, crusty plaques, and tumors
  - Squamous cell carcinoma may arise in chronic lesions
- Histology:
  - Fibrous tissue is dispersed between large numbers of giant cells and histiocytes, parakeratosis, and acanthosis; round or lemon-shaped organisms joined in a chain
- Treatment: surgical excision

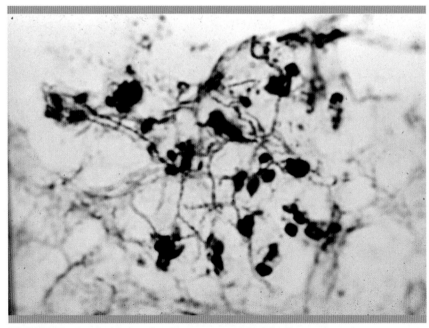

FIGURE 4-12 *Nocardia. (Courtesy of Mark LaRocco.)*

DIMORPHIC FUNGI

- See Table 4-8
- Different anamorphic forms or phases
- Regulated by several biologic and physical factors, the most important being temperature
  - 25°C fungi grow as molds: saprophytic or environmental phase
  - 35–37°C fungi grow as yeasts or yeastlike: tissue or parasitic phase
- Disease characteristics
  - Portal of entry: respiratory tract
    - Infection is acquired via inhalation of conidia produced by the mold phase
    - Primary infections occur most commonly in the respiratory tract
    - Can progress to serious pulmonary or disseminated disease with multiorgan involvement
    - Tissue phase not transmissible, no person-to-person spread of infection
  - Extent of disease is regulated by the immunologic response of the host
    - Humoral response
      - ▲ Minimal role in protection
      - ▲ Sometimes increases disease severity (hypersensitivity responses)
      - ▲ Measurement of antibody titers is useful occasionally for diagnosis and prognosis (see below)
    - Cell-mediated response (T cells, cytokines, activated macrophages)
    - Primary protective mechanism and major determinant of disease severity

Coccidioidomycosis (San Joaquin Valley Fever, Desert Rheumatism)

- Acquired by inhalation of arthroconidia of *Coccidioides* spp
- Lower Sonoran desert, southwestern United Sates, a soil inhabitant

TABLE 4-8 List of Dimorphic Fungi

Blastomyces dermatitidis
Coccidioides immitis
Histoplasma capsulatum and *duboisii*
Paracoccidiodes brasiliensis
Sporothrix schenckii
Penicillium manerfeii

- *Coccidioides immitis* (San Joaquin Valley, CA)
- *C. posadasii* (Texas, Arizona, outside the United States.)
- Clinical
  - Up to 60 percent of cases may be asymptomatic
  - Another 35 percent present as mild flulike illness with fever, chest pain, and arthralgia
  - Allergic manifestations are often the first presenting symptoms of infection (erythema nodosum, erythema multiforme)
  - Extrapulmonary disease is rare (<5 percent of cases) but serious; usually involves central nervous system, skin, and pericardium
  - Disseminated disease may spread hematogenously from lungs
  - Increased risk in immunosupressed patients, Mexicans, blacks, pregnant women, and Filipinos
- Mycology
  - Mold phase
    - Culture: white to tan fluffy colony matures in 5–10 days
    - Microscopic: Hyphae will fragment into barrel-shaped arthroconidia, separated by disjunctor cells (Fig. 4-13) arthroconidia are very infectious, can cause lab-acquired disease
  - Tissue phase
    - Microscopic: multinucleated spherules filled with endospores (produced by repeated internal cleavage) (Fig. 4-14)
    - Mature spherule ruptures, releases endospores that develop into new spherules
- Chest x-ray: eggshell cavities
- Therapy
  - Benign pulmonary disease: none
  - Extrapulmonary disease: itraconazole, fluconazole, amphotericin B

Histoplasmosis (Darling's Disease)

- *Histoplasma capsulatum* and *duboisii*
  - Associated with bird and bat droppings Mississippi and Ohio River valleys
  - Inhalation of microconidia
- Clinical
  - Self-limiting pulmonary disease, severity related to dose of conidia
    - Endemic histoplasmosis: flulike symptoms; benign, self-healing pulmonary exposure; calcification on chest x-ray
    - Epidemic histoplasmosis: acute pulmonary infection after plentiful exposure
  - Occasionally progressive pulmonary disease and/or disseminated infection (immunosupressed, AIDS)
    - Can involve any organ system, typically bone marrow, spleen, skin, gastrointestinal, CNS

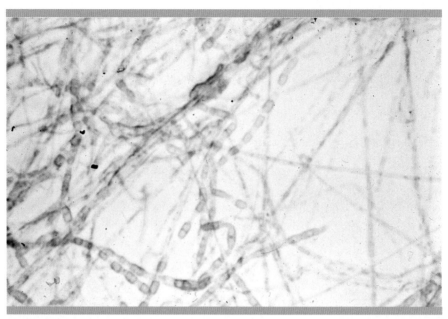

FIGURE 4-13 *Coccidioides immitis* mold phase. *(Courtesy of Mark LaRocco.)*

- Acute: splenic calcification, anemia, Addison's disease
- Chronic: granulomatous oral/rectal ulcerations, nonspecific skin lesions; risk factors: HIV, hematogenous malignancy
- African histoplasmosis
  - *H. duboisii*
  - Involves mucocutaneous, bone, lymph nodes, lungs
  - Skin lesions can resemble molluscum contagiosum
- Mycology
  - Mold phase
    - Culture: white cottony colony after 2–4 weeks of incubation (Fig. 4-15)
    - Microscopic: septate hyphae, formation of microconidia (infectious) and tuberculated macroconidia (diagnostic) (Fig. 4-16)

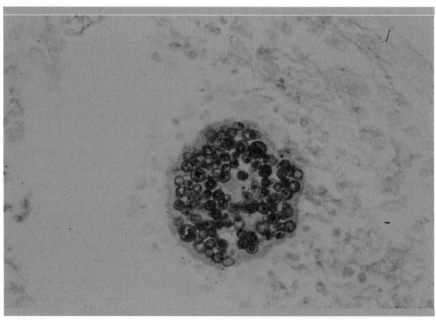

FIGURE 4-14 *C. immitis* tissue. *(Courtesy of Mark LaRocco.)*

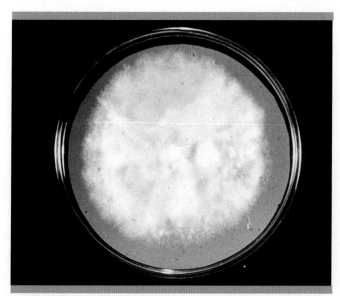

FIGURE 4-15 *Histoplasma* colony. *(Courtesy of Mark LaRocco.)*

- Tissue phase
  - Parasitized histiocytes: small (4–6 μm), oval yeasts, usually found in monocytes and macrophages of the blood, lungs, and reticuloendothelial system (Fig. 4-17)
- Therapy
  - Benign pulmonary disease in immunocompetent patient: none
  - Moderate disease: itraconazole
  - Extrapulmonary/disseminated in immunocompromised host: amphotericin B

Blastomycosis (Gilchrist's Disease)

- *Blastomyces dermatitidis*
- Mississippi River valley, southeastern United States
- Acquired by inhalation of microconidia
- Clinical
  - Pulmonary disease occurs, but extrapulmonary presentation is more common with chronic infection of the skin and bones
  - Skin lesions
  - Characterized by microabscess formation, papulopustular nodules, and crusty verrucous granulomas of the hands, face and mucocutaneous areas, cribiform scars
  - Systemic blastomycosis
    - Pulmonary spread to skin, bones (osteolytic lesions), genitourinary tract, and CNS
    - Pulmonary disease is similar to tuberculosis
  - Inoculation blastomycosis is a rare and mild form of cutaneous disease in lab workers
- Mycology
  - Mold phase
    - Septate hyphae, white colony in 3–4 weeks
    - Formation of oval microconidia
  - Tissue phase
    - Large, thick-walled yeast with broad-based bud (Fig. 4-18)
- Therapy: itraconazole, amphotericin B

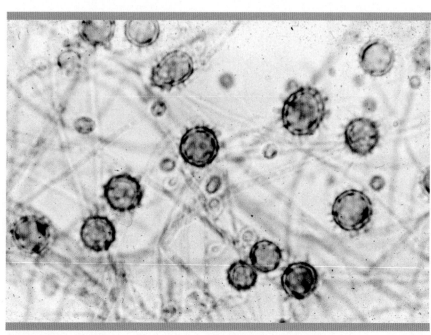

FIGURE 4-16 *H. capsulatum*, mold phase. *(Courtesy of Mark LaRocco.)*

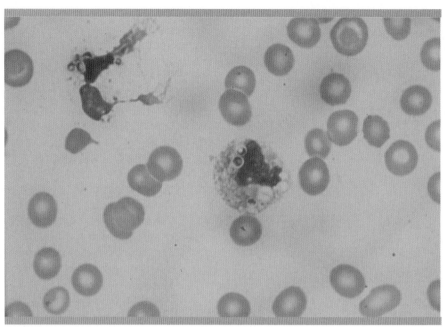

FIGURE 4-17 *H. capsulatum,* yeast phase within histiocytes in peripheral blood. *(Courtesy of Mark LaRocco.)*

Paracoccidioidomycosis (South American Blastomycosis)

- *Paracoccidioides brasiliensis*
- Chronic granulomatous disease
- Clinical
  - Begins as a pulmonary infection and disseminates
- Forms ulcerative granulomata and mulberry-like erosions of buccal, nasal, and occasionally the gastrointestinal mucosa
- Lymph node involvement (commonly cervical) with extension to cutaneous tissue
- Systemic involvement of multiple organ systems is a rare complication

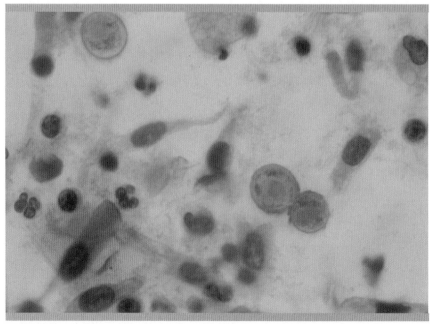

FIGURE 4-18 *Blastomyces dermatitidis,* yeast phase in tissue. *(Courtesy of Mark LaRocco.)*

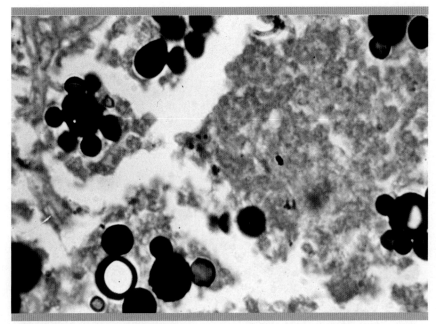

FIGURE 4-19 *Paracoccidioides brasiliensis,* yeast phase in tissue. *(Courtesy of Mark LaRocco.)*

- Male-to-female ratio 8:1 (estrogen may inhibit the hyphae to yeast transformation)
- Mycology
  - Mold phase
    - Culture: white to tan colony, growth in 2–4 weeks
    - Microscopic: septate hyphae, oval microconidia indistinguishable from *B. dermatitidis* (must observe tissue phase)
  - Tissue phase
    - Thin-walled yeast with multiple buds arranged in a "ship's wheel" configuration; thin points of attachment of buds to mother cell (Fig. 4-19)
- Treatment: itraconazole, ketoconazole, amphotericin B

OPPORTUNISTIC MYCOSES

Candidiasis

- Five or six significant human pathogens:
  - *Candida albicans* (most common)
  - *C. glabrata* (increasing in frequency)
  - *C. tropicalis*
  - *C. parapsilosis*
  - *C. kruseii*
- *C. albicans* (most common)
  - Oval, 3- to 6-μm yeast that reproduces by budding

- Organism is part of normal enteric flora
- Infection is usually of endogenous origin
- Buds that fail to detach from mother cell may elongate to form pseudohyphae
- Clinical
  - Initiation of disease due to abnormalities in the host
  - Infection usually of endogenous origin, part of normal flora
  - Predisposing factors for *Candida* infection
  - Steroids and anticancer agents (immunosuppressive, cytotoxic)
  - Antibiotics (inhibition of normal bacterial flora leads to yeast overgrowth)
  - Iatrogenic infection (long-term percutaneous catheterization)
  - Metabolic abnormalities (diabetes, hypoparathyroidism)
  - Mucocutaneous candidiasis: (Fig. 4-20)
  - Thrush, denture stomatitis, perleche, leukoplakia, median rhomboid glossitis, black hairy tongue, balanitis
  - Cutaneous candidiasis
    ▲ Intertrigo, diaper dermatitis, erosio interdigitalis blastomycetica, *Candida* miliaria, folliculitis, paronychia (Fig. 4-21)
  - Congenital candidiasis
    ▲ Benign in first 24 hours of life; may have transient respiratory distress; associated with chorioamnionitis

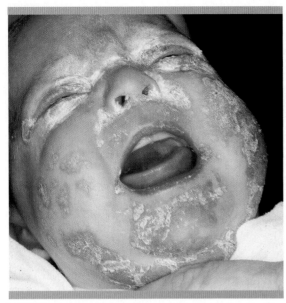

FIGURE 4-20 Mucocutaneous candidiasis. *(From Wolff K et al: Fitzpatrick's Color Atlas & Synopsis of Clinical Dermatology, 5th ed. New York: McGraw-Hill, 2005, p. 728.)*

- Disseminated candidiasis
  ▲ Organisms gain access from the oropharynx or gastrointestinal tract; hemorrhagic papulonodules on the trunk and extremities; associated with thrombocytopenia, fever, myalgias

- Infections of species of *Candida* other than *C. albicans*
  - Endocarditis due to *C. tropicalis* and *C. parapsilosis* found in intravenous drug abusers
- Microscopic: pseudohyphae or true septate hyphae (Fig. 4-22)
- Culture: Colonies are white and creamy on Sabouraud dextrose agar after 24–48 hours of incubation at 35°C (Fig. 4-23)
- Treament
  - Topicals (nystatin, miconazole, clotrimazole) for uncomplicated cutaneous disease
  - Amphotericin B, liposomal AMB, fluconazole, voriconazole, caspofungin for invasive and/or disseminated disease

Cryptococcosis

- *Cryptococcus neoformans* is the major human pathogen (United States and Europe)
  - Four serotypes described (A, B, C, and D)
  - Pigeons are a major reservoir for the fungus
  - Allows survival in dry environments
  - *C. neoformans* is found in bird droppings
  - *C. gatti* (tropics including Africa)
  - Found in leaf and bark debris from red gum trees
- Clinical
  - Pulmonary portal of entry but primary infection is usually subclinical

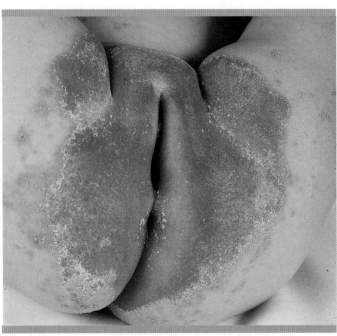

FIGURE 4-21 *Candida* diaper. *(From Wolff K et al: Fitzpatrick's Color Atlas & Synopsis of Clinical Dermatology, 5th ed. New York: McGraw-Hill, 2005, p. 721.)*

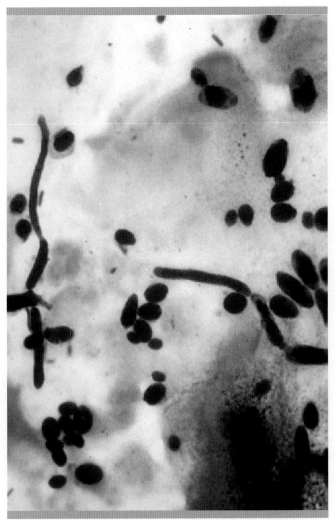

FIGURE 4-22 *C. albicans,* microscopic view. *(Courtesy of Mark LaRocco.)*

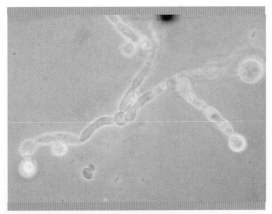

FIGURE 4-23 *C. albicans* colony. *(From Wolff K et al: Fitzpatrick's Color Atlas & Synopsis of Clinical Dermatology, 5th ed. New York: McGraw-Hill, 2005, p. 717.)*

- Stains with mucicarmine; best seen with PAS or GMS
- India ink smear for CSF
- Therapy
  - Amphotericin B
  - Amphotericin B + 5-fluorocytosine
  - Fluconazole

Aspergillosis

- Ubiquitous to most environments
- *Aspergillus flavus*:
  - Most common primary cutaneous pathogen; affects intravenous sites in immunosuppressed patients
- *A. fumigatus*:
  - Most common pathogen overall, affecting primarily the lung
- *A. niger*:
  - Associated with burn wounds
- Clinical
  - Infection acquired by inhalation of conidia
  - Allergic bronchopulmonary aspergillosis
    - Hypersensitivity response to conidiospores; no tissue invasion
    - Aspergilloma (fungus ball); cavities in lungs (tuberculosis, sarcoidosis)
  - Invasive pulmonary aspergillosis
    - Parenchymal invasion with hyphal progression along vascular pathways
  - Disseminated aspergillosis
    - Involvement of two or more non-contiguous organ systems
  - Mycotoxicoses
    - Ingestion of food contaminated with toxins produced by some aspergilli (aflatoxins)

- Fungus has a predilection for the central nervous system
- Skin lesions: widespread papules, acneiform pustules around the nose and mouth, subcutaneous abscesses may ulcerate and form granulomatous, eroded areas
- Serious, life-threatening disease seen in patients with impaired cellular defenses (AIDS, lymphoma)
- Cryptococcosis is the number one cause of fatal fungal infection in AIDS patients
- Can have hematogenous spread to lungs, bones, and viscera
- Mycology
  - Encapsulated 4- to 8-μm yeast that produces by single or double buds surrounding clear halo; no pseudohyphae formed (Fig. 4-24)
  - Polysaccharide capsule: serves as a virulence trait of the fungus

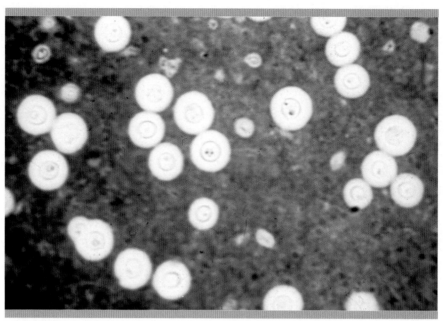

FIGURE 4-24 *Cryptococcus neoformans,* India ink preparation. *(Courtesy of Mark LaRocco.)*

- Invasive and/or disseminated aspergillosis
  - Often fatal disease in immunosupressed patients; predisposing factors or conditions include
    - ▲ Neutropenia
    - ▲ Neoplasm
    - ▲ Organ transplantation
    - ▲ Chemotherapy, especially steroids
- Cutaneous infection
  - Necrotic ulcers or embolic lesions with black eschar
- Mycology
  - Rapidly growing monomorphic molds
  - Mycelium consists of septate hyaline hyphae
  - Conidiophores with terminal vesicle and phialides produce chains of conidia; different species have different conidial color, size and spatial arrangements (Fig. 4-25)
- Diagnosis
  - Microscopic examination of tissue
  - GMS, PAS, or calcofluor stains
  - Look for septate hyphae with 45-degree angle branching (Fig. 4-26)
- Culture
  - Growth of hyaline mold in 1–2 days on routine fungal media incubated at 25°C. (Fig. 4-27)
  - Conidial pigmentation differs according to species (*A. fumigatus* = green)
- Serologic tests

- Antibody tests available for allergic disease and aspergilloma, no good for invasive disease (patients often can't produce antibodies)
- Galactomannan antigenemia test available; results variable
- Therapy
  - Allergic disease: steroids
  - Aspergilloma: none, surgical resection
  - Invasive disease: amphotericin B, liposomal AMB, itraconazole, voriconazole, caspofungin

Zygomycosis (Mucormycosis)

- Order *Mucorales*
- Fungi are ubiquitous in nature.
- Found as common bread molds
  - *Rhizopus* spp
  - *Mucor* spp
  - *Absidia* spp
- Clinical
  - Respiratory portal of entry, occasionally ear
  - Rhinocerebral infection (most common)
    - Rapidly progressive infection of sinuses, orbits, and brain, with infarction and necrosis
    - Associated with ketoacidotic diabetes
    - Sinus pain, proptosis, unilateral palsy, facial edema, purulent drainage, meningitis
  - Thoracic infection
    - Pleural disease produces chest pain, cough
  - Abdominal, gastric infection

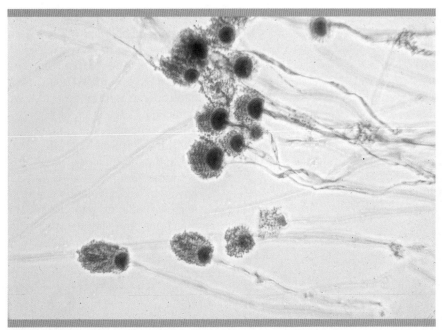

FIGURE 4-25 *Aspergillus,* microscopic view. *(Courtesy of Mark LaRocco.)*

- Skin infection (burn patients)
- Associated with vascular occlusion, infarction, hemorrhage
- Mycology
  - White cottony mold, rapid growth (1–2 days) at 25°C on standard fungal media; colony turns dark on sporulation
- Microscopic

- Hyphae are hyaline broad, ribbon-like, and nonseptate; branch at 90-degree angle
- Asexual reproduction by production of sporangia and sporangiospores
- Differentiation of *Rhizopus, Absidia,* and *Mucor*
  - Based on the presence of rhizoids and their spatial relation to sporangia
  - Rhizoids directly opposite sporangia = *Rhizopus*

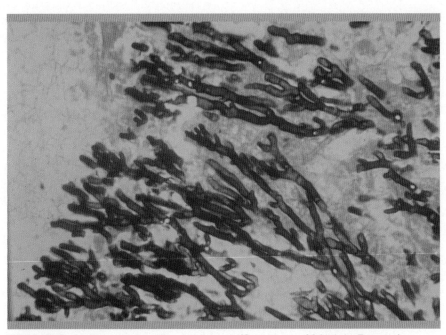

FIGURE 4-26 *Aspergillus* in tissue. *(Courtesy of Mark LaRocco.)*

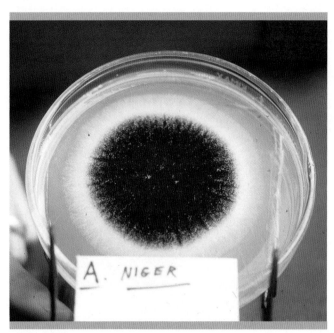

FIGURE 4-27 *Aspergillus* colony. *(Courtesy of Mark LaRocco.)*

- Rhizoids between two sporangia (internodal) = *Absidia*
- No rhizoids present = *Mucor*
- Diagnosis
  - Direct examination: see broad nonseptate hyphae with 90-degree-angle branching (differs from *Aspergillus*)
  - Culture: rapid grower on fungal media; species determined by observing sporulation and rhizoid pattern
  - Serology: none available
- Therapy
  - Lipid preparations of amphotericin B (some efficacy, mortality still high)
  - Surgical resection

Penicilliosis

- *Penicillium marneffei*; endemic in Southeast Asia
  - Clinical
    - Umbilicated papules (molluscum-like)
    - Prominent lymphadenopathy, localized pulmonary lesions in disseminated disease
  - Mycology
    - Histology: histiocytes with intracellular yeastlike cells divided by a septum
  - Culture: Green or gray mold with diffusible apricot red pigment
    - Microscopic: Hyphae have paintbrush or broom look

Fusarium

- Common in soil and dead or living plants
- Most common of these are *Fusarium solani*, *F. oxysporum*, and *F. chlamydosporum*
- Immunocompromised hosts, particularly in neutropenic and transplant patients
- Clinical
- Infection begins after trauma
- Central venous catheter infections, septic arthritis, disseminated infections, and fungemia
- Keratitis, endophthalmitis, otitis media, onychomycosis, cutaneous infections particularly of burn wounds, mycetoma, sinusitis, pulmonary infections, endocarditis, peritonitis
- Neutropenic or burn patients
- Culture: Colonies are usually fast growing, pale or brightly colored (depending on the species), and may or may not have a cottony aerial mycelium
- Microscopic: sickle-shaped "banana" multiseptated macroconidia
- Treatment
- Very drug-resistant fungi
- Intrinsically resistant to the novel glucan synthesis inhibitors, caspofungin, anidulafungin, and micafungin; can try amphotericin B, voriconazole, and natamycin

OTHER

Pneumocystosis

- Formerly classified as parasite, but recent molecular evidence (16S and 5S rRNA) indicates that *Pneumocystis jiroveci* is phylogenetically related to fungi
- Organism has several forms.
  - Trophic form (1–5 μm)
  - Uninucleated sporocyst (4–5 μm)
  - Mature spore case containing eight oval to fusiform spores (1–3 μm)
- Disease
  - Respiratory tract is portal of entry
  - Subclinical infection probably common
  - Hallmark of infection is interstitial pneumonitis and plasma cell infiltration
- Diagnosis
  - Morphologic identification of *P. jiroveci* in lung tissue, bronchial washings,and sputum
  - Gomori methenamine silver stain (stains cyst wall)
  - Giemsa stain (stains troph nuclei)
  - Immunofluorescent antibody stain (more sensitive)

- Therapy
  - Primary: trimethoprim-ulfamethoxazole or dapsone
  - Secondary: clindamycin, pentamidine, primaquine, atovaquone
  - Concomitant use of corticosteroids in acutely ill, immunosuppressed patients

Protothecosis

- *Prototheca wickerhamii*
- Achloric algae in stagnant, brackish water
- Ubiquitous in nature
- Infection follows trauma to the skin; low virulence
- Clinical
  - Skin
    - Most common site of infection
    - Ill-defined plaque or nodule that may have a verrucous surface
  - Periarticular bursae
    - Causing olecranon bursitis
- Diagnosis

- Histology: "morula"; sporangia with a central rounded endospore surrounded by a corona of molded endospores
- Culture: creamy yeastlike colonies at 30°C, inhibited by cycloheximide

REFERENCES

Elewski BE: *Cutaneous Fungal Infections,* 2nd Ed. Marden, Massachusetts: Blackwell Publishers; 1998. (Translated into Polish 2000).

Freedberg IM et al. *Fitzpatrick's Dermatology in General Medicine,* 6th Ed. New York: McGraw-Hill; 2003.

Kyle AA, Dahl MV: Topical therapy for fungal infections. *Am J Clin Dermatol* 2004;5(6):443–451.

Loo DS: Cutaneous fungal infections in the elderly. *Dermatol Clin* 2004;22(1):33–50.

McKee PH. *Pathology of the Skin: With Clinical Correlations.* London: Mosby-Wolfe; 1996.

Ribes JA, Vanover-Sams CL, Baker DJ: Zygomycetes in human disease. *Clin Microbiol Rev* 2000;13(2):236–301.

Vander Straten MR, Hossain MA, Ghannoum M: Cutaneous infections dermatophytosis, onychomycosis, and tinea versicolor. *Infect Dis Clin North Am* 2003;17(1):87–112.

CHAPTER 5

CUTANEOUS INFESTATIONS

MELISSA A. BOGLE
ASRA ALI

Parasite

- An organism that lives on or within another organism (*host*)
- Relationship may be one of mutual benefit (mutualism) or one in which the host derives no benefit but is not injured by the relationship (commensalism)
- Host, in addition to providing a steady food source, provides warmth and shelter
- *Definitive* host: Parasite becomes sexually mature and undergoes reproduction
- *Reservoir* hosts are those in which parasites that are pathogenic to other animals or to humans
- *Vector*: agent by which a parasite is transmitted to the host (e.g., arthropod, mollusk)

ARTHROPODA

- Bites usually result in localized, cutaneous reactions and pruritus
- Some of these organisms are medically important: Fleas, lice, and ticks can transmit lethal epidemic disorders
- Many of these vector-transmitted diseases are endemic in various regions of the world
- Four classes of arthropods are of dermatologic interest and are covered in this chapter:
  - Chilopoda: including centipedes
  - Diplopoda: including millipedes
  - Insecta: including caterpillars, moths, bedbugs, lice, flies, mosquitoes, beetles, bees, wasps, hornets, fire ants, and fleas
  - Arachnida: including ticks, mites, scorpions, and spiders
- Organisms from the arhropod classes Arachnida and Insecta have a hard-jointed exoskeleton and paired, jointed legs

- Class Insecta: a group of organisms with six legs and three body segments: head, thorax, and abdomen
  - *Siphonaptera:* fleas
  - *Anoplura:* head and body lice
  - *Pthiridae:* crab louse
  - *Diptera:* two-winged flies, mosquitos, midges
  - *Hemiptera:* true bugs
  - *Lepidoptera:* butterflies, moths, and their caterpillars
  - *Hymenoptera:* ants, wasps and bees
- Class Arachnida: a group of organisms with eight legs and two body segments: head and abdomen
  - *Ixodidae:* hard ticks
  - *Argasidae:* soft ticks
  - *Araneae:* spiders
- Centipedes and millipedes

INSECTA

Siphonaptera (Fleas)

- Wingless, laterally compressed insects with a hard, shiny integument
- The body has three regions: head, thorax, and abdomen
- Mouthparts are modified (paired maxillary palpi) for piercing and sucking
- Survive months without feeding
- Order *Siphonaptera* contains only two flea families of medical importance:
  - *Pulicidae:* (human, cat, dog, and bird fleas)
  - *Sarcopsylidae* (also called *Tungidae*): the sand flea
- In humans, the flea is only a transient visitor for the purpose of feeding
- Fleas jump, on average, about 20 cm
- One flea can bite two to three times over a small area
- It is not uncommon to see three flea bites in a row—described as breakfast, lunch, and dinner

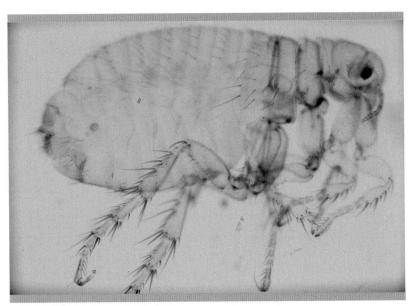

FIGURE 5-1 *Pulex irritans* (human flea).

- Bites produce irregular, pruritic, red wheals up to 1 cm in diameter
- Patients may present with a surrounding halo with a central papule, vesicle, or bulla or with hemorrhagic macules, papules, vesicles, or bullae
1. *Pulex irritans* (human flea) (Fig. 5-1)
   - Farms, urban areas
2. *Tunga penetrans* (chigoe flea)
   - Tropical and subtropical regions of North and South America, Africa
   - Intense itching and local inflammation
   - Causes tungiasis
     - Female sand flea, which burrows into human skin at the point of contact, usually the feet
     - Head is down into the upper dermis feeding from blood vessels
     - Caudal tip of the abdomen is at the skin surface
     - Nodule (usually on the foot) that slowly enlarges over a few weeks
   - Treatment
     - Occlusive petrolatum suffocates the organism.
     - Lindane, dimethyl phthalate, or dimethyl carbamate
3. *Xenopsylla cheopis* (Oriental rat flea)
   - Plague (*Yersinia pestis*)
   - Endemic (murine) typhus (*Rickettsia typhi*)

Anoplura

PEDICULIDAE

- After attaching to the skin, these flattened, wingless insects feed on human blood and can cause intense itching

- They will die of starvation if kept off the body for more than 10 days
- They are also killed by washing in water at 53.5°C for 5 minutes
- Life span of a louse is about 30 to 45 days
1. *Pediculus humanus corporis* (body louse)
   - Up to 5 mm long
   - Vector for
     - Epidemic typhus (*Rickettsia prowazekii*)
     - Trench fever, bacillary angiomatosis, bacillary peliosis (*Bartonella quintana*)
     - Relapsing fever (*Borrelia recurrentis, Borrelia duttoni*)
   - Crowded, unsanitary conditions
   - Lives in clothing and moves to body to feed
   - Pyoderma involving areas covered by clothing, most notably the trunk, axillae, and groin; erythematous macules, papules, and wheals, as well as excoriations, also may be seen
   - Treatment: dichlorodiphenyltrichloroethane (DDT) powder, lindane 1% powder, or malathion 1% powder
2. *Pediculus humanus capitus* (head louse) (Fig. 5-2)
   - Whitish in color and up to 3 mm long
   - Confined to the scalp
   - Lice and their eggs can withstand vigorous washing and combing
   - Nits: cementing of white eggs to the hair; usually found in the warm areas of the scalp such as behind the ears and on the posterior neck
   - Eggs hatch in approximately 7 to 9 days
   - Treatment: requires that both the adult lice and the nits be killed

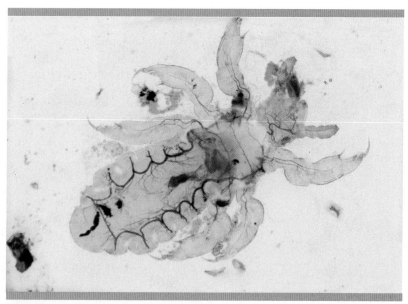

FIGURE 5-2 *Pediculus humanus capitus* (head louse).

- Two treatments a week apart are recommended because nits hatch in 7 days
- Lindane, gamma-benzene hexachloride
- Malathion lotion
- Natural and synthetic pyrethrin products
- Nits are best removed with a comb after soaking the hair in a vinegar solution

Pthiridae

Pthirus pubis (Fig. 5-3)
- Pubic louse, crab louse
- Short, broad body with rather stout claws on the middle and hind legs
- Grayish white to reddish in color
- Sexually transmitted
- Rarely involves facial (eyelashes), chest, or axillary hair
- Patients can remain asymptomatic for up to a month before pruritus develops; nits, similar to those in pediculosis capitis, are seen
- Blue macules (maculae ceruleae) are often seen on the surrounding skin and are believed to be produced by louse saliva acting on blood products
- Treatment: lotions or shampoos containing 1% lindane, 0.3% pyrethrins, or 5% permethrin
- Infestation of the eyelashes: petrolatum

Diptera

- Two-winged, biting insects
- All require a blood meal at some time in their development
- Bites can manifest as immediate urticarial papules, delayed erythematous papules, or both

FLIES

- Number of infectious diseases can be transmitted by biting flies
- A variety of flies commonly bite humans
- Common housefly does not bite but rather feeds on the surface of the skin

DERMATOBIA HOMINIS (BOTFLY)

- Most common cause of furuncular myiasis
- Occurs when fly larvae (maggots) invade tissue
- Wound myiasis: Eggs are deposited on an open wound
- Furuncular myiasis: Eggs are deposited beneath the skin via a puncture
- Raised, erythematous papule develops at the site of the bite, most frequently on the distal extremity or scalp
- Enlarges to become an indurated nodule with a central punctum, which is the breathing hole for the larva
- Treatment
  - Surgical excision; may be lured out by bacon fat
  - Block air supply with petroleum jelly

SAND FLIES (PHLEBOTOMUS AND LUTZOMYIA SPECIES)

- Vectors for bartonellosis, Oroya fever, Carrion's disease (*Bartonella bacilliformis*)
- Leishmaniasis
- *Leishmania:* protozoan infection
- *Leishmania* transform to the *promastigote* (or flagellate) form in the gut of the vector
  - Promastigote is a slender organism with a flagellum

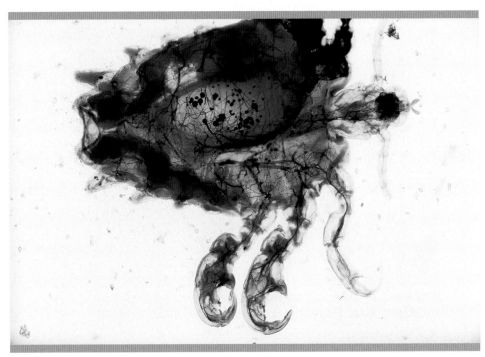

FIGURE 5-3 *Pthirus pubis* (pubic louse).

- After replicating, the promastigotes migrate to the sandfly's proboscis, from which they are regurgitated into the next host as the sandfly feeds
- Become internalized by means of complement receptors on mature macrophages
- Assuming that the amastigote forms, the *Leishmania* replicate, causing the cell to rupture, which releases amastigotes that then infect other cells
- Located within reticuloendothelial cells of infected tissues, *Leishmania* exist in an amastigote (nonflagellate) form
  - Round or oval in shape
- Intracellular parasites infect the mononuclear phagocytes
- Vector: sand fly (*Phlebotomus* and *Lutzomyia* species)
- Clinical
  - Cutaneous
  - Nontender, firm, red papule at bite
  - Lesion widens with central ulceration, serous crusting, and granulomas
  - Lesions may be wet or dry and become fibrotic or hyperkeratotic with healing
- Mucocutaneous
  - Excessive tissue obstructing the nares, septal granulation, and perforation
  - Gingivitis, periodontitis, and localized lymphadenopathy
- Visceral
  - Recurrent high fevers, wasting, anorexia, night sweats, diarrhea, and malaise

- *Leishmaniasis recidivans*
  - Occur years after a localized cutaneous lesion has healed
  - New ulcers and papules form over the edge of the old scar
- After kala-azar
  - Multiple, hypopigmented, erythematous macules
- Old World
  - Middle East, Indian subcontinent, Asia, Mediterranean, East Africa, and republics of the former Soviet Union
  - Visceral leishmaniasis (kala-azar/black fever)
    - Systemic infection of the liver, spleen, and bone marrow
    - *L. donovani* and *L. infantum*
  - After kala-azar:
    - *L donovani* and *L infantum*
  - Cutaneous lesions
    - *L. tropica* and *L. major*
    - Multiple lesions
  - Mucocutaneous disease (espundia)
    - *L. aethiopica*
  - Leishmaniasis recidivans
    - *L. tropica*
  - Diffuse cutaneous leishmaniasis
    - *L. aethiopica*
- New World
  - Throughout the Americas
  - Visceral disease
    - *L. chagasi*

- Cutaneous lesions
  - *L. mexicana*
  - Solitary nodule
- Mucocutaneous disease (espundia)
  - *L. braziliensis*
- *Leishmaniasis recidivans*
  - *L. viannia braziliensis*
- Diffuse cutaneous leishmaniasis
  - *L. mexicana*
  - *L. amazonensis*
- Post–kala-azar leishmaniasis
  - *L. donovani chagasi*
- Diagnosis
  - Culture
  - Direct agglutination test, immunofluorescence assay, or enzyme-linked immunosorbent assay (ELISA)
  - Montenegro skin test: determines delayed-type hypersensitivity reactions
- Treatment
  - Pentavalent antimony, administered intravenously or intramuscularly
  - Amphotericin B and pentamidine

TSETSE FLY (GLOSSINA), GLOSSINIDAE FAMILY

- Vector for African trypanosomiasis (sleeping sickness)
- Trypanosomes are ingested during a blood meal by the tsetse fly from a human reservoir, develop into epimastigotes, and are reinfected into human hosts
- Extensive antigenic variation of parasite surface glycoproteins
- West African (*T. brucei gambiense*)
- Slow progression
- East African (*T. brucei rhodesiense*)
- Rapid progression (within a week)
- Stage 1
  - Chancre
  - Hypersensitivity reaction: urticaria, pruritus, facial edema, fever, arthralgias, Winterbottom's sign (posterior cervical lymphadenopathy)
  - Kerandel's sign: delayed sensation to pain or a sensation of hyperesthesia
- Stage 2: Central nervous system (CNS) changes
  - Headaches, behavioral changes, seizures in children
- Laboratory studies
  - Anemia, hypergammaglobulinemia, elevated erythrocyte sedimentation rate (ESR), thrombocytopenia, and hypoalbuminemia
  - Wet smear of unstained blood, bone marrow, spinal fluid, skin lesions: parasite is visualized
  - Card agglutination test for trypanosomiasis (CATT)
- Treatment

- Early stages: suramin, pentamidine
- CNS stage: intravenous melarsoprol B, eflornithine

CHRYSOPS (DEER FLY)

- Vector for loaisis (see below)

MOSQUITOS

- Belong to the family *Culicidae*
- Delicate winged insects with long proboscises and long, thin legs
- Require water to mature through the larval and pupal stages
- Can be the vector for filariasis, yellow fever, dengue fever, and malaria
- Cutaneous reactions to bites include urticarial wheals, delayed papules, bullous lesions, hemorrhagic necrotic lesions, excoriations, eczematous patches, and granulomatous nodules

CULEX

- Vector for
  - Japanese encephalitis
  - Murray Valley encephalitis virus
  - Rift Valley fever
  - Ross River virus
  - *Sindbis* virus
  - St. Louis encephalitis (*Flaviviridae*)
  - West Nile fever: arthropathy, muscle weakness, rash
  - Filariasis (*Wuchereria bancrofti*)
  - Dirofilariasis: *Dirofilaria immitus* (dog heart worm), *Dirofilaria tenuis* (raccoons), *Dirofilaria repens* (dogs), *Dirofilaria ursi* (bears)

ANOPHELES

- Vector for malaria (*Plasmodium falciparum, P. malariae, P. vivax, P. ovale*)

AEDES AEGYPTI

- Yellow fever (*Flaviviridae*)

BEETLES

- Blister beetles cause cutaneous injury when a potent vesicating agent, cantharidin, is released from their bodies and contacts human skin
- *Lytta vesicatoria*, also known as "Spanish fly," is the source of cantharidin
- Two species, *Epicauta vittata* and *E. pennsylvanica*, are found in the southern and southwestern United States
- Blisters develop within a day and then dry up and desquamate in about a week
- Treatment: Affected skin should be washed immediately with alcohol, acetone, ether, or soap to dissolve or dilute the cantharidin

Hemiptera (True Bugs)

CIMEX LECTULARIUS (BED BUG)

- Feeds nocturnally on human blood
- Adult can survive more than a year without feeding
- 8 mm long, reddish brown, and wingless, with a greatly flattened body
- Linear arrangement of large wheals, often >1 cm, which are accompanied by itching and inflammation
- Bullous eruptions can occur
- Transmission of hepatitis B, ricketts, and leishmaniasis by these bugs is possible

Reduviid Bug (Kissing Bug, Assassin Bug)

- Vector for Chagas' disease (American trypanosomiasis) caused by *T. cruzi*
- 15 mm long, dark brown in color
- *Reduviid* bug ingests the trypomastigote while feeding on infected animals; it then divides and transforms in the gut of the bug into metacyclic trypomastigotes
- Bug ventures out at night to feed on exposed skin; 80 percent enter through conjuntiva, deposit stool when biting
- Transform into amastigotes after ingestion by macrophages; *T. cruzi* burst from the macrophages as trypomastigotes and disseminate widely to invade most human tissues
- Lymphatic spread then carries the organism to regional lymph nodes
- Chagoma: red nodule at site of bite; lasts only a few days to a couple of weeks
- Ramaña's sign: Bite near the eye causes unilateral periorbital conjunctivitis and edema
- Hematogenous dissemination: Acute phase with fever to 104°F, vomiting, diarrhea, cough, hepatosplenomegaly, edema, myocarditis, seizures, and meningoencephalitis
- Latent phase: Myocardial heart disease, with fibrosis, conduction defects
- Cardiac involvement: congestive heart failure
- Gastrointestinal system affected: dysphagia and abdominal pain, constipation secondary to megacolon (owing to destruction of the parasympathetic ganglion)
- Sequelae of myocardial damage, megacolon, megaesophagus
- Diagnosis: Parasites are relatively numerous initially and easily demonstrable on peripheral blood smear
- Treatment: Benzimidazole, nifurtimax

Lepidoptera (Caterpillars)

1. *Automeris io* (family *Saturniidae*)
   - Io moth
   - East of the Rocky Mountains from Canada to Mexico
   - Feed on deciduous (broadleaf) trees and herbaceous plants

- Yellow-green with red and white lateral stripes
- Urticating spines
2. *Megalopyge opercularis* (puss caterpillar, asp caterpillar) (Fig. 5-4)
   - Broad and flat
   - Dense covering of long, silky, gray to reddish brown hairs
   - Urticating spines dispersed among the hairs
3. *Sibine stimulea* (saddleback caterpillar)
   - Brown at both ends
   - Green around the middle "saddle blanket"
   - Purple-brown oval-spot "saddle"
   - Urticating spines along the sides and at the front and rear of the body

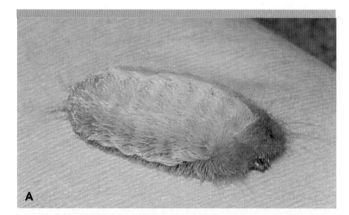

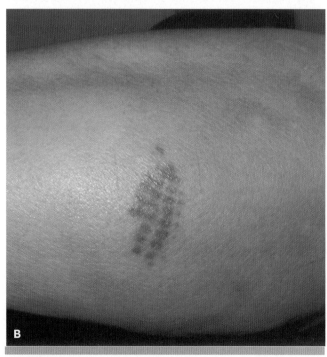

FIGURE 5-4 *Megalopyge opecularis* (puss catepillar, asp catepillar). *(From Freedberg IM et al: Fitzitzpatrick's Dermatology in General Medicine, 6th ed. New York: McGraw-Hill, 2003, p. 2297.)*

4. Hagmoth: brown with nine pairs of variable-length lateral processes with urticating hairs
5. Buck moth
   - Purple-black with a reddish head
   - Pale-yellow dots scattered over the body with reddish to black branches
   - Stinging spines arising from tubercles

Hymenoptera

- Known for producing a painful sting that rarely may result in anaphylaxis and death
- Reactions produced by *Hymenoptera* stings
- Local: erythema, edema, and pain at the site of the sting
- Wells' syndrome, consisting of erythematous, edematous plaques composed histologically of eosinophilic granulomatous dermatitis
- Systemic toxic venom
- From multiple stings
- Constitutional symptoms
- Systemic allergic
- Immunoglobulin (Ig) E antibodies cause degranulation and the release of vasoactive substances: urticaria and angioedema
- Other: serum sickness, acute renal failure, possible Guillain-Barré syndrome

SUBORDER: APOCRITA—ANTS, WASPS AND BEES

1. *Formicidae:* ants
- *Solenopsis* (fire ant)
  - Alkaloid venom contains phospholipase and hyalurinidase
  - May be red or black and live in ground colonies
  - Sting by first biting the victim with their powerful set of pincer jaws and then swiveling about their attached head and stinging in a circular pattern
  - Pustules, burning itch
2. *Vespidae:* yellowjackets, hornets, paper wasps
- Paper wasps build hives under the eaves of buildings
- Yellow jackets are ground-nesting
- Hornets reside in shrubs and trees
3. *Apoidea* family
- Bumble bees and honey bees
- Honeybees feed on flowering plants
- Stinger contains a barb, causing it to be left on the victim along with the venom sac
- This act eviscerates and kills the bee

ARACHNIDA

- Composed of arthropods
- Adult forms have four pairs of legs, six-legged larvae; the eight legged nymphs may cause human injury by

biting, burrowing in, and feeding on skin, stinging, and delivering toxic venom that may cause two syndromes:
- Tick-bite alopecia
  - Patchy alopecia at the site of tick attachment
  - Hair loss begins about 1 week after the tick is removed
- Tick paralysis
  - Ascending flaccid paralysis
  - Symptoms usually disappear rapidly if the tick is found and removed
  - Tick-bite pyrexia
- While the tick feeds, the host may develop fever, chills, headache, abdominal pain, and vomiting
- Natural parasites of many different animals, including mammals, birds, reptiles, and amphibians
- Vectors for numerous infectious diseases
- Two families of ticks:
  - Hard ticks (*Ixodidae*)
    - Hard chitinous dorsal shield
    - Can endure cold, humid weather
  - Soft ticks (*Argasidae*)
    - Lack a dorsal shield
    - Prefer drier environments
- Most ticks fast for long periods because they cannot live on vegetable matter; blood meal is acquired mostly by chance
- Feeding is usually complete within 6 to 7 days, but the tick can remain attached to the host for an unspecified period
- Ticks require a blood meal before they can lay eggs
- Body of mites and ticks
  - Divided into two regions
  - Anterior: cephalothorax (or prosoma)
  - Posterior: abdomen (or opisthosoma)

Cheyletiella (Fig. 5-5)

- "Walking dandruff": caused by movement of mite under scales
- Live on keratin layer of small mammals (dogs, cats, rabbits)
- Pruritic dermatitis in humans who handle pets

Liponyssoides (Formerly Allodermanyssus Sanguineus)

- House mouse mite
- Rickettsial pox (*Rickettsia akari*)

Ornithonyssus Sylviarum

- Found in birds and domestic fowl
- Bird handlers are bitten most commonly

Dermanyssus Gallinae and Ornithonyssus Bursa

- Can infest domestic poultry

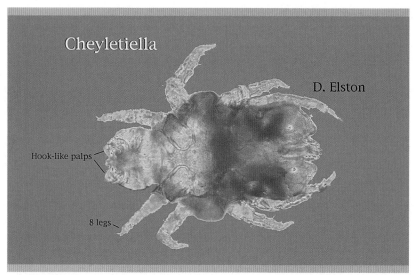

FIGURE 5-5 *Cheyletiella. (From Lesher JL: An Atlas of Microbiology of the Skin. Pearl River, NY: Parthenon, 2000, p. 49.)*

Dermatophagoides (Family Pyroglyphidae)

- House dust mite
- Tiny, translucent mites, generally less than 0.2 mm long
- Cause severe asthma and other allergic complaints in humans
- Humidity levels below 60 percent appear to support fewer mites

Mange Mites (Family Demodicidae)

DEMODEX FOLLICULORUM (FIG. 5-6)

- Elongate, microscopic mites
- Live in hair follicles and sebaceous glands
- Generally asymptomatic
- May cause folliculitis
- Associated with rosacea

Harvest Mites (Family Trombidiidae)

TROMBICULIDAE (CHIGGER, "RED MITE")

- Only the six-legged larval form parasitizes other animals
- Attach to a host, feed for 2 to 3 days, molt to the nymphal stage, and then leave the host
- Skin lesions develop 3 to 24 hours later when an allergic reaction to mite saliva develops
- Pruritic red papules grouped about the waist, thighs, and legs
- Can persist for several weeks
- *Eutrombicula alfreddugesi* most common variety in the United States
- *Neotrombicula autumnalis* most common variety in Europe
- Scrub typhus (*Rickettsia tsutsugamushi*)

Scabies or Itch Mites (Family Sarcoptidae)

SARCOPTES SCABEI (FIG. 5-7)

- Globular, semitranslucent mites, less than 0.3 mm long
- Adult mites copulate on the skin, after which the female will burrow, laying her eggs along the way
- Six-legged larvae hatch and take 10 to 14 days before becoming adults
- Will survive off the human body for only 2 to 3 days
- Symptoms take 30 days after an immune response develops to the mites or their excrement (scybala)
- Spread by close personal contact
- Hands and wrists are affected most often
- Burrows, which are produced by the adult female mite, and erythematous papules
- In adult patients, the scalp and face are uninvolved
- Pruritus of scabies generally is severe and most noticeable at night
- Diagnosis: mites, eggs, larvae, or scybala on microscopical examination of lesional skin scrapings
- Nodular scabies
  - Erythematous, firm nodules that persist for weeks to months after treatment
  - Long after the rest of the eruption has resolved
- Norwegian scabies
  - Seen in immunocompromised or debilitated patients
  - Thick, scaling, crusted plaques that are found most commonly on the hands, feet, and scalp but may be generalized in distribution
  - Lesions contain thousands of mites
- Treatment
  - Lindane: Avoid in young children and pregnant women owing to reports of neurotoxicity
  - 5% to 10% precipitated sulfur in petrolatum

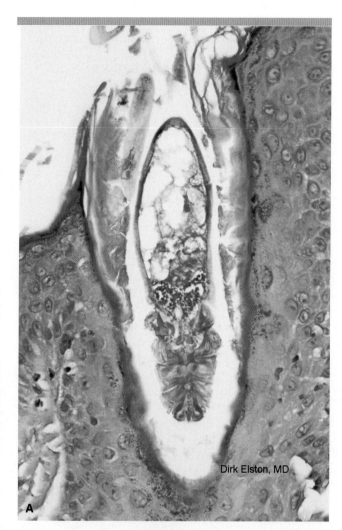

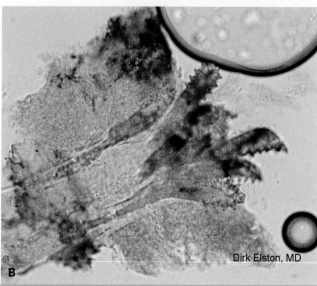

FIGURE 5-6 *Demodex folliculorum. (From Lesher JL: An Atlas of Microbiology of the Skin. Pearl River, NY: Parthenon, 2000, p. 49.)*

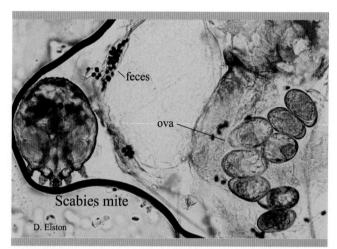

FIGURE 5-7 *Sarcoptes scabei. (From Lesher JL: An Atlas of Microbiology of the Skin. Pearl River, NY: Parthenon, 2000, p. 48.)*

- 5% permethrin
- 25% crotamiton
- Nodular scabies: topical or intralesional injection of a corticosteroid
- Norwegian scabies: oral ivermectin

Hard or Shield Ticks (Family Ixodidae)

- Wingless arthropods
- No true head
- Eight-legged as adults, six-legged larva
- Flattened dorsoventrally
- Often teardrop-shaped from dorsal view
- Scutum (shield) on the dorsal surface

1. *Ixodes* tick
   - *I. scapularis:* eastern United States
   - *I. pacificus:* in California
   - *I. ricinus:* in Europe
   - Vector for
     - Lyme disease (*Borrelia burgdorferi*)
     - Babesiosis
     - Ehrlichiosis
2. *Amblyoma americanum* (lone star tick) (Fig. 5-8)
   - Prominent white dot on the back of the adult female
   - Primarily found in the southwestern United States
   - Vector for
     - Rocky Mountain spotted fever (*Rickettsia rickettsii*)
     - Ehrlichiosis (*Ehrlichia chaffeensis*)
     - Tularemia (*Francisella tularensis*)
   - *Amblyomma maculatum* (Gulf Coast tick): tick paralysis
3. *Dermacentor* (Fig. 5-9)
   - Rocky Mountain spotted fever
   - Ehrlichiosis

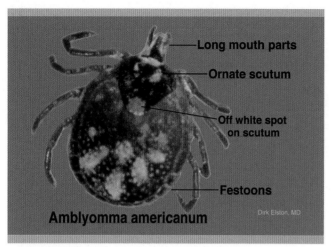

FIGURE 5-8 *Amblyoma americanum* (lone star tick). *(From Lesher JL: An Atlas of Microbiology of the Skin. Pearl River, NY: Parthenon, 2000, p. 52.)*

- Tularemia
- Colorado tick fever
  - Causative agent, an RNA virus of the genus *Orbivirus* of the family Reoviridae
  - Limited to *D. andersoni*
- *D. andersoni*
  - Wood tick
  - Western United States
  - Adults are generally brown but become slate gray when engorged
  - Commonly involved with tick paralysis
  - Female: dark reddish brown with a white shield covering the front third of the body
  - Male: grayish-white shield area on top of the body
- *D. variabilis*
  - Dog tick

- Eastern United States
- Commonly involved in cases of tick paralysis

Soft or Leathery Ticks (Family Argasidae)

- *Ornithodoros hermsi, O parkeri, O turicata*
- Light gray and leathery in appearance
- Mouthparts are hidden underneath the body
- Transmits relapsing fever: *Borrelia duttoni, Borrelia recurrentis*

Araneae (Spiders)

- All spiders have a cephalothorax from which extend eight legs and an abdomen
- A pair of jaws (chelicerae) are found at the anterior end of the cephalothorax
- Jaws terminate in sharp, chitinized fangs from which venom is ejected

Lactrodectus Mactans (Black Widow) (Fig. 5-10)

- Eastern and central regions of the United States
- Black with a globose abdomen that has the characteristic red hourglass-like marking on the ventral surface
- Prefer a warm, dry environment and can be found both outdoors and inside buildings
- Only the female of the species is capable of envenomating humans
- Neurotoxin (α-latrotoxin)
- Causes release of acetylcholine and catecholamines at neuromuscular junction
- Ca^{2+}-dependent release of neurotransmitters down the concentration gradient ensues
- No reuptake of the neurotransmitters
- Bite: Two tiny red puncta; urticarial with white halo, local piloerection; little local damage

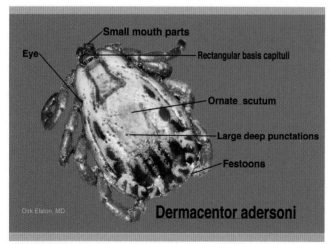

FIGURE 5-9 *Dermacentor. (From Lesher JL: An Atlas of Microbiology of the Skin. Pearl River, NY: Parthenon, 2000, p. 51.)*

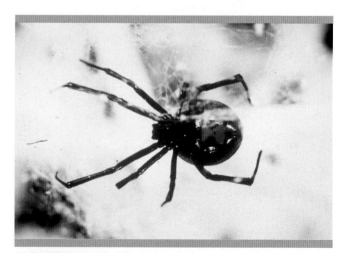

FIGURE 5-10 *Lactrodectus mactans* (black widow). *(From Freedberg IM et al: Fitzitzpatrick's Dermatology in General Medicine, 6th ed. New York: McGraw-Hill, 2003, p. 2295.)*

- Systemic symptoms begin within an hour, peak at 1 to 6 hours, and can last 1 to 2 days
- Severe myalgias and muscle cramping regionally and then through the body
- Abdominal musculature is involved and may simulate an acute surgical abdomen
- Painful lymphadenopathy, hypertension, profuse sweating, nausea, and tremors
- Treatment: symptomatic—narcotics, muscle relaxants, and intravenous calcium gluconate
- Spider antivenin

Loxosceles Reclusa (Brown Recluse) (Fig. 5-11)

- Violin-like marking on dorsal aspect of the cephalothorax
- Yellow to brown cephalothorax and a tan abdomen
- From 1 to 1.5 cm in length
- South central part of the United States; they avoid daylight
- Necrotic arachnidism
- Phospholipase (sphingomyelinase D) causes platelet aggregation, thrombosis, and massive neutrophil infiltration
- Initial bite is often painless and unnoticed by the patient; central papule and associated erythema
- Flag sign
  - Central blue-gray area due to thrombosis
  - Blanched halo from arterial spasm
  - A large surrounding area of reactive erythema
  - Progression to eschar formation, dermal necrosis, and stellate ulceration
- Systemic: hematuria, anemia, constitutional symptoms, rash, cyanosis, and severe intravascular hemolysis

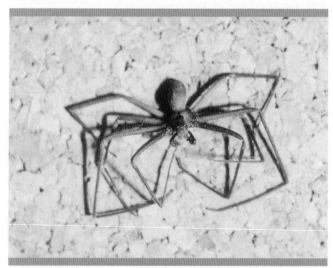

FIGURE 5-11 *Loxosceles reclusa* (brown recluse). *(From Freedberg IM et al: Fitzitzpatrick's Dermatology in General Medicine, 6th ed. New York: McGraw-Hill, 2003, p. 2293.)*

- Treatment
  - Tetanus toxoid
  - Dapsone, 100 mg daily, is effective in limiting the cutaneous necrosis
  - Cold compresses, simple analgesics
  - Antibiotics if superficial infection develops

Scorpions

- *Centruroides sculpturatus* most common in United States
- Large arachnids with an elongated abdomen that terminates in a stinger
- Abdominal glands that release both neurotoxic and hemolytic venom into the stinger
- Nocturnal and hide during the daytime in dark places
- Pain and swelling at the site of sting
- Neurotoxin can result in: localized numbness, fasciculation, lacrimation, salivation, profuse sweating, urinary urgency, nausea, tongue paresthesia, restlessness, convulsions, and an increase in extraocular muscle activity
- Treatment
  - Remove the stinger; apply a tourniquet
  - Cool the site with ice; antivenin
  - Barbiturates or diazepam for the central nervous system hyperactivity
  - Atropine for cholinergic side effects of the neurotoxin

CENTIPEDES AND MILLIPEDES

American Centipedes

- Slender, segmented body that ranges in color from yellow to green to brown or black and may vary in length from 1 to 30 cm
- Nocturnal carnivores and prefer a dark, moist environment like that found under rocks and logs
- *Scutigera* species
  - Found in the eastern United States
  - Does not sting humans
- *Scolopendra* species
  - Western United States and Hawaii
  - Can inflict a painful sting
  - Immediate reaction consists of local burning pain
  - A pair of hemorrhagic puncta surrounded by erythema and edema at the sting site
  - Occasionally, local necrosis, regional lymphangitis, and lymphadenopathy
- Treatment
  - Cleanse the wound
  - Inject a local anesthetic into the wound
  - Tetanus prophylaxis
  - Systemic antihistamines

Millipedes

- Multisegmented, with a hard, often brightly colored exoskeleton
- Nocturnal vegetarians that prefer dark, moist environments
- When disturbed, millipedes will coil into a tight spiral and then secrete a toxic liquid from repugnatorial glands located on the sides of each segment
- Causes an immediate burning sensation when it contacts human skin
- Skin then becomes yellow-brown and in 24 hours develops intense erythema and often vesiculation
- Treatment: immediate lavage of the area with alcohol or water

CESTODA

Tape Worms

- Long, segmented worms
- Include
  - Cysticercosis
  - Echinococcosis
  - Sparganosis
  - Coenurosis
- Life cycle
  - Eggs passed from the primary host and ingested by an intermediate host, where eggs hatch
  - Larvae encyst within tissues
  - Infection of the primary host occurs by ingesting the cyst-infested flesh of the intermediate host

Cysticercosis

- *Taenia solium*
- Most common helminth infection in the United States
- Eggs in undercooked pork ingested and penetrate bowel to enter muscle, brain, and eyes where they develop into larvae
- Seizures, mass lesions, nodules
- Treatment: surgical excision, albendazole, praziquantel

Echinococcosis

- *Echinococcus* species (*E. granulosus:* dog; *E. multilocularis:* fox)
- Eggs from animal feces are ingested; larvae hatch and penetrate gut wall
- Hydatid cyst in the abdomen
- Treatment: surgical excision, mebendazole

Sparganosis

- *Spirometra* species
- Larvae from undercooked fish are ingested
- Enlarging subcutaneous nodule
- Treatment: surgical excision

Coenurosis

- *Taenia* species (*multiceps, serialis, brauni*)
- Eggs in host feces (dogs, fox, wolf)
- Ingested by herbivores (cows) and penetrate bowel to enter muscle, brain, and eyes, where they develop into larvae
- Seizures, mass lesions, subcutaneous nodules
- Treatment: surgical excision

PROTOZOA

Cutaneous Amebiasis

- *Entamoeba histolytica*
- Humans are the only reservoir
- Clinical presentation includes an acute dysenteric form and a less symptomatic nondysenteric intestinal form
- Life cycle: Cysts travel to the small intestine after ingestion from fecally contaminated food or water
- Trophozoites are released, and two outcomes can occur
- They reencyst and produce asymptomatic infection (resolves spontaneously within 12 months) or parasite causes symptomatic amebiasis
- Intestinal disease: acute proctocolitis (dysentery)
- Extraintestinal disease: brain and liver amebic abscesses, peritonitis, pericarditis, cutaneous lesions of amebiasis seem to be extremely rare (direct extension of intestinal disease): with painful ulcerations that may enlarge rapidly
- Diagnosis: indirect hemagglutination, immunofluorescence, and ELISAs
- Treatment: metronidazole, iodoquinol, paromomycin

HELMINTHIC INFECTIONS

- *Helminth* is derived from the Greek word *helmins*, meaning "worm"
- Categorized as
  - Annelids (i.e., phylum Annelida, the segmented worms)
  - Nematodes (i.e., phylum Nematoda, the roundworms)
  - Platyhelminths (i.e., phylum Platyhelminthes, the flatworms)
  - Trematodes (i.e., flukes) and cestodes (i.e., tapeworms)

SOIL-MEDIATED HELMINTHIC INFECTIONS

NEMATODES (ROUNDWORMS)

- Hookworm: *Ancylostoma* and *Necator*
- Strongyloidiasis

- Ascariasis
- Enterobiasis
- Trichinosis
- Dracunculiasis
- Filariasis: loiasis, onchocerciasis
- Hookworms: caused by the roundworms

ANCYLOSTOMA DUODENALE, NECATOR AMERICANUS

- Ground itch
- Life cycle: Female worms, residing in the host's small intestine, release eggs that are passed in the feces
- Larvae in soil penetrate foot and migrate to lungs through the venous system
- Larvae are then coughed up and swallowed, and they end up in intestine and mature into adults
- Pruritic, erythematous, edematous, linear, threadlike tracts marking larval migration in the skin
- Gastrointestinal bleeding, iron-deficiency anemia, hypoproteinemia
- Treatment: mebendazole, albendazole

CUTANEOUS LARVA MIGRANS (CREEPING ERUPTION) (FIG. 5-12)

- *Ancylostoma braziliensis,* hookworm of wild and domestic dogs and cats
- Most common cause of cutaneous larva migrans; human is a dead-end host
- Eggs are passed from animal feces into warm, moist, sandy soil, where the larvae hatch
- Larva penetrate skin directly but cannot penetrate basement membrane
- Larvae migrate slowly (2 cm/day) in skin, lack the ability to invade further, and complete their life cycle
- Produce raised, threadlike, serpiginous, pruritic, erythematous tracks
- Treatment: topical thiabendazole, ivermectin, albendazole

STRONGYLOIDES (LARVA CURRENS, "RACING LARVA")

- *Strongyloides stercoralis* (known as threadworm)
- Nematodes live in the small intestine
- Eggs hatch into larvae (rhabditiform), which are passed in the feces
- Larvae can penetrate skin of the host (quick migration rate of 5 to 10 cm/h) and then penetrate basement membrane to affect lungs and the gastrointestinal tract
- Larvae subsequently are swallowed and reach the small intestine
- Intense pruritus, purpura, serpentine urticarial streaks
- Autoinfection: transformation of noninfective larvae (rhabditiform) into infective larvae (filariform)
- Chronic strongyloidiasis
- Serpiginous wheals beginning perianally and extending to the buttocks, upper thighs, and abdomen

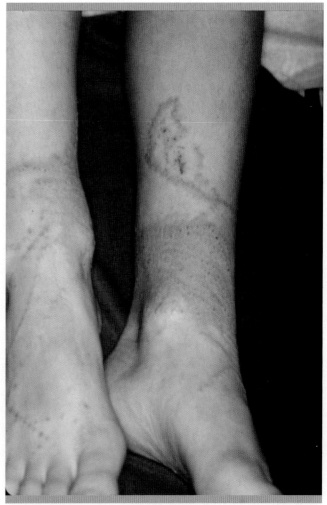

FIGURE 5-12 Cutaneous larva migrans (creeping eruption). *(From Freedberg IM et al: Fitzitzpatrick's Dermatology in General Medicine, 6th ed. New York: McGraw-Hill, 2003, p. 2270.)*

- Hemorrhagic pneumonia can result
- Stool for ova and parasites
- Enterotest (string test) or duodenal aspiration to examine duodenal fluid
- Blood cultures
- Enzyme immunoassay (EIA), indirect fluorescent antibody (IFA)
- Chest radiograph to reveal possible patchy alveolar infiltrate
- Sputum examination
- Loefler's syndrome: eosinophilia, pneumonitis
- Treatment: thiobendazole, albendazole, ivermectin

ASCARIASIS

- *Ascaris lumricoides*
- Adult worms live in the small intestine; eggs are laid and then passed out in the feces
- Eggs may remain viable in soil up to 17 months

- Larvae develop within the eggs
- Eggs re ingested or inhaled from soil; larvae hatch and move to heart, lungs, and pharynx
- Swallowed larvae mature into adults in intestine
- Urticaria
- Gastrointestinal symptoms/obstruction
- Cough, dyspnea, asthma, and chest pain
- Stool examination for ova and parasites
- Treatment: mebendazole, pyrantel pamoate

ENTEROBIASIS (PINWORM DISEASE)

- *Enterobius vermicularis*
- Most common helminth infection in industrialized countries
- After ingestion, eggs usually hatch in the duodenum within 6 hours
- Female worm migrates to the rectum after copulation and, if not expelled during defecation, migrates to the perineum (often at night)
- Pruritus ani, bruxism
- Diagnosis
  - Transparent tape is pressed against the perineum at night
  - Identify eggs under the low-power lens of microscope (Fig. 5-13)
- Treatment: pyrantel

TRICHINOSIS

- *Trichinella spiralis*
- Larval cysts ingested from undercooked meat (usually pork)
- Acidity and enzymatic activity of the human digestive system disrupt the cyst, releasing large numbers of newborn larvae that penetrate the gut wall, enter the systemic circulation, and migrate to various tissues
- Larvae usually persist only in striated skeletal muscle cells, transformed into nurse cells
- Calcified cysts in muscle, elevated muscle enzymes
- Fever, myalgias, and periorbital edema (increased interstitial fluid)
- Vasculitis: splinter hemorrhages in nails and eyes
- Diagnosis
  - Enzyme immunoassay (EIA) or the bentonite flocculation (BF) test
  - Elevated creatine kinase (CK) and lactate dehydrogenase (LDH)
  - Stool examination: Charcot-Leyden crystals from eosinophils may be found in stools
- Treatment
  - Trichinosis is usually a self-limited illness
  - Prednisone
  - Mebendazole and albendazole
  - Proper cooking of meat is the most effective method to prevent infection

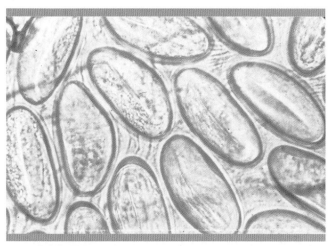

FIGURE 5-13 *Enterobius* eggs under the microscope. *(From Freedberg IM et al: Fitzitzpatrick's Dermatology in General Medicine, 6th ed. New York: McGraw-Hill, 2003, p. 2239.)*

DRACUNCULIASIS

- *Dracunculus medinesis*, guinea fire worm; nematode
- Ingested larvae reside in an intermediate host, a tiny freshwater crustacean or copepod
- Migrates from the gastrointestinal tract to a location in the lower extremity (most commonly the foot), causing a bulla that ruptures to release the larvae back into water
- Clinical: presence of the adult worm in the subcutaneous tissue, usually lower extremity
- Constitutional symptoms
- Treatment
  - Slowly wind worm around stick
  - Metronidazole, thiabendazole

FILARIAE

- Eight species of roundworm belonging to the family Filarioidea develop to adulthood in humans
- Larvae or microfilariae are ingested by a feeding insect vector
- Larvae are then inoculated into the vertebral host for the final stages of development
- Cutaneous group (listed below)
  - *Loa loa*
  - *Onchocerca volvulus*
  - *Mansonella streptocerca*
- Lymphatic group
  Wuchereria bancrofti: causes Bancroftian filariasis
    - Genital disease: edema of scrotal skin, funiculitis, epididymitis, orchitis, and hydrocele
    - Distinctive lymphangitis of the arms or legs characterized by a unique retrograde spread or extension

- Starting in a single node, erythematous patches of subcutaneous edema or diffuse erythema and edema develop and progress distally
- Treatment: diethylcarbamazine
- *Brugia malayi:* causes Malayan filariasis
- *Brugia timori:* causes Timorian filariasis
  - Clinical manifestations of Malayan filariasis and Timorian filariasis
  - Axillary or inguinal lymphadenitis, lymphangitis, and fever are common
  - Lymphatic abscesses and resulting scarring

Body cavity group
- *Mansonella streptocerca:* causes streptocerciasis
- Central and West Africa
- Transmitted by the midge *Culicoides grahami*
- Adult worms are found in the dermis of the patient's upper trunk
- Microfilariae are found in the dermis and lymph nodes
- Treatment: diethylcarbamazine
- Loiasis (*Loa loa*)
- Vector: *Chrysops* (deer fly)
- Rain forests of Central and West Africa
- Diurnal periodicity: Microfilariae are found in the bloodstream in highest numbers during the day
- Clinical manifestations
  - Transient, nontender areas of angioedema and urticaria are the major signs and symptoms
  - Calabar swellings: transient subcutaneous swellings on the extremities
  - Worm migration across conjunctiva or bridge of nose
  - Localized pain, pruritus, and urticaria
  - Arthritis, breast calcification, meningoencephalopathy, endomyocardial fibrosis, peripheral neuropathy, pleural effusions, and retinopathy

Treatment: diethylcarbamazine
  - Mazzotti reaction: stroke or meningoencephalitis from release of dead microfilariae in blood and cerebrospinal fluid (CSF) after treatment with diethylcarbamazine (DEC); it may occur without drug therapy
- Onchocerciasis (river blindness, hanging groins, leopard skin, or sowdah)
- *Onchocerca volvulus*
- Vector: *Simulium* species of blackflies
- Tropical Africa
- Microfilariae found in the dermis, eyes, and regional lymph nodes
- Clinical manifestations
  - Pruritus, subcutaneous lumps, lymphadenitis, and blindness
  - Onchocercoma: Subcutaneous nodules common over bony prominences

- Ocular: punctate keratitis, pannus formation, corneal fibrosis, iridocyclitis, glaucoma, choroiditis, and optic
- "Lizard skin," "hanging skin": Fibrosis and atrophy may cause lymph nodes or portions of bowel to hang in pockets of skin
- Hypopigmented patches in Africans ("leopard skin")
- Hyperpigmented patches in Arabics (sowdah)
- Facial edema/pruritus in Mexico and Guatemala (erysipela de la Costa)
- Diagnosis
  - Slit-lamp examination: microfilariae in the eye
  - Biopsy of a nodule will reveal an adult worm
- Treatment: ivermectin (does not produce a significant Mazzotti reaction)
- Mansonelliasis
- Vectors: midge species *Culicoides austeni* and *Culicoides grahami*
- *Mansonella streptocerca*
- Subcutaneous infection in humans

TOXOCARIASIS

- Visceral larva migrans
- Caused by the roundworm of the dog and cat: *Toxocara canis* and *T. catis*
- Eggs ingested from soil; larvae penetrate bowel and lodge in organs and blood vessels
- Hemorrhage, necrosis, urticaria
- Ocular larva migrans: Penetrating larva can become ecysted, leading to the fomation of a large granuloma

Snail-Mediated Helminthiasis

TREMATODES (FLUKES)

- Phylum Platyhelminthes contains the dorsoventrally flattened worms
- Schistosomiasis (bilharziasis)
- Life cycle
  - Eggs passed in urine (*S. haematobium*) or feces (*S. japonicum* and *S. mansoni*), hatch in water
  - From eggs, miracidia hatch into the water, where they penetrate into snails; in the snails they develop into cercariea that penetrate the host skin
  - Enter the portal venous system of the liver and travel to heart, lungs, and finally the bladder or the mesenteric vessels
- Schistosomiasis organisms (blood flukes):
  - *S. mansoni*
    - South America
    - Portal hypertension, found in large intestine and liver, eggs shed in stool
    - Location of spine on ova: lateral
  - *S. japonicum*
    - Asia
    - Portal hypertension; found in small intestine and liver; eggs shed in stool
    - Location of spine on ova: no spine

- *S. haematobium*
  - Africa, Middle East
  - Found in bladder, pelvic/urogenital venules; eggs shed in urine
  - Location of spine on ova: apical
- Clinical
  - Cercarial dermatitis (swimmer's itch):
    - Pruritus, dermatitis
    - Skin exposure to fresh or salt water
    - Macular eruption, pruritic
    - Spares clothing-covered skin
  - Acute syndrome, Katayama fever: spiking afternoon fevers, chills, bronchitis, pneumonitis, headache, lymphadenopathy, hepatosplenomegaly, joint pain, diarrhea, urticaria, eosinophilia, leukocytosis, and an elevated erythrocyte sedimentation rate
  - Late hypersensitivity reaction: generalized urticaria, pruritus, lichenified papules, or dermatographism
- Treatment: antihistamines plus topical steroids

REPTILES

Snakes

- United States: rattlesnake, cottonmouth moccasin, and copperhead (family *Crotalidae*) account for the vast majority of bites

Elapidae Family

- Coral snake
  - Round eyes
  - Red and yellow or white bands
  - Nonvenomous mimics tend to have red and black bands
  - Neurotoxic
  - Muscle fasciculations, later flaccid paralysis
- Viperidae family (pit viper)
  - Copperhead, rattlesnake, cottonmouth (water moccasin)
  - Triangular head distinct from the body
  - Elliptical "cat's eye" pupils
  - Venom with hydrolases; anticoagulant in the venom causes hemolysis and capillary leakage
  - Pain, edema, ecchymosis, vesiculation, petechiae, and tissue necrosis can develop at the site of the bite
  - Damage to vascular endothelium, hypotension

MISCELLANEOUS

1. *Chironex fleckeri*
   - Box jellyfish (Australia)
   - Venom causes death from circulatory and respiratory failure
2. Seabather's eruption
   - Larvae from coelenterates become trapped under clothing and discharge irritating nematocysts
   - Pruritic popular eruption under swimwear
3. Fascioliasis
   - *Fasciola hepatica*
   - Metacercariae on plants are ingested by sheep or humans; larvae migrate to the bile duct
   - Hepatomegaly, right upper quadrant pain, jaundice, urticaria
   - Treatment: surgery, bithionel, triclabendazole
4. Gnathostomiasis (Wandering swelling, Yangtse river edema)
   - *Gnathostoma spinigerum*
   - Humans eat fish that contain larvae, or larvae penetrate the skin directly
   - Migrating erythematous swelling, pain, pruritus
   - Treatment: surgery, ivermectin, albendazole

REFERENCES

Buxton, PK: ABC of dermatology. Insect bites and infestations. *Br Med J* 1988;296:489–491.

Chaudhry AZ, Longworth DL: Cutaneous manifestations of intestinal helminthic infections. *Dermatol Clin* 1989;7:275–290.

Freedberg IM et al. *Fitzpatrick's Dermatology in General Medicine*, 6th Ed. New York: McGraw-Hill; 2003.

Mackey SL, Wagner KF: Dermatologic manifestations of parasitic diseases. *Infect Dis Clin North Am* 1994;8:713–743.

McGinley-Smith DE, Tsao SS: Dermatoses from ticks. *J Am Acad Dermatol* 2003;49;363–392.

McKee PH. *Pathology of the Skin: With Clinical Correlations.* London: Mosby-Wolfe; 1996.

Meinking TL, Burkhart CN, Burkhart CG: Changing paradigms in parasitic infections: common dermatological helminthic infections and cutaneous myiasis. *Clin Dermatol* 2003;21: 407–416.

Metry DW, Hebert AA: Insect and arachnid stings, bites, infestations, and repellents. *Pediatr Ann* 2000;29(1):39–48.

Normann SA: Venomous insects and reptiles. *J Fla Med Assoc* 1996;83:183–186.

Rosen T: Caterpillar dermatitis. *Dermatol Clin* 1990;8:245–252.

Wilson DC, King LE Jr: Spiders and spider bites. *Dermatol Clin* 1990;8:277–286.

CHAPTER 6

CONTACT DERMATITIS

MELISSA A. BOGLE
RAJANI KATTA

CONTACT DERMATITIS

- Inflammatory response of the skin to an antigen or irritant
- Allergic contact dermatitis (ACD)
  - Delayed hypersensitivity reaction
  - Individuals previously sensitized to the contactant
  - Acute ACD: Lesions appear within 24 to 96 hours of exposure to the allergen
- Irritant contact dermatitis (ICD)
  - Irritant produces direct local cytotoxic effect on the cells of the epidermis
  - Subsequent inflammatory response in the dermis
  - Caused mostly by chemicals
  - Two types
    - Mild irritants: require prolonged or repeated exposure before inflammation is noted
    - Strong irritants
      - ▲ Strong acids, alkalis
      - ▲ Can produce immediate reactions similar to thermal burns
- Clinical changes
  - Acute contact dermatitis: clear fluid–filled vesicles or bullae that appear on bright red edematous skin
  - Subacute contact dermatitis: less edema and formation of papules
  - Chronic contact dermatitis
    - Minimal edema
    - Scaling, skin fissuring, and lichenification
- Histology
  - Dermis with lymphocytes and other mononuclear cells
  - Epidermal edema
  - Chronic ACD: acanthosis with hyperkeratosis and parakeratosis

CONTACT URTICARIA

- An immunoglobulin E (IgE)–mediated immediate hypersensitivity reaction (type I)
- Immediate release of inflammatory mediators, resulting in a wheal-and-flare reaction
- Rubber latex currently is the most important source of allergic contact urticaria

PHOTODERMATITIS

- Diagnosed by the presence of lesions limited to sun-exposed body areas

PHOTOSENSITIVITY INDUCED BY EXOGENOUS AGENTS

- Photoallergic reaction
  - Delayed-type hypersensitivity
  - Onset delayed as long as 24 to 72 hours after exposure to the drug and light
  - Amount of drug required to elicit photoallergic reactions is considerably smaller than that required for phototoxic reaction
  - Irradiation of certain substances by ultraviolet light results in the transformation of the substance into allergens
  - Reactions resemble allergic contact dermatitis, with a distribution limited to sun-exposed areas of the body
  - When the reactions are severe or prolonged, they may extend into covered areas of skin
  - Examples of agents that can cause a photoallergic reaction (Tables 6-1 and 6-2).
    - Sunscreens
    - Padimate A, padimate O

TABLE 6-1 Topical Photoallergens

Group	INCI Name/Chemical Name/Trade Name*

Sunscreens	*UVB absorbers:*
	  para-Aminobenzoic acids (PABA):
	    Amyl dimethyl PABA (*Padimate A; Escalol 506*)[†]
	    PABA (*Pabanol*)[†]
	    Ethylhexyl dimethyl PABA (octyl dimethyl PABA; *Padimate O; Escalol 507*)[†]
	  Cinnamates:
	    Cinoxate (2-ethoxyethyl-*p*-methoxycinnamate; *Phiasol*)
	    Ethylhexyl methoxycinnamate (octyl methoxycinnamate; *Parsol MCX; Escalol 557*)
	  Salicylate:
	    Homosalate (metahomomenthyl salicylate; *Eusolex HMS*)
	UVA absorbers:
	  Anthranllate:
	    Menthyl anthranilate (cyclohexanol; *Trivent MA*)
	  Benzophenones:
	    Benzophenone-3 (oxybenzone; *Escalol 567*)[†]
	    Benzophenone-4 (sulisobenzone; *Escalol 577*)[†]
	  Dibenzoylmethane:
	    Butyl methoxydibenzoylmethane (avobenzone; *Parsol 1789*)[†]

Fragrances	6-Methylcoumarin[†] Musk ambrette[†] Sandalwood oil
Antibacterials	Dibromosalicylanilide (dibromsalan; DBS)[†] Tetrochlorosalicylanilide (TCSA; *Impregon; Irgasan BS200*)[†] Tribromosalicylanilide (tribromsalan; TBS)* Chlorhexidene (*Hibiclens*) Dimethylol-dimethyl hydantoin Hexachlorophene (*pHisoHex*) Bithionol (thiobisdichlorophenol; bisphenol; *Actamar*)[†] Dichlorophene (G4) Triclosan (*Irgasan DP300*)
Antifungals	Fentichlor (thiobischlorophenol)* Jadit (butylchlorosalicylamide; buclosamide) Multifungin (bromochlorosalicylanilide; BCSA)
Others	Chlorpromazine (*Thorazine*)* Clioquinol Ketoprofen (*Orudis*) Olaquindox Promethazine (*Phenergan*)* Quinidine (*Cardioquin; Quinidex*) Thiourea (thiocarbamide)

*INCI: International Nomenclature of Cosmetic Ingredients.
[†]Commonly reported photoallergens.
Source: Freedberg IM et al: *Fitzpatrick's Dermatology in General Medicine*, 6th ed. New York: McGraw-Hill, 2003, p. 1305.

TABLE 6-2 Systemic Photoallergens

Property	Generic Name (U.S. Trade Name)
Antifungal	Griseofulvin (*Fulvicin-U/F*)
Antimalarial	Quinine
Antimicrobials	Quinolone: Enoxacin (*Penetrex*) Sulfonamides
Cardiac medication	Quinidine (*Quinaglute, Quinidex*)
Nonsteroidal	Ketoprofen (*Orudis, Oruvall*)
	Piroxicam (*Feldene*)
Vitamin	Pyridoxine hydrochloride (vitamin B$_6$)

Source: Freedberg IM et al: *Fitzpatrick's Dermatology in General Medicine,* 6th ed. New York: McGraw-Hill, 2003, p. 1305.

- *para*-Aminobenzoic acid (PABA)
- Cinnamates
- Benzophenones
- Salicylates
- Fragrances
  - ▲ Musk ambrette
  - ▲ 6-Methylcoumarin
- Phototoxic reaction (Tables 6-3 and 6-4).
  - Often occur within minutes or hours of light exposure
  - Chemically induced nonimmunologic acute skin irritation
  - Does not require prior sensitization
  - Active chemical may enter the skin via topical administration or via ingestion, inhalation, or parenteral administration
  - Damaging effects of light-activated compounds on cell membranes

- Most compounds are activated by wavelengths within the ultraviolet A (UV-A) (320–400 nm) range
- Clinical appearance of an exaggerated sunburn reaction
- Common inducing agents include tars, furo-coumarins, (limes, celery, parsley) and 8- and 5-methoxypsoralen
- Photopatch test
  - Used to find causative agent of photoallergic reaction
  - Photopatch testing protocol
    - Day 1: Determine minimal erythema doses (MEDs), and apply two sets of patches
    - Day 2: Read MEDs
    - Day 2: Remove patches, read, and irradiate one set (10 J/cm^2 UV-A)
    - Day 4: First reading
    - Days 5–9: Second reading

TABLE 6-3 Topical Phototoxic Agents

Agent	Exposure
Rose bengal	Ophthalmologic examination
Furocoumarins	Occur naturally in plants, fruits and vegetables (lime, lemon, celery, fig, parsley, and parsnip); used in perfumes and cosmetics; used for topical photochemotherapy
Tar	Topical therapeutic agent; roofing materials

Source: Freedberg IM et al: *Fitzpatrick's Dermatology in General Medicine,* 6th ed. New York: McGraw-Hill, 2003, p. 1301.

TABLE 6-4 Systemic Phototoxic Agents

Property	Generic Name (U.S. Trade Name)	Property	Generic Name (U.S. Trade Name)
Antianxiety drugs	Alprazolam (*Xanax*) Chlordiazepoxide (*Librax; Librium; Limbitrol*)		Prochlorperazine (*Compazine*)* Thioridazine (*Mellaril*) Trifluoperazine (*Stelazine*)
Anticancer drugs	Dacarbazine (*DTIC-Dome*) Fluorouracil (*Adrucil*) Methotrexate (*Rheumatrex*) Vinblastine (*Velban*)	Cardiac medications	Amiodarone (*Cordarone; Pacerone*)* Quinidine (*Quinaglute; Quinidex*)
Antidepressants	Tricyclics: Amitriptyline (*Elavil; Limbitrol; Triavil*) Desipramine (*Norpramin*) Imipramine (*Tofranil*)	Diuretics	Furosemide (*Lasix*)* Thiazides: Bendroflumethiazide (*Corzide*) Chlorothiazide (*Aldoclor; Diuril*)* Hydrochlorothiazide (*Accuretic; Aldactazide; Aldoril; Atacana Avalide; Capozide; Dlovan; Dyazide; HydroDIURII*)*
Antifungal	Griseofulvin (*Fulvicin; Grifulvin V; Gris-PEG*)		
Antimalarials	Chloroquine (*Aralen*) Quinine		
Antimicrobials	Quinolones: Ciprofloxacin (*Cipro*) Enoxacin (*Penetrex*) Gemifloxacin Lomefloxacin (*Maxaquin*)* Moxifloxacin (*Avelox*) Nalidixic acid (*NegGram*)* Norfloxacin (*Chibroxin; Noroxin*) Ofloxacin (Floxin; Ocuflox) Sparfloxacin (*Zagam*)* Suifonamides Tetracyclines Demeclocycline (*Declomycin*)* Doxycycline (*Monodox; Periostat; Vibramycin*)* Minocycline (*Dynacin; Minocin*) Tetracycline (*Helidac; Sumycin*) Trimethoprim (*Bactrim; Polytrim; Primsal; Septra*)	Dye	Fluorescein (*AK-Fluor; Fluor; Fluor-I-Strip Fluorescite*) Methylene blue (*Urised*)
		Furocoumarins	Psoralens: 5-Methoxypsoralen* 8-Methoxypsoralen (*Oxsoralen-Ultra 4,5',8-Trimethylpsoralen*)
		Hypoglycemics	Sulfonylureas: Acetohexamide Chlorpropamide (*Diabinase*) Glipizide (*Glucotrol*) Glyburide (*DiaBeta; Glucovance Glynase Pres Tab; Micronase*) Tolazamide (*Tolinase*) Tolbutamide (*Orinase*)*
Antipsychotic drugs	Phenothiazines: Chlorpromazine (*Thorazine*)* Perphenazine (*Triavil; Trilafon*)	NSAIDs	Acetic acid derivative: Diclofenac (*Arthrotec; Cataplan Voltaren*) Anthranilic acid derivative: Mefenamic acid (*Ponstel*) Enolic acid derivative: Piroxicam (*Feldene*)*

TABLE 6-4 (Continued)

Property	Generic Name (U.S. Trade Name)	Property	Generic Name (U.S. Trade Name
	Propionic acid derivatives: Ibuprofen (*Advil; Motrin; Nuprin Vicoprofen*) Ketoprofen (*Orudis; Oruvail*) Naproxen (Aleve; Naprelan; Naprosyn)* Oxaprozin (*Daypro*) Tiaprofenic acid Salicyclic acid derivative: Diflunisal (*Dolobid*) Others: Celecoxib (*Celebrex*) Nabumetone (*Relafen*)*	Retinoids	Acitretin (*Soriatane*) Isotretinoin (*Accutane*) Etretinate
		Other	Flutamide (*Eulexin*) Hypericin Pyridoxine (vitamin B6) Ranitidine (*Zantac*)
Photodynamic therapy agents	Porfimer (*Photofrin*)* Verteporfin (*Visudyne*)*		

*Commonly reported
Source: Freedberg IM et al: *Fitzpatrick's Dermatology in General Medicine,* 6th ed. New York: McGraw-Hill, 2003, p. 1302.

FRAGRANCE-RELATED ALLERGENS

1. Balsam of Peru
   - Wood extract derived from *Myroxolon balsamum* tree
   - Contains
     - Cinnamein (cinnamic acid, cinnamyl cinnamate, benzyl benzoate, benzoic acid and vanillin)
     - Polymers of coniferyl alcohol with benzoic acid and cinnamic acid
   - Fragrances, flavorings/spices (cola), pharmaceuticals (antifungal and antibacterial properties), diaper powders and ointments, cough medicines, aperitifs
   - Cross-reacts with colophony, turpentine, benzoin, wood tar
2. Bergamot
   - Berloque dermatitis (see "Plants Related Allergens")
3. Cinnamic aldehyde
   - Fragrance and flavor agent; constituent of cinnamon oil
   - Toothpaste, mouthwash, gum: perioral dermatitis, tongue swelling, mouth ulceration
   - Flavoring in beverages (cola)
   - Spices: hand dermatitis in bakers
   - Essential oils: balsam of Peru, hyacinth, myrrh, patchouli, ceylon, cassia oil
4. Lily of the valley
   - Allergen: hydroxycitronellal (synthetic)
   - Found in perfumes, soaps, cosmetics, eye cream, aftershaves
   - Also used in insecticides and antiseptics

5. Musk ambrette
   - Fixative in perfumes
   - Photoallergen
6. Oak moss absolute
   - *Evernia prunastri:* lichen oak moss
   - Main allergen: atranorin
   - Essential oil from lichens can contain the following other allergens: evernic acid and fumarprotocetaric acid
   - "Masculine" odor in aftershaves
7. Geraniol
   - *Sweet floral* odor of rose
   - Constitutes a large portion of rose and palmarose oil, geranium oil, lavender oil, jasmine oil, and citronella oil
   - Most widely used fragrance in perfumes, colognes, facial makeup, and skin-care products
8. Eugenol
   - Powerful spicy odor of clove with a pungent taste
   - Found in oils of clove and cinnamon leaf
   - Also found in roses, carnations, hyacinths, and violets
   - Fragrance in perfume, cosmetics; flavoring in toothpaste, mouthwash; and food flavorings, dental cement, insecticidal and fungicidal properties—used to preserve meats and other foods

HAIR-RELATED ALLERGENS

1. Paraphenylenediamine (PPD)
   - Blue-black aniline dye

- Dark permanent hair dye: hand dermatitis in hairdressers, scalp/hairline dermatitis in clients
- Dyed furs, photographic developers, photocopy, printing ink, dark cosmetics, black rubber (rubber antioxidant), leather processing
- Cross-reacts with PABA, ester anesthetics, sulfa medications, azo dyes (textile dermatitis; blue dyes 106 and 124 can be used as screening agents)
- Synthetic henna: Formulations are available that contain PPD and sometimes lead to an allergic reaction (Type IV hypersensitivity)
  - Natural henna is derived from the *Lawsonia alba* plant and does not usually lead to ACD
- Patch test with PPD
2. Glycerol thioglycolate (GTG)
   - Acidic (salon) permanent wave solutions and hair straighteners
   - Chemical remains in hair shaft for months: chronic dermatitis in hairdressers and clients
   - Note: Alkaline (home) permanent solutions contain ammonium thioglycolate (ATG) and are also irritating
3. Ammonia persulfate
   - Peroxide hair bleaches
   - Bleached baking flour
   - Contact urticaria and anaphylactoid reactions
4. Cocamidopropyl betaine
   - Allergen may be dimethylaminopropylamine (produced in synthesis)
   - Surfactant
   - Shampoo (dermatitis in hair dressers), liquid soaps

MEDICINE-RELATED ALLERGENS

1. Tixocortol pivalate
   - Used to test for allergy to group A steroids (e.g., prednisone, hydrocortisone)
   - Short-chain esters
2. Budesonide
   - Screening agent for allergy to groups B (e.g., triamcinolone) and D (e.g., HC-17 butyrate) steroids
   - Long-chain steroids
3. Ethylenediamine dichloride
   - Stabilizer in topical creams, medicines, dyes, rubber, resin, waxes, insecticides, asphalt, fungicides
   - Previously found in nystatin cream
   - Cross-reacts with aminophylline, antihistamines (hydroxyzine), meclizine (antivert)
4. Gluteraldehyde
   - Cold sterilizing solution (medical/dental equipment)

- Embalming fluid, electron microscopy, cosmetics, waterless hand cleansers, wallpaper, liquid fabric softener, leather tanning
5. Wool alcohols
   - Lanolin and lanolin alchol
   - From the sebum of sheep
   - Lanolin consists of 95 Percent wool esters: alcohols (52 Percent) and acids (48 Percent)
   - Wool alcohols are used to test for lanolin allergy
   - Topical creams (e.g., Eucerin), cosmetics, adhesives, topical steroids
6. Propylene glycol
   - A dimer alcohol used to make drugs more soluble
   - Vehicle base in pharmaceuticals (Valium, ECG and lubricant jelly), cosmetics, food, and topical medications (corticosteroid creams, ointments, foams, gels, and solutions)
   - Brake fluid, tobacco formulations, antifreeze
7. Thimerosol
   - Mercury-containing organic compound (an organomercurial)
   - Made from the combination of ethyl mercuric chloride, thiosalicylic acid, sodium hydroxide, and ethanol
   - Preservative in vaccines: Influenza (flu) vaccines and tetanus and diphtheria vaccines (Td and DT) are not available without thimerosol
   - Also found in antitoxins, immunoglobulins
   - False-positive intradermal testing (e.g., to tuberculosis) can occur if material is preserved with thimerosol
   - Eye/ear drops, nasal sprays, contact lens solutions: conjunctivitis, eyelid dermatitis
   - Cosmetics, liquid soap, oral hygiene products, pesticides
   - Cross-reacts with piroxicam, mercury
8. Neomycin sulfate
   - Antibiotic in the aminoglycoside group
   - Used topically in ointments, creams, ear drops, and eye drops
   - Cross-reacts with gentamycin, tobramycin, streptomycin, or any systemic aminoglycoside
   - Often cosensitivity to bacitracin
9. Triclosan
   - Antibacterial agent
   - Soap, shampoo, mouthwash
10. Benzocaine
    - Topical anesthetic (remedies for hemorrhoids, sunburn, toothaches, sore throats, athlete's foot)
    - Cross-reacts with ester anesthetics, PABA, paraphenylenediamine, sulfa medications
    - Patch test with Caine mix: benzocaine, dibucaine hydrochloride, and tetracaine hydrochloride

NAIL-RELATED ALLERGENS

1. Ethyl cyanoacrylate
   - Instant glue ("superglue"), artificial nail glue
   - Liquid bandages, sealant for ileostomy appliances
   - Electronic circuit boards, aircrafts, automobiles
2. Methyl methacrylate
   - Clear, rigid plastic (artificial nails, hard contact lenses, hearing aids, dentures, dental fillings/sealants)
   - Glue for surgical prostheses/artificial joints: dermatitis in orthopedic surgeons
   - Cross-reacts with ethyl methacrylate
3. Toluene-sulfonamide (tosylamide) formaldehyde resin
   - Used in nail polishes
   - Nail polish: eyelid, face, neck, finger dermatitis

PLANT-RELATED ALLERGENS

1. *Pinaceae*
   - Pine trees (ie, *Pinus* species) and spruce trees
   - Source of colophony (or wood rosin)
     - Main allergens of colophony are oxidation products of abietic acid and its isomer primaric acid
     - Found in medical adhesives, cosmetics, athletic grip aids, dental cement, violin bow rosin, newsprint/magazine paper, soldering materials, nail coating (construction workers)
     - Cross-reacts with balsam of Peru
   - Source of turpentine, oleoresin also contains irritants, such as alpha-pinene, and allergens, such as delta-3-carene
2. *Alliaceae*
   - Genus *Allium*
   - Includes onions, garlic, and chives
   - Allergens: diallyldisulfide, allylpropyl disulfide, and allicin
   - Fresh garlic is both an allergen and a potent irritant
   - Causes second- and third-degree burns when applied to injured skin
   - Most common cause of fingertip dermatitis in housewives and caterers
3. Lichens
   - Allergens: usnic acid, atranorin, evernic acid, fumarprotocetraric acid
   - Forest workers, gardeners, woodcutters
   - Lichen extracts (oak moss, tree moss): dermatitis from aftershave products
4. *Primulaceae* (Fig. 6-1).
   - *Primula obconica*: primrose
   - Allergen is primin
   - Highly allergenic petals and sepals
   - May cross-react with other quinones: orchids or tropical woods, such as teak, rosewood
5. Family *Asteraceae* (previously *Compositae* family) (Fig. 6-2).
   - Ragweed, chrysanthemum, feverfew and carrot weed, daisy, sunflower, dandelion, artichoke, lettuce, and endives
   - Gardeners, florists, farmers, cooks: airborne or summer-exacerbated dermatitis
   - Allergen: *Sesquiterpene lactones*

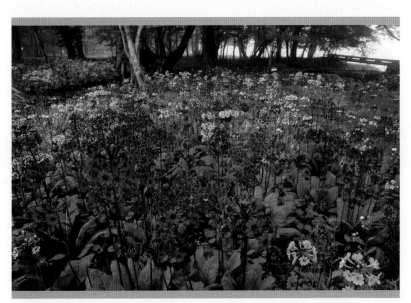

FIGURE 6-1 *Primulaceae. (Courtesy of Kiyoshi Isono.)*

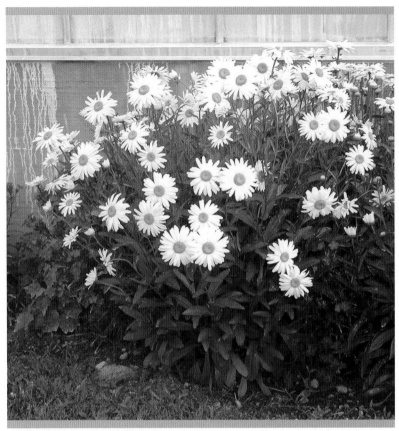

FIGURE 6-2 Family *asteraceae.*

- Found in the leaves, stems, flowers, and some pollen
- Cross-reactivity occurs randomly
- Patch-test mix (ie, alantolactone, dehydrocostus lactone, costunolide) is not very sensitive
- Ragweeds (*Ambrosia* species)
  - Oleoresin is thought to cause airborne contact dermatitis
  - Typically occurs in atopic patients
- Feverfew and carrot weed (*Parthenium hysterophores*)
- Chrysanthemum (*Dendranthema grandiflorum* cv.): most common *Asteraceae* plants that cause occupational contact dermatitis
- Sunflower (*Helianthus annuus*)
  - 1-0-methyl 1-4,5-dihydroniveusin A
  - Trichomes, or small hairs, on the surfaces of the leaf secrete the allergen
  - Windblown trichomes from dry plants can cause airborne contact dermatitis
- Dandelion (*Taraxacum officinale*)
  - Airborne allergic contact dermatitis
  - Allergen is taraxinic acid (1-0-*b*-glucopyranoside)

6. Toxicodendron
   - Species (*Rhus*); family (*Anacardiaceae*)
   - Allergens are pentadecylcatechols, found in the plant sap
     - Urushiol (milky secretion)
     - Oleoresin (dry resin)
     - Cathecols are soluble in rubber.
     - Particles suspended in smoke can carry urushiol.
     - Blister fluid does not contain urushiol
     - Nonleaf portions of the plant can induce dermatitis
   - Most common cause of contact dermatitis in children
   - Poison ivy
     - *T. radicans:* climbing vine, eastern United States
     - *T. rydbergii:* nonclimbing dwarf shrub, the northwestern United States (Fig. 6-3)
   - Poison oak
     - *T. diversilobum,* western United States
     - *T. toxicarium,* eastern United States (Fig. 6-4)
   - Poison sumac: *T. vernix*

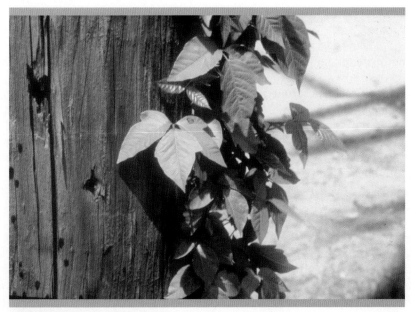

FIGURE 6-3 Poison ivy.

- Identification
  - Poison ivy and poison oak: three to five leaflets per compound leaf
  - Poison sumac, 7 to 13 leaflets per leaf; have smooth edges

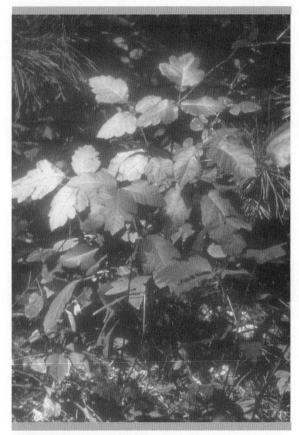

FIGURE 6-4 Poison oak.

- Cross-reacting substances
  - Cashew nut tree: entire tree except for the cashew nut
  - Indian marking tree: black juice
  - Japanese laquer tree: viscous sap that is used for varnishing wood; polymerized urushiol persists in the lacquer
  - Brazilian pepper tree: sap and crushed berries
  - Mango tree: Skin of the fruit and the leaves, bark, and stems of the plant contain sensitizing resorcinols; pulp of the fruit is nonallergenic
  - Ginkgo tree: anacardic acid, which is present in the seed pulp
7. *Liliaceae*
   - Tulips, hyacinths, and asparagus
   - Tulip fingers
   - Combined allergic and irritant contact dermatitis
   - Allergen: Tuliposide A is converted to tulipalin A, the allergen, by means of acidic hydrolysis
8. *Alstroemeriaceae* family (Peruvian lily)
   - Tuliposide A and B are found in virtually all portions of the plant
   - Flowers contain more allergen than the stems; the leaves have the smallest amount of allergen
   - Most common cause of allergic hand dermatitis in florists
9. Phytophotodermatitis
   - Berloque dermatitis is due to bergamot oil
   - UV light reacts with bergapten (a furocoumarin) and induces melanogenesis
   - Phytophotodermatitis results in hyperpigmentation

- Plant families *Umbiliferae* (most common), *Rutaceae*, and *Moraceae*
- Celery, lime, lemon, parsley, figs, fennel, grapefruit, bergamot, parsnip, mokihana (Hawaiian leis)
- Perfumes and fragrances, cosmetics, toiletries, soap, household cleaners, detergents, air fresheners
10. Contact urticaria from plants
    - Roasted chili peppers: capsaicin
    - *Urticaceae* family: stinging nettle (*Urtica dioica*)
      - Irritant chemicals, which include acetylcholine, histamine, and 5-hydroxytryptamine
11. Chemical irritant dermatitis
    - Most common dermatitis in florists
    - *Dieffenbachia picta* (*Araceae*), also known as dumb cane: calcium oxalate
    - Daffodil itch: calcium oxalate in the sap

Rubber Allergens

1. Latex
   - Milky fluid derived from rubber tree *Hevae brasiliensis*
   - Composed primarily of *cis*-1,4-polyisoprene
   - Reaction can involve irritant dermatitis, immediate (type I) hypersensitivity; rarely may cause delayed (type IV) hypersensitivity
   - Multiple episodes of contact urticaria with scratching can lead to clinical appearance of chronic dermatitis.
   - Gloves, condoms, balloons, rubber adhesives
   - Corn starch powder—with which gloves are dusted—is a potent carrier of latex proteins
   - Health care workers, rubber industry workers, children with spina bifida or urogenital abnormalities
   - In vitro tests: radioimmunoassay tests (RAST) for IgE
   - Cross-reaction
     - Food: bananas, avocados, chestnuts, kiwis
     - Shared IgE epitopes: ragweed, grasses, and *Ficus* trees
2. Rubber accelerators
   - Rubber accelerators are chemicals used to speed up the manufacturing process of rubber (vulcanization); sulfur cross-links the polymer chains in the latex
   - Carbamates (carba mix)
     - Rubber accelerator
     - Rubber dermatitis in bleached fabrics (waistbands, bra straps)
     - Consumer rubber products (condoms, swimwear, makeup sponges, eyelash curlers, gloves, shoes)

- Crosss-reacts with thiurams
- Mercaptobenzothiazole (MBT, mercapto mix)
  - Rubber accelerator
  - Most common cause of allergic shoe dermatitis
  - Rubber products: gloves, makeup sponges, rubber in undergarments/clothing, swimwear
  - Also in tires, condoms, antifreeze, fungicides, flea and tick powders, photographic film emulsions, adhesives, bactericides, and is an anticorrosive agent in cutting oils and greases
- Thiuram mix
  - Most common rubber additives to cause a type IV reaction
  - Almost all rubber products
  - Also in shoes, gloves, condoms, elastic bands, and ingredients of pesticides, insect repellents, antiscabies medication, fungicides, wood preservatives, paint additives, lubricating oils, and the drug disulfiram (Antabuse)

Antioxidants

- Added to decrease the rate of rubber degradation
- Substituted phenols are used for latex gloves

PRESERVATIVES

1. Formaldehyde
   - Released from the proallergen N-hydroxymethyl succinimide
   - cleaved into succinimide and formaldehyde when it comes in contact with the transepidermal water on the surface of the skin
2. Formaldehyde is the active allergenic compound
   - Textile resins
     - Permanent press or wrinkle-resistant textiles
   - Cosmetics, household products, ink, latex paint, pathology fixatives, fertilizer, embalming solution, insulation
   - *Formaldehyde resins*
     - *p-tert*-butylphenol
       ▲ Leather adhesive
       ▲ Other uses: waterproof glues and finishes
   - Formaldehyde-releasing preservatives
     - Quaternium-15 (most common): cosmetics, lotions, creams, shampoos and soaps, polishes, cleaners, cutting fluids, and paints
     - Imidazolidinyl urea (Germall 115, Euxyl K200)
     - Diazolidinyl urea (Germall II)
     - DMDM hydantoin
     - 2-Bromo-2-nitropane-1,3-diol (Bronopol)
3. Non-formaldehyde-releasing preservatives
   - Methyldibromo glutaronitrile (MDBGN)
   - Parabens
     - Most used topical preservatives worldwide

- Medical creams, lotions, pastes, and several cosmetics and skin care products; food preservatives; industrially in oils, fats, and glues
- Isothiazolinones
  - Kathon CG: combination of methylchloroisothiazolinone and methylisothiazolinone
  - Cosmetics and commercial household products such as shampoos, creams, lotions, cleaners, and washing materials; it is also a widely used industrial preservative for cutting fluids

METAL ALLERGENS

1. Nickel
   - Most common cause of allergic contact dermatitis overall in clinical studies
   - Jewelry, clothing (snaps, zippers, and buttons), coins, keys, other metals; gold less than 18 carats can contain nickel
   - Also used for nickel plating, to color ceramics, to make some batteries
   - Foods naturally high in nickel include chocolate, soybeans, nuts, and oatmeal
   - Chocolate, orange pekoe tea, barley, baking powder
   - Dimethylglyoxime test is used to detect nickel
     - Rub on the item; if solution turns color (pink to reddish), it indicates a positive reaction
     - Indicates the presence of nickel in a concentration of at least 1:10,000

2. Potassium dichromate
   - Chromates (chrome)
   - Usually found as chrome salts
   - Cement, leather tannin, ceramics, paint, match heads, suture, bleach/detergents, numerous industrial chemicals, green felt of card tables, glues
   - Green tattoo and cosmetic pigments
   - Green textile dyes (military green, green pool table felt)

COLORS AND DYE ALLERGENS

Tattoos

- Ink particles are found within large phagosomes in the cytoplasm of both keratinocytes and phagocytic cells
- Allergic reactions to red tattoo pigments are the most common (Table 6-5)
- Photoaggravated reactions: most commonly yellow dye
- Foreign-body reaction: most commonly red (mercury)
- Tattoo-induced pseudolymphoma: most commonly red

ADHESIVES

Epoxy Resin

- Two-component adhesives
- Most common allergens: bisphenol A and epichlorohydrin

TABLE 6-5 Tattoo Components

Tattoo Color	Component
Blue	Cobalt aluminate
Brown	Ferric oxide
Green	Chromic oxide, lead chromate, phthalocyanine dyes
Red	Cinnabar (mercuric sulfide), sienna (ferric hydrate), sandalwood, brazilwood, organic pigments (aromatic azo compounds)
Yellow	Cadmium sulfide
Black	Carbon (India ink), iron oxide, Iogwood
Purple	Manganese, aluminum
White	Titanium oxide, zinc oxide

- Glue, laminates, eyeglass frames, vinyl gloves, handbags, plastic necklaces, dental bonding agents, microscopy immersion oil, floor coverings

OTHER ALLERGENS

Sodium Hypochlorite

- Chlorinated swimming pools
- Bleach

PATCH TESTING

- T.R.U.E. Test (allergen patch test) (Table 6-6)
  - Ready-to-use contact allergen test
  - Contains 23 allergens and allergen mixes
  - Test also contains one negative control: uncoated polyester patch
  - Allergen mixes incorporated into hydrophilic gels attached to a waterproof backing
  - Perspiration and transepidermal water loss rehydrate the dried gel layer, thereby releasing the allergens onto the skin
  - T.R.U.E. Test is removed after 48 hours.
  - Reactions are interpreted at 72 to 96 hours after test application

- Fragrance mix
  - Contains eight allergens
  - Geraniol, cinnamaldehyde, hydroxycitronellal, cinnamyl alcohol, eugenol, isoeugenol, *a*-amylcinnamaldehyde, and oak moss
- Mercapto mix
  - Composed of three chemical accelerators: benzothiazole sulfenamide derivatives
  - *N*-Cyclohexylbenzothiazyl-sulfenamide, dibenzothiazyl disulfide, and morpholinylmercaptobenzothiazole
- Thiuram mix
  - Composed of four substances in equal parts
  - Tetramethylthiuram monosulfide, tetramethylthiuram disulfide, disulfiram, dipentamethylenethiuram disulfide
- Black rubber mix: *N*-Isopropyl-*N'*-phenylparaphenylenediamine, *N*-cyclohexyl-*N'*-phenyl paraphenylene-diamine, *N, N'*-diphenyl paraphenylenediamine
- Carba mix
  - Chemicals used to stabilize rubber products
  - Diphenylguanidine, zincdibutyldithiocarbamate, and zincdiethyldithiocarbamate in equal parts
- Repeat open application test (ROAT)
  - For individuals who develop weak or 1 + positive reactions to a chemical in the T.R.U.E Test

TABLE 6-6 True Test Panels

Panel 1.1	Panel 2.1
1. Nickel sulfate	13. *p-tert*-Butylphenol formaldehyde resin
2. Wool alcohols	14. Epoxy resin
3. Neomycin sulfate	15. Carba mix
4. Potassium dichromate	16. Black rubber mix
5. Caine mix	17. Cl + Me-isothiazolinone
6. Fragrance mix	18. Quaternium-15
7. Colophony	19. Mercaptobenzothiazole
8. Paraben mix	20. *p*-Phenylenediamine
9. Negative control	21. Formaldehyde
10. Balsam of Peru	22. Mercapto mix
11. Ethylenediamine dihydrochloride	23. Thimerosal
12. Cobalt dichloride	24. Thiuram mix

- Useful in determining whether the reaction is significant
- Consists of rubbing in the product twice daily for several days to the skin of the upper arm or forearm
- If no reaction, then the patch test probably was a false-positive reaction, and no further action is necessary
- A reaction often consists of erythematous papules
- Samples of the individual ingredients used by the cosmetic manufacturer may be requested and tested on the individual
- Finn chamber system
  - Allows for customized patch testing and flexibility
  - Employs a multiwell aluminum patch
  - Most common size is 8-mm chamber applied to Scanpor tape in two rows of five
  - Each well is filled with a small amount of the allergen being tested, and the patch is taped to normal skin on the patient's upper back
  - After 48 hours, the patch is removed, and an initial reading is taken
- Second reading is made a few days later; each 8-mm chamber holds 20 μl

REFERENCES

Antezana M, Parker F: Occupational contact dermatitis. *Immunol Allergy Clin North Am* 2003;23:269–290.

Baran R: Nail cosmetics: allergies and irritations. *Am J Clin Dermatol* 2002;3:547–555.

Chan EF, Mowad C: Contact dermatitis to foods and spices. *Am J Contact Dermat* 1998 Jun;9(2):71–79.

Fisher A, Rietschel R, Fowler J: *Fisher's Contact Dermatitis*, 4th ed. Baltimore: Williams & Wilkins, 1995.

McCleskey PE, Swerlick RA: Clinical review: thioureas and allergic contact dermatitis. *Cutis* 2001;68:387–396.

Scheinman PL: Allergic contact dermatitis to fragrance: a review. *Am J Contact Dermat* 1996;7:65–76.

Scheman A: Adverse reactions to cosmetic ingredients. *Dermatol Clin* 2000;18:685–698.

Thiboutot DM, Hamory BH, Marks JG Jr: Dermatoses among floral shop workers. *J Am Acad Dermatol* 1990;22:54–58.

Van der Walle HB, Brunsveld VM: Dermatitis in hairdressers. *Contact Dermatitis* 1994;30:217–221.

CHAPTER 7

DERMATOLOGIC MEDICATIONS

MELISSA A. BOGLE
NOR CHIAO
STEPHEN E. WOLVERTON

SYSTEMIC MEDICATIONS

Glucocorticoids

- Mechanism of action
  - Form complexes with intracellular receptors
  - Modulate transcription rate of specific genes that lead to an increase or decrease in the levels of specific proteins: decreased transcription of AP-1 and NF-κB (nuclear factor-κB)
  - Decreased synthesis of proinflammatory molecules: cytokines, interleukins, adhesion molecules, and proteases
- Other effects
  - Increase blood glucose by promoting gluconeogenesis
  - Stimulate protein catabolism (except in liver), leading to negative nitrogen balance
  - Increase plasma fatty acids and ketone body formation via increased lipolysis and decreased glucose uptake into fat cells
  - Decrease plasma adrenocorticotropic hormone (ACTH)
  - Decrease fibroblasts production of collagen
  - Stimulate acid and pepsin secretion in stomach
  - Increase surfactant production in fetal lungs
- Adverse effects
  - Osteoporosis, hyperglycemia, hypertension, increased infection risk, poor wound healing, muscle weakness and tissue loss, increased appetite, Cushingoid features, peptic ulcers, euphoria, psychoses, adrenal suppression
  - Pregnancy category C

Sulfones

DAPSONE

- Mechanism of action
  - Competitive antagonists of dihydropterate synthetase and para-aminobenzoic acid prevent

formation of folic acid, inhibiting bacterial growth, neutrophil chemotaxis
- Adverse effects: Dapsone hypersensitivity/ mononucleosis-like syndrome, hepatitis, hemolytic anemia, photosensitivity, agranulocytosis in G6PD deficiency, lupus erythematosus, hypoalbuninemia, hypothyroidism
  - Causes dose-related hemolysis in all patients and methemoglobinemia (in patients with methemoglobin reductase deficiency)
  - Hepatitis on idiosyncratic basic
  - Peripheral neuropathy (predominantly motor; however, sensory defects can occur)
  - Toxic epidermal necrolysis
  - Monitor complete blood counts (CBCs), recommended weekly to biweekly for first month of therapy and monthly to bimonthly thereafter for the next 5 months
  - Check baseline liver function tests and every 3 months thereafter
  - Screen patients for glucose 6 phosphate dehydrogenase deficiency
  - Pregnancy category C
- Interactions
  - May inhibit anti-inflammatory effects of clofazimine; hematologic reactions may increase with folic acid antagonists
  - Probenecid increases dapsone toxicity; trimethoprim with dapsone may increase toxicity of both drugs
- Contraindications: documented hypersensitivity; known G6PD deficiency or methemoglobin reductase deficiency

Aminoquinolones (Derived from Quinine)

HYDROXYCHLOROQUINE/CHLOROQUINE/ QUINACRINE

- Mechanism of action

- Inhibits chemotaxis of eosinophils and locomotion of neutrophils; impairs complement-dependent antigen-antibody reactions
- Adverse effects
  - Crosses placenta and may cause ocular, CNS, or ototoxicity in fetus; do not use in breast-feeding mothers
  - Premaculopathy, reversible; true retinopathy, irreversible: Perform regular ophthalmologic exams (including visual acuity, slit lamp, funduscopic, and visual field tests)
  - Hemolytic anemia in patients with G6PD deficiency
  - Blue/gray mucocutaneous pigmentation; quinacrine may cause yellow pigmentation
  - Worsening of psoriasis, mainly chloroquine
- Interactions
  - Cimetidine may increase serum levels of chloroquine
  - Magnesium trisilicate may decrease absorption of 4-aminoquinolones
  - Pregnancy category C

Cytotoxic and Antimetabolic Agents

- Antimetabolites: mimic natural molecules and are most active while DNA is being synthesized in the S phase
  - Require a target-cell population that is proliferating in order to exert their effect
  - Side effects are most prominent in cells with an innately high proliferative index (e.g., bone marrow)
- Alkylating agents interact with preformed DNA molecules
  - Affect proliferating populations of cells and cells that are not actively synthesizing DNA
  - Have a greater propensity for mutagenicity

METHOTREXATE

- Mechanism of action
  - Inhibits dihydrofolate reductase to interfere with folate metabolism; inhibits thymidylate synthetase to block DNA synthesis
  - Adverse effects: gastrointestinal distress, renal failure, liver cirrhosis/hepatotoxicity, abortifacient, pancytopenia, pulmonary fibrosis, neprotoxicity, phototoxicity, acral erythema, ultraviolet light recall, lymphoma, ulcerative stomatitis
  - Potentially deadly pancytopenia when administered with trimethoprim-sulfamethoxazole (TMP-SMX) or some nonsteroidal anti-inflammatory drugs (NSAIDs) (some relatively safe NSAIDs that can be used in combination include ketoprofen, flurbiprofen, piroxicam, and celecoxib)

- Monitor: liver function tests, CBC, lipid panel, pregnancy, periodic liver biopsy (most suggest 1.5 g after every methotrexate)
- Leucovorin (folinic acid) given for acute toxicity
- Pregnancy category C
- Folic acid supplementation can decrease gastrointestinal side effects

FLUCYTOSINE (5-FC)

- Mechanisms of action
  - Enters fungal cell via cytosine-specific permease (not in mammalians)
  - 5-FC then converted to 5-FdUMP, which inhibits thymidylate synthetase, thus depriving the organism of thymidylic acid, an essential DNA component
  - Also metabolized into 5-FUTP and disrupts nucleic acid and protein synthesis
  - Amphotericin B allows more flucytosine to penetrate the cell—synergistic
  - Synthetic pyrimidine antimetabolite used only in combination with amphotericin B owing to quick buildup of resistance when used alone
- Resistance: mutations in cytosine permease or cytosine deaminase (resistance common)
- Adverse effects
  - Selective toxicity owing to human cells inefficiently converting flucytosine into 5-fluorouracil, so uptake by human cells is poor
  - Gastrointestinal intolerance; depresses bone marrow, resulting in dose-related and reversible anemia, leukopenia, thrombocytopenia
  - Pregnancy category C

HYDROXYUREA

- Inhibits ribonucleotide diphosphate reductase and leads to inhibition of DNA synthesis
- Adverse effects: pancytopenia, alopecia, radiation recall, photosensitivity, leg ulcers, hyperpigmentation, antinuclear antibody (ANA)–positive dermopathy
- Monitor: CBC, urinalysis (UA), liver function tests (LFTs) at least monthly
- Interactions: Avoid other myelosuppressive agents because of the potential for additive bone marrow toxicity
- Pregnancy category D

AZATHIOPRINE

- Three enzymes involved in metabolism:
  - Hypxanthine-guanine phosphoribosyl transferase (HGPRT)
  - Xanthine oxidase (XO)
  - Thiopurine methyl transferase (TPMT)
- Azathiorine is a prodrug that is metabolized to 6-mercaptopurine

- 6-Mercaptopurine is converted to active analogues by HGPRT; the analogues (including 6-thioguanine) block purine synthesis
- 6-Mercaptopurine is also oxidized to inactive metabolites by xanthine oxidase and thiopurine methyl transferase (TPMT)
- Adverse effects: gastrointestinal distress, pancytopenia, lymphoma, hypersensitivity syndrome, hepatitis, pancreatitis, teratogenicity
- Patients with thiopurine methyltransferase deficiency are at an increased risk for myelosuppression
- Patients with Lesch-Nyhan syndrome lack HGPRT and are resistant to the cytotoxic effects of the drug
- Monitor: LFTs, CBC, pregnancy
- Pregnancy category D

MYCOPHENYLATE MOFETIL AND MYCOPHENOLIC ACID (MPA)

- Antibmetabolite that noncompetitively inhibits inosine monophosphate dehydrogenase (IMPDH) and suppresses de novo purine synthesis: conversion of inosine-5-phosphate and xanthine-5-phosphate to guanosine-5-phosphate
- MPA is cytotoxic for cells that rely predominantly on de novo purine biosynthesis, such as lymphocytes (T and B)
- Adverse effects: gastrointestinal distress, dysuria/urinary frequency, leukopenia, lymphoma, increased risk for infection, increased toxicity in patients with renal impairment, caution in active peptic ulcer disease
- Pregnancy category B
- Drug interactions: may elevate levels of acyclovir and ganciclovir; antacids and cholestyramine decrease absorption, reducing MPA levels (do not administer together); probenecid may increase levels; salicylates may increase toxicity

CYCLOPHOSPHAMIDE

- Alkylating agent, cell-cycle-nonspecific cytotoxic drug
- Chemically related to nitrogen mustards
- As an alkylating agent, the mechanism of action of the active metabolites may involve DNA cross-linking, which may interfere with growth of healthy and neoplastic cells.
- Adverse effects: teratogenicity, gastrointestinal distress, leukopenia, hemorrhagic cystitis, thrombocytopenia, anemia, acral erythema, pneumonitis/pulmonary fibrosis, alopecia
- Monitor: chemistry panel, CBC, LFTs, UA
- Pregnancy category D

Retinoids

- Small molecular hormones that possess vitamin A activity (synthetic forms also available)

- Function in the regulation of cellular proliferation and differentiation and the modulation of immune function and cytokine function
- Mechanisms of action
  - Mediated via two main families of intracellular receptors:
    - Retinoic acid receptor (RAR; bound and activated by all-*trans* retinoic acid)
    - Retinoid X receptor (RXR; 9-*cis* retinoic acid is the proposed ligand)
- Each family has three receptor subtypes: alpha, beta, and gamma
- Retinoid receptors are members of the steroid-receptor family and act by modulating transcription of specific genes
- Elicit biologic effects by
  - Activating nuclear receptors
  - Regulating gene transcription: contain both positive and negative gene regulatory activities; can stimulate gene transcription directly and inhibit gene transcription indirectly
    - Direct gene transcription effects are mediated through so-called retinoic acid response elements
    - Indirect effects of retinoids result from their ability to regulate negatively certain genes
    - Antagonize effects of transcription factors activating protein 1 (AP1) and nuclear factor-interleukin-6 (NF-IL6) (upregulated in a variety of hyperproliferative and inflammatory conditions)

ISOTRETINOIN (13-*CIS*-RETINOIC ACID)

- Isomer of naturally occurring tretinoin (*trans*-retinoic acid)
- Decreases sebaceous gland size and sebum production; may inhibit sebaceous gland differentiation and abnormal keratinization
- Absorption increased with food intake
- Dose 1–2 mg/kg range
- Pregnancy category X

BEXAROTENE

- Binds to retinoic X receptor; 100-fold stronger than RAR
- Absorption increased by fatty meals.
- Monitoring: Perform fasting blood lipid determinations before therapy is initiated and weekly until lipid response to the drug is established; obtain and serially monitor baseline CBC, LFTs, and thyroid function tests; advise patients to limit vitamin A supplements and minimize exposure to sunlight and artificial ultraviolet (UV) light
- Pregnancy category X

ACITRETIN/ETRETINATE

- Second-generation rctinoids (aromatic retinoids)
- Acitretin: derived from etretinate, has a terminal half-life in plasma of only 2 days
- Following oral absorption, acitretin undergoes extensive metabolism and interconversion by simple isomerization to its 13-*cis* form (*cis*-acitretin)
- Etretinate has a longer half-life than acitretin owing to greater storage of etretinate in adipose tissue; can be formed with concurrent ingestion of acitretin and ethanol
- Oral absorption of acitretin is optimal when given with food
- Pregnancy category X

SIDE EFFECTS OF ORAL RETINOIDS

- Mucocutaneous: cheilitis, dry skin, pruritus, epistaxis
- Acitretin: palm, sole, and fingertip desquamation; recommended that women who take acitretin avoid pregnancy for at least 3 years after discontinuing therapy
- Increased serum triglycerides owing to inhibited lipoprotein lipase
- Ophthalmologic: blepharoconjunctivitis, blurred vision, abnormal night vision
- Teratogenicity: retinoic acid embryopathy, central nervous system abnormalities (hydrocephalus, microcephaly), external ear abnormalities (anotia, small or absent external auditory canals), cardiovascular abnormalities (septal wall and aortic defects), facial dysmorphia, eye abnormalities (microphthalmia), thymus gland abnormalities, and bone abnormalities
- Monitor BHCG monthly
- Isotretinoin has a terminal half-life in plasma of 10 to 20 hours and is completely cleared from the body within 1 month after the drug is stopped
- Etretinate stored in body fat deposits; terminal elimination half-life in plasma of about 100 days; detected in serum in trace amounts for as long as 3 years after cessation of therapy
- Skeletal: long bones, decalcification, progressive calcification of ligaments and tendon insertions, cortical hyperostosis, periosteal thickening, premature epiphyseal closure, and possible osteoporosis
- Myalgias and arthralgias: sometimes associated with high creatinine kinase levels
- Neurologic: headache, fatigue, lethargy, pseudotumor cerebri
- Psychologic: reported anxiety and depression
- Lipids: increase in plasma lipids (dose-dependent), especially triglycerides; increase in cholesterol levels
- Gastrointestinal: Elevated LFTs, most commonly the transaminases, can occur in approximately

15 percent of patients; nausea, diarrhea, abdominal pain

Antihistamines

- Competitive inhibitors of histamine at tissue receptor sites
- Binding is reversible
- H_1 receptors distributed in brain, most smooth muscle cells, endothelial cells, adrenal medulla, and heart
- Affect smooth muscle contraction, stimulation of nitric oxide formation, endothelial cell contraction, and increasing vascular permeability
- Central nervous system effects are due to blockade of central muscarinic receptors
- H_1 blockers
  - HEA
  - Tricyclic dibenzoxepins
    - Doxepin HCl
  - Ethanolamine
    - Diphenhydramine
  - Short-acting alkylamines
    - Pheniramine
    - Chlorpheniramine
    - Dextrochlorpheniramine
  - Piperazine
    - Hydroxizine
  - Piperidines
    - Cyproheptadine HCl
  - Phenothiazines
    - Promethazine
    - Trimeprazine
  - Ethylenediamine
    - Mepyramine maleate
- H_1 blockers (second-generation agents)
  - Less lipid soluble and only cross the blood-brain barrier in small amounts; also have longer half-lives, allowing for less frequent dosing
    - Piperazines
      - ▲ Loratadine
      - ▲ Fexophenadine
  - H_2 receptors (H_2Rs): cause cAMP accumulation in the gastric cells, cardiac tissues, smooth muscle cells, and immune cells; H_2R agonists have been proven to be effective for acid peptic disorders of the gastrointestinal tract
  - H_2 blockers
    - Cimetidine
    - Ranitidine
    - Famotidine
    - Nizatidine

DIPHENHYDRAMINE

- Antagonizes H_1 receptors in periphery
- Adverse effects: may exacerbate angle-closure glaucoma, hyperthyroidism, peptic ulcer disease, and

urinary tract obstruction; may cause sedation; anticholinergic adverse effects (especially in elderly patients)
- Pregnancy category B

HYDROXYZINE

- Antagonizes H_1 receptors in periphery
- Adverse effects: clinical exacerbation of porphyria (may not be safe for patients with porphyria); electrocardiographic (ECG) abnormalities (alterations in T waves) may occur; drowsiness
- Pregnancy category C

DOXEPIN

- Inhibits histamine and acetylcholine activity
- Adverse effects: conduction disturbances, seizure disorders, urinary retention, hyperthyroidism
- Pregnancy category C

CETIRIZINE

- Forms complex with histamine for H_1-receptor sites in blood vessels, gastrointestinal tract, and respiratory tract
- Adverse effects: Caution in hepatic or renal dysfunction; doses >10 mg/d may cause drowsiness; anticholinergic effects may occur
- Pregnancy category B

FEXOFENADINE

- Competes with histamine for H_1 receptors in gastrointestinal tract, blood vessels, and respiratory tract
- Pregnancy category C

LORATADINE

- Selectively inhibits peripheral histamine H_1 receptors
- Adverse effects: Initiate therapy at lower dose in patients with liver impairment
- Pregnancy category B

DESLORATADINE

- Antagonist selective for H_1 receptors
- Major metabolite of loratadine, which is metabolized to active metabolite 3-hydroxydesloratadine
- Adverse effects: decrease dose in hepatic impairment; rarely causes pharyngitis or dry mouth
- Drug interactions: Erythromycin and ketoconazole increase desloratadine and 3-hydroxydesloratadine plasma concentrations, but no increase in clinically relevant adverse effects, including no increase in QTc, is observed
- Pregnancy category C

Leukotriene Inhibitors

- Leukotriene receptor antagonists or inhibition of leukotriene production

- Zafirlukast, montelukast: bind CysLt1 receptor
- Zileuton: competitive inhibitor of lipoxygenase—inhibits leukotriene formation (LTB1, LTC1, LTD1, LTE1)
- Adverse effects: possible association with Churg-Strauss vasculitis (zileuton), may increase liver enzymes
- Monitor LFTs
- Pregnancy category B, except for zileuton: category C

Antibiotics

BETA-LACTAM ANTIBIOTICS

- Include penicillins and cephalosporins
- Active against many gram-positive, gram-negative, and anaerobic organisms

PENICILLINS

- Mechanism of action
  - Inhibit bacterial cell wall synthesis
  - Active against gram-positive organisms and spirochetes
  - Penicillinase-resistant penicillins (i.e., dicloxacillin, nafcillin, and oxacillin)
  - Adverse effects: hemolytic anemia, nephritis, anaphylaxis, TEN (toxic epidermal necrolysis), erythema nodosum, cutis laxa
  - Beta-lactamase inhibitor; ampicillin-sulbactam, amoxicillin-clavulanic acid: use in the treatment of bite wounds; active against oral anaerobes, streptococci, anaerobes, and staphyloccoci
  - Pregnancy category B

CEPHALOSPORINS

- Mechanism of action: inhibit bacterial cell wall synthesis by interfering with peptidoglycan synthesis
- Grouped into four generations according to the spectrum of antibacterial activity
  - First generation: *Streptococci*, methicillin-sensitive *Staphylococcus aureus,* some gram-negative bacilli
  - Second generation: increased activity against gram-negative bacilli; all are less active against gram-positive bacteria than first-generation drugs
  - Third generation: mostly IV (intravenous)
    - Most active cephalosporins against gram-negative organisms: *Escherichia coli, Proteus mirabilis, Klebsiella,* indole-positive *Proteus*
    - Increased activity (relative to earlier generations) against *Pseudomonas aeruginosa*
  - Fourth generation: comparable to third generation but more resistant to some chromosomal beta-lactamases; penetrates well into CSF; good for *P. aeruginosa*
- Adverse effects: Hypersensitivity, cross-reactivity with penicillins immunologic studies (up to 20 percent), clinical reports (5 to 10 percent), diarrhea, nausea, vomiting, abdominal pain, dizziness,

Stevens-Johnson syndrome, toxic epidermal necrolysis, cefaclor: serum sickness–like reaction, *Clostridium difficile* colitis
- Pregnancy category D

TETRACYCLINES: TETRACYCLINE, DOXYCYCLINE, AND MINOCYCLINE

- Mechanism
  - Bacteriostatic
  - Binds to 30S subunit of bacterial ribosome, interfering with protein synthesis
  - Active against *Mycoplasma pneumoniae*, chlamydiae, rickettsiae, *Propionibacterium acnes* and *vibrio* spp., *Borrelia burgdorferi*, *Mycobacterium marinum*
- Adverse effects: photosensitivity, gastrointestinal disturbances, enamel dysplasia in children (younger than 12 years of age), lupus erythematosus, photoonycholysis, blue-gray pigmentation (minocycline), postacne osteoma cutis, vertigo, pseudotumor cerebri, esophageal ulceration; neurologic changes: dizziness, vertigo; minocycline: autoimmune hepatitis, systemic lupus erythematosus
- Reduce dose in renal impairment
- Pregnancy category D

MACROLIDES: ERYTHROMYCIN, AZITHROMYCIN, CLARITHROMYCIN

- Bacteriostatic
- Bind to 50S bacterial ribosomal subunit to inhibit protein synthesis
- Active against gram-positive organisms (most streptococci and *S. aureus*)
- Adverse effects: gastrointestinal distress, eosinophilia, oral mucosal lesions, xerosis; estolate formulation may cause cholestatic jaundice (caution in liver disease)
- Pregnancy category B

FLUOROQUINOLONES

- Ciprofloxacin, ofloxacin, gatifloxacin, levofloxacin, moxifloxacin, sparfloxacin, grepafloxacin
- Mechanism of action
- Bacteriocidal
- Inhibit bacterial DNA gyrase
- Active against gram-positive organisms (*S. aureus*, streptococci, except ciprofloxacin and ofloxacin) and gram-negative organisms (mycobacteria, *Neisseria gonorrhoeae*)
- Adverse effects: photosensitivity, flushing, hyperhidrosis, possible cartilage erosions in children
- Pregnancy category C

LINCOSAMIDES: CLINDAMYCIN, LINCOMYCIN

- Mechanism of action
- Bacteriostatic

- Inhibit 50S bacterial ribosomal subunit to inhibit protein synthesis
- Active against gram-positive organisms (*Staphylococcus aureus*, streptococci) and anerobes (*Propionibacterium acnes*), aerobic and anaerobic streptococci (except enterococci)
- Adverse effects: photosensitivity, diarrhea, pseudomembranous colitis (owing to overgrowth of *Clostridium difficile*), hepatic dysfunction, morbilliform rash
- Pregnancy category B

SULFAPYRIDINE

- Competitive antagonist of para-aminobenzoic acid
- Adverse effects: Idiosyncratic reactions (e.g., hypersensitivity pneumonitis, lupus-like syndrome, pancreatitis, and toxic hepatitis) may occur; agranulocytosis occurs rarely; nephrolithiasis may occur as with other sulfa drugs
- Pregnancy category B

CHLORAMPHENICOL

- Mechanism of action
- Binds to 50S subunit of bacterial ribosomes and inhibits peptidyl transferase
- Used to treat *Salmonella*, *Haemophilus*, and pneumococcal and meningococcal meningitis in penicillin-sensitive patients; treats verruga peruana
- Adverse effects: gray baby syndrome, gastrointestinal disturbances, anemia
- Pregnancy category C

AMINOGLYCOSIDES

- Mechanism of action
- Gentamicin, tobramycin, and amikacin
- Bind to 30S subunit of bacterial ribosomes to inhibit protein synthesis
- Active against aerobic gram-negative organisms
- Adverse effects: ototoxicity, nephrotoxicity, neuromuscular blockade, injection-site necrosis
- Pregnancy category D

SULFONAMIDES (TRIMETHOPRIM-SULFAMETHOXAZOLE)

- Mechanism of action
- Interfere with folic acid synthesis by inhibiting synthesis of dihydrofolate reductase and dihydropteroate synthetase
- Gram-positive (*S. aureus*) and gram-negative organisms, *Chlamydia*, *Nocardia*
- Adverse effects: TEN, Stevens-Johnson syndrome; high doses may cause bone marrow depression (if signs occur, give 5 to 15 mg/day leucovorin); caution in folate deficiency hemolysis may occur in individuals with G6PD deficiency
- Pregnancy category C

VANCOMYCIN

- Mechanism of action
- Inhibits bacterial cell wall synthesis and causes secondary damage to the cytoplasmic membrane
- Active against gram-positive organisms
- Adverse effects: linear IgA bullous dermatosis, bullous eruptions, red-man syndrome, ototoxicity, nephrotoxicity, thrombophlebitis at injection site; erythema, histamine-like flushing, and anaphylactic reactions may occur when administered with anesthetic agents; when taken concurrently with aminoglycosides, risk of nephrotoxicity; neuromuscular blockade may be enhanced when coadministered with nondepolarizing muscle relaxants
- Use with caution in patients with renal impairment or with nephrotoxic or ototoxic drugs; facial flushing from histamine release (e.g., red-man syndrome); usually resolves by slowing IV infusion over 2 hours and by giving antihistamines; adjust daily dosing frequency in renal impairment
- Pregnancy category C

METRONIDAZOLE

- Mechanism of action
- Forms toxic metabolites in bacteria that inhibit nucleic acid synthesis
- Active against anaerobes, protozoa
- Adverse effects: glossitis, stomatitis, disulfiram-like reactions with ethanol, mucosal xerosis, vestibular dysfunction
- Pregnancy category B

OXAZOLIDINONES (LINEZOLID)

- Mechanism of action: binds to a site on the bacterial 23S ribosomal RNA of the 50S subunit and prevents the formation of a functional 70S initiation complex
- Adverse effects: thrombocytopenia depending on duration of therapy (generally greater than 2 weeks of treatment), nausea, headache, diarrhea, vomiting, pseudomembranous colitis
- Activity: bacteriostatic against enterococci and staphylococci and bactericidal against most strains of streptococci
- Pregnancy category C

Antiviral Agents

ACYCLOVIR

- Mechanism of action: inhibits DNA synthesis by competing with deoxyguanosine triphosphate for viral DNA polymerase; initial phosphorylation of acyclovir to acyclovir monophosphate is catalyzed by virus-induced thymidine kinase; selective activation of the drug in infected cells

- Activity: human herpes viruses, varicella-zoster virus (VZV), Epstein-Barr virus (EBV), and to a lesser extent, cytomegalovirus (CMV) (Cytomegalovirus does not produce thymidine kinase, and so the antiviral activity of acyclovir in cytomegalovirus-induced infections is poor)
- Pharmakokinetics: Bioavailability of oral acyclovir is low (15 to 30 percent of an oral dose is absorbed)
- Adverse effects: nephrotoxicity, phlebitis, and encephalopathy with IV infusion, seizures
- Resistant herpes simplex virus (HSV) mutants: *thymidine kinase negative (tk–)* or *tk* mutant and hence do not phosphorylate and activate acyclovir; have an altered DNA polymerase that is not as greatly inhibited by the phosphorylated drug
- Pregnancy category B

FAMCICLOVIR

- Mechanism of action: prodrug of the antiviral agent penciclovir; converted to active form via deacetylation and oxidation
- Action similar to acyclovir: activated by viral thymidine kinase to inhibit viral DNA polymerase
- Activity: HSV, VZV, CMV
- Pharmakokinetics: Bioavailability of penciclovir is 77 percent
- Adverse effects: nephrotoxicity with IV infusion, seizures
- Pregnancy category B

VALACYCLOVIR

- Mechanism of action
- Valacyclovir (a prodrug) is the L-valine ester of acyclovir and exerts its action after being transformed into acyclovir during its first pass through the intestine and liver.
- Activated by viral thymidine kinase to inhibit viral DNA polymerase
- Bioavailability is three to five times greater than acyclovir
- Activity against HSV, VZV, and CMV
- Adverse effects: nephrotoxicity with IV infusion, seizures
- Pregnancy category B

GANCICLOVIR

- Mechanism of action: nucleoside analogue that competes with deoxyguanosine for incorporation into viral DNA; hydroxymethylated derivative of acyclovir
- Initially phosphorylated by virus-encoded kinases
- Ganciclovir triphosphate competitively inhibits herpes virus DNA polymerase and inhibits elongation of the nascent DNA chain

- HSV and VZV with thymidine kinase deficiency or with viral DNA polymerase mutations may be resistant to gancyclovir
- Activity: more active than acyclovir against CMV, especially CMV retinitis in immunocompromised patients
- Adverse effects: mucositis, hepatic dysfunction, seizures, granulocytopenia and thrombocytopenia; may not be totally reversible after cessation
- Pregnancy category C

VALGANCICLOVIR

- L-valyl ester of ganciclovir
- Acts as a prodrug for ganciclovir; converted to active drug by intestinal and hepatic esterases
- Adverse effects similar to parent compound
- Activity: CMV retinitis in patients with AIDS

FOSCARNET

- Phosphonoformate: analogue of pyrophosphate
- Mechanism of action: noncompetatively inhibits viral DNA polymerase and HIV-1 reverse transcriptase by binding directly to the enzymes' pyrophosphate-binding sites
- Does not require phosphorylation for antiviral activity
- Activity: acyclovir-resistant HSV infections in AIDS patients and CMV retinitis in immunocompromised patients
- Adverse effects: nephrotoxicity, electrolyte imbalances, genital and oral ulcerations
- Pregnancy category C

AMANTADINE AND RIMANTADINE

- Mechanism of action
- Both inhibit the uncoating of viral RNA within infected host cells, thereby preventing virus replication; effective when administered orally
- Activity: influenza A and C viruses (but not influenza B), rubella
- Adverse effects: ataxia, hypertrichosis, livedo reticularis, photosensitivity, peripheral edema, alopecia, anticholinergic reactions, gastrointestinal disturbances; effects less likely with rimantidine
- Pregnancy category C

INTERFERONS (INTERFERON-α-2B)

- Mechanism of action: protein product manufactured by recombinant DNA technology
- Induces differential gene transcription; inhibits viral replication; antiviral and immunomodulatory effects by suppressing cell proliferation; direct antiproliferative effects against malignant cells and modulation of host immune response

- Adverse effects: flulike symptoms, cardiovascular arrythmias, eyelash hypertrichosis, spastic diplegia, rhabdomyolysis
- Pregnancy category C

RIBAVIRIN

- Mechanism of action: inhibits viral RNA polymerase
- Purine nucleoside analogue that is phosphorylated by host cells
- Activity: respiratory scyncytial virus (RSV), influenza A and B, measles
- Adverse effects: exanthem
- Pregnancy category X

CIDOFOVIR

- Mechanism of action: nucleoside analog of deoxycytidine monophosphate
- Converted by host cell enzymes to cidofivir diphosphate, which competitively inhibits viral DNA polymerase
- Cidofovir is independent of thymidine kinase activation
- Adverse effects: renal toxicity (renal tubular damage), granulocytopenia may occur; with topical application, local irritation, pain
- Pregnancy category C

Antiretroviral Agents

NUCLEOSIDE REVERSE TRANSCRIPTASE INHIBITORS

- Zidovudine (AZT, ZDV)
  - Mechanism of action: thymidine analogue; acts as a chain terminator
  - Resistance: due to mutations in the reverse transcriptase gene
  - Adverse effects: myelosuppression; results in anemias and/or neutropenia
  - Pregnancy category C
- Didanosine: (ddI)
  - Mechanism: similar to zidovudine
  - Adverse effects: peripheral neuropathy and potentially fatal pancreatitis
  - Pregnancy category B
- Lamivudine (3TC), stavudine (d4T), and zalcitabine (ddC)
  - Mechanism of action: similar to zidovudine
  - Adverse effects: flulike symptoms, lipodystrophy, acneiform eruption, mucosal ulcers, pruritus, melanonychia, hyperpigmentation, eyelash hypertrichosis
  - Pregnancy category C
- Abacavir (ABC)
  - Mechanism of action: similar to zidovudine
  - Adverse effects: Alcohol increases levels 41 percent; hypersensitivity reaction (which can be fatal)
  - Pregnancy category C

- Emtricitabine (FTC)
  - Mechanism of action: similar to zidovudine
  - Adverse effects: minimal toxicity; lactic acidosis with hepatic steatosis (rare)
  - Pregnancy category B

NONNUCLEOSIDE REVERSE TRANSCRIPTASE INHIBITORS

- Nevirapine, delavirdine, efavirenz
- Bind directly to HIV-1 reverse transcriptase and noncompetitively inhibit cDNA synthesis
- Adverse effects: Rash is common (especially with nevirapine)
- Pregnancy category C

PROTEASE INHIBITORS (PIs)

- Mechanism of action: inhibit HIV protease activity, blocking Gag and Gag-Pol cleavage required for assembly of progeny virions
- Saquinavir, indinavir, nelfinavir, amprenavir and ritonavir, atazanavir, lopinavir
- Adverse effects: nephrolithiasis (indinavir), severe diarrhea (nelfinavir), hepatotoxicity associated with concurrent use of other HIV agents and with comorbid hepatitis C, lipodystrophy, osteopenia, insulin resistance, severe lipid abnormalities
- Pregnancy category C

NUCLEOTIDE ANALOGUES: TENOFOVIR

- Mechanism of action: inhibits reverse transcriptase
- Adverse effects: peripheral wasting, facial wasting, breast enlargement, and cushingoid appearance; gastrointestinal complaints
  - Monitor: changes in serum creatinine and serum phosphorus in patients at risk or with history of renal dysfunction
- Pregnancy category B

Antifungal Agents

ALLYLAMINES

- Examples: butenafine, naftifine, terbinafine
- Mechanism of action: inhibits first step of ergosterol synthesis by blocking the activity of squalene epoxidase
- Adverse effects: hepatocellular injury, delayed gastric emptying, dysgeusia (metallic taste), reversible agranulocytosis, lupus erythematosus; terbinafine can cause gastrointestinal disturbance and nausea
- Pregnancy category B

AZOLES

- Class members
  - Imidazoles: Azole ring contains two nitrogen atoms
    - Ketoconazole, clotrimazole, miconazole

- Triazoles: Azole ring contains three nitrogen atoms
  - Fluconazole, itraconazole, voriconazole
- Mechanism of action: blocks ergosterol synthesis by binding to and inhibiting the fungal CYP-dependent enzyme lanosterol 14-α-demethylase (converts lanosterol to ergosterol; see Table 7-1)
- Fungistatic drugs in vitro
- Adverse effects
  - Hepatitis (greatest risk with ketoconazole), congestive heart failure (CHF) (itraconazole)
  - Ketoconazole: endocrine effects (gynecomastia, infertility, menstrual irregularities)
  - Miconazole: thrombophlebitis after IV administration
  - Voriconazole: visual disturbances in 30 percent of patients: altered/enhanced visual perception, blurred vision, color vision change, and or photophobia–effects clear after discontinuation of medication
- Pregnancy category C

POLYENES

- Amphotericin B
- Mechanism of action: binds to ergosterol (a component of fungal cell membranes) and forms amphotericin B–associated membrane pores, altering the membrane's permeability and causing leakage of intracellular Na^+, K^+, and H^+ ions, leading to cell death
- Adverse effects:
  - Amphotericin B binds cholesterol (mammalian cell membranes) to a far lesser extent than ergosterol
  - Hepatitis, infusion reactions, anemia, fever, flushing/generalized erythema, nephrotoxicity, hypotension
- Resistance: develops when binding of the drug to ergosterol is impaired or when ergosterol concentration in the membrane is decreased
- Pregnancy category B

GLUCAN SYNTHESIS INHIBITORS/ECHINOCANDINS

- Caspofungin
- IV administration
- Mechanism of action: inhibits glucan synthesis (essential polysaccharide of the fungal cell wall)
- Activity: primarily *Candida, Aspergillus*
- Pregnancy category C

GRISEOFULVIN

- Mechanism of action: interferes with microtubule function, causing metaphase arrest
- Produced by *Penicillium griseofulvum*
- Activity: fungistatic for dermatophytes

TABLE 7-1 Examples of CYP3A4 Subfamily Substrates, Inducers, and Inhibitors*

CYP3A4 Substrates	CYP3A4 Inducers	CYP3A4 Inhibitors
Alprazolam	Carbamazepine	Cimetidine
Atorvastatin	Cortisol	Clarithromycin
Buspirone	Dexamethasone	Diltiazem
Busulfan	Griseofulvin	Erythromycin
Cyclosporine	Nevirapine	Felfinavir
Digoxin	Omeprazole	Fluconazole (high dose)
Didanosine	Pantoprazole	Fluoxetine
Docetaxel	Phenobarbital	Fluvoxamine
Dofetilide	Phenylbutazone	Gestodene
Erythromycin	Phenytoin	Grapefruit
Felodipine	Prednisone	Indinavir
Fluconazole (antifungal)	Primdone	Itraconazole
Glyburide	Rifabutin	Ketoconazole
Indinavir	Rifampicin	Miconazole
Itraconazole (antifungal)	Rifampin	Mibefradil
Ketoconazole (antifungal)	Troglitazone	Nefazodone
Loratadine (antihistamine)		Nifedipine
Lovastatin (statins)		Omeprazole
Metformin		Prophoxyphene
Miconazole (antifungal)		Ritonavir
Midazolam		Saquinavir
Nifedipine		Verapamil
Pimozide		
Prednisone		
Quinidine		
Rifampin		
Ritonavir		
Saquinavir		
Sildenafil		
Simvastatin (statins)		
Tacrolimus		
Triazolam		
Verapamil		
Vincristine		
Warfarin		

* This is not a complete list, and readers should refer to the manufacturer's individual package insert for current information.
Source: Freedberg IM et al: *Fitzpatrick's Dermatology in General Medicine,* 6th ed. New York: McGraw-Hill, 2003, p. 2445.

- Adverse effects: gastrointestinal irritation, photosensitivity, granulocytopenia, hepatotoxicity, teratogenic
- Pregnancy category C

Immunosuppressive Agents

CYCLOSPORINE

- Binds to an immunophilin called *cyclophylin A* (CyPA)
- This complex binds to calcineurin and inhibits it's actions

- Calcineurin regulates the transcription factor NFAT (nuclear factor of activated T cells) by dephosphorylating the cytoplasmic component (NFATc); NFATc transloctes into the nucleus, where it binds NFATn
- NFATn regulates cytokine-encoding genes, including interleukin 2 (IL-2) and interferon-γ (IFN-γ)
- Pregnancy category C
- Adverse effects: hypertension, renal toxicity, hypertrichosis, gingival hyperplasia, metabolic

abnormalities, neurotoxicity (headache, tremor, paresthesias), lymphoma (especially in transplant patients), increased incidence of skin cancer, osteoporosis, hyperuricemia, decreased magnesium
- Monitor: chemistry panel, magnesium, lipid panel, blood pressure, lymph nodes; serum creatinine in long-term cyclosporin A therapy is a poor predictor of altered renal function (check creatinine clearance); oral retinoids may decrease incidence of skin cancer

IMMUNOBIOLOGICALS

- Antibodies as the active agent
  - Murine monoclonals
  - Chimeric monoclonals
  - Humanized monoclonals
  - Primatized monoclonals
  - Human sequenced monoclonals
- Antibody-like fusion proteins: composed of ligand-binding domains of human cellular receptors linked to hinge and CH2/CH3 constant-region domains of human IgG
- Cytokines
- Small proteins synthesized based on human gene sequences

ETANERCEPT

- Mechanism of action: recombinant human receptor fusion protein comprised of a dimer of the external domain of tumor necrosis factor-α (TNF-α) receptor linked to the Fc portion of human IgG1 receptor
- Competitively binds to free and receptor-bound TNF, inhibiting the normal action of TNF
- Self-administered by subcutaneous injection
- No pretreatment, laboratory evaluation, purified protein derivative (PPD) test is helpful
- Adverse effects: multiple sclerosis, positive antinuclear antibody ANA (11 percent), injection-site reaction, exacerbation of CNS demyelinating disorders, worsening of heart failure, rare reports of pancytopenia
- Pregnancy category B

INFLIXIMAB

- Mouse-human chimeric IgG1 monoclonal antibody specific for TNF-α (human antibody constant regions and murine antibody variable region)
- Acts by binding to soluble and transmembrane forms of TNF-α molecules, thus inhibiting its binding to TNF-α receptors
- IV infusion 3–10 mg/kg, 4- to 8-week intervals
- Adverse effects: reactivation of tuberculosis, positive ANA, serum sickness, and infusion reactions

- Contraindicated in patients with tuberculosis (a PPD test is required prior to initiating therapy)
- Pregnancy category C

EFALIZUMAB

- Mechanism of action: humanized form of a murine antibody against CD11a
- Blocks human leukocyte function antigen-1 (LFA-1) interactions with intercellular adhesion molecules 1 and 2 (ICAM-1 and ICAM-2, respectively)
- LFA-1 is expressed on endothelial cells, epidermal keratinocytes, and leukocytes, and although T cells are not unique in their expression, they depend on LFA-1 for both successful extravasation and antigen presentation
- Subcutaneous injection given weekly; conditioning dose recommended
- Worsening of psoriasis can occur during or after discontinuation
- Adverse effects: sepsis and opportunistic infections, lymphoma, thrombocytopenia for first 6 months, hypersensitivity reaction
- Monitoring: platelet counts monthly
- Pregnancy category C

ALEFACEPT

- Mechanism of action: fully human dimeric fusion protein
- Consists of the extracellular CD2-binding portion of the LFA-3 linked to the Fc (hinge, CH2 and CH3 domains) portion of human IgG1
- LFA-3 binds CD2 on the T-cell surface, inhibiting T-cell activation and proliferation
- IgG1 segment binds to accessory cells, triggering apoptosis of selected memory T cells expressing high levels of CD2 on the surface
  - Intramuscular injection contains 15 mg alefacept per 0.5 ml of reconstituted solution
- Dosing: given weekly for 12 weeks, followed by 12-week observation peroid
- Adverse effects: lymphopenia, malignancies (most commonly skin cancer), infections, hypersensitivity reactions, injection-site reactions
- Monitoring: CD4+ T-lymphocyte counts should be monitored weekly during the 12-week dosing period (this guides dosing); dose should be held if CD4+ T-lymphocyte counts fall below 250 cells/μl; medication should be discontinued if counts remain below 250 cells/μl for 1 month
- Pregnancy category B

ADALIMUMAB

- Mechanism of action: fully human monoclonal antibody to TNF-α blocks TNF-α interaction with the P55 and P75 cell surface TNF receptors

- Dosing: 40 mg subcutaneous injection every other week or weekly
- Potential adverse effects: sepsis and opportunistic infections, demyelinating disorders, lymphoma, exacerbation or new-onset CHF, injection site reactions, positive ANA
- Monitor: check initial PPD

DENILEUKIN DIFTITOX

- Mechanism of action: Diphtheria toxin and the receptor-binding domain of human IL-2 are fused
- Drug binds to the IL-2 receptor [cluster of differentiation 25 (CD25)]
- Internalized by receptor-mediated endocytosis
- Inhibits protein synthesis by translocation of the active portion of diphtheria toxin into the cytosol
- Fifty percent of patients with mycosis fungoides or Sézary syndrome have malignant cells that express CD25; patient's malignant cells should be tested for CD25 expression
- Pregnancy category C
- Adverse effects: hypersensitivity/vascular leak syndrome: characterized by two or more of the following three symptoms: hypotension, edema, and hypoalbuminemia; usually occurs within the first 2 weeks of infusion and may persist or worsen after the cessation of denileukin diftitox; hypoalbuminemia: occurs after 1 to 2 weeks (serum albumin levels should be at least 3.0 g/dl); infectious complications

THALIDOMIDE

- Mechanism of action: TNF-α and IL-12 suppressor, antiangiogenic; downregulates adhesion molecules
- Adverse effects: sedation, constipation, peripheral (sensory) neuropathy, teratogenicity, leukopenia, bradycardia, rash and fever (mainly in HIV patients), severe birth defects; malformations of extremities, microphthalmia, neural tube defects, cardiac and renal malfomations, esophageal fistulas, duodenal atresia, vaginal obstruction
- System for Thalidomide Educational Prescribing Safety (STEPS): monitoring program created by the Food and Drug Administration (FDA): (1) controls access to drug, (2) educates prescribing physicians, pharmacists, and patients, and (3) monitors compliance.
- Monitoring: baseline and monthly neurologic examinations; CBC
- Serum pregnancy testing 24 hours prior to starting medication, then every week for first month, then monthly thereafter; contraception, testing, and drug therapy compliance survey by patient
- Pregnancy category X

Antimycobacterial Agents

ISONIAZID

- Mechanism of action: disrupts mycobacterial cell walls, inhibits mycolic acid synthesis
- Bacteriostatic at most concentrations
- Elimination mainly acetylation
- Fast and slow acetylation of patient affects elimination half-life: fast = 70 min, slow = 180 min
- Adverse effects: neurotoxic, hepatotoxic, hemolysis in G6PD deficiency, lupus erythematosus, acneiform eruption, onycholysis, pellagra-like eruption, photosensitivity, pyridoxin (B_6) deficiency with high doses
- Pyridoxine supplementation can decrease risk of peripheral neuritis
- Pregnancy category C

RIFAMPIN

- Mechanism of action
- Macrocyclic antibiotic derived from *Streptomyces mediterranei* of action
- Mechanism: bactericidal; inhibits DNA-dependent RNA polymerase, interfering with bacterial RNA synthesis
- Activity: *Mycoplasma tuberculosis,* many gram-negative organisms, many chlamydiae
- Adverse effects: orange-red discoloration of skin, urine, tears; glossodynia
- Monitoring: CBCs and baseline clinical chemistries prior to and during therapy; interruption of therapy and high-dose intermittent therapy associated with thrombocytopenia (reversible if therapy is discontinued as soon as purpura occurs)
- Pregnancy category C
- Rifapentine, a second generation of rifampin, has a much longer half-life than rifampin and can be given weekly
- Rifabutin: semisynthetic rifampin

CLOFAZIMINE

- Red, fat-soluble, crystalline dye
- Mechanism of action: inhibits mycobacterial growth by binding preferentially to mycobacterial DNA
- Adverse effects: skin discoloration; secretions discolored: red urine; ichthyosis; severe abdominal symptoms, splenic infarction (rare), bowel obstruction, and gastrointestinal bleeding; crystalline deposits of clofazimine in tissues, including intestinal mucosa, spleen, liver, and mesenteric lymph nodes
- Pregnancy category C

ETHAMBUTOL

- Mechanism of action: inhibits metabolite synthesis in susceptible bacteria, resulting in impaired cellular metabolism and cell death

- Bacteriostatic
- Useful for organisms resistant to streptomycin and isoniazid (no cross-resistance)
- Adverse effects: dose-dependent visual disturbances, neurotoxicity, hyperhidrosis, gout
- Pregnancy category B

PYRAZINAMIDE (PZA)

- Mechanism of action: is not known
- Bacteriostatic or bactericidal against *M. tuberculosis* depending on concentration of drug attained at site of infection
- Adverse effects: photosensitivity, myalgias, hyperuricemia, gastrintestinal irritation, red-brown change in skin color, alopecia, flushing, hepatic injury (most common and serious side effect); gout can be precipitated by inhibition of excretion of urate, resulting in hyperuricemia
- Pregnancy category C

STREPTOMYCIN

- Mechanism of action
- Bactericidal antibiotic; interferes with normal protein synthesis
- Added as a fourth drug for *M. tuberculosis* treatment
- Given by injection
- Adverse effects: renal tubular damage, vestibular damage, and ototoxicity; caution with myasthenia gravis, hypocalcemia, and conditions that depress neuromuscular transmission
- Pregnancy category D

Miscellaneous

PENICILLAMINE

- Mechanism of action
- Metal chelator used to treat arsenic poisoning
- Forms soluble complexes with metals excreted in urine
- Adverse effects: thrombocytopenia; agranulocytosis; aplastic anemia, elastosis perforans serpiginosa
- Pregnancy category D

COLCHICINE

- Mechanism of action
- Decreases leukocyte motility and phagocytosis in inflammatory responses
- Adverse effects: renal failure, hepatic failure, permanent hair loss, bone marrow suppression, numbness or tingling in hands and feet, disseminated intravascular coagulopathy, decreased sperm count, dose-dependent gastrointestinal upset common
- Pregnancy category C

SULFASALAZINE

- Mechanism of action

- Induces neutrophil apoptosis and enhances adenosine release at sites of inflammation
- Adverse effects: gastrointestinal upset, fatigue, headache, drug eruption and photosensitivity; slow acetylators are prone to toxicity

AURANOFIN

- Mechanism of action
- Gold is taken up by macrophages, which in turn inhibit phagocytosis and lysosomal membrane stabilization
- Alters immunoglobulins, decreasing prostaglandin synthesis and lysosomal enzyme activity
- Precautions: discontinue therapy if platelet counts fall to less than $100,000/mm^3$, white blood cell count to less than $4000/mm^3$, granulocytes to less than $1500/mm^3$
- Pregnancy category B

INTRAVENOUS IMMUNE GLOBULINS

- Adverse effects: increases in creatinine and blood urea nitrogen
- Contraindications: documented hypersensitivity; IgA deficiency; anti-IgE/IgG antibodies
- Pregnancy category C

SPIRONOLACTONE

- Mechanism of action
- Aldosterone antagonist
- Potassium-sparing diuretic
- Potent competitive inhibitor of dihydrotestosterone (DHT) at its receptor sites at pilosebaceous units
- Adverse effects: hyperkalemia; menstrual irregularities, hyperkalemia, hyponatremia, potential teratogenicity as an antiandrogen
- Pregnancy category D

PHOTOTHERAPY

- Ultraviolet B (UV-B): 290–320 nm
- Narrow band UV-B (311 nm)
- Goeckerman regimen: coal tar followed by UV-B exposure
- Ingram method: anthralin application following a tar bath and UV-B treatment
- Psoralen and ultraviolet A (PUVA) photochemotherapy (wavelengths 320–400 nm)
- Mechanism of action: uses the photosensitizing drug methoxsalen (8-methoxypsoralens) in combination with ultraviolet A (UV-A) irradiation
- Interferes with DNA synthesis by inhibiting mitosis and binding covalently to pyrimidine bases in DNA when photoactivated by UV-A
- Decreases cellular proliferation, and also induces apoptosis of cutaneous lymphocytes leading to a localized immunosuppression
- Pregnancy category C

- Adverse effects of PUVA therapy include nausea, pruritus, and burning; known to be carcinogenic, with risk being dose-dependent; minimize exposure to outdoor or bright indoor light for 24 hours after each dose due to photosensitivity
- Contraindications: diseases associated with photosensitivity
- Pregnancy category C

TOPICAL TREATMENTS

Vehicles in Dermatologic Therapy

- Cream: a semisolid emulsion of oil in water; contains a preservative to prevent overgrowth of microorganisms; stabilized by an aqueous emulsifier
- Gel : a semisolid, transparent, nongreasy emulsion
- Lotion: liquid vehicle, aqueous or alcohol-based, that may contain a salt in solution
- Ointment: a semisolid grease/oil, sometimes also containing powder, but little or no water; the active ingredient is suspended; usually no preservative needed
- Paste: an ointment with a high proportion of powder that gives a stiff consistency
- The whole body requires 20 to 30 g of ointment per single dose. In an adult:
  - Face or neck: 1 g
  - Trunk (each side): 3 g
  - Arm: $1\frac{1}{2}$ g
  - Hand: $\frac{1}{2}$ g
  - Leg: 3 g
  - Foot: 1 g

Acne Preparations

BENZOYL PEROXIDE

- Antibacterial effect
- Adverse effects: skin irritation and drying; contact allergy (1 percent)

AZELAIC ACID

- Mechanism of action
- Dicarboxylic acid
- Reduces production of keratin and inhibits growth of *Propionibacterium acnes,* antityrosinase activity
- Adverse effects: may produce hypopigmentation, skin irritation
- Pregnancy category B

SALICYLIC ACID

- Keratolytic
- Adverse effects: erythema and peeling, salicylism (effects marked by tinnitus, nausea, and vomiting)

SULFUR

- Comedolytic, Keratolytic, mild antibacterial dose 5–10%
- Adverse effects: odor, application site reaction
- Lotion 5% sulfur, 22% alcohol
- Combination: sulfur–sodium sulfacetamide
- Lotion 50 mg sulfur, 100 mg sulfacetamide

RETINOIDS

- Mechanism of action: regulation of cellular proliferation and differentiation and modulation of immune function and cytokine function
- Help normalize hyperkeratinization and have anti-inflammatory effects
- See systemic section for further detail
- Tretinoin (all-*trans* retinoic acid)
  - Binds with approximately equal affinity to all three RARs and also can be converted to forms that activate the RXRs
  - Adverse effects: tenderness, erythema, and burning; also increased risk of sunburn
  - Pregnancy category C
- Adapalene
  - Retinoid properties from a synthetic naphtholic acid derivative
  - Selectivity for the nuclear RAR β/γ receptors
  - Pregnancy category C
- Tazarotene
  - Prodrug is hydrolyzed rapidly in tissues to the active metabolite tazarotenic acid
  - Mainly binds to RAR-γ and RAR-β nuclear receptor; also can bind to RAR-α; does not bind to RXRs
  - Pregnancy category X
- Alitretinoin (9-*cis*-retinoic acid): binds to and activates both RXRs and RARs
  - Naturally occurring endogenous retinoid
- Arotinoids: adverse-effect profile offers little, if any, improvement over previously developed retinoids

Alpha-Hydroxy Acids (see Chap. 14)

Topical Antibiotics

See above for mechanisms of other antibiotics

MUPIROCIN

- Produced by fermentation of *Pseudomonas fluorescens*
- Mechanism of action: inhibition of bacterial protein synthesis
- Pregnancy category B

SILVER SULFADIAZINE

- Mechanism of action: inhibiting DNA replication and modification of the cell membrane adverse effects—early luekopenia (in post burn patients)

Bleaching Agents

HYDROQUINONE

- Inhibit tyrosinase: inhibits enzymatic oxidation of tyrosine to 3, 4-dihydroxyphenylamine
- Prepared 2%, 3%, and 4% concentrations
- Adverse events: exogenous ochronosis
- Pregnancy category C

KOJIC ACID

- Mechanism of action: inhibits tyrosinase
- Adverse effects: contact sensitivity

MEQUINOL

- Mechanism of action: exact action unknown Monomethyl ether of hydroquinone, substrate for tyrosinase and a competitive inhibitor of formation of melanin precursors
- Pregnancy category X when used with tretinoin

Topical Anesthetics (see Chaps. 13 and 14)

Topical Immunosuppressives

TACROLIMUS AND PIMECROLIMUS

- Mechanism of action: macrolide lactone/calcineurin inhibitors
- Binds to FK-binding protein (receptor within cytoplasm)
- The drug-protein complex inhibits calcineurin (a calcium-dependent phosphatase enzyme)
- Without the phosphatase activity of calcineurin, nuclear factor of activated T-cells (NF-AT) cannot translocate to the nucleus and activate transcription of proinflammatory cytokines
- IL-2, IL-3, IL-4, IL-5, IL-10, GM-CSF, and TNF-α
- Reduction in the activity of T-lymphocytes in the immune system
- Adverse effects: minimally absorbed into the blood; application site stinging
- Pregnancy category C

Topical Antivirals

IMIQUIMOD 5% CREAM

- Imidazoquinoline amine
- Mechanism of action: induction of cytokines after binding to a transmembrane receptor: Toll-like receptor 7 (an innate immunity response)
- Stimulation of the cellular arm of acquired immunity through induction of IFN-α, IFN-γ, and IL-12; T memory cells are created after activation from dendritic cells
- Adverse effects: local skin irritation
- Pregnancy category C

ACYCLOVIR, PENCICLOVIR

- Mechanism of action and side effects: See oral section above

DOCOSANOL 10% CREAM

- Mechanism of action: inhibits fusion between the plasma membrane and the herpes simplex virus (HSV) envelope
- Adverse effects: headache
- Pregnancy category B

Antifungals

ZINC PYRITHIONE

- Mechanism of action: inhibitor of membrane transport in fungi
- Adverse effects: allergic contact dermatitis
- Azoles, allylamines, polyenes: see oral section

SELENIUM SULFIDE

- Mechanism of action: increase fungal shedding by decreasing comeocyte production; sporocidal
- Adverse effects: skin irritation, hair loss

CICLOPIROX

- Mechanism of action: chelation of polyvalent metal cations (e.g., Fe^{3+} and Al^{3+}); inhibits metal-dependent enzymes, responsible for the degradation of peroxides within microbial cells
- Adverse effects: contact dermatitis and pruritus
- Pregnancy category B

Androgenetic Alopecia Treatment

MINOXIDIL

- Mechanism of action
- Relaxes arteriolar smooth muscle, causing vasodilation, mechanism for hair growth not known
- Adverse effects: may exacerbate angina pectoris; caution in pulmonary hypertension, congestive heart failure, coronary artery disease, and significant renal failure
- Pregnancy category C

FINASTERIDE

- Mechanism of action: inhibits conversion of testosterone to dihydrotestosterone by inhibiting competitive inhibition of type II 5α-reductase
- Adverse effects: decreased libido or erectile dysfunction (2%)
- Pregnancy category X

Excessive Hair Treatment

EFLORNITHINE HCL 13.9% CREAM

- Mechanism of action: inhibits enzyme ornithine decarboxylase (ODC)
- Metabolic activity in the hair follicle decreases, and hairs grow in more slowly
- Adverse effect: mild skin irritation
- Pregnancy category C

Sunscreens

- Chemical absorbers
- Aromatic compounds conjugated with a carbonyl group

ULTRAVIOLET FILTERS B

- Aminobenzoic acid and derivatives
- Padimate O
  - Most potent UV-B absorber
  - *para*-Aminobenzoic acid (PABA): high incidence of hypersensitivity
  - 290–315 nm
- Cross-sensitivity with PABA
  - Artificial sweeteners (e.g., saccharin, sodium cyclamate); ester-type anesthetics, Azo dyes (e.g., aniline, paraphenylenediamine), sulfonamide antibiotics, sulfonamide-based oral hypoglycemics, or thiazide diuretics
- Cinnamates
- Octyl methoxycinnamate
  - Second most potent UV-B absorber compared with padimate O
  - 290–320 nm
  - Cross sensitivity to cinnamon derivatives (balsam of Peru, balsam of Tolu, Cassia, cinnamic acid, cinnamic alcohol, cinnamic aldehyde, cinnamon oil, coca leaves)
- Salicylates
  - Octyl salicylate
  - Used to augment the UV-B protection in a sunscreen
  - 280–320 nm
  - Weak UV-B absorbers
- Octocrylene
  - May be used in combination with other UV absorbers
  - 250–360 nm
  - Phenylbenzimidazole sulfonic acid
  - Selective UV-B filter

ULTRAVIOLET FILTERS A

- Benzophenones Oxybenzone
  - Absorbs well through UV-A II (benzophenone-3) wavelengths
  - Benzophenones are primarily UV-B absorbers
  - 270–350 nm
- Anthranilates
  - Menthyl anthranilate
  - absorb mainly in the near UV-A portion
  - 260–380 nm
- Dibenzoylmethanes
- Avobenzone (Parsol 1789)
  - 320–400 nm

- Dioxybenzone
  - 250–390 nm

PHYSICAL BLOCKERS

- Titanium dioxide
  - 290–700 nm
- Zinc oxide
  - 290–700 nm
- SPF 15 product filters out more than 93% of UV-B
- SPF 30 product filters out less than 97% of UV-B

Parasiticidals

MALATHION

- Mechanism of action: irreversible cholinesterase inhibitor hydrolyzed (and therefore detoxified) rapidly by mammals, but not by insects
- Binds to hair and may provide some residual protection after therapy
- Adverse effects: Alcohol may irritate excoriated skin; the lotion is flammable; take care to avoid mucosal surfaces, eyes; do not apply to lashes
- Pregnancy category B

NATURAL PYRETHRIN

- Mechanism of action: Neurotoxin

PERMETHRIN

- Mechanism of action: synthetic pyrethrin
- Neurotoxin that causes paralysis and death in ectoparasites
- Adverse effects: lack of safety data on children younger than 2 months, pregnant and breast-feeding women
- Pregnancy category B

LINDANE 1% (GAMMA-BENZENE HEXACHLORIDE)

- Mechanism of action: neurotoxin that causes seizures and death in parasitic arthropods
- Adverse effects: do not use in infants, small children, patients with a history of seizure, or lactating or pregnant women

Topical Steroids

- Anti-inflammatory, immunosuppressive, and antiproliferative properties
- Bind to a receptor in the cytoplasm of cells and transported to the nucleus
- Affect gene transcription multiple proteins
- Decrease inflammation by suppressing migration of polymorphonuclear leukocytes and reversing increased capillary permeability
- Efficacy of an individual topical corticosteroid is related to its potency
- Class 1—superpotent

- Class 2—potent
- Class 3—upper midstrength
- Class 4—midstrength
- Class 5—lower midstrength
- Class 6—mild
- Class 7—least potent
- Adverse effects: acne, tachyphylaxis, skin atrophy (striae, telangiectasia and purpura), may suppress hyperthalmic-pituitary-adrenal (HPA) axis (rare)
- Risk factors for adverse effects
  - Young age
  - Liver disease
  - Renal disease
  - Amount of topical steroid applied
  - Potency of topical steroid
  - Use of occlusion
  - Location of topical application

Topical Chemotherapy Agents

NITROGEN MUSTARD

- Mechanism of action: cytotoxic to cancer cells via DNA alkylation
- Adverse effects: Delayed hypersensitivity (35 to 60 percent) can be overcome with use of topical steroids or desensitization; less common with use of ointment; associated with an increased risk of nonmelanoma skin cancers
- Pregnancy category D

5-FLUOROURACIL

- Mechanism of action: inhibits thymidylate synthetase, leading to inhibition of DNA synthesis and cell death
- Adverse effects: local pain, pruritus, hyperpigmentation, irritation, inflammation and burning at the site of application, allergic contact dermatitis, scarring, soreness, tenderness, suppuration, scaling and swelling
- Pregnancy category D

Other

Castellani Paint

- Resorcinol (8 g), acetone (4 ml), magenta (0.4 g), phenol (4.0 g), boric acid (0.8 g), industrial methylated spirit 90% (8.5 ml), and water (100 ml) a fungicidal and bactericidal
- Pregnancy category C
- Adverse effects: magenta can stain clothing and skin; may be toxic in children because of phenol content; may cause irritation

PHOTODYNAMIC THERAPY (PDT)

- Mechanism of action
- Topical application of aminolevulinic acid HCl on skin leads to the accumulation of the endogenous photosensitizer protoporphyrin IX (PpIX) in epidermal cells
- Conversion of ALA to PpIX occurs in skin cells by enzymes in the heme biosynthetic pathway
- Rapidly proliferating skin cells convert more ALA to PpIX than do less rapidly proliferating normal epidermal cells
- Subsequent illumination of the lesion with noncoherent red light (570–670 nm) 3 to 6 hours after ALA application causes ALA to be enzymatically converted into the active endogenous photosensitizer PpIX
- Methyl 5-aminolevulinate also can be used instead of ALA
- Apoptotic cell death and vascular injury for PDT-mediated tissue ablation
- Adverse effects: burning pain, stinging, or itching restricted to the illuminated area; erythema and mild edema of the treated area; action spectrum for PDT-induced phototoxicity lies within the visible spectrum range; strict avoidance of sunlight and excessive indoor light, generalized cutaneous photosensitivity, photophobia, and/or ocular discomfort, residual hyperpigmentation and hypopigmentation
- Pregnancy category C

CALCIPOTRIENE

- Mechanism of action
- Vitamin D derivative
- Alters keratinocyte proliferation and keratinocyte differentiation
- Reduction in concentration of calcipotriene by UV-A
- Adverse effects: Hypercalcemia: use should not exceed 100 g per week
- Pregnancy category C

ANTHRALIN

- Mechanism of action
- Synthetic derivative of a tree bark extract
- Naturally occurring saturated dicarboxylic acid–possessing antibacterial, comedolytic, and anti-inflammatory activities
- Inhibits cell growth and restores cell differentiation
- Prolonged contact method uses 0.5%–1.0% preparations applied for several hours; short contact method uses higher concentrations of anthralin (0.5%–1.0%) but usually applied for only 1 hour or less
- Adverse effects: Irritating to normal skin
- Applications in excessive amounts may stain clothing; long-term corticosteroid treatment withdrawal may cause complications of rebound phenomenon
- Pregnancy category C

Antiperspirants
ALUMINUM SALTS

- Mechanism of action: unknown, possibly secondary to blockage of the sweat duct or atrophy of secretory cells
- Aluminum chloride 10% to 30% in distilled water or 60% alcohol
- Pregnancy category C
- Mechanism of action: increase the permeability of the sweat ducts resulting in complete dermal resorption of the sweat

Botulinum Toxin (see Chap. 14)
Diclofenac Sodium Gel 3%

- Mechanism: non steroidal anti-inflammatory
- Adverse effects: localized contact dermatitis
- Pregnancy category B

PREGNANCY CATEGORIES (TABLE 7-2)

- Classification system indicating the level of safety of a particular drug during pregnancy
- All drugs are classified into the following categories
- A. Controlled studies show no risk
  - Adequate, well-controlled studies in pregnant women have failed to demonstrate risk to fetus
- B. No evidence of risk in humans
  - Either animal findings show risk but human findings do not, or if no adequate human studies have been done, animal findings are negative
- C. Risk cannot be ruled out
  - Human studies are lacking, and the animal studies are either positive for fetal risk or lacking as well. However, potential benefits may justify the potential risk
- D. Positive evidence for risk
  - Investigational or postmarketing data show risk to fetus. Nevertheless, potential benefits may outweigh the potential risk
- X. Contraindicated in pregnancy
  - Studies in animals or humans or investigational or postmarketing reports have shown fetal risk that clearly overweighs any possible benefit to the patient

Antifungal

- Category A: Nystatin
- Category B
  - Amphotericin B
  - Naftifine
  - Cicloprox
  - Oxiconazole nitrate
  - Terbinafine

Antiacne

- Category B: Azelaic acid
- Category C: Benzoyl peroxide

Antibiotic

- Category A: Bacitracin
- Category B
  - Clindamycin
  - Erythromycin
  - Meclocycline
  - Metronidazole gel or cream
  - Mupirocin

Bleaching

- Category B: Hydroquinone

Antiscabetic

- Catergory A
  - Permethrin B
  - Antihistamines
- Category B
  - Chlorpheniramine
  - Dexchlorpheniramine
  - Diphenhydramine
  - Brompheniramine
  - Cetirizine
  - Cyproheptadine
  - Clemastine
  - Azatadine
  - Loratadine
- Category C
  - Azelastine
  - Hydroxyzine
  - Promethazine

DRUG SIDE EFFECTS

- Acanthosis nigricans: NODES: nicotinic acid/niacin, oral contraceptives, dilantin, estrogens, steroids
- Acne (pimples)
  - Phenytoin
  - Isoniazid, iodides
  - Moisturizers
  - Phenobarbitol
  - Lithium
  - Ethionamide
  - Steroids
- Acral erythema
  - Ara-C
  - Bleomycin
  - Doxorubicin
  - Etoposide
  - 5-FU
  - Hydroxyurea
  - Mercaptopurine
  - Methotrexate

TABLE 7-2 Pregnancy Categories

Drug	Pregnancy Category
Systemic Medications	
Glucocorticoids	C
Sulfones	C
Aminoquinolones	C
Cytotoxic/Antimetabolic Agents	
Methotrexate, 5-FC	C
Hydroxyurea, azathioprine, cyclophosphamide	D
MPA	B
Retinoids	X
Antihistamines	
Diphenhydramine, cetirizine, loratadine	B
Hydroxyzine, doxepin, fexofenadine, desloratidine	C
Leukotriene inhibitors	B
Leukotriene inhibitors (zileuton)	C
Antibiotics	
Penicillins, macrolides, lincosamides, sulfapyridine, metronidazole	B
Cephalosporins, tetracyclines, aminoglycosides	D
Fluoroquinolones, chloramphenicol, sulfonamides, vancomycin, oxazolidinones	C
Antiviral agents	
Acyclovir, famciclovir, valacyclovir	B
Ganciclovir, foscarnet, amantadine, rimantadine, interferons, cidofovir	C
Valganciclovir, ribavirin	?
Antiretroviral agents	
NRTI/zidovudine, lamivudine, abacavir	C
NRTI/didanosine, emtricitabine	B
non-NRTI	C

(Continued)

TABLE 7-2 Pregnancy Categories *(Continued)*

Drug	Pregnancy Category
Protease inhibitors	C
Nucleotide analogues/tenofovir	B
Antifungal agents	
Allylamines, polyenes	B
Azoles, glucan synthesis inhibitors, griseofulvin	C
Immunosuppressive agents	
Cyclosporine, infliximab, efalizumab, denileukin biftitox	C
Immunobiologicals, adalimumab	?
Etanercept, Alefacept	B
Thalidomide	X
Anitimycobacterial agents	
Isoniazid, rifampin, clofazimine, PZA	C
Ethambutol	B
Streptomycin	D
Miscellaneous	
Penicillamine, spironalactone	D
Colchicine, intravenous immunoglobulins, phototheraphy	C
Sulfasalazine	?
Auranofin	B
Topical Treatments	
Therapeutic vehicles	?
Acne preparations	
Benzoyl perozide, salicylic acid, sulfur	?
Azelaic acid	B
Retinoids (Tretinoin, adapalene)	C
Retinoids (Tazarotene)	X
Retinoids (alitretinoin, arotinoids, ALAs)	?

TABLE 7-2 Pregnancy Categories *(Continued)*

Drug	Pregnancy Category
Topical antibiotics	
Mupirocin	B
Silver sulfadiazine	?
Bleaching agents	
Hydroquinone	C
Kojic acid	?
Mequinol	X (when used with tretinoin)
Topical anesthetics	Chap. 14
Topical immunosuppressives	
Tacrolimus/pimecrolimus	C
Topical antivirals	
Imiquimod 5% cream	C
Acyclovir/penciclovir, docosanol 10% cream	?
Antifungals	
Azoles, allylamines, polyenes	See oral section
Zinc pyrithione, selenium sulfide	?
Ciclopirox	B
Androgenetic alopecia treatments	
Minoxidil	C
Finasteride	X
Excessive hair treatments	
Eflornithine HCL 13.9% cream	C
Sunscreens	
UVB, UVA, physical blockers	?
Parasiticidals	
Malathion, permethrin	B
Lindane	?
Topical steroids	?
Castellani paint	C

(Continued)

TABLE 7-2 Pregnancy Categories *(Continued)*

Drug	Pregnancy Category
Topical chemotherapy agents	
Nitrogen mustard, 5-FU	D
Other	
PDT	C
Calcipotriene	C
Anthralin	C
Antiperspirants (aluminum salts)	C
Antiperspirants (Botulinum toxin)	See cosmetic chapter
Diclofenac sodium gel 3%	B

- Acral sclerosis: Bleomycin
- Acute generalized exanthematous pustulosis
  - Penicillin
  - Macrolide antibiotics
- Alopecia
  - Chemotherapy agents
  - Anticoagulants
  - Hormones
  - Anticonvulsants
  - Amantidine
  - Captopril
  - Cholesterol-lowering drugs
  - Accutane/isotretinoin
  - Ketoconazole
  - Propranolol
  - Cimetidine
- Blue-gray hyperpigmentation
  - Desipramine
  - Amiodarone
  - Antimalarials/anticonvulsants
  - Minocycline
  - Imipramine
  - Thorazine
- Bullous eruptions
  - Lasix
  - Penicillamine
  - Thiols (Captopril)
  - Penicillin
  - Sulfonamides
  - PUVA
- Cutis laxa: Penicillin
- Dental abnormalities: Tetracycline (gray, discolored teeth)

- Dermatomyositis
  - Hydroxyurea
  - Penicillamine
- Elastosis perforans serpiginosa: Penicillamine
- Erythema nodosum
  - OCP
  - Antibiotics (sulfonamides, tetracycline, penicillin)
  - 13-*cis* retinoic acid
  - Gold
  - Opiates
  - Halogens
- Eyelash growth: Interferon
- Fixed drug eruptions
  - NSAIDs (pigmented)
  - Sulfonamides (pigmented)
  - Pseudoephedrine (nonpigmented)
  - Phenopthaleine laxatives
  - OCP
  - Tetracycline
  - Aspirin
  - Barbiturates
  - Carbamazepime
- Gingival hyperplasia
  - Calcium channel blockers
  - Cyclosporine
  - Dilantin
- Gray baby syndrome: Chloramphenicol
- Hypertrichosis
  - Cyclosporine (but *not* Prograf)
  - Diazoxide
  - Danazol
  - Minoxidil

- Spironolactone
- Psoralen
- Ichthyosis: Nicotinic acid
- Leg ulcers: Hydroxyurea
- Lichenoid Eruptions
  - Lasix
  - Penicillamine
  - Gold
  - Thiazides
  - Chlorpropamide
  - Antimalarials
  - Methyldopa
  - Phenylthiazides
  - Beta blockers
- Linear IgA: Vancomycin
- Lipodystrophy: Crixivan ("crix belly")
- Livedo reticularis
  - Quinidine (photodistributed)
  - Amantadine
- Lupus
  - CCLE
  - Smoking
  - SCLE
  - D-Penicillamine
  - HCTZ
  - Lamisil
  - Sulfonureas
  - Griseofulvin
  - Naproxen
  - Diltiazem
  - Procainamide
  - PUVA
  - Minocycline
- Systemic lupus erythematosus (D-CHIPS)
  - Dilantin
  - Chlorpropamide
  - Hydralazine
  - Isoniazid
  - Procainamide
  - Sprouts (alfalfa sprouts/L-canavanine)
- Melanonychia striata
  - AZT (zidovudine)
- Neutrophilic eccrine hidradenitis
  - Ara-C
  - Bleomycin
- Optic neuritis: Ethambutal
- Pellagra-like eruption
  - Isoniazid
  - Azathioprine
  - 5-FU
- Pemphigus vulgaris
  - Penicillamine
  - Thiols (captopril)
- Penile ulcers: Foscarnet
- Photoallergic drug reaction
  - Griseofulvin
  - NSAIDs
  - Phenothiazines
  - Quinidine
  - Sulfonamide
  - Sulfa drugs
  - Thiazide diuretics
  - *para*-Amino benzoic acid
  - *para*-Phenylene diamine
- Photoonycholysis
  - Tetracycline
  - 8-MOP
- Phototoxic drug reaction
  - Amiodarone
  - Nalidixic acid
  - NSAIDS
  - Phenothiazines (chlorpromazine)
  - Tetracyclines
- Pityriasis rosea-like eruptions
  - Barbiturates/Bismuth
  - Omeprazole
  - Beta blockers
  - Captopril
  - Clonidine
  - Griseofulvin
  - Isotretinoin
  - Metronidazole
  - Penicillin
- Porphyria cutanea tarda
  - Griseofulvin
  - Rifampin
  - Antimalarials/alcohol
  - Busulfan/benzenes
  - Hormones
  - Iron
  - Phenols
  - Sulfonylurea
- Pseudolymphoma
  - Anticonvulsants (dilantin, phenobarbitol)
  - Antihypertensives (beta blockers, ACE inhibitors, calcium channel blockers)
  - Tricyclic antidepressants
  - Allopurinol
- Pseudomembranous colitis: Clindamycin
- Pseudoporphyria
  - Tetracycline
  - Accutane
  - Naproxen
  - Naldixic acid
  - Piroxican
  - Lasix
  - Sulfonamides
  - Hemodialysis for chronic renal failure
- Pseudotumor cerebri
  - Accutane

- Tetracycline
- Steroids
- Pseudoxanthoma elasticum: Penicillamine
- Psoriasis
  - GCSF
  - INH
  - NSAIDs
  - Steroids
  - Lithium
  - ACE inhibitors/antimalarials
  - Beta blockers
  - Penicillamine
  - OCP
- Pulmonary fibrosis
  - Methotrexate
  - Interferon-α
  - Gold
  - Imuran
  - Cyclophosphamide, cytoxan
  - Bleomycin
  - Raynaud's
  - Bleomycin
  - Vincristine
- Red-orange body fluids (tears/urine): Rifampin
- Sweet's syndrome
  - Neupogen
  - OCP
  - Minocycline
  - All trans retinoic acid
  - TMP-SMZ
  - Celebrex
- Toxic epidermal necrolysis
  - Sulfonamides
  - Penicillin
  - Allopurinol
  - NSAIDs
  - Anticonvulsants (phenytoin, phenobarbitol, carbamazepime)
  - Pentamidine

- Urticaria
  - Aspirin
  - NSAIDs
  - Antibiotics (penicillin, sulfonamides, rifampin, vancomycin)
  - Opiates
  - Barbiturates
  - Contrast dye
  - ACE inhibitors (captopril)
- Vasculitis
  - Ampicillin
  - Sulfonamides
  - Thiazides
  - Lasix
  - NSAIDs
  - Cimetidine
  - ACE inhibitors
- Vestibular toxicity: Aminoglycosides

REFERENCES

Dukes MNG, Aronson JK, eds. *Meyler's Side Effects of Drugs,* 14th Ed, Amsterdam: Elsevier; 2000.

Hardman JG, Limbird LE, eds. *Goodman & Gilman's The Pharmacological Basis of Therapeutics,* 10th Ed. New York: McGraw-Hill; 2001.

Litt JZ, ed. *Drug Eruption Reference Manual 2002.* New York: The Parthenon Publishing Group, Inc.; 2002.

McEvoy GK, ed. *American Hospital Formulary Service Drug Information 2002.* Bethesda, Maryland: American Society of Health-System Pharmacists; 2002.

Medical Economics Staff and Physicians, eds. *Physicians' Desk Reference,* 57th Ed. Montvale, New Jersey: Thomson Healthcare; 2002.

Wolverton SE, ed. *Comprehensive Dermatologic Drug Therapy.* Philadelphia: W.B. Saunders; 2001.

CHAPTER 8

PEDIATRIC DERMATOLOGY

ADRIENNE M. FEASEL
DENISE W. METRY

DISORDERS OF PIGMENTATION

Mongolian Spot (Fig. 8-1)

- Presentation
  - Blue-gray patches present at birth or early infancy
  - Usually buttocks, lumbosacral back
  - Common in black, Hispanic, and Asian races
  - Color due to Tyndell effect (scattering of light as it strikes dermal melanin)
- Course
  - Usually resolves by early to late childhood
  - Extensive Mongolian spots (dermal melanocytosis) with dorsal/ventral distribution, indistinct borders, and persistent and/or "progressive" behavior may be a sign of underlying lysosomal storage disease (most commonly GM1 gangliosidosis type 1 and Hurler disease)

Nevus of Ota (Fig. 8-2)

- Also known as oculodermal melanocytosis, nevus fuscoceruleus ophthalmomaxillaris
- Presentation
  - Unilateral bluish gray discoloration of facial skin
  - Affects region supplied by trigeminal nerve V_1 and V_2 ± ipsilateral eye
  - Congenital or acquired by second decade
  - More common in black or Asian races, females
- Treatment: pigmented lesion lasers
- Course
  - Persists; both this and nevus of Ito may increase in size/intensity over time
  - Ocular involvement: risk of glaucoma

Nevus of Ito (Fig. 8-3)

- Also known as nevus fusoceruleus acromiodeltoides
- Presentation: similar to nevus of Ota but localized to unilateral shoulder, lateral neck, scapula, and/or deltoid

- Course: persists
- Treatment: pigmented lesion lasers

Mosaic Hypopigmentation (Fig. 8-4)

- Includes hypomelanosis of Ito (incontinentia pigmenti acromians), nevus depigmentosus (achromic nevus)
- Presentation
  - Benign, hypopigmented oval or round patches, bands, or swirls
  - May be localized or extensive
  - Arranged along one or more Blaschko lines
  - No preceding vesicular or inflammatory stage
  - Incidence of systemic manifestations highest with most extensive lesions
  - Most commonly CNS, musculoskeletal, and eyes depending on particular chromosome defect and level of mosaicism
- Course: persists

VASCULAR DISORDERS

Blueberry Muffin Baby (Fig. 8-5)

- Presentation
  - Multiple, dark blue to magenta, small, nonblanching papules and macules
  - Present at birth or by first day of life
- Etiology
  - Extramedullary hematopoiesis
  - Associated with congenital infections (TORCH viruses, most commonly cytomegalovirus), hemolytic disease of the newborn, hereditary spherocytosis, twin-twin transfusion syndrome
- Differential
  - Includes neoplastic-infiltrative disease (lesions typically larger, more nodular, and fewer in number):

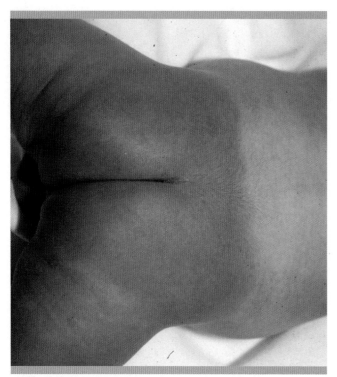

FIGURE 8-1 Mongolian spot. *(Courtesy of Dr. Adelaide Hebert.)*

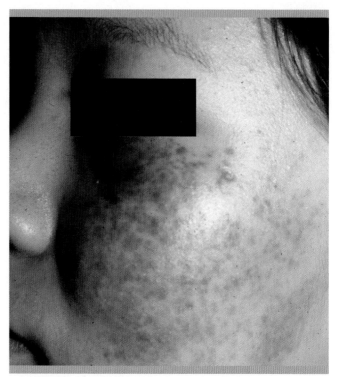

FIGURE 8-2 Nevus of Ota. *(Courtesy of Dr. Adelaide Hebert.)*

- Neuroblastoma, rhabdomyosarcoma, Langerhans' cell histiocytosis (especially congenital self-healing histiocytosis, also known as Hashimoto-Pritzker disease), congenital leukemia (especially myelogenous)
- Course
  - Skin lesions involute spontaneously in 2 to 6 weeks

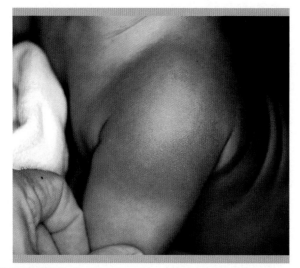

FIGURE 8-3 Nevus of Ito. *(From Weinberg S et al. Color Atlas of Pediatric Dermatology, 3rd ed. New York: McGraw-Hill, 1998, p. 229.)*

- Evaluation may include complete blood count (CBC), viral cultures, TORCH serologies, Coombs' test; skin biopsy if neoplastic infiltration suspected
- Therapy: directed toward underlying cause

Acute Hemorrhagic Edema of Infancy (Finkelstein's Disease) (Fig. 8-6)

- Presentation
  - Acute form of leukocytoclastic vasculitis
  - Children under 2 years
  - Often history of preceding infection
  - Rapid onset
  - Fever, edema, and "cockade" or targetoid purpuric lesions on face, ears, distal extremities
  - Children generally appear well despite alarming appearance of skin lesions
- Systemic symptoms: renal, joint, gastrointestinal (GI) involvement exceptional (important difference from adult Henoch-Schonlein purpura)
- Course: clinical improvement in 1 to 3 weeks

Henoch-Schonlein Purpura (Anaphylactoid Purpura) (Fig. 8-7)

- Presentation
  - Triad: characteristic skin lesions, abdominal pain, and hematuria
  - Children and young adults
  - Often preceding upper respiratory infection

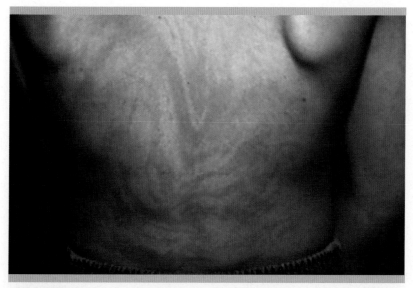

FIGURE 8-4 Hypomelanosis of Ito. *(Courtesy of Dr. Adelaide Hebert.)*

- Pink or erythematous papules that become purpuric on extensor extremities, buttocks
- Develop in crops
- Systemic symptoms
  - Abdominal pain
  - Arthralgias
  - Hematuria
  - Nephritis; rare progressive glomerular disease
- Course
  - Most resolve in 6 to 16 weeks
  - May recur

- Severe/prolonged disease more common in older children/adolescents
- Nephritis may manifest up to 3 years after initial onset; important to monitor urinalyses (UAs)
- Treatment: supportive care

Nevus Anemicus (Fig. 8-8)

- Presentation
  - Congenital vascular abnormality, asymptomatic
  - Most commonly occurs as a single patch of skin pallor on the trunk

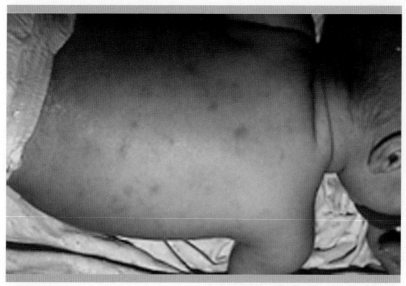

FIGURE 8-5 Blueberry muffin baby. *(Courtesy of Dr. Adelaide Hebert.)*

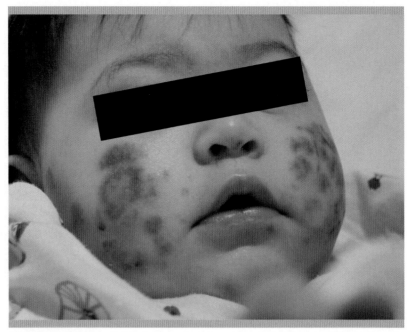

FIGURE 8-6 Acute hemorrhagic edema of infancy. *(Courtesy of Dr. Denise Metry.)*

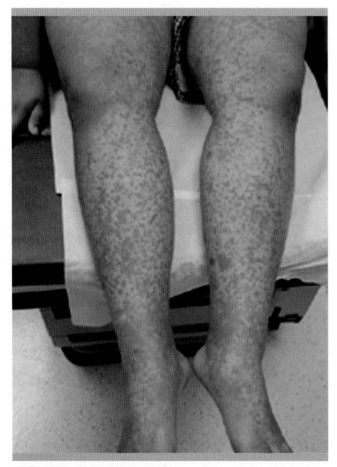

FIGURE 8-7 Henoch-Schonelin purpura. *(Courtesy of Dr. Denise Metry.)*

- Localized vascular hypersensitivity to catecholamines
- Catecholamine sensitivity produces increased vasoconstriction and skin pallor
- Diagnosis
  - Diascopy: when pressure is applied to the border of the patch with a clear glass slide; the border between lesion and normal skin disappears
  - Rubbing the affected area causes erythema of the surrounding skin, but the lesion itself remains unchanged
  - Histopathology is normal
- Treatment: none

INFECTIONS

Molluscum Contagiosum (Fig. 8-9)

- Presentation
  - Skin-colored, umbilicated papules
  - Children commonly affected
  - Contagious, with autoinoculation
- Causative organism
  - Pox virus
  - Large DNA virus (200–300 nm)
- Diagnosis
  - Usually clinical
  - Histology: Henderson-Patterson bodies (cytoplasmic viral inclusion bodies) on path
- Course: Individual lesions last several weeks; total course may last several months to years
- Treatment

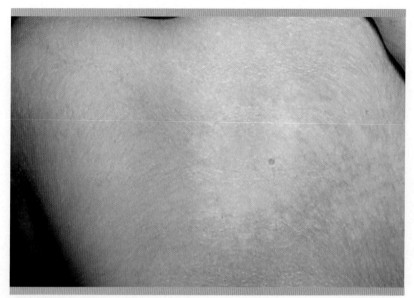

FIGURE 8-8 Nevus anemicus. *(Courtesy of Dr. Denise Metry.)*

- Not required because lesions will resolve spontaneously
- Destructive options include cantharidin, curettage, cryotherapy, and topical irritants (retinoic acid, imiquimod)

Eczema Herpeticum (Kaposi's Varicelliform Eruption) (Fig. 8-10)

- Presentation
  - Herpes simplex virus (HSV) infection within preexisting dermatitis (atopic dermatitis, severe seborrheic dermatitis, scabies, bullous disorders)

  - Sudden onset of grouped, uniformly sized vesicles and/or pustules that evolve into crusted erosions
  - Fever, lymphadenopathy
- Diagnosis
  - Tzanck smear
  - Biopsy
  - Rapid HSV immunofluorescence
- Treatment
  - First episode most serious because of risk of systemic involvement
  - Oral or intravenous acyclovir

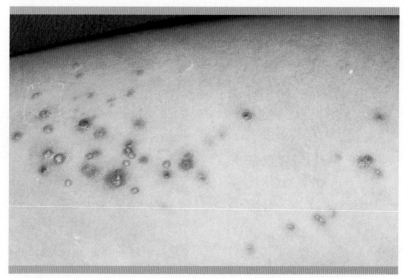

FIGURE 8-9 Molluscum contagiosum. *(From Freedberg IM et al: Fitzpatrick's Dermatology in General Medicine, 6th ed. New York: McGraw-Hill, 2003, p. 2115.)*

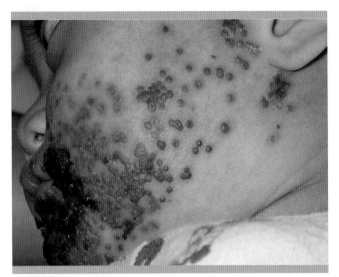

FIGURE 8-10 Eczema herpeticum. *(Courtesy of Dr. Denise Metry.)*

Unilateral Laterothoracic Exanthem (Asymmetric Periflexural Exanthem of Childhood)

- Presentation
  - Erythematous papules develop close to a flexure (typically axilla)
  - Papules coalesce and spread to involve the adjacent trunk and extremity
  - Lymphadenopathy common
  - Contralateral involvement occurs occasionally
  - Typically affects children younger than 10 years of age
- Causative organism
  - Etiology unknown
  - Viral cause suspected owing to high incidence of preceding upper respiratory infection or gastroenteritis
- Diagnosis
  - Mainly clinical
  - Histology: lymphocytic infiltrate around eccrine ducts
- Treatment: resolves spontaneously in 2 to 6 weeks

Scabies (Fig. 8-11)

- Presentation
  - Pruritic papules, vesicles, burrows of web spaces, flexures, genitals
  - Often excoriated, impetiginized
  - Spread by close contact
  - Norwegian scabies (Fig. 8-12)
    - Heavily crusted lesions with many mites
    - Immunodeficient, debilitated patients
  - Nodular scabies (Fig. 8-13)
    - Persistent red nodules; represents hypersensitivity to mites

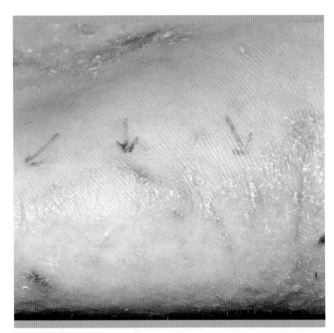

FIGURE 8-11 Scabies. *(From Freedberg IM et al: Fitzpatrick's Dermatology in General Medicine, 6th ed. New York: McGraw-Hill, 2003, p. 2283.)*

- Causative organism
  - Sarcoptes scabei
  - Female mite burrows and deposits eggs in stratum corneum
- Diagnosis
  - Clinical
  - Microscopic examination of mite, ova, or feces (scutula) on skin scraping
- Treatment
  - Topical 5% permethrin is treatment of choice (approved down to 2 months of age)

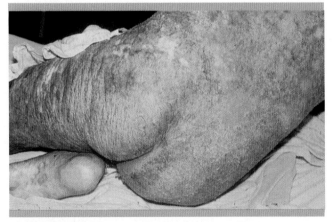

FIGURE 8-12 Norwegian scabies. *(From Freedberg IM et al: Fitzpatrick's Dermatology in General Medicine, 6th ed. New York: McGraw-Hill, 2003, p. 2284.)*

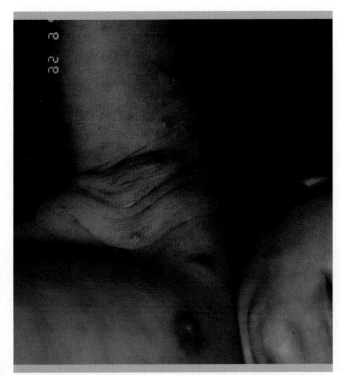

FIGURE 8-13 Nodular scabies. *(Courtesy of Dr. Adelaide Hebert.)*

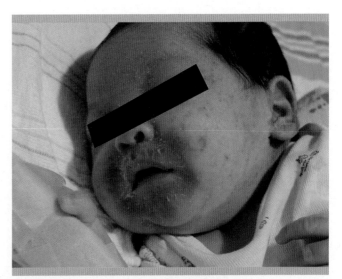

FIGURE 8-14 Staphylococcal scalded skin syndrome. *(Courtesy of Dr. Denise Metry.)*

- For newborn infants or pregnant/nursing women, 6% to 10% sulfur in petrolatum (permethrin is pregnancy category factor B)

Staphylococcal Scalded Skin Syndrome (Ritter's Disease) (Fig. 8-14)

- Presentation
  - Acute onset of tender erythema
  - Rapid development of superficial blistering in periorificial and flexural distribution
  - Subsequent desquamation and fissuring around mouth/eyes produces classic "sad old man" facies.
  - Usually young children (younger than age 2) or adults with predisposing conditions (immunosuppression, renal impairment, overwhelming sepsis)
  - Nikolsky sign present
  - Resolves without scarring
- Causative organism: epidermolytic toxin of *Staphylococcus* phage group II (desmoglein 1 target)
- Diagnosis
  - May isolate *Staphylococcus* from nasopharynx (most common), blood, urine, umbilicus, conjunctivae (not skin)
  - Histology: shows split at granular layer
- Treatment
  - Penicilinase-resistant penicillin
  - Supportive measures

DERMATOSES

Seborrheic dermatitis ("Cradle Cap") (Fig. 8-15)

- Presentation
  - Yellowish, scaling dermatitis of scalp

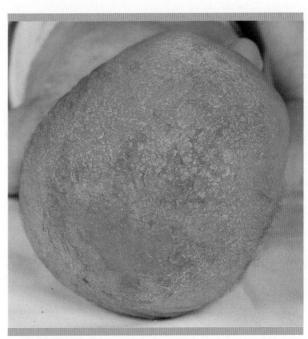

FIGURE 8-15 Seborrheic dermatitis of scalp: infantile type. Erythema and yellow-orange scales and crust on the scalp of an infant ("cradle cap"). Eczematous lesions are also present on the arms and trunk. *(From Wolff K et al. Fitzpatrick's Color Atlas & Synopsis of Clinical Dermatology, 5th ed. New York: McGraw-Hill, 2005, p. 51.)*

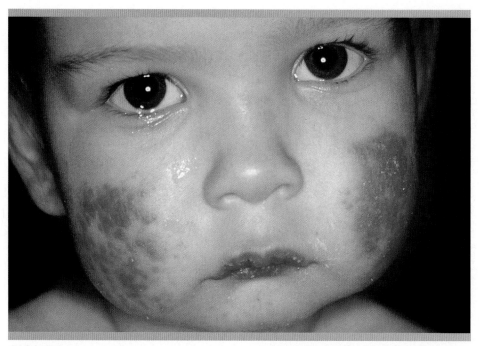

FIGURE 8-16 Gianotti-Crosti syndrome. *(From Kane K et al. Color Atlas & Synopsis of Pediatric Dermatology. New York: McGraw-Hill, 2002, p. 595.)*

- Greasy, salmon-colored patches on face (central forehead, glabella, eyebrows, nasolabial folds), retroauricular, intertriginous areas
  - Blepharitis may be present
- Etiology: possible role of *Pityrosporum ovale* (*Malassezia furfur*)
- Course
  - Generally resolves by 1 year of age
  - Postinflammatory hypopigmentation characteristic of darker-skinned infants
- Treatment
  - Low-potency topical corticosteroids
  - Antiseborrheic shampoos
  - Topical antifungals

Gianotti-Crosti Syndrome (Papular Acrodermatitis of Childhood) (Fig. 8-16)

- Presentation
  - Monomorphic papules or papulovesicles
  - Symmetrically distributed on the face, buttocks, extremities of children (generally starts on thighs/buttocks and then goes to arms and then face)
  - Lesions tend to cluster on knees and elbows
  - Usually spares the trunk
  - Lesions koebnerize
  - Constitutional symptoms: low-grade fever, lymphadenopathy, splenomegaly
- Pathology: associated with viral infections: Epstein-Barr virus (most common association in the United States), hepatitis B virus, cytomegalovirus (CMV), respiratory syncitial virus (RSV)
- Course: resolves spontaneously in 3 to 8 weeks
- Treatment: symptomatic

Acropustulosis of Infancy (Infantile Acropustulosis) (Fig. 8-17)

- Presentation
  - Crops of pruritic vesiculopustules on the hands and feet of infants/young children
  - Occurs in crops every 2 to 4 weeks
  - Scabies prep negative
- Etiology: may be reactive to previous scabies exposure
- Pathology: subcorneal and intraepidermal neutrophilic abscesses
- Treatment
  - Potent topical steroids
  - Oral antihistamines
  - Oral erythromycin
  - Dapsone reserved for exceptionally severe cases
- Course: resolves in 1 to 2 years

Transient Neonatal Pustular Melanosis (TNPM)

- Presentation
  - Very superficial vesicles, sterile pustules
  - Seen at birth in up to 4 percent of healthy, term newborns
  - Rupture/desquamation leaves characteristic residual hyperpigmented macules generally within first 2 days of life

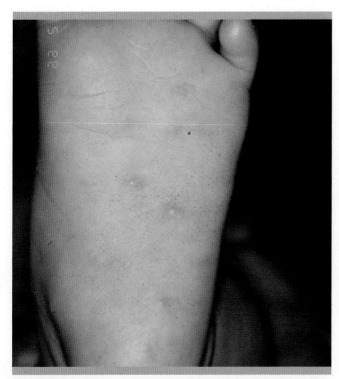

FIGURE 8-17 Acropustulosis of infancy. *(Courtesy of Dr. Adelaide Hebert.)*

- Pathology: intracorneal and subcorneal neutrophilic spongiosis (few if any eosinophils)
- Treatment
  - Self- limited
  - Postinflammatory pigmentation fades in weeks to months

Erythema Toxicum Neonatorum (ETN) (Fig. 8-18)

- Presentation
  - Common; affects half of full-term newborns
  - "Flea-bitten rash" of few to hundreds of erythematous macules, wheals, papules, and pustules
  - Occurs in the first 24 to 48 hours of life
  - Both TNPM and ETN almost always spare the palms and soles (important distinguishing clinical feature from congenital candidiasis)
- Histology: folliculitis with eosinophils (few neutrophils, no spongiosis)
- Treatment: resolves within 1 to 2 weeks

Lichen Striatus (Fig. 8-19)

- Presentation
  - Linear band of erythematous to flesh-colored papules
  - Develops over several weeks
  - Follows Blaschko's lines
  - Affects children and young adults

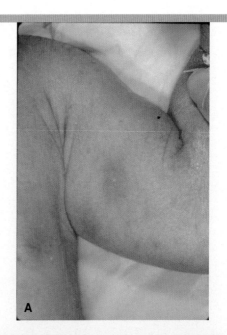

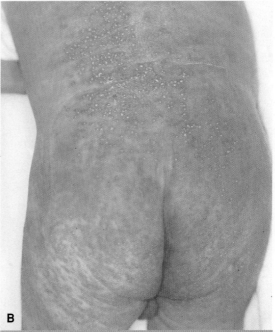

FIGURE 8-18 Erythema toxicum. *(From Freedberg IM et al: Fitzpatrick's Dermatology in General Medicine, 6th ed. New York: McGraw-Hill, 2003, p. 1368.)*

- Resolves within 1 to 2 years with postinflammatory hypopigmentation that resolves slowly
- Initially may be mildly pruritic
- Pathology
  - Spongiotic or lichenoid dermatitis with necrotic keratinocytes
  - Lymphocytic infiltrate around eccrine coils

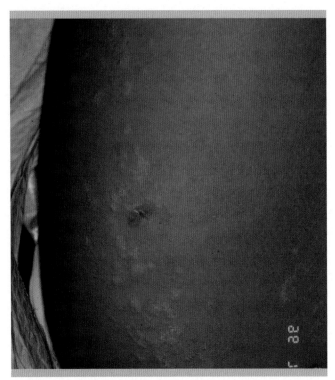

FIGURE 8-19 Lichen striatus. *(Courtesy of Dr. Adelaide Hebert.)*

- Treatment: topical anti-inflammatories useful for pruritus; may hasten resolution of inflammatory lesions

CUTANEOUS NEOPLASMS AND MALFORMATIONS

Epstein's Pearls (Bohn's Nodules)

- Presentation: white to yellow mobile papules at the hard palate (Epstein's pearls) or gum margin (Bohn's nodules) of newborns
- Etiology/pathology: milia
- Treatment
  - No treatment required
  - Resolves within weeks

Pseudoverrucous Papules and Nodules (Fig. 8-20)

- Presentation: shiny, moist, flat-topped erythematous papules of diaper area or surrounding urostomy/colostomy sites
- Etiology/pathology: form of severe irritant contact dermatitis resulting from incontinence, encopresis, severe diaper dermatitis
- Treatment: protection of skin by barrier creams

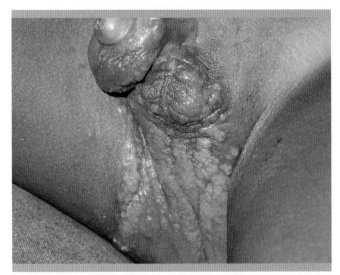

FIGURE 8-20 Pseudoverrucous papules and nodules. *(Courtesy of Dr. Denise Metry.)*

Perianal (or Perineal) Pyramidal Protrusion (Fig. 8-21)

- Presentation
  - Triangular-shaped, flesh-colored to erythematous nodule on the perineal median raphe, anterior to the anus
  - More than 90 percent of cases occur in female infants
  - Average age at presentation: 14 months
- Etiology/pathology: related to constipation, possibly lichen sclerosus et atrophicus
- Course: resolves spontaneously over several months to 1 to 2 years
- Treatment: Treating associated constipation may hasten resolution

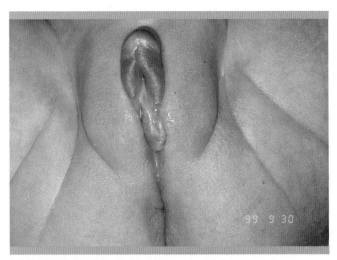

FIGURE 8-21 Perianal pyramidal protrusion. *(Courtesy of Dr. Adelaide Hebert.)*

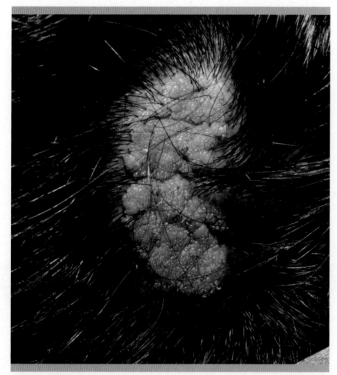

FIGURE 8-22 Nevus sebaceous. *(Courtesy of Dr. Adelaide Hebert.)*

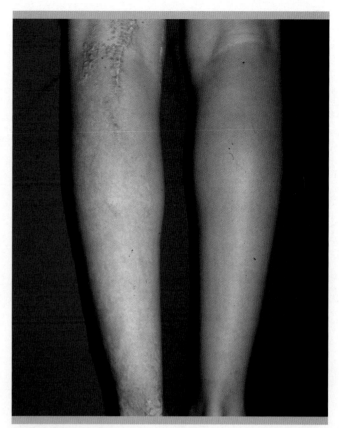

FIGURE 8-23 Linear epidermal nevus. *(Courtesy of Dr. Adelaide Hebert.)*

Nevus Sebaceous of Jadassohn (Fig. 8-22)

- Presentation
  - Congenital hairless, yellow to orange plaque on the scalp (usually round), face, or neck (usually linear)
  - Pebbly, velvety, or verrucous surface, although often flat at birth
- Etiology/pathology
  - Early: increased numbers of immature sebaceous glands and hair follicles
  - Postpubertal: Papillomatosis, hyperkeratosis, and hypergranulosis accompany lobules of sebaceous glands and ectopic apocrine glands
- Course/therapy
  - Prepubertal excision often recommended due to low risk of secondary tumor growth later in life
  - Most commonly associated malignant neoplasm: basal cell carcinoma (BCC)
  - Most common benign neoplasm: syringocystadenoma papilliferum

Schimmelpenning's Syndrome

- Presentation: large nevus sebaceous associated with ocular lesions, intracranial masses, mental retardation, seizures, and skeletal and pigmentary abnormalities

Linear Epidermal Nevus (Fig. 8-23)

- Presentation
  - Verrucous pink to brown papules following Blaschko's lines
  - Generally presents at birth or within first year of life, sometimes later in childhood or adolescence
  - Systematized epidermal nevus (Fig. 8-24): extensive, bilateral lesions
  - Ichthyosis hystrix/nevus unius lateris: unilateral lesion
  - Inflammatory linear verrucous epidermal nevus (ILVEN)
    - Inflammatory variant with erythema, pruritus
    - Often on an extremity or perineum in girls
- Etiology/histology
  - Hyperplasia of epidermal structures with hyperkeratosis, acanthosis, papillomatosis, some with epidermolytic hyperkeratosis
  - Accompanying parakeratosis and inflammation (with ILVEN)
- Course/therapy
  - Destruction by excision, laser ablation, cryotherapy, dermabrasion, chemical peels, topical retinoids
  - Recurrence is common
  - Pruritus with ILVEN often refractory to treatment

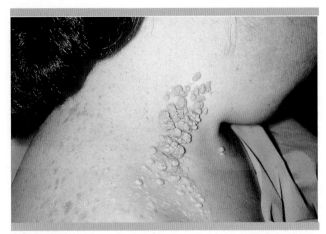

FIGURE 8-24   Epidermal nevus. *(From Freedberg IM et al: Fitzpatrick's Dermatology in General Medicine, 6th ed. New York: McGraw-Hill, 2003, p. 2508.)*

Aplasia Cutis Congenita (Fig. 8-25)

- Presentation
  - Well-demarcated ulceration or erosion often with thin, glistening membrane-like surface
  - Present at birth
  - Most commonly on vertex
  - Seventy percent solitary
  - Rare association with other developmental abnormalities
  - Irregular, large, stellate defects of the scalp associated with trisomy 13 and underlying cerebrovascular malformations

- Large, bilateral, truncal stellate defects associated with fetus papyraceus (placental infarction after the death of a twin fetus) and gastrointestinal atresia
- Etiology/pathology
  - Sporadic or autosomal dominant inheritance with variable penetrance
  - Localized absence of the epidermis, dermis ± subcutis
- Course/therapy
  - Protection form trauma and infection
  - Most heal within several months, leaving scar
  - MRI/MRA and radiographs for large scalp defects; abdominal imaging for large truncal defects

MASTOCYTOSIS

Solitary Mastocytoma (Fig. 8-26)

- Presentation
  - One to several pink, yellowish, or brown nodule(s)
  - Presents within first 6 months of life
  - Often on trunk, upper extremities, neck
  - Darier's sign: When stroked, lesion urticates.
  - May develop bullae in infancy
  - Spontaneous regression within several years
- Treatment: Topical anti-inflammatories can be used for symptoms; otherwise, treatment is unnecessary

Urticaria Pigmentosa

- Presentation
  - Most common form of mastocytosis

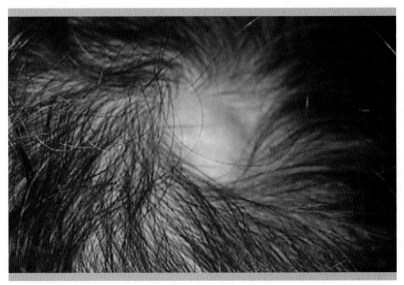

FIGURE 8-25   Aplasia cutis congenita. *(Courtesy of Dr. Denise Metry.)*

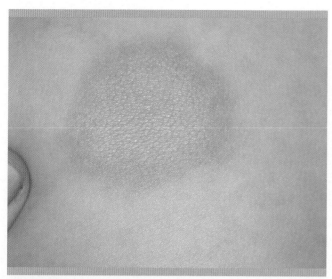

FIGURE 8-26 Solitary mastocytoma. *(Courtesy of Dr. Denise Metry.)*

- Develops at between 3 and 9 months of life
- Persistent, pruritic red-brown-yellow macules, papules, or nodules
- Lesions most common on the trunk
- Positive Darier's sign
- Pruritus induced by rubbing, exercise, heat, mast-cell degranulators (EtOH, opiates)
- Etiology: *Hymenoptera* stings, rubbing, or histamine-releasing drugs may cause severe symptoms, anaphylaxis
- Treatment
  - H_1 antagonists for pruritus, urticaria, flushing
  - H_2 antagonists for gastrointestinal symptoms
  - Diarrhea may be controlled with cromolyn (disodium chromoglycate)
  - Calcium channel blockers may inhibit mast cell degranulation
  - Epi-Pen for patients with a history of anaphylaxis
  - Seventy percent of patients markedly improved by age 10

Diffuse Cutaneous Mastocytosis

- Presentation
  - Rare
  - Presents at birth or within first few weeks of life
  - Skin diffusely infiltrated by mast cells
  - Leathery, orange-peel appearance (*peau d' orange*), especially in the flexures
  - Widespread spontaneous blistering with erosions and crusts, erythroderma, pruritus
- Etiology: systemic involvement in up to 10 percent of children (greater in adults)

Systemic Mastocytosis

- Presentation
  - Rare mast cell accumulation in one or more organs other than the skin, especially bone marrow
  - The presence of systemic symptoms does not make a diagnosis of systemic mastocytosis
  - Invasive diagnostic procedures for
    - Patients with hematologic abnormalities
    - Persistent, localized bone pain and severe gastrointestinal symptoms
    - Evidence of hepatic insufficiency
- Signs and symptoms
  - Flushing
  - Osteoporosis or sclerosis
  - Lymph node involvement
  - Hepatomegaly, splenomegaly, may have increased heparin with bleeding
  - Pancytopenia
  - Heart, kidneys, GI tract, or lung may be affected
  - Mast cell leukemia (rare) portends poor prognosis
  - Other leukemias or lymphomas may develop
- Diagnosis (of cutaneous mastocytosis)/etiology
  - Histology
    - Accumulation of mast cells in skin
    - Dense dermal aggregate of mast cells
    - Mast cells stains: Leder, toluidine blue, Giemsa
  - Mutation of c-*kit* protooncogene receptor that codes for transmembrane tyrosine kinase (also in piebaldism)
  - Urinary histamine metabolites are increased (not specific)

REFERENCES

Eichenfield L, Esterly N, Frieden (eds): *Textbook of Neonatal Dermatology*. Philadelphia: Saunders, 2001.

Fleet SL, Davis LS. Infantile perianal pyramidal protrusion: report of a case and review of the literature. *Pediatr Dermatol* 2005 Mar–Apr; 22(2):151–152.

Freedberg IM et al. *Fitzpatrick's Dermatology in General Medicine*, 6th Ed. New York: McGraw-Hill; 2003.

Heide R, Tank B, Oranje AP: Mastocytosis in childhood. *Pediatr Dermatol* 2002 Sep–Oct; 19(5):375–381.

Kane KS, Bissonette J, Baden HP, et al.: *Color Atlas & Synopsis of Pediatric Dermatology*. New York: McGraw-Hill, 2002.

McKee PH. *Pathology of the Skin: With Clinical Correlations*. London: Mosby-Wolfe; 1996.

Verbov J: *Essential Pediatric Dermatology*. Cliften, UK, Clinical Press, 1988.

Weinberg S, Prose NS, Kristal L: *Color Atlas of Pediatric Dermatology*, 3rd Ed. New York: McGraw-Hill, 1998.

CHAPTER 9

VASCULAR TUMORS AND MALFORMATIONS

DENISE W. METRY
ASRA ALI

OVERVIEW

- Vascular tumors: dynamic lesions that clinically demonstrate proliferation and are characterized histologically by endothelial cell hyperplasia
- Vascular tumors of infancy and childhood
  - Hemangioma of infancy
  - "Congenital hemangiomas" (noninvoluting, or NICH; rapidly involuting, or RICH)
  - Kaposiform hemangioendothelioma
  - Tufted angioma
  - Pyogenic granuloma
- Vascular tumors of adulthood
  - Kaposi sarcoma
  - Angiolymphoid hyperplasia with eosinophilia
  - Intravascular papillary endothelial hyperplasia (Masson's tumor)
  - Low-grade angiosarcomas
    - Endovascular papillary angioendothelioma (Dabska's tumor)
    - Epithelioid hemangioendothelioma
    - Spindle cell hemangioendothelioma
    - Retiform hemangioendothelioma
  - Angiosarcoma
- Vascular malformations
  - Almost always present at birth (although they may not manifest until later in childhood)
  - Arise from dysmorphogenesis
  - Exhibit normal cellular turnover
  - Are static or undergo slow expansion over time
  - Can be further subdivided on the basis of
    - Flow rate
      - ▲ Slow flow: capillary, venous, or lymphatic
      - ▲ Fast flow: arteriovenous fistulas and arteriovenous malformations
    - Resemblance to vessel type: capillary, lymphatic, venous, or arteriovenous; can occur alone or in combination
      - ▲ Capillary
        - △ Salmon patch

- △ Port wine stain
- △ Phakomatosis pigmentovascularis
- △ Telangiectasia
- △ Cutis marmorata telangiectatica congenita
- △ Unilateral nevoid telangiectasia
- △ Angiokeratomas
- ▲ Lymphatic: microcystic, macrocystic. or combined
- ▲ Venous
  - △ Blue rubber bleb nevus syndrome
  - △ Glomuvenous malformations: glomus tumors, glomangiomas, and glomangiomatosis
- ▲ Arterial
  - △ Arteriovenous fistula
  - △ Arteriovenous malformation
- ▲ Combined
  - △ Klippel-Trenaunay syndrome (capillary-lymphaticovenous malformation)
  - △ Parkes-Weber syndrome (capillary-arteriovenous fistula and capillary-arteriovenous malformation)

VASCULAR TUMORS OF INFANCY AND CHILDHOOD

Hemangiomas of Infancy (HOIs)

- Characteristics
  - Most common tumor of infancy
  - Characterized by endothelial cell proliferation
  - GLUT-1 (glucose transporter) is an immunohistochemical stain specific for HOI in all phases of growth and involution
  - Positive staining occurs *only* with HOI and *not* with any other vascular tumor or malformation
  - Proliferative phase: 6 to 18 months
  - Involution phase: gradual over 2 to 12 years
  - Risk factors: Caucasians, females, low birth weight, multiple gestations

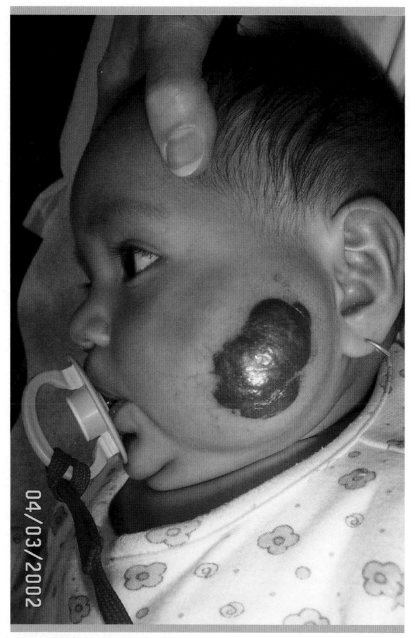

FIGURE 9-1 Combined HOI. *(Courtesy of Adelaide Hebert, MD.)*

- Location: More than 60 percent occur on head or neck, most commonly midcheek, lateral upper lip, and upper eyelid
- Types
  - Superficial, deep, or combined
    - Superficial
      ▲ Most common
      ▲ Raised, bright-red papule, nodule or plaque
    - Deep: soft, flesh-colored nodule that often demonstrates a bluish hue and/or central telangiectasias
    - Combined: often resembles "fried egg" (Fig. 9-1)
  - Localized, segmental, or multiple
- Classification by morphology

- Localized: papules or nodules that appear to arise from a single focal point and demonstrate clear spatial containment
- Segmental (Fig. 9-2)
  - Plaquelike and show a linear and/or geographic pattern over a cutaneous territory
  - Much more likely to be complicated, require more intensive and prolonged therapy, and have a poorer overall outcome
- Multifocal
  - Generally defined as five or more small, localized lesions
  - Multiple hemangiomas are associated with multiple births

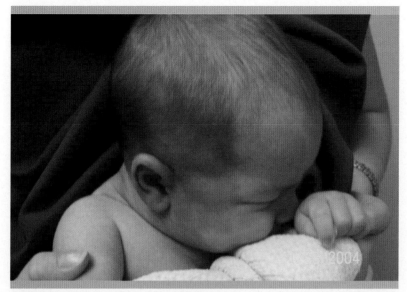

FIGURE 9-2 Segmental facial HOI. *(Courtesy of Adelaide Hebert, MD.)*

- Complications
  - Ulceration
    - Most common in proliferative phase
    - Often leads to pain, scarring, bleeding, secondary infection
    - Favors HOI in trauma-prone sites: lip, perineum, intertriginous, posterior scalp, back
  - Scarring
    - More common with segmental HOI, localized HOI of superficial, raised morphology with sharp "cliff drop" border, ulcerated HOI
    - High-risk locations: lip, nasal tip, ear
  - Vital organ compromise
    - Visual obstruction
      ▲ Amblyopia from stimulus deprivation or astigmatism
      ▲ Most common when HOI involves upper eyelid (Fig. 9-3)
      ▲ Refer to ophthalmology
    - Airway (especially subglottic) HOI
      ▲ Associated with segmental HOI in a cervicofacial or "beard" distribution
      ▲ Watch for development of stridor
      ▲ Endoscopy for definitive diagnosis
  - Visceral HOI
    - Associated with multifocal *and* segmental HOI
    - Liver most worrisome site
    - Gastrointestinal HOI can lead to significant bleeding
    - Brain involvement can lead to mass effects/neurologic sequelae
  - Lumbosacral HOI
    - Segmental lesions that span the midline and often are flat or telangiectatic in appearance are of greatest concern

- Risks: spinal dysraphism (especially tethered cord; supragluteal cleft deviation is an especially concerning clinical sign), anorectal anomalies, bony anomalies of the sacrum, abnormal genitalia, renal abnormalities, lipomeningomyelocele
    - MRI best study for spinal dysraphism
  - Developmental anomalies
    - PHACE syndrome
      ▲ *Posterior fossa* (Dandy-Walker) brain malformations, *h*emangioma (segmental, usually cerviofacial), *a*rterial anomalies, *c*ardiac defects/coarctation of the aorta, *e*ye anomalies
      ▲ Sometimes referred to as PHACES when ventral developmental defects such as sternal clefting and supraumbilical raphe are present
      ▲ Structural cerebral and cerebrovascular anomalies: most common and potentially devastating manifestations
      ▲ Cerebrovascular anomalies can lead to progressive vasculopathies causing stroke in early childhood
      ▲ Workup
        △ MRI/MRA of brain
        △ Cardiac echo or MRI/MRA of chest
        △ Eye examination
- Diagnosis
  - Generally clinical
  - Surgical biopsy (±GLUT-1 staining) warranted if any suspicion for malignancy
  - Imaging studies cannot generally be relied on to distinguish a benign from malignant vascular tumor

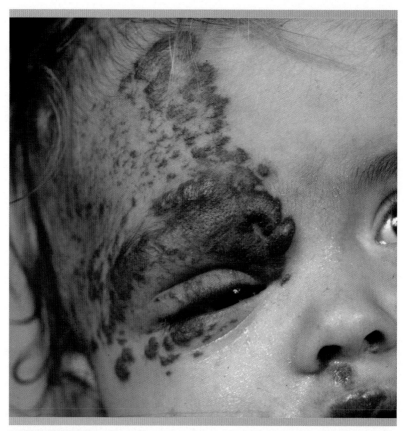

FIGURE 9-3 Segmental hemangioma involving the upper eyelid. *(From Wolff et al.: Fitzpatrick's Color Atlas and Synopsis of Clinical Dermatology, 4th ed. New York: McGraw-Hill, 2005, p. 183.)*

- Treatment
  - Most common indications: ulceration, vital organ compromise, to improve the ultimate cosmetic outcome
  - Options
    - Meticulous wound care for ulceration
    - Corticosteroids: topical, intralesional, or systemic
    - Vincristine is second-line agent for serious cases
    - Interferon also second line because of 20 percent risk of spastic diplegia
    - Excisional or laser surgery in select patients

"Congenital" Hemangiomas
- Types: noninvoluting (NICH), rapidly involuting (RICH)
  - Uncommon
  - Fully developed at birth and GLUT-1-negative
- RICH
  - Gray-violaceous tumor
  - Most common on an extremity
  - Undergoes rapid involution during the first year of life with characteristic atrophy
- NICH
  - Most commonly presents on the trunk

- Oval to round plaque with coarse, central telangiectasias and a surrounding rim of pallor
- Often feels warm to palpation and may have a slight bruit
- Path is hybrid between a vascular tumor and malformation

Kaposiform Hemangioendothelioma
- Characteristics
  - Rare
  - Histologically benign but clinically aggressive tumor
  - Most commonly affects children younger than 2 years of age and is often present at birth
  - Male-female incidence equal
  - Generally solitary
  - Favors the skin (particularly trunk, extremities) or retroperitoneum
  - Grows rapidly
  - Early on develops distinct violaceous color as a clue to underlying Kasabach-Merritt phenomenon
  - Kasabach-Merritt phenomenon = life-threatening thrombocytopenia as a result of platelet trapping within the tumor

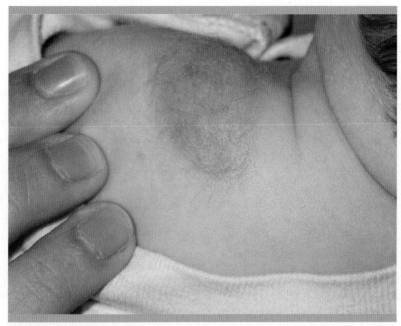

FIGURE 9-4 Tufted angioma. *(Courtesy of Denise Metry, MD.)*

- Consumption coagulopathy with very low platelet counts and low fibrinogen levels
- Does not occur with Hemangioma of infancy
- Pathology: densely infiltrated nodules composed of spindle cells with minimal atypia and infrequent mitoses and slitlike vessels containing hemosiderin; GLUT-1-negative
- Treatment
  - Corticosteroids often used as first-line therapy but rarely effective alone
  - Complete surgical excision if feasible
  - Interferon-α, vincristine
  - Platelets and heparin should be avoided

Tufted angioma (Angioblastoma of Nakagawa) (Fig. 9-4)

- Characteristics
  - Uncommon, histologically benign tumor
  - Presents during infancy or early childhood; presence at birth uncommon
  - Most common on trunk, extremities
  - Slow, lateral extension occurs from a few months to several years
  - Spontaneous regression may occur
  - Variable presentation
    - Large, infiltrated plaque
    - Sometimes with overlying vellus hair growth, tenderness
    - Surrounding may occur
    - Port-wine stain–like areas with a cobblestone surface sometimes seen

- Associated with KMP much less commonly than the kaposiform hemangioendothelioma
- Histology: tufts of capillaries throughout dermis, "cannonball" pattern

Pyogenic Granuloma (Fig. 9-5)

- Characteristics
  - Can be seen at any age, but majority occur during childhood
  - Prior history of trauma in minority
  - Most common on head and neck; mucosal lesions more common in females, especially during pregnancy

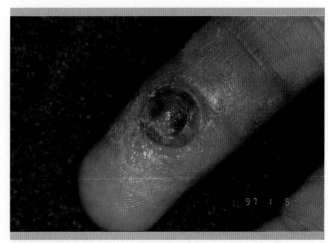

FIGURE 9-5 Pyogenic granuloma. *(Courtesy of Adelaide Hebert, MD.)*

- Usually presents as rapidly growing, bright-red papule or nodule
- Bleeds repeatedly and profusely; generally does not regress
- Umbilical granulomas seen in neonates have similar clinical appearance, but if persistent, may represent umbilical remnant
- Histology: well-circumscribed lobular proliferation of capillaries; possible erosion of epidermis
- Treatment
  - Depends on location/size
  - Most small lesions can be shave excised or curetted with light electrodessication to the base
  - Alternatives: excision, pulsed-dye or carbon dioxide laser, cryotherapy
- Course: recurrence more common with larger lesions

VASCULAR TUMORS OF ADULTHOOD

Kaposi Sarcoma

- Associated with human herpesvirus type 8
- Subtypes
  - Classic KS
    - Males, older than 50 years of age, predominant in Mediterranean and Jewish populations
    - Increased risk of lymphoreticular neoplasms
    - Violaceous macules with slow progression to plaques
    - Distal lower extremities, unilateral involvement with centripedal spread to a disseminated and multifocal pattern
    - Oral cavity and GI tract (90 percent); possible involvement of lung, spleen, and heart
    - Benign course owing to slow progression
  - African endemic KS
    - Black Africans, males > females, third to fourth decades
    - In childeren, the disease runs a fulminant course with rapid dissemination
    - Clinicopathologic subvariants
      - ▲ Nodular: benign, similar to classic KS
      - ▲ Florid or vegetating type: nodules extend into deep dermis, subcutis, muscle, and bone
      - ▲ Infiltrative: like florid/vegetating type but more aggressive
      - ▲ Lymphadenopathic: affects children and young adults, usually confined to lymph nodes but may affect skin and mucous membranes
  - KS in iatrogenically immunocompromised patients
    - Presents in organ-transplant, autoimmune, and cancer patients
    - Discontinuation of therapy may cause regression of KS lesions

- Epidemic HIV-associated KS
  - Oral mucosa (palate most common) is initial site of presentation in 10 to 15 percent
  - Early lesions appear as small pink/reddish macules or dermatofibroma-like papules
  - Extracutaneous sites: lymph nodes, gastrointestinal tract (80 percent of AIDS patients, usually duodenum and stomach), and lungs (bronchospasm, cough, respiratory insufficiency)
- Histology
  - Patch stage: proliferation of spindle-shaped cells in upper dermis; neoplastic cells outline irregular, bizarre slits and clefts
  - Plaque stage: multiple dilated and angulated vascular spaces outlined by attenuated endothelium, solid cords, and fascicles of spindle cell arranged between jagged vascular channels
  - Tumor stage: spindle cells in interlacing fascicles in dermis; lack of pronounced pleomorphism and nuclear atypia, slitlike vascular spaces with extravasated red blood cells (RBCs)
- Treatment
  - Ionizing radiation
  - (Poly)chemotherapy: vinblastin or vincristin; combination with actinomycin D, adriamycin, bleomycin, and dacarbazine; liposomal encapsulated doxorubicin and daunorubicin
  - Interferon-α in combination with antiretrovirals (zidovudine)
  - Topical tretinoin gel
  - Intralesional injections of β-human chorionic gonadotropin (β-hCG)

Angiolymphoid Hyperplasia with Eosinophilia

- Characteristics
  - Occurs mainly in the West
  - Thought to be inflammatory or reactive process
- Location: head, trunk, extremities
- Presentation
  - Peripheral eosinophilia
  - Papules or nodules
  - Young adults, females > males
- Diagnosis/pathology
  - Irregular vessels lined by plump endothelial cells with "hobnail" appearance
  - Infiltrate of lymphocytes, histiocytes, and eosinophils

Kimura's Disease

- Characteristics
  - Occurs mainly in Asia
  - Classified as cutaneous lymphoid hyperplasia
- Location: head
- Presentation
  - Solitary or multiple nodules
  - Young to middle-aged adults

- Almost exclusively male
- Peripheral eosinophilia and lymphadenopathy
- Diagnosis/pathology
  - Hyperplasia of small vessels lined with plump endothelial cells within the dermis or subcutis
  - Dense infiltrates of lymphocytes, plasma cells, histiocytes, and eosinophils
  - Multiple lymphoid follicles with germinal centers

Intravascular Papillary Endothelial Hyperplasia (Masson's Pseudoangiosarcoma)

- Characteristics
  - Reactive hyperplasia after intravascular thrombosis
  - As a focal change in a preexisting vascular lesion (hemangioma, pyogenic granuloma, or vascular malformation)
  - Small (<2 cm in diameter), firm, blue or purple nodule
  - Located on extremities, usually fingers
- Histology
  - Papillated vascular structures extending from the wall within vascular lumina are lined by single layer of plump endothelial cells
  - Occluded by thrombus
- Treatment: simple excision

Low-Grade Angiosarcoma

- Types
  - Endovascular papillary angioendothelioma (Dabska's tumor)
  - Epithelioid hemangioendothelioma
  - Retiform hemangioendothelioma
- Location
  - Skin or soft tissue of extremities
  - Extremities > scalp
- Presentation
  - Solitary tender nodule
  - Plaques and nodules
- Complications
  - Frequent recurrence but low metastatic rate
  - Greater than 50 percent with metastasis die of disease

Dabska's Tumor (Papillary Intralymphatic Angioendothelioma)

- Characteristics
  - Low-grade angiosarcoma
  - Slow-growing, painless, intradermal nodule that grows to 2 to 3 cm
- Laboratory studies
  - Immunoreactivity for factor VIII–related antigen, *Ulex europaeus* agglutinin I, vimentin, blood group isoantigens, and C2.1 antibody
  - Histology:
    - Multiple vascular channels that interconnect

- Lined by atypical endothelial cells; vacuolated cytoplasm, and hyperchromatic eccentric nuclei
- Weibel-Palade bodies may be present
- Treatment: wide local excision is the treatment of choice; regional lymph node dissection if clinically necessary
- Prognosis: favorable prognosis; however, they can be locally invasive and have the potential to metastasize

Hemangioendothelioma (Epithelioid and Spindle)

- Characteristics
  - Poorly circumscribed, usually biphasic proliferation of venous or capillary vessels
  - Minimal dysplasia, few mitotic figures, and minimal differentiation toward a vascular lumen or channel
  - A third of epithelioid hemangioendotheliomas develop metastases in regional lymph nodes
  - Red/blue nodules that may be multiple and are usually superficial
  - Distal extremities (particularly the hands)
  - Second and third decades of life
- Types
  - Epithelioid hemangioendothelioma: vessels are intermixed with solid sheets of epithelioid cells
  - Spindle cell hemangioendothelioma: spindle-shaped mesenchymal cells; this can occur at any age; thought to represent a reactive vascular tumor arising in conjunction with malformed vasculature (primarily lymphatic); can be associated with Maffucci's syndrome
- Histology: slitlike vascular channels, mild extravasation of erythrocytes, and hemosiderin deposition; epithelioid cells have abundant eosinophilic cytoplasm; spindle cell variant has bland bipolar mesenchymal fibroblast-like cells that may contain vacuoles that stain with *Ulex europaeus* and cytoplasmic factor VIII–associated antigen
- Treatment
  - Wide surgical excision
  - Greater than 50 percent of cases recur at the operative site or several centimeters distant

Retiform Hemangioendothelioma

- Characteristics
  - Slowly growing exophytic or plaquelike tumor is usually noted in young adults, predominantly on the lower limbs
  - May be associated with radiotherapy or chronic lymphedema
- Histology: arborizing vessels; focal solid areas composed of spindle and epithelioid; vessels lined by "hobnail" endothelial cells, prominent stromal lymphocytic infiltrate

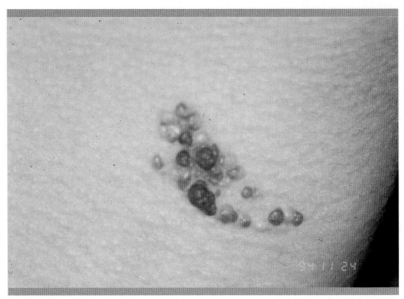

FIGURE 9-6 Angiosarcoma. *(Courtesy of Adelaide Hebert, MD.)*

Angiosarcoma (Fig. 9-6)

- Characteristics: subtypes
  - Idiopathic angiosarcoma
    - Elderly patients
    - Purpuric macule, plaque, nodule, or ulceration
    - Location: scalp, upper forehead
  - Lymphedema-associated angiosarcoma
    - Edematous arm of women after mastectomy on side with lymph adenectomy
    - Bluish plaques, nodules, and vesicles
  - Postirradiation angiosarcoma: years after radiotherapy
- Diagnosis
  - Histology
    - Irregular anastomosing vascular channels
    - Lined by hyperchromatic, pleomorphic endothelial cells; mitosis prominent
  - Immunohistochemistry: CD31, CD34, and factor VIII–related antigen are less specific

VASCULAR MALFORMATIONS

Capillary

SALMON PATCH (NEVUS SIMPLEX) (FIG. 9-7)

- Characteristics
  - Best classified as capillary malformation
  - Prognosis generally differs from port-wine stain
  - Thought to represent persistent fetal circulatory patterns in the skin
  - Disappears when the autonomic innervation of these vessels matures during infancy
  - Present in nearly half of all newborns

- Slow flow
- Location: nape of neck > eyelid > glabella ("angel's kiss") > nasolabial region
- Presentation
  - Pink to red patch
  - Usually fades by 1 to 2 years of age, although lesions of the nape and forehead may persist

PORT-WINE STAIN (NEVUS FLAMMEUS) (FIG. 9-8)

- Characteristics
  - Capillary malformation
  - Slow flow
- Location: variable
- Presentation
  - Present at birth as a well-demarcated vascular stain
  - Persists throughout life
  - With age (predominantly with facial lesions), can develop a dark red or deep purple color and thicken into nodules and/or pyogenic granuloma-like lesions
- Complications/associations
  - Bony and soft tissue hypertrophy, especially in the V2 and V3 facial distributions
  - Sturge-Weber syndrome (encephalotrigeminal angiomatosis)
    - Triad
    - Facial port-wine stain
      - ▲ Usually trigeminal V1 dermatome: forehead and upper eyelid
      - ▲ Approximately 10 percent of infants with port-wine stain in trigeminal V1 location will have Sturge-Weber syndrome
    - Ipsilateral ocular vascular anomalies: can lead to retinal detachment, glaucoma, and blindness

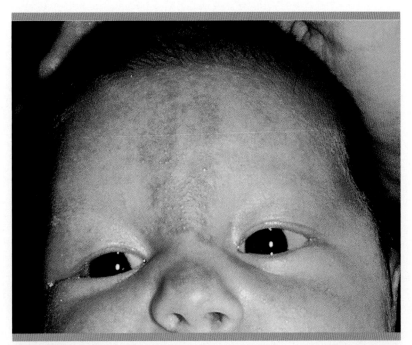

FIGURE 9-7 Nevus simplex. *(From Kane et al.: Color Atlas and Synopsis of Pediatric Dermatology. New York: McGraw-Hill, 2001, p. 183.)*

- – Leptomeningeal vascular anomalies: can lead to early-onset seizures
- • Midline facial stains have been associated with Beckwith-Wiedemann syndrome
- • Diagnosis/pathology: dilated, mature capillaries in the superficial dermis
- • Treatment
  - • Flashlamp-pumped, pulsed-dye laser (585 and 595 nm)
    - – Low risk of scarring
    - – Multiple treatments required
    - – Most patients achieve lightening but not complete clearance
    - – V2 and distal extremity lesions respond less well
  - • Cosmetic camouflage

PHAKOMATOSIS PIGMENTOVASCULARIS

- • Characteristics
  - • Coexistence of port-wine stain with a melanocytic or epidermal lesion (dermal melanocytosis, nevus

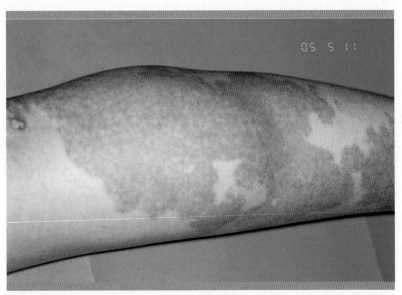

FIGURE 9-8 Port-wine stain. *(Courtesy of Adelaide Hebert, MD.)*

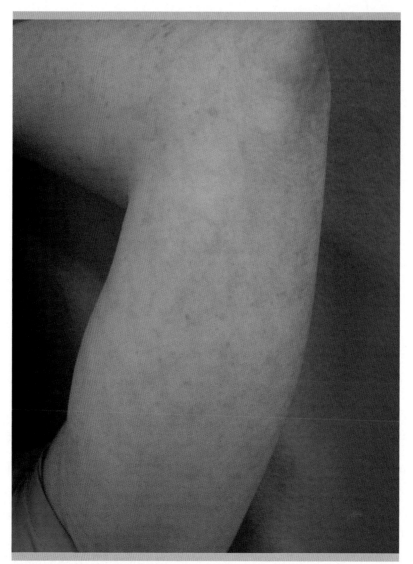

FIGURE 9-9 Cutis marmorata telangiectatica congenita.
(Courtesy of Adelaide Hebert, MD.)

spilus or speckled lentiginous nevus, nevus anemicus)
- Hereditary disorder thought to be explained by the "twin spot" phenomenon

CUTIS MARMORATA TELANGIECTATICA CONGENITA (FIG. 9-9)
- Characteristics
  - Congenital, with reticulate purple network
  - Most cases occur sporadically
  - Associated atrophy and/or ulceration
  - Limb +/− trunk
  - Limb girth discrepancy: common; other associated anomalies probably less common
- Diagnosis: generally clinical
- Treatment: no treatment is needed unless associated anomalies

UNILATERAL NEVOID TELANGIECTASIA (UNT)
- Characteristics
  - Congenital or acquired patches of superficial telangiectases in a unilateral linear distribution
  - May result from a somatic mutation during embryologic development
  - Third and fourth cervical dermatomes are the most common sites, but the thoracic dermatomes and scattered distant sites also may be involved
  - Pathogenesis of UNT remains unknown, possibly related to hormonal causes
- Histology: dilated capillaries in the superficial dermis
- Treatment: pulsed-dye lasers

ANGIOKERATOMA
- Characteristics
  - Slow flow

- Capillary ectasia in the papillary dermis
- May produce papillomatosis, acanthosis, and hyperkeratosis of the epidermis
- Types
  - Angiokeratomas of Fordyce
    - Uncommon
    - 2- to 4-mm red-to-blue domed papules with keratotic surface
    - Peak incidence after the third decade; more common in males
    - Most often on the scrotum and vulva
    - Lesions number from one to many (>100)
  - Angiokeratoma circumscriptum
    - Uncommon
    - Small red macules coalesce to form large acanthokeratotic plaques
    - Usually occurs in childhood; equally common in males and females
    - Often found on the extremities
    - Associated with vascular malformations and atrophy or hypertrophy of regional soft tissue and bone
  - Angiokeratoma corporis diffusum (Fabry's disease)
    - Rare
    - X-linked inherited disorder
    - Caused by a deficiency of the lysosomal enzyme α-galactosidase
    - Unremitting deposition of neural glycosphingolipids in the lysosomes of: vascular endothelium, fibroblasts, and pericytes of the dermis, heart, kidneys, and autonomic nervous system
    - Clinical findings:
      - ▲ Skin: verrucous papules, deep red to blue-black in color, between the umbilicus and the knees, with a predilection for the scrotum, penis, lower back, thighs, hips, buttocks
      - ▲ Ocular: corneal opacities, posterior capsular cataracts
      - ▲ Neurologic: burning, tingling paresthesias, hemiplegia, hemianesthesia, balance disorders, and personality changes
      - ▲ Extremities: chronic edema of the feet, arthritis of the distal interphalangeal joints
      - ▲ Cardiac: Infiltration results in angina, myocardial infarction, mitral valve prolapse, congestive heart failure, hypertension, mitral insufficiency, and ventricular hypertrophy
      - ▲ Urinalysis: urinary maltese crosses of lipid globules
  - Angiokeratoma of Mibelli
    - Uncommon
    - Multiple 3- to 5-mm dark red papules with verrucous surface
    - Most often affects females younger than 20 years
    - Most often found on dorsa of fingers and toes; less commonly observed on elbows, knees, shoulders, and earlobes
    - Associated with recurrent chilblains and acrocyanosis
    - Autosomal dominant inheritance with variable penetrance
  - Solitary angiokeratoma (Fig. 9-10)
    - Most common type
    - 2- to 10-mm nonkeratotic dark papules or plaques that keratinize and turn blue-black
    - Peak incidence during third to fourth decades of life; more common in males
    - Presents most often on the lower extremities
- Treatment
  - Either ablation (after a firm diagnosis is established) or excision (when the diagnosis is uncertain) can be performed
  - Erbium or carbon dioxide laser to remove the hyperkeratotic-acanthotic epidermis, followed by the use of lasers that target hemoglobin
  - Cryotherapy

Lymphatic Malformation (Fig. 9-11)

- Characteristics
  - Slow flow
  - Microcystic (lymphangioma circumscriptum, lymphangioma)
  - Macrocystic (cystic hygroma)
  - Combined
- Location
  - Macrocystic
    - Neck, axilla, groin, or chest wall
    - Large lesions documented on fetal ultrasound may be associated with Down or Turner syndrome
  - Microcystic: axillary folds, shoulders, neck, proximal limbs, perineum, tongue, floor of mouth
- Presentation
  - May become evident at birth or become so in early childhood
  - Microcystic lymphangiomas of the skin
    - Consist of grouped, clear vesicles ("frog spawn")
    - May contain blood, giving lesions a pink, purple, or black color
    - May have overlying hyperkeratosis
- Complications/associations: numerous, depending on location, but disfigurement, infection, bleeding most common

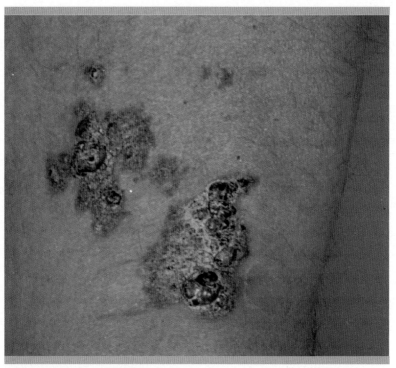

FIGURE 9-10 Solitary angiokeratoma. *(From Freedberg IM et al: Fitzpatrick's Dermatology in General Medicine, 6th ed. New York: McGraw-Hill, 2003, p. 1015.)*

- Diagnosis
  - Histology
    - Ectatic thin-walled channels filled with lightly eosinophilic lymph
    - Lymphatic endothelial marker: D2-40
  - MRI: best means of determining lesion extent

- Treatment
  - Surgery and/or sclerotherapy: mainstay of therapy, although cure rarely achieved
  - OK-432
    - Killed strain of group A *Streptococcus pyogenes*

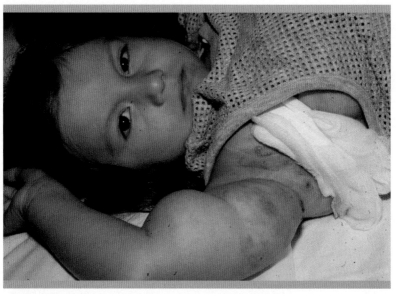

FIGURE 9-11 Lymphatic malformation. *(Courtesy of Adelaide Hebert, MD.)*

– New sclerotherapeutic agent useful for macrocystic lesions
- Laser photocoagulation: can be temporizing measure for microcystic cutaneous lesions
- Elastic compression stockings for extremity lesions

VENOUS MALFORMATION: GENERAL

- Characteristics: slow flow
- Location: skin, subcutaneous tissues, mucosa
- Presentation
  - Present, though not always evident, at birth
  - Usually solitary, localized
  - Soft, deep-blue masses that are easily compressible and slowly refill on release
  - Swell with dependency or activity
  - Undergo slow expansion over time
  - Phleboliths (progressive calcifications) are a hallmark of venous malformation and a common source of localized pain
  - Pain and stiffness on morning awakening and dull aching are other common complaints
- Associated conditions
  - Blue-rubber bleb nevus syndrome: autosomal dominant
    - Clinical
      ▲ Skin (most commonly trunk, palms and soles) and bowel venous malformations
      ▲ Latter commonly leads to chronic gastrointestinal bleeding
    - Diagnosis
      ▲ Histology: anomalous, dilated veins with irregularly thickened walls

  ▲ MRI best means of determining lesion extent
- Treatment
  ▲ Elastic support stockings of affected extremity
  ▲ Low-dose aspirin may be useful for painful thrombosis
  ▲ Sclerotherapy and/or surgery reserved for lesions causing significant functional compromise or cosmetic deformity
- Glomuvenous malformations: also known as glomus tumors, glomangiomas, or glomangiomatosis (Fig. 9-12)
  - Characteristics
    ▲ Solitary tumors most common in adults, sporadically inherited
    ▲ Multiple more common in childhood generally autosomal dominant (linked to chromosome 1p21-22)
    ▲ Solitary, extremely tender lesions most common on upper extremities, especially in nail beds
    ▲ Multiple lesions may be scattered or grouped, often in a segmental distribution
    ▲ Congenital lesions tend to be large and plaquelike and are bluish purple with a "cobblestone" and/or hyperkeratotic appearance
    ▲ Resemble venous malformation but lack tendency toward mucosal or deep muscle involvement, are firmer and less compressible, and frequently tender to palpation

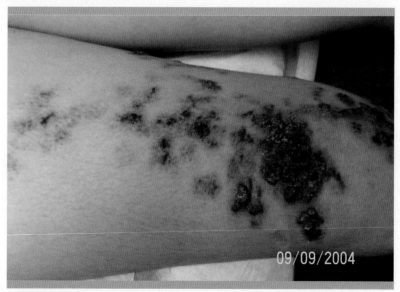

FIGURE 9-12 Glomuvenous malformation. *(Courtesy of Adelaide Hebert, MD.)*

– Histology: shows overlapping features of capillary-venous malformation and glomus cell tumor
– Treatment: surgical excision only reliable treatment

Arteriovenous Malformation and Fistula

- Characteristics: fast flow, the most dangerous type of vascular anomaly
- Presentation
  - Present at birth but may manifest later.
  - Early lesions may appear as a faint vascular stain that is often mistaken for a capillary malformation
  - Will eventually manifest itself, often following trauma or with the onset of puberty, as a warm, pulsatile mass with draining veins and deepening of color
  - End stage lesion: ulceration, bleeding, intractable pain, disfigurement
  - Location: intracranial > extremities > trunk > viscera
- Treatment
  - Always complex and difficult
  - Generally should not be considered until significant symptoms develop
  - Embolization
  - Surgery

Maffucci Syndrome

- Inheritance: sporadic
- Clinical
  - Triad of dyschondrodysplasia of one or more limbs, multiple enchondromas, and vascular lesions
  - Vascular lesions include venous malformations and spindle cell hemangioendotheliomas
  - Enchondromas, exostoses, recurrent fractures
  - Neurologic deficits result from cerebral enchondromas.
  - Risk of chondrosarcoma (15 to 20 percent), angiosarcoma, fibrosarcoma, osteosarcoma, lymphangiosarcoma, intracranial tumors

Cobb Syndrome (Cutaneomeningospinal Angiomatosis)

- Inheritance: sporadic
- Clinical
  - Arteriovenous malformation (AVM) of the spinal cord with overlying cutaneous "blush" of the posterior thorax
  - Neurologic problems secondary to cord compression by the AVM or spinal subarachnoid hemorrhage
  - May result in pain, subarachnoid hemorrhage, motor or sensory deficit
- Treatment: see AVM

Complex Vascular Malformation Syndromes

KLIPPEL-TRENAUNAY-WEBER SYNDROME

- Inheritance
  - Sporadic, males > females
  - Most common vascular malformation syndrome
- Clinical
  - Triad of port-wine stain, venous and/or lymphatic malformation, and bony and/or soft tissue hypertrophy
  - Typically limited to a single extremity
  - Lymphatic component common, evidenced by lymphedema or cutaneous lymphatic vessels
  - Overgrowth of affected limb apparent at birth or occurs within the first few months to years of life
- Treatment
  - Compression hose
  - Regular visits to clinically and radiographically assess for limb length discrepancy; if significant, refer to orthopedics
  - See VM, LM, CM

PROTEUS SYNDROME

- Inheritance: sporadic
- Clinical
  - Disproportionate overgrowth of multiple tissues in association with various cutaneous and subcutaneous mesodermal hamartomas, including vascular malformations
  - Changes can be present at birth of develop over time
  - Striking cerebriform hyperplasia of the plantar feet
  - Associated with mutations in PTEN tumor-suppressor gene

BECKWITH-WIEDEMANN SYNDROME

- EMG (exomphalos-macroglossia-gigantism) syndrome
- Capillary malformation at midforehead
- Inheritance: sporadic
- Clinical
  - Macroglossia
  - Exomphalmos
  - Linear earlobe creases; circular depression on helix
  - Gigantism
  - Organomegaly (big baby, big tongue, big organs)
  - Wilm's tumor, adrenal cortical carcinoma, rhabdomyocarcoma, hepatoblastoma
  - Omphalocele; intestinal malrotation

REFERENCES

Buckmiller LM: Update on hemangiomas and vascular malformations. *Curr Opin Otolaryngol Head Neck Surg* 2004 Dec; 12(6):476–487.

Freedberg IM et al. *Fitzpatrick's Dermatology in General Medicine,* 6th Ed. New York: McGraw-Hill; 2003.

Gampper TJ, Morgan RF: Vascular anomalies: hemangiomas. *Plast Reconstr Surg* 2002 Aug;110(2):572–585.

Marler JJ, Mulliken JB: Current management of hemangiomas and vascular malformations. *Clin Plast Surg* 2005 Jan; 32(1):99–116, ix.

McKee PH. *Pathology of the Skin: With Clinical Correlations.* London: Mosby-Wolfe; 1996.

Metry D: Update on hemangiomas of infancy. *Curr Opin Pediatr* 2004;16(4):373–377.

Metry DW: Potential complications of segmental hemangiomas of infancy. *Sem Cut Med Surg* 2004;23(2):107–115.

Mulliken JB, Fishman SJ, Burrows PE: Vascular anomalies. *Curr Probl Surg* 2002;37(8):517–584.

Spring MA, Bentz ML: Cutaneous vascular lesions. *Clin Plast Surg* 2005 Apr;32(2):171–186.

Werner JA, Dunne AA, Lippert BM, et al.: Optimal treatment of vascular birthmarks. *Am J Clin Dermatol* 2003;4(11): 745–756.

CHAPTER 10

AUTOIMMUNE BULLOUS DISEASES

KELLY L. HERNE
ROBERT E. JORDON
SYLVIA HSU

TERMINOLOGY

Indirect Immunofluorescence

- Detects circulating autoantibodies
- Antibodies do not have the fluorescent dye attached
- Using serum with fluorescein-conjugated human anti-immunoglobulin against a mucosal substrate such as monkey esophagus or rat bladder

Direct Immunofluorescence

- Detects antibody deposited within the patient's tissue
- Antibodies have the fluorescent dye attached
- Fluorescein-conjugated antibodies directed against complement fractions and immunoglobulins (IgG, IgM, and IgA) are placed on frozen sections of patient tissue

Direct Immunofluorescence (DIF) on Salt-Split Skin

- Incubate the patient's skin biopsy sample in 1 mol/liter salt prior to performing the DIF technique; induces cleavage through the lamina lucida
- Helps differentiate autoimmune diseases with similar DIF by where IgG localizes
- Dermal roof pattern found in bullous pemphigoid
- Dermal floor pattern found in sera of patients with
  - Bullous systemic lupus erythematosus (SLE)
  - Antiepiligrin cicatricial pemphigoid (with autoantibodies to laminin-5 and laminin-6)
  - Anti-p105 pemphigoid (with autoantibodies to a 105-kDa lower lamina lucida protein)
  - Epidermolysis bullosa acquisita (EBA)

Nikolsky's Sign

- Lateral pressure applied to edge of bulla
- Positive test if bulla extends laterally with pressure

- Suggests epidermis detaches from skin
- Common causes
  - Staphylococcal scalded skin syndrome (Ritter disease)
  - Toxic epidermal necrolysis
  - Pemphigus vulgaris

AUTOIMMUNE BULLOUS DISEASES

Bullous Pemphigoid (Fig. 10-1)

- Clinical
  - Autoimmune, subepidermal, blistering skin disease
  - May start initially as an urticarial eruption
  - Tense blisters and bullae; affects older patients over age 60
  - Most common locations are abdomen, flexor forearms, and inner thighs
  - No scar formation noted following the lesions, but milia may appear at sites of previously involved skin
  - Nikolksky's sign negative
  - Rarely involves mucous membranes: 10 to 35 percent
  - Drugs associated with bullous pemphigoid include furosemide, ibuprofen and other nonsteroidal anti-inflammatory agents, captopril, penicillamine, and antibiotics
- Diagnosis
  - Histology: subepidermal blistering process with prominent eosinophil infiltration
  - Antigens
    - Bullous pemphigoid antigen 1 (BPAgI)
      ▲ 230 kDa
      ▲ Intracellular portion of hemidesmosome plaque

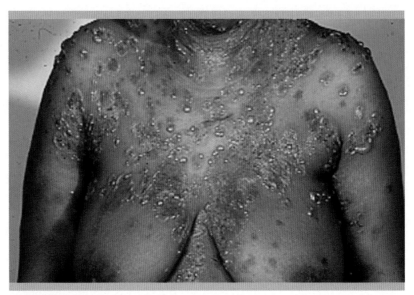

FIGURE 10-1 Bullous pemphigoid. *(Courtesy of Robert Jordon.)*

- – Bullous pemphigoid antigen 2 (BPAgII)
  - ▲ 180 kDa, type XVII collagen
  - ▲ Transmembranous protein with a collagenous extracellular domain
- Direct immunofluorescence (DIF) (Fig. 10-2)
  - Optimal location for DIF testing is normal-appearing perilesional skin
  - False-negative results can be observed when it is performed on lesional skin
  - Linear band of C3 (90 to 100 percent of patients) and IgG (70 to 90 percent of patients) at basement membrane zone (BMZ)

- DIF on salt-split skin reveals IgG on the blister roof
- Indirect immunofluorescence (IIF):
  - Circulating IgG to BMZ in 70 to 80 percent of patients
  - Serum levels of autoantibodies against BPAgII are reportedly correlated with disease activity
- Prognosis
  - Self-limited disease with good prognosis
  - Fifty percent enter remission within 2 to 6 years
- Therapy: topical steroids or oral prednisone alone or in combination with tetracycline, azathioprine,

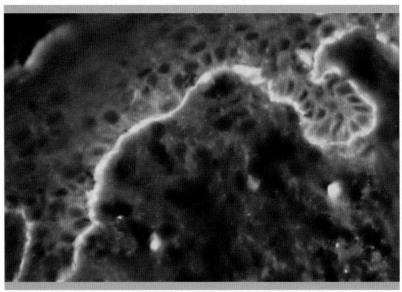

FIGURE 10-2 Bullous pemphigoid immunofluorescence. *(Courtesy of Robert Jordon.)*

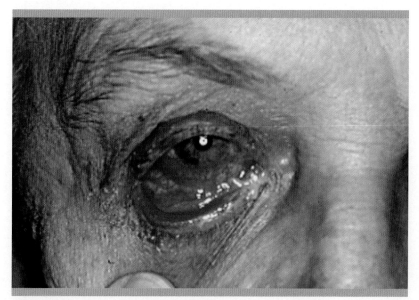

FIGURE 10-3 Cicatricial pemphigoid. *(Courtesy of Robert Jordon.)*

cyclophosphamide, dapsone, methotrexate, plasmapheresis, and intravenous immunoglobulin (IVIG)

Cicatricial Pemphigoid (Fig. 10-3)

- Clinical
  - Erosive lesions of the skin and mucous membranes
  - Skin involvement occurs in one-third of patients
    - Usually on scalp, face, and upper trunk
    - Heals with scars
  - Bullae are tense and located on an erythematous or urticarial base
  - Mucosal involvement
    - Oral mainly; may present with hoarseness or dysphagia
    - Can include the nasopharynx, larynx, esophagus, genitalia, and rectal mucosa
    - May lead to esophageal stenosis requiring dilatation procedures
    - Ocular lesions
      - ▲ Characterized by chronic conjunctivitis progressing to keratinization of the corneal epithelium
      - ▲ Progressive corneal injury secondary to trichiasis (ingrown eyelashes)
      - ▲ Decreased vision, photosensitivity, and scarring (symblepharon) that eventually can cause blindness
  - Brunsting-Perry (Fig. 10-4)
    - Variant of cicatricial pemphigoid without mucosal involvement
    - Small blisters or erosions that heal with scarring
    - Head and neck area, scalp typically involved
- Diagnosis
  - Histology
    - Similar or identical to bullous pemphigoid
    - Blisters are subepidermal with a mixed inflammatory cell infiltrate
  - Antigens
    - Bullous pemphigoid antigen 2 (BPAG2)
    - Bullous pemphigoid antigen 1 (BPAG1)
    - B4 integrin—pure ocular
    - Epiligrin (laminin-5) or the EBA antigen (type VII collagen)
  - Direct immunofluorescence (DIF)
    - Biopsy unaffected and perilesional skin
    - Reveals linear deposition of C3 and IgG continuously along the basement membrane
    - IgA and IgM also may be detected
  - Indirect immunofluorescence (IIF)
    - Assay reveals circulating IgG in 20 percent of patients, typically a low titer
    - Antiepiligrin cicatricial pemphigoid circulating autoantibodies bind to the dermal side of salt-split skin
    - Patients with cicatricial pemphigoid associated with reactivity to BPAG2 binding to the epidermal roof
- Course
  - Chronic progressive
  - Intermittent exacerbations and waning of disease activity

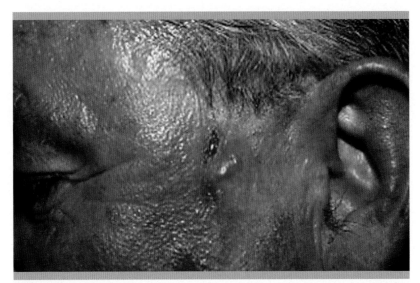

FIGURE 10-4 Cicatricial pemphigoid Brunsting-Perry. *(Courtesy of Robert Jordon.)*

- Therapy
  - Topical glucocorticoids
  - Oral prednisone alone or in combination with tetracycline, azathioprine, cyclophosphamide, dapsone, methotrexate, plasmapheresis, and IVIG

Bullous Lupus Erythematosus

- Clinical
  - Blistering in the setting of the autoimmune disease systemic lupus erythematosus (SLE)
  - May coincide with the activity of the patient's preexisting SLE or may be the initial presenting cutaneous eruption of SLE
  - Patients may exhibit any of the symptoms associated with SLE
  - Extensive vesiculobullous eruption develops suddenly
    - Arises either on erythematous areas or on clinically normal skin
    - Bullae are tense and range from herpetiform vesicles to large hemorrhagic bullae
    - Not associated with skin fragility or healing of lesions with scars and milia
    - Tends to favor the upper part of the trunk and the proximal upper extremities
- Antigens: noncollagenous domain of type VII collagen (similar to patients with epidermolysis bullosa acquisita)
- Histology
  - Subepidermal separation
  - Neutrophil-predominant inflammatory infiltrate in the upper dermis
  - Perivascular lymphocytic or mixed infiltrate

- Thickened and hyalinized BMZ
- Vacuolar degeneration of basal keratinocytes
- Direct immunofluorescence (DIF)
  - Perilesional skin
  - Linear or granular BMZ granular IgG/C3 deposits along BMZ
  - Salt-split skin: dermal-side staining
- Indirect immunofluorescence (IIF): subdivided immunohistologically into type 1 and type 2 depending on the presence or absence, respectively, of identifiable circulating and/or tissue-bound antibodies to type VII collagen
- Course: Course of bullous lupus often is remitting, and the disorder may resolve spontaneously in less than 1 year
- Therapy
  - Dapsone
  - Systemic steroids
  - Hydroxychloroquine
  - Azathioprine
  - Methotrexate
  - Cyclophosphamide

Herpes Gestationis (Pemphigoid Gestationis) (Fig. 10-5)

- Clinical
  - Rare autoimmune dermatosis of pregnancy
  - No relationship to the herpesvirus infection
  - Usually occurring during second and third trimesters
  - In 25 percent of patients, the lesions appear immediately after delivery
  - Extremely pruritic polymorphic bullous dermatosis

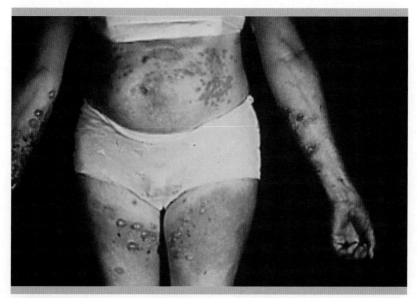

FIGURE 10-5 Herpes gestationis. *(Courtesy of Robert Jordon.)*

- Hive-like plaques differ from true urticaria because of their relatively fixed nature
- Lesions commonly start on abdomen
- Rash spreads peripherally, often sparing the face, palms, soles, and mucous membranes
- Umbilical (pruritic urticarial papules and plaques of pregnancy typically spares the umbilicus)
- Exacerbations immediately after delivery common
- Relapses with first few menses and reinitiation of oral contraceptives and with subsequent pregnancies
- Infants
  - Transient blistering or papular lesions (several weeks after delivery)
  - Greater incidence of premature and small-for-gestational-age babies
- Diagnosis
  - Histology
    - Subepidermal blister with an eosinophil-predominant infiltrate
    - Keratinocyte necrosis and dermal edema
    - Antigens
    - Extracellular domain of BP antigen II—180 kDa
      - ▲ Type XVII collagen
      - ▲ Transmembrane protein
  - Complement fixation assay: serum herpes gestationis factor: heat-stable IgG that binds normal human complement to the BMZ of healthy human skin in a complement fixation assay
  - Direct immunofluorescence (DIF)
    - Normal skin and perilesional skin

- Linear band of almost exclusively C3 deposited along the BMZ
- Indirect immunofluorescence (IIF): specific for IgG in 20 percent of patients
- Course
  - Maternal mortality rate is unaffected
  - Regresses without scarring within days after delivery
  - May recur in subsequent pregnancies and may be precipitated by menses and the use of oral contraceptives
- Therapy
  - Goal is to control pruritus and suppress extensive blistering
  - Topical steroids
  - Oral prednisone

Pemphigus Vulgaris (Fig. 10-6)

- Clinical
  - Bullous disease involving the skin and mucous membranes
  - Fatal if not treated appropriately
  - Flaccid blisters rapidly progressing to erosions
  - Nikolsky's sign present
  - Lesions usually start in the oral mucosa, followed by the appearance of skin lesions months later
  - Primary skin lesion is a flaccid blister that ruptures easily
  - Drug-induced pemphigus foliaceus associated with penicillamine, nifedipine, or captopril or medications with a cysteine-like chemical structure

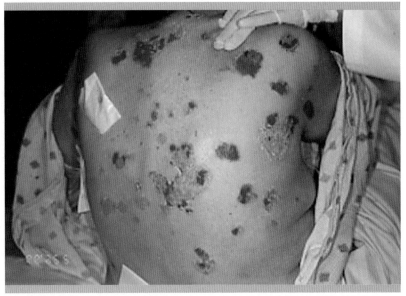

FIGURE 10-6   Pemphigus vulgaris. *(Courtesy of Robert Jordon.)*

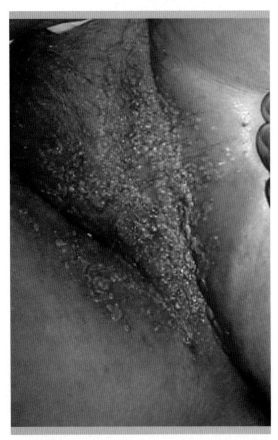

FIGURE 10-7   Pemphigus vegetans.
(Courtesy of Robert Jordon.)

- Vegetating pemphigus vulgaris pemphigus
  vegetans (Fig. 10-7)
  - Ordinary pemphigus vulgaris erosions may
    develop excessive granulation tissue and crusting
  - Lesions in skin folds readily form vegetating
    granulations
  - Can be more resistant to therapy
- Antigens
  - Desmoglein 3
    - 130-kDa glycoprotein, member of cadherin
      supergene family
    - Desmosomal core protein
  - Less commonly
    - Plakoglobin: 85-kDa plaque protein found in
      desmosomes
    - Desmoglein 1: seen in patients with oral and
      cutaneous disease
- Histology
  - Biopsy the margin of a bulla
  - Suprabasilar blister with acantholysis
- Direct immunofluorescence (DIF) (Fig. 10-8)
  - Intercellular deposits of IgG and C3 in a net-like
    pattern throughout the epidermis of perilesional
    skin
  - Monkey esophagus is best substrate
- Indirect immunofluorescence (IIF)
  - Circulating IgG to keratinocyte cell surfaces in
    greater than 75 percent of patients with active
    disease
  - Titers generally do correlate with disease
    activity

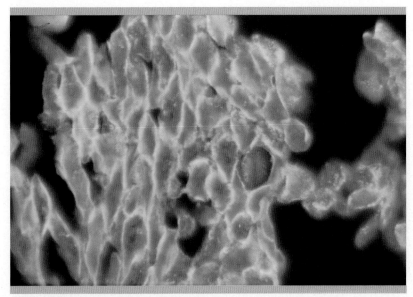

FIGURE 10-8 Pemphigus vulgaris immunofluorescence. *(Courtesy of Robert Jordon.)*

- Course: Common cause of death is infection secondary to the immunosuppression required to treat the disease
- Therapy
  - Corticosteroids are the mainstay of treatment; prednisone (1 mg/kg per day), with or without other immunosuppressive agents
  - Azathioprine
  - Methotrexate
  - Cyclophosphamide
  - Mycophenolate mofetil
  - Plasmapheresis may be required in severe cases
  - IVIG

Paraneoplastic Pemphigus

- Clinical
  - Tumor antigens are hypothesized to evoke an immune response that leads to the development of oral erosions or ulcerations
  - Leukemia or lymphoma most often
  - Three other associated neoplasms: (malignant and benign): Waldenström's macroglobulinemia, sarcomas, thymomas, and Castleman's disease
  - Cutaneous lesions: highly variable
    - Diffuse erythema, vesiculobullous lesions, papules, scaly plaques, exfoliative erythroderma, erosions, or ulcerations
    - 100 percent have mucosal involvement
- Histology
  - Biopsy from noninvolved, perilesional skin

- Suprabasilar acantholysis, basal cell vacuolation, lymphocytic exocytosis, and dyskeratotic keratinocytes
- Antigens
  - Desmoplakin I (250 kDa)
  - BPAG I (230 kDa)
  - Desmoplakin II (210 kDa)
  - Envoplakin (210 kDa)
  - Periplakin (190 kDa)
  - HD1/plectin (500 kDa)
  - Unidentified 170-kDa protein
  - Desmoglein I and desmoglein III antigens
- Direct immunofluorescence (DIF) (Fig. 10-9): IgG and C3 deposits within the intercellular spaces and along the BMZ
- Indirect immunofluorescence (IIF)
  - Binding to rat bladder transitional epithelium separates it from pemphigus vulgaris and pemphigus foliaceus because desmogleins are present in stratified squamous epithelium only and not in transitional epithelium
  - IgG autoantibodies are directed against above-mentioned antigens
- Course
  - Mortality rate is estimated at 75 to 80 percent.
  - Both the presence of an underlying neoplasm and the adverse effects of the potent medications required to treat the disease add to both the morbidity and the mortality
- Treatment: prednisone, azathioprine, cyclosporine, cyclophosphamide, IVIG

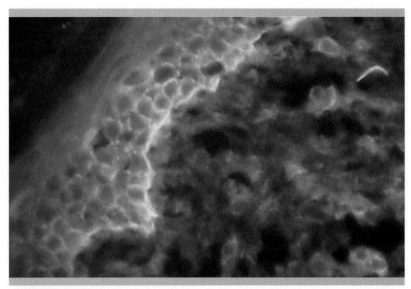

FIGURE 10-9 Paraneoplastic pemphigus immunofluorescence. *(Courtesy of Robert Jordon.)*

Pemphigus Foliaceus (Fig. 10-10)

- Clinical
  - Shallow, flaccid blisters rapidly progressing to scaling, crusted erosions on erythematous base
  - Localized or generalized
  - Often coalesce into large denuded areas with marginated or serpiginous borders
  - Rare mucous membrane involvement; sun and/or heat exacerbates disease
  - Nikolsky sign present
  - Fogo selvagem
    - Endemic pemphigus foliaceus
    - Occurs along Brazilian river beds
    - Possible relation to black fly *Simulium nigrimanum*
    - More common in children than nonendemic pemphigus foliaceus
  - Pemphigus erythematosus (Senear and Usher)
    - Localized form of pemphigus foliaceus
    - Starts as erythematous patches with vesiculation
    - On the cheeks and forehead, with similar patches on the sternal and interscapular skin
    - May have positive antinuclear antibody (ANA) but rarely concomitant lupus erythematosus
    - Can generalize to pemphigus foliaceus
    - Crusted plaques may appear in the healing phase
- Antigens
  - Desmoglein 1
    - 160 kDa
    - Transmembrane glycoprotein of desomosomes
    - Member of cadherin superfamily
    - Expressed mainly in the granular layer of the epidermis
  - Plakoglobin—85-kDa desmosomal plaque protein
- Histology
  - Intraepidermal blister just below stratum corneum and in granular layer
  - Bulla may form showing acantholysis at both the roof and the floor
  - Dermal lymphocytic infiltrate occurs, often with the presence of eosinophils
  - Direct cell surface immune deposits are often present throughout the entire epidermis
- Direct immunofluorescence (DIF):
  - Typically cannot distinguish from pemphigus vulgaris
  - Intercellular IgG, C3
- Indirect immunofluorescence (IIF): Based on substrate; guinea pig esophagus is best substrate for DIF
- Therapy
  - Topical glucocorticosteroids
  - Immunosuppressants, including systemic corticosteroids, cyclophosphamide, and cyclosporine; plasmapheresis in patients with recalcitrant disease

Dermatitis Herpetiformis (Fig. 10-11)

- Associated with HLA B8-DR3-DQ2
- Clinical
  - Intensely pruritic, chronic skin disease
  - Onset tends to be between 20 and 40 years of age but may occur at any age, including childhood

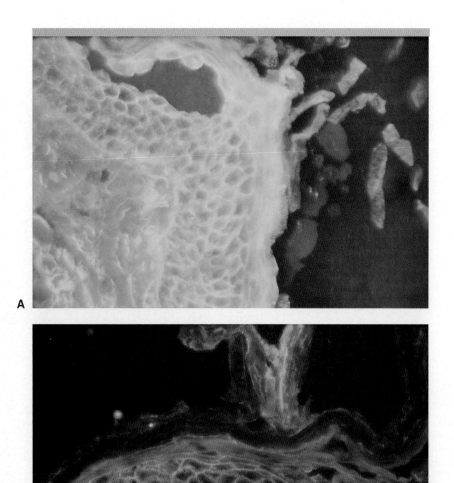

FIGURE 10-10 Pemphigus foliaceus. *(Courtesy of Robert Jordon.)*

- Intensely pruritic, chronic, grouped papules/vesicles giving a "herpetiform" appearance
- Symmetrically distributed on extensor surfaces, as well as buttocks, hairline and nuchal areas
- Oral lesions rare
- Eruption commonly preceded by burning or itching
- Associated with a gluten (wheat, barley, rye ± oats)–sensitive enteropathy
- Can lead to steatorrhea, abnormal D-xylose absorption, and anemia
- NSAIDs and iodine can induce eruptions
- Patients with increased incidence of other autoimmune disorders: thyroid disease, type 1 diabetes mellitus, systemic lupus erythematosus, vitiligo, and Sjögren's syndrome

- Antigens
  - IgA antibodies to gliadin (a portion of wheat protein), reticulum, and smooth muscle endomysium
  - IgA antiendomysial antibodies (tissue transglutaminase antibodies) that bind to intermyofibril substance in smooth muscle cells correlate with severity of intestinal disease and adherence to gluten-free diet
  - IgA endomysial antibodies are most specific for gluten sensitivity
  - Found in patients with dermatitis herpetiformis and those with isolated gluten sensitive enteropathy
- Histology
  - Subepidermal blister at level of lamina lucida
  - Neutrophilic microabscesses in dermal papillae

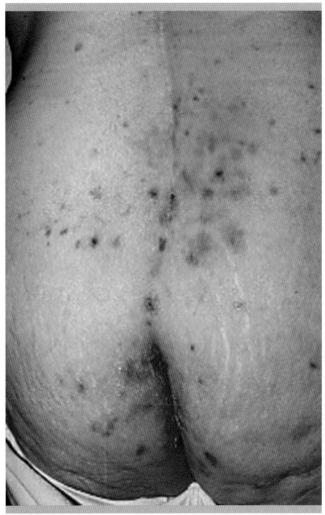

FIGURE 10-11 Dermatitis herpetiformis. *(Courtesy of Robert Jordon.)*

- Dermal infiltration of neutrophils
- Direct immunofluorescence (DIF) (Fig. 10-12)
  - Granular IgA1 deposits in dermal papillae of normal and lesional skin
  - Disappears with gluten-free diet, but does not disappear with dapsone
- Course
  - Disease persists indefinitely
  - Waxes and wanes without treatment
- Therapy
  - Dapsone or sulfapyridine (does not treat the gastrointestinal symptoms)
  - Gluten-free diet: protein present in barley, rye, and wheat but not in rice
  - Avoid iodine and NSAIDs

Linear IgA Dermatoses/Chronic Bullous Disease of Childhood (Fig. 10-13)

- Clinical
  - Linear IgA dermatosis

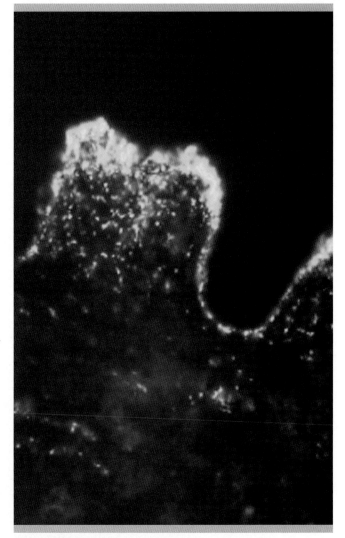

FIGURE 10-12 Dermatitis herpetiformis immunofluorescence. *(Courtesy of Robert Jordon.)*

- – Most commonly presents in patients older than 30 years of age
- – Annular or grouped papules, vesicles, and/or bullae symmetrically distributed on extensor surfaces: "cluster of jewels"
- – Most commonly involves perioral/perineal areas
- – Lesions are clinically indistinguishable from dermatitis herpetiformis.
- – Seventy percent have oral involvement
- Chronic bullous disease of childhood
  - – Occurs in young children, usually presenting in those younger than 5 years of age
  - – Abrupt onset of tense bullae on an inflamed, erythematous base
  - – Oral ulcers are noted in 50 percent
  - – Characteristic "collarettes" of blisters often form as new lesions arise in the periphery of old lesions

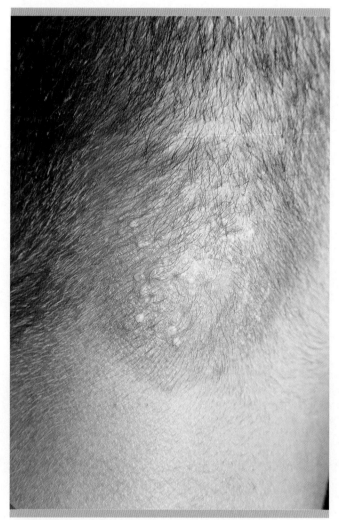

FIGURE 10-13 Chronic bullous disease of childhood. *(Courtesy of Robert Jordon.)*

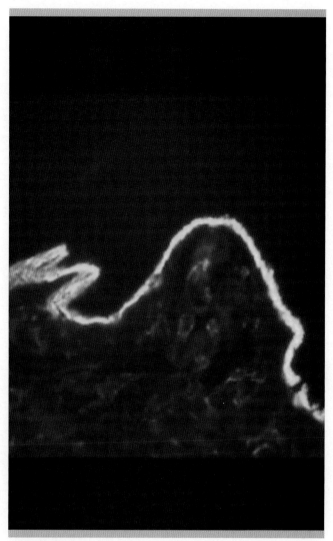

FIGURE 10-14 Linear IgA immunofluorescence. *(Courtesy of Robert Jordon.)*

- Drug associations: vancomycin, lithium, diclofenac
- Antigens
  - 97-kDa extracellular portion of BP antigen II
  - 120-kDa antigen also described
  - 97- and 120-kDa antigens may represent cleaved fragments of BPAgII
- Histology
  - Bullae are subepidermal
  - Collections of neutrophils along the basement membrane
- Direct immunofluorescence (Fig. 10-14): IgA in a linear pattern is noted along the basement membrane (occasionally IgG and C3)
- Course
  - Variable and unpredictable
  - Disease may remit spontaneously in some cases

- May last for years with few episodes of remission in chronic bullous disease of childhood
- Resolution occurring within 2 years of onset in most cases
- Treatment: dapsone or sulfapyridine

Epidermolysis Bullosa Acquisita (EBA)
- Clinical
  - Chronic autoimmune subepidermal blistering disease
  - Primarily involves the skin, but it also can affect mucous membranes
  - Trauma-prone areas of the skin: extensor surfaces of elbows, knees, ankles, and buttocks most commonly
  - Nail destruction and hair loss
  - Oropharyngeal mucous membrane involvement: periodontal disease, oral mucosal erosions

TABLE 10-1 Revised Classification of Inherited Epidermolysis Bullosa, Based on Clinical Phenotype and Genotype, for the Most Commonly Observed and Well-Characterized Variants or Subtypes of This Disease

Major EB Type	Major EB Subtype	Protein/gene Systems Involved
EBS ("epidermolytic EB")	EBS-WC	K5, K14
	EBS-K	K5, K14
	EBS-DM	K5, K14
	EBS-MD	Plectin
JEB	JEB-H	Laminin-5*
	JEB-nH	Laminin-5; type XVII collagen
	JEB-PA[†]	$\alpha_6\beta_4$ Integrin[‡]
DEB ("dermolytic EB")	DDEB Type VII	Collagen
	RDEB-HS	Type VII collagen
	RDEB-nHS	Type VII collagen

DDEB, dominant dystrophic EB; *EBS-DM,* EBS, Dowling-Meara; *EBS-K,* EBS, Köbner; *EBS-MD,* EBS with muscular dystrophy; *EBS-WC,* EBS, Weber-Cockayne; *JEB-H,* JEB, Herlitz; *JEB-nH,* JEB, non-Herlitz; *JEB-PA,* JEB with pyloric atresia; *RDEB-HS,* recessive dystrophic EB, Hallopeau-Siemens; *RDEB-nHS,* RDEB, non-Hallopeau-Siemens.
*Laminin-5 is a macromolecule composed of 3 distinct (α_3, β_3,γ_2) laminin chains; mutations in any of the encoding genes result in a JEB phenotype.
[†]Some cases of EB associated with pyloric atresia may have intraepidermal cleavage or both intralamina lucida and intraepidermal clefts.
[‡]$\alpha_6\beta_4$ Integrin is a heterodimeric protein; mutations in either gene have been associated with the JEB-PA syndrome.

- Antigen: IgG autoantibodies targeting the noncollagenous (NC1) domain of type VII collagen
- Histology
  - Biopsy from edge of a new blister
  - Subepidermal blister, mixed inflammatory cell dermal infiltrate

- Direct immunofluorescence
  - Thick band of IgG and to a lesser extent C3 deposited linearly at the BMZ
  - Salt-split skin: Antibodies bind to the dermal floor

TABLE 10-2 Genetic Modes of Transmission in Inherited Epidermolysis Bullosa*

Major EB Type	Usual Mode(s) of Transmission	Rare Modes of Transmission
EBS[†]	Autosomal dominant	Autosomal recessive
JEB	Autosomal recessive	—
DEB	Autosomal dominant	Autosomal dominant/autosomal recessive heterozygosity
	Autosomal recessive	

*Excluding de novo mutations, which have been reported to occur in most forms of inherited EB.
[†]An X-linked recessive disorder, referred to as Mendes da Costa disease, which was once included among the many variants of EBS, is no longer considered to be a subtype of any form of inherited EB.

TABLE 10-3 Ultrastructural Findings Among Major Types and Selected Subtypes of Inherited Epidermolysis Bullosa

EB Type or Subtype	Ultrastructural Site of Skin Cleavage	Other Ultrastructural Findings
EBS		
EBS-WC	Intrastratum basale	Split may spread to the suprabasilar layer
EBS-DM	Intrastratum basale, just superficial to the HD	Dense, circumscribed clumps of keratin filaments (most commonly observed within lesional biopsy sites)
EBS-MD	Predominantly in the stratum basale, above the level of the HD attachment plaque	Lack of integration of keratin filaments with HD
EBS-AR	Intrastratum basale	Absent keratin filaments within basal keratinocytes
EBSS	Intrastratum granulosum	—
JEB		
JEB-H	Intralamina lucida	Markedly reduced or absent HD; absent SBDP
JEB-nH	Intralamina lucida	Variable numbers or rudimentary appearance of HDs
JEB-PA	Both intralamina lucida and lower stratum basale, above the level of the HD plaque	Small HD plaques often with attenuated SBDP, and reduced integration of keratin filaments with HD
DDEB		
DDEB	Sublamina densa	Normal or decreased numbers of AF
DDEB-TBDN	Sublamina densa	Electron-dense stellate bodies within stratum basale; reduced AF
RDEB		
RDEB-HS	Sublamina densa	Absent AF
RDEB-nHS	Sublamina densa	Reduced or rudimentary-appearing AF

AF, anchoring fibril; *HD,* hemidesmosome; *SBDP,* subbasal dense plate; for explanation of other abbreviations, see footnote to Table 10-1.
Modified from the J-D, Smith LT. Non-molecular diagnostic testing of inherited epidermolysis bullosa: Current Techniques, major findings, and relative sensitivity and specificity, In Fine J-D, Bauer EA, McGuire J, Moshell A (eds.), *Epidermolysis Bullosa: Clinical, Epidemiologic, and Laboratory Advances, and the Findings of the National Epidermolysis Bullosa Registry.* Baltimore: Johns Hopkins University Press, 1999, p. 52.

- Indirect immunofluorescence: IgG circulating autoantibodies in the patient's serum that target the skin basement membrane component, type VII collagen
- Course: chronic inflammatory disease with periods of partial remissions and exacerbations
- Treatment: oral corticosteroids and immunosuppressants, including systemic corticosteroids, cyclophosphamide, and cyclosporine; plasmapheresis in patients with recalcitrant disease

Inherited Epidermolysis Bullosa

- See Tables 10-1 to 10-3

REFERENCES

Amagai M: Pemphigus. In: Bolognia JL, Jorizzo JL, Rapini RP (eds). *Dermatology.* New York: Mosby, 2003, pp. 449–462.

Bickle K, Roark TR, Hsu S: Autoimmune bullous dermatoses: a review. *Am Fam Physician* 2002; 65(9):1861–1870.

Borradori L, Bernard P. Pemphigoid group. In: Bolognia JL, Jorizzo JL, Rapini RP, (eds.) *Dermatology.* New York: Mosby, 2003, pp. 463–477.

Freedberg IM et al. *Fitzpatrick's Dermatology in General Medicine,* 6th Ed. New York: McGraw-Hill; 2003.

Herron MD, Zone JJ. In: Bolognia JL, Jorizzo JL, Rapini RP, (eds). *Dermatology* New York: Mosby, 2003, pp. 479–489.

McKee PH. *Pathology of the Skin: With Clinical Correlations.* London: Mosby-Wolfe; 1996.

CHAPTER 11

RADIOLOGIC FINDINGS

MELISSA A. BOGLE
ASRA ALI

METABOLIC DISORDERS

1. Alkaptonuria
   - Autosomal recessive
   - Deficiency of homogentisic acid oxidase
   - Blue-black discoloration of sclera and cartilage, dark sweat/urine/cerumen, arthropathy (large joints)
   - Deafness, renal stones, prostate concretions
   - Radiologic findings: aortic and vertebral disk calcification (Fig. 11-1)
2. Gaucher disease
   - Autosomal recessive
   - Deficiency in glucocerebrosidase
   - Type I: manifests in adults as hyperpigmentation, hepatosplenomegaly, lymphadenopathy, pancytopenia
   - Type II: manifests in infancy as hepatosplenomegaly, rapid neurologic deterioration, chronic aspiration, pneumonia
   - Radiologic findings: fractures, Erlenmeier flask deformity of long bones, osteopenia, periosteal new bone formation
   - Bone marrow: Gaucher cells ("crumpled tissue paper")
3. Lipoid proteinosis (hyalinosis cutis et mucosae, Urbach-Wiethe disease)
   - Autosomal recessive
   - Hoarse cry at birth
   - Early bullae with later pearly papules on face, eyelid, neck, mucosa, and extremities; alopecia, parotiditis, large wooden tongue, abnormal teeth, seizures
   - Radiologic finding: "bean bag" hippocampal calcifications
4. Albright's hereditary osteodystrophy
   - X-linked or autosomal dominant
   - Brachydactyly
   - Dimpling over the metacarpophalangeal joints (Albright's sign)

GENETIC/CONGENITAL SYNDROMES

1. Bushke-Ollendorf
   - Autosomal dominant disorder
   - Dermatofibrosis lenticularis disseminata, juvenile elastomas
   - Radiologic finding: asymptomatic osteopoikilosis (may be mistaken for bone metastases)
     - Oval opacities on x-ray
2. Cockayne syndrome
   - Autosomal recessive
   - Defect in DNA helicase
   - "Cachectic dwarf": long limbs, contractures, cool acral extremities, photosensitivity, progressive neural degeneration, deafness, retinitis pigmentosum, cataract, dental caries
   - Radiologic finding: intracranial calcifications (Fig. 11-2)
3. Conradi-Hunermann
   - X-linked dominant
   - Defect in *PEX7* (peroxisomal enzyme)
   - Ichthyosiform erythroderma in Blashko's lines, patchy alopecia, asymmetric focal cataracts
   - Radiologic findings: stippled epiphyses (chondrodysplasia punctata), unilateral limb shortening, scoliosis
4. DiGeorge syndrome
   - Zinc finger anomaly
   - Congenital absence of thymus and parathyroid
   - Abnormal aorta, hypocalcemia, tetany
   - Recurrent fungal and viral infections
   - Cardiac problems most common cause of death
   - Radiologic finding: absent thymic shadow
5. Gardner's syndrome
   - Autosomal dominant
   - Defect in *APC* gene (β-catenin)
   - Radiologic findings: osteomas, odontomas/supernumerary teeth

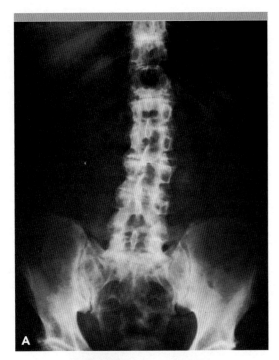

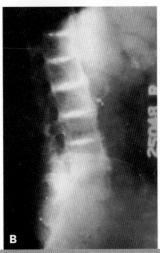

FIGURE 11-1 Radiologic findings in an alkaptonuric patient showing aortic and vertebral disk calcification. *(From Freedberg IM et al: Fitzpatrick's Dermatology in General Medicine, 6th ed. New York: McGraw-Hill, 2003, p. 1425.)*

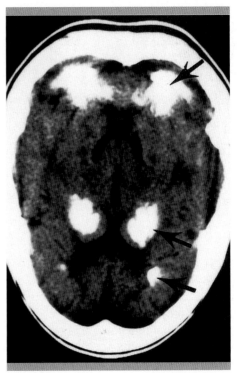

FIGURE 11-2 Intracranial calcifications. *(From Freedberg IM et al: Fitzpatrick's Dermatology in General Medicine, 6th ed. New York: McGraw-Hill, 2003, p. 1516.)*

6. Goltz syndrome (focal ectodermal dysplasia)
   - X-linked dominant
   - Radiologic findings: osteopathia striata, lobster claw deformity of the hand, asymmetric trunk and limbs
7. Gorlin-Goltz (basal cell nevus syndrome) (See also Chap. 23)
   - Autosomal dominant
   - Defect in *PATCHED* gene
   - Basal cell carcinomas, palmoplantar pits, frontal bossing
   - Meduloblastoma, ovarian fibromas, fibrosarcoma
   - Radiologic findings: odontogenic jaw cysts
   - Calcification of falx cerebri (Fig. 11-3)
   - Albright's sign: short fourth metacarpal (Fig. 11-4)
   - Rib deformities, bifid ribs
   - Kyphoscoliosis
   - Long bone cysts
8. Junctional epidermolysis bullosa (Herlitz/Letalis)
   - Autosomal recessive
   - Defect in $\alpha_6\beta_4$-integrin
   - Generalized bullae, perioral granulation tissue, absent/shed nails, dysplastic teeth, respiratory edema
   - Radiologic finding: pyloric atresia
9. Klippel-Trenaunay-Weber
   - Most common vascular malformation syndrome
   - Capillary malformation, usually on lower extremity
   - Underlying bone and soft tissue hypertrophy, varicosities, thromboses

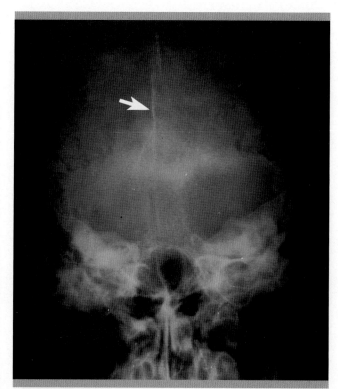

FIGURE 11-3 Calcification of falx cerebri. *(From Freedberg IM et al: Fitzpatrick's Dermatology in General Medicine, 6th ed. New York: McGraw-Hill, 2003, p. 759.)*

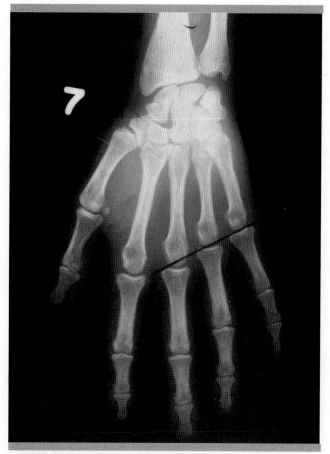

FIGURE 11-4 Albright's sign. *(From Freedberg IM et al: Fitzpatrick's Dermatology in General Medicine, 6th ed. New York: McGraw-Hill, 2003, p. 759.)*

- Radiologic findings: destructive bone lesions, limb hypertrophy
- Parkes-Weber variant: artrioventricular fistulas, high-output heart failure

10. Maffucci's syndrome (enchondromatosis with cavernous hemangiomas)
   - Grapelike superficial and deep venous malformations (rarely malignant)
   - Radiologic findings: multiple enchondromas (phalanges, long bones), fractures, bowing, limb-length discrepancies
   - Between 15 and 30 percent of enchondromas transform to chondrosarcoma
   - Ollier's disease: multiple enchondromas of tubular and flat bones without hemangiomas

11. McCune-Albright syndrome
   - "Coast of Maine" café-au-lait macules, precocious puberty, endocrine abnormalities (hyperthyroidism)
   - Radiologic findings: polyostotic fibrous dysplasia, recurrent fractures, bowing of the limbs, limb-length discrepancies, bone cysts, sclerosis at the skull base

12. Nail patella syndrome
   - Autosomal dominant
   - Defect in *LMX1B* gene
   - Dysplastic nails (triangular lunula), nephropathy (may be subclinical), Lester iris
   - Radiologic findings: hypoplastic or absent patellae, posterior iliac horns

13. Neurofibromatosis I
   - Autosomal dominant
   - Defect in neurofibromin
   - Radiologic findings
     - Sphenoid wing dysplasia
     - Cortical thinning of long bones
     - Bowing of the tibia (Fig. 11-5)
     - Tibial pseudoarthrosis
     - Scoliosis
   - Optic glioma
     - Diagnose with MRI
     - Occurs during the first 4 years of life; bilateral in 4 percent
     - Most common intracranial tumor associated with neurofibromatosis type 1

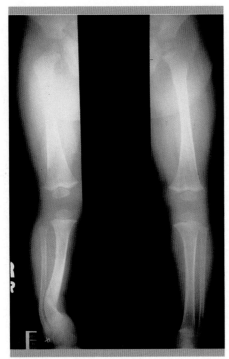

FIGURE 11-5 Tibial bowing. *(From Freedberg IM et al: Fitzpatrick's Dermatology in General Medicine, 6th ed. New York: McGraw-Hill, 2003, p. 1829.)*

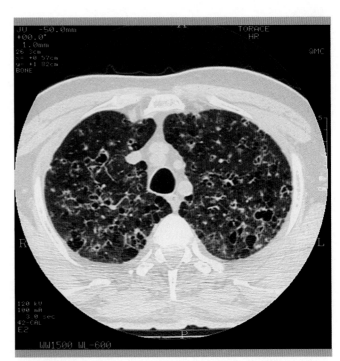

FIGURE 11-6 Letterer-Siwe disease. *(From Freedberg IM et al: Fitzpatrick's Dermatology in General Medicine, 6th ed. New York: McGraw-Hill, 2003, p. 1583.)*

14. Papillon-Lefèvre syndrome
    - Autosomal recessive
    - Defect in cathepsin C
    - Palmoplantar keratoderma, psoriasiform hyperkeratotic plaques on elbows and knees, periodontitis
    - Decreased neutrophilic phagocytosis and lymphocyte responsiveness
    - Radiologic findings: calcification of dura mater
15. Sturge-Weber
    - Facial capillary malformation, underlying soft tissue and skeletal hypertrophy, seizures, hemiparesis, choroidal malformations, glaucoma
    - Radiologic finding: tram track calcifications
16. Tuberous sclerosis
    - Autosomal dominant
    - Defect in hamartin (chromosome 9) or tuberin (chromosome 16)
    - Radiologic findings: phalangeal cysts, periosteal thickening, paraventricular calcifications, cortical tubers, subependymal hamartomas
17. Fanconi's syndrome (familial pancytopenia)
    - Pigment abnormalities
    - Severe anemia, thrombocytopenia, hyperreflexia, retinal hemorrhage, testicular hypoplasia

- Radiologic findings: aplasia of the radius, absent thumbs
18. Langerhans' cell histiocytosis
    - Letterer-Siwe
        - Honeycomb lung involvement with cystic cavities (Fig. 11-6)
        - Floating teeth, osteolytic bone lesions
    - Hand-Schüller-Christian:
        - "Punched out" osteolytic skull lesions (Fig. 11-7)
    - Eosinophilic granulomas: granulomatous bone lesion (Fig. 11-8)
19. Dyskeratosis congenita
    - X-linked
    - Pulmonary fibrosis
20. Ehlers-Danlos syndrome
    - Congenital dislocation of the hip (types I, IV, VIIA and VIIB)
    - Mitral valve prolapse and aortic root dilatation
21. Marfan's syndrome
    - Kyphoscoliosis
    - Pectus excavatum: depression of sternum
    - Pectus carinatum: projection of sternum
    - Mitral valve prolapse and aortic root dilation

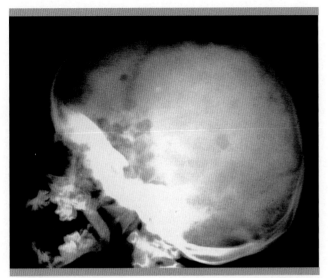

FIGURE 11-7 Hand-Schüller-Christian disease. *(From Freedberg IM et al: Fitzpatrick's Dermatology in General Medicine, 6th ed. New York: McGraw-Hill, 2003, p. 1583.)*

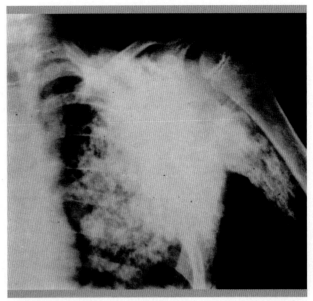

FIGURE 11-9 Dermatomysitis. *(From Freedberg IM et al: Fitzpatrick's Dermatology in General Medicine, 6th ed. New York: McGraw-Hill, 2003, p. 1701.)*

RHEUMATOLOGIC DISORDERS

1. Dermatomyositis (Fig. 11-9)
   - Cutaneous findings with proximal muscle weakness
   - Gottron's papules, heliotrope rash, periungual telangiectasias
   - Radiologic findings: osteoporosis, calcinosis
2. Morphea
   - Localized scleroderma
   - Radiologic finding: melorheostosis (dense linear pattern of hyperostosis)
3. Reiter's syndrome
   - Reactive arthritis, seronegative spondyloarthritidies
   - Develops after enteric infections
   - Enthesopathy
   - Bone lucency
   - New bone formation
   - Sacroiliitis
   - Spondyloarthritis

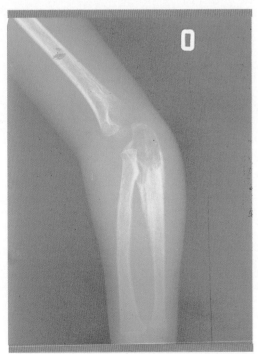

FIGURE 11-8 Eosinophilic granulomas. *(From Freedberg IM et al: Fitzpatrick's Dermatology in General Medicine, 6th ed. New York: McGraw-Hill, 2003, p. 1584.)*

INFECTIOUS

1. Congenital syphilis
   - Early
     - Epiphysitis of long bones (pain on motion, Parrot's pseudoparalysis)
     - Osteochondritis

- Sawtooth lesion on x-ray in the metaphysis
  - Onion-peel periosteum sign—multiple layers of new bone
- Late
  - Knee perisynovitis (Clutton's joints)
  - Bulldog jaw: mandibular protuberance
  - Gummas (skull, long bones)
  - Saber shins: anterior bowing of tibia
  - Higoumenaki's sign (unilateral hyperostosis of the medial clavicle)
  - Scaphoid scapulae: concavity of vertebral border of scapulae
2. Mycetoma
   - Fungal or bacterial infection of the subcutaneous tissue
   - Radiologic finding: honeycomb bone destruction in the foot
3. SAPHO syndrome
   - Eponym for the combination of *s*ynovitis, *a*cne, *p*ustulosis, *h*yperostosis, and *o*steitis

- Hyperostosis, osteitis, "bullhead" sign in sternocostoclavicular region on bone scan
4. Kawasaki's syndrome
   - Echocardiogram—coronary artery aneurysm

OTHER

1. Sarcoidosis
   - Granulomatous multisystem disorder
   - Radiologic findings: bilateral hilar adenopathy, interstitial pulmonary infiltrates, osteolytic lesions

SUMMARY

See Table 11-1.

TABLE 11-1 Radiological Findings in Skin Diseases and Related Conditions

Albright hereditary osteodystrophy
Heterozygous inactivating mutations of the *GNAS1* gene Polyostotic fibrous dysplasia: lytic lesions are seen in the affected bones Sclerosis of the basilar or temporal skull Pituitary adenoma Thyroid nodules, ovarian cysts
Ataxia-teleangiectasia
Cerebellar atrophy Absent thymic shadow, decreased mediastinal lymphoid tissue Decreased or absent adenoidal tissue in the nasopharynx
Ectodermal dysplasia
Jaw radiographs: hypodontia or dental abnormalities
Focal dermal hypoplasia syndrome
Osteopathia striata; linear vertical opacities in metaphyses of the bones
Gardner syndrome
Osteomas or hyperostosis Thyroid tumors Osteomas of mandible Colonic adenomatous polyps
Hypomelanosis of Ito
Cerebral atrophy Musculoskeletal abnormalities Mediastinal tumors

TABLE 11-1 (Continued)

Incontinentia pigmenti

    Hypoplasia and partial agenesis of corpus callosum

Proteus syndrome

    Pulmonary cystic malformations
    Bony overgrowth of the cranium of facial structures

Pseudoxanthoma elasticum

    Mitral valve insufficiency
    Artery calcification
    Coronary artery disease

Fungal Infections

Aspergillosis

    Aspergilloma: pulmonary cavitary lesions
    Alveolar infiltrates

Blastomycosis

    Alveolar infiltrates (reticulonodular pattern)
    Pleural effusion

Coccidioidomycosis

    Infiltrates, nodules, cavity, mediastinal or hilar adenopathy, pleural effusion

Cryptococcosis

    Patchy pneumonitis, granulomas

Histoplasmosis

    Patchy pulmonary infiltrates
    Upper lobe cavitations
    Healed lesions that appear as residual pulmonary nodules

Mucormycosis

    Sinus disease, bone erosion

Nocardiosis

    Pulmonary lesion

Paracoccidioidomycosis

    Confluent nodular infiltrates

Lipidoses, histiocytoses

Multicentric reticulohistiocytosis

    Resorption of subchondral bone
    Arthritis mutilans

(Continued)

TABLE 11-1 (Continued)

Metabolic diseases
Calcinosis cutis
Visceral and nonvisceral calcification
Gout
Erosions with sclerotic borders   Tophi may calcify
Hepatolenticular degeneration

Cortical atrophy
   Ventricular enlargement
   Dual energy x-ray absorptiometry (DEXA) scan: osteoporosis

Menkes syndrome
Elongated and tortuous vessels   Subdural hematomas
Tumors and cysts of the epidermis and epidermal appendages
Cowden disease
Mammograms   Barium swallow, upper and lower GI endoscopy
Dermoid cyst
MRI to diagnose intracranial or intramedullary cysts
Epidermal nevus syndrome
MRI: cerbral atrophy, dilated ventricles, hemimegalencephaly
Tumors of fibrous and vascular tissue
Blue rubber nevus syndrome
GI lesions with endoscopy   Fractures, bony overgrowth, and articular derangement
Osler-Weber-Rendu disease
Autosomal dominant   CT scan: pulmonary arteriovenous malformations, liver, kidney, and splenic lesions
Peutz-Jeghers syndrome

Autosomal dominant
   Mutation of *STK11*
   Intestinal hamartomatous polyps in association with mucocutaneous melanocytic macules
   Esophagogastroduodenoscopy
   Colonoscopy

REFERENCES

Freedberg IM et al. *Fitzpatrick's Dermatology in General Medicine,* 6th Ed. New York: McGraw-Hill; 2003.

Houser OW, Gomez MR. CT and MR imaging of intracranial tuberous sclerosis. *J Dermatol* 1992;19(11):904–908.

Kimonis VE, Mehta SG, Digiovanna JJ, Bale SJ, Pastakia B. Radiological features in 82 patients with nevoid basal cell carcinoma (NBCC or Gorlin) syndrome. *Genet Med* 2004;6(6): 495–502.

McKee PH. *Pathology of the Skin: With Clinical Correlations.* *London:* Mosby-Wolfe; 1996.

Spitz JL. *Genodermatoses: A Full-Color Clinical Guide to Genetic Skin Disorders.* New York: Lippincott Williams & Wilkins; 1996.

Verhelst H, Van Coster R. Neuroradiologic findings in a young patient with characteristics of Sturge-Weber syndrome and Klippel-Trenaunay syndrome. *J Child Neurol* 2005;20(11): 911–913.

Yanardag H, Pamuk ON. Bone cysts in sarcoidosis: what is their clinical significance? *Rheumatol Int* 2004;24(5):294–296. Epub 2003 Aug 20.

CHAPTER 12

ELECTRON MICROSCOPY

ASRA ALI

1. Langerhans cell (Fig. 12-1)
   - Bone marrow–derived
   - Antigen-processing and -presenting cells
   - Indented nucleus
   - Rod- and racket-shaped cytoplasmic granules (Birbeck granules)—form when membrane-bound antigen is internalized by endocytosis
   - Cytoplasm contains dispersed vimentin intermediate filaments
2. Merkel cell (Fig. 12-2)
   - Slowly adapting type I mechanoreceptors located in sites of high tactile sensitivity
   - Present among basal keratinocytes
   - Nucleus is lobulated
   - Cytoplasm is electron-lucent with prominent Golgi
   - Margins of cells project cytoplasmic spines toward keratinocytes
   - Dense core granules (80 to 200 nm) contain neurotransmitter-like substances
   - Intermediate filaments are numerous and assume a parallel or whorled arrangement near the nucleus (dotlike pattern)
3. Lamellar granules (Fig. 12-3)
   - In the intercellular space and cytoplasm of the granular cell
   - 0.2 to 0.3 nm in diameter
   - Membrane-bound secretory organelles containing a series of alternating thick and thin lamellae (folded sheets/disk-like/liposome-like structures)
   - Contain glycoproteins, glycolipids, phospholipids, free sterols, acid hydrolases, and glucosylceramides
4. Dermal-epidermal junction (Fig. 12-4)
   - Interface between epidermis and dermis
   - LL = lamina lucida
   - LD = lamina densa
   - AFib = anchoring fibrils
   - AFil = anchoring filaments
   - HD = hemidesmosome
   - KF = keratin filaments

5. Desmosome (Fig 12-5)
   - Calcium-dependent cell surface structures that function to promote adhesion of epidermal cells and aid in resistance to mechanical stresses
   - Components of desmosome
     - Desmosomal plaque
     - Transmembrane glycoproteins (part of cadherin family)
     - Desmosomal core
6. Melanocyte (Fig. 12-6)
   - Contains melanosomes in cytoplasm
   - Melanosome (stage IV): striated organelle enriched in melanin
   - Melanosomes become elongated and form ordered striations in stage II of development
   - Melanocytes project dendrites to adjacent keratinocytes to transfer melanosomes
   - Melanocytes can be distinguished from keratinocytes by the absence of keratin filaments
7. Macrophage (Fig. 12-7)
   - Part of the mononuclear phagocytic system
   - Derived from precursor cells of bone marrow that differentiate into monocytes in the blood
   - Skin macrophages express CDIIc, CD6, and KiM8 antigens
   - On electron microscopy: melanosomes within phagosomes
8. Mast cell (Fig. 12-8)
   - Specialized secretory cells: originate in bone marrow from CD34 positive stem cells
   - Proliferation depends on *c-kit* receptor and the stem cell factor (SCF) ligand
   - Round/ovoid nucleus
   - Granules can be secretory or lysosomal (0.2 to 0.5 nm)
   - Mediators can be preformed and stored in granules (histamine, heparin, tryptase, chymase)
   - Lattice-like structure of granules: found in mast cells of skin and intestinal submucosa

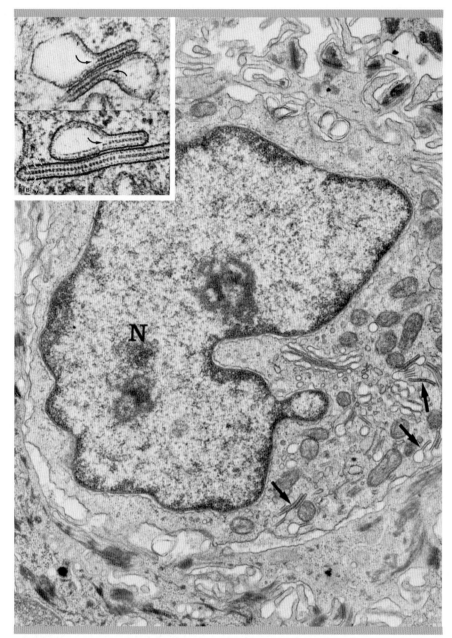

FIGURE 12-1 Langerhans cell. *(From Freedberg IM et al: Fitzpatrick's Dermatology in General Medicine, 6th ed. New York: McGraw-Hill, 2003, p. 256.)*

- Scroll-like structure of granules: found in mast cells of lung and intestinal mucosa
9. Collagen (Fig. 12-9)
  - Fibers have regular banding pattern at approximately 70-nm intervals
  - Regularly oriented fibers composed of fibrils and microfibrils

- Fibrils are aligned in a parallel manner, resulting in a pattern of cross-striations
10. Elastic tissue (Figs. 12-10 and 12-11)
  - Amorphous branching structures forming continuous sheets in some connective tissues
  - Fibers composed of elastin with an electron-lucent core surrounded by thin, electron-dense microfibrils (see Fig. 12-11)

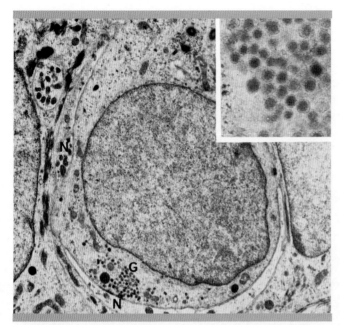

FIGURE 12-2 Merkel cell. *(From Freedberg IM et al: Fitzpatrick's Dermatology in General Medicine, 6th ed. New York: McGraw-Hill, 2003, p. 67.)*

- F = fibroblast; E = elastic tissue; C = collagen fibers (see Fig. 12-10)

11. Eosinophil (Fig. 12-12)
    - Granules contain electron-dense core surrounded by a lucent matrix
    - Granules that contain the eosinophil basic proteins
      - Major basic protein (MBP)—only protein located in core
      - Eosinophilic cationic protein (ECP)—located in matrix
      - Eosinophil-derived neurotoxin (EDN)—located in matrix
      - Eosinophil peroxidase (EPO)—located in matrix

12. Fabry's disease (Fig. 12-13)
    - Concentric lamellar inclusions in lysosomes of fibrocytes
    - Deficient activity of lysosomal enzyme and galactosidase-A
    - Accumulation of glycosphingolipids in most visceral tissues and body fluids

13. Pox virus (Fig. 12-14)
    - Single molluscum contagiosum virus virion
    - Size = 240 × 300 nm, no envelope
    - dsDNA virus, capsid assembly in cytoplasm
    - Also known to cause Orf, milker's nodules, variola, and vaccinia

14. Herpes virus (Fig. 12-15)
    - Varicella virus
    - Size = 120 to 200 nm
    - Icosahedral, enveloped dsDNA
    - Replicates in nucleus
    - Herpes simplex (types 1 and 2), varicella-zoster, cytomegalovirus, Epstein-Barr virus

15. Papillomavirus (Fig. 12-16)
    - Multiple nonenveloped virions
    - Size: 50 to 55 nm, icosahedral with capsid subunits (capsome)
    - Nonenveloped dsDNA replicates in nucleus

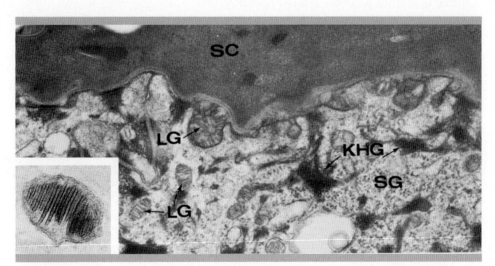

FIGURE 12-3 Lamellar granules. *(From Freedberg IM et al: Fitzpatrick's Dermatology in General Medicine, 6th ed. New York: McGraw-Hill, 2003, p. 62.)*

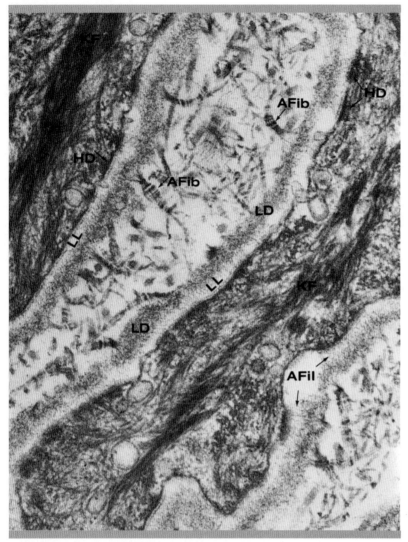

FIGURE 12-4   Dermal-epidermal junction. *(From Freedberg IM et al: Fitzpatrick's Dermatology in General Medicine, 6th ed. New York: McGraw-Hill, 2003, p. 70.)*

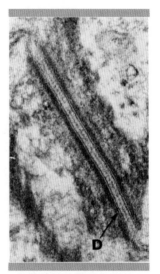

FIGURE 12-5
Desmosome. *(From Freedberg IM et al: Fitzpatrick's Dermatology in General Medicine, 6th ed. New York: McGraw-Hill, 2003, p. 62.)*

16. Sézary cell (Fig. 12-17)
    • CD4+ T-helper lymphocytes
    • Convoluted nucleus
17. Granular cell tumor
    • Cytoplasmic granules = lysosomes, contain granular and membranous debris

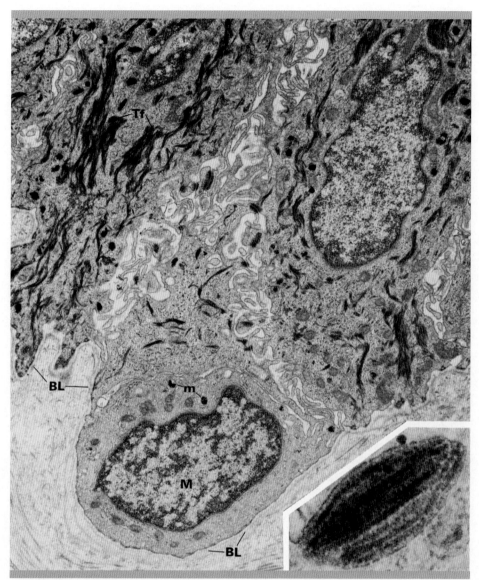

FIGURE 12-6 Melanocyte. *(From Freedberg IM et al: Fitzpatrick's Dermatology in General Medicine, 6th ed. New York: McGraw-Hill, 2003, p. 61.)*

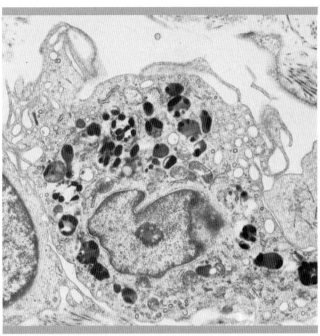

FIGURE 12-7 Macrophage. *(From Freedberg IM et al: Fitzpatrick's Dermatology in General Medicine, 6th ed. New York: McGraw-Hill, 2003, p. 74.)*

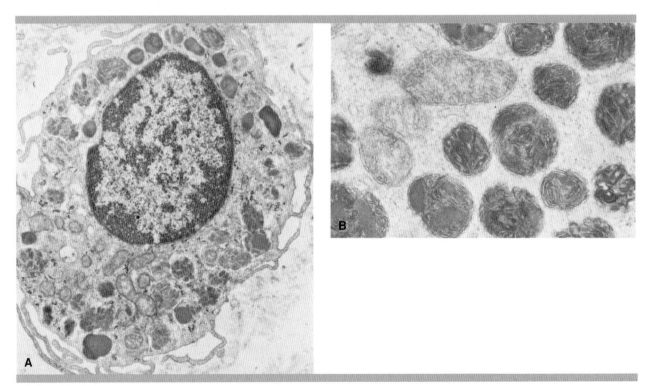

FIGURE 12-8 Mast cell. *(From Freedberg IM et al: Fitzpatrick's Dermatology in General Medicine, 6th ed. New York: McGraw-Hill, 2003, p. 75.)*

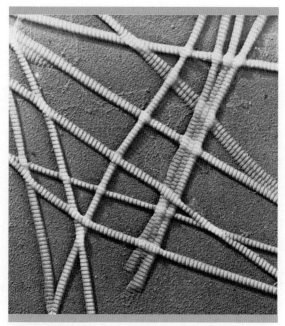

FIGURE 12-9 Collagen. *(From Freedberg IM et al: Fitzpatrick's Dermatology in General Medicine, 6th ed. New York: McGraw-Hill, 2003, p. 165.)*

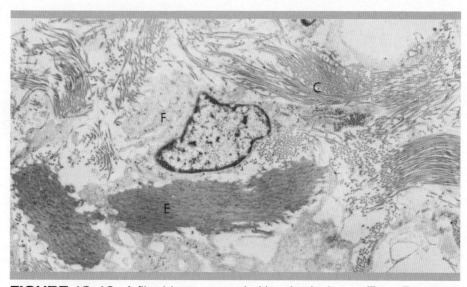

FIGURE 12-10 A fibroblast surrounded by elastic tissue. *(From Freedberg IM et al: Fitzpatrick's Dermatology in General Medicine, 6th ed. New York: McGraw-Hill, 2003, p. 181.)*

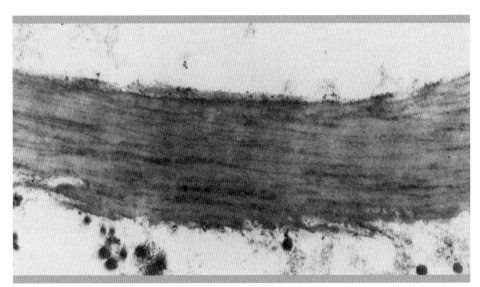

FIGURE 12-11 Elastic fibers in normal human skin. *(From Freedberg IM et al: Fitzpatrick's Dermatology in General Medicine, 6th ed. New York: McGraw-Hill, 2003, p. 181.)*

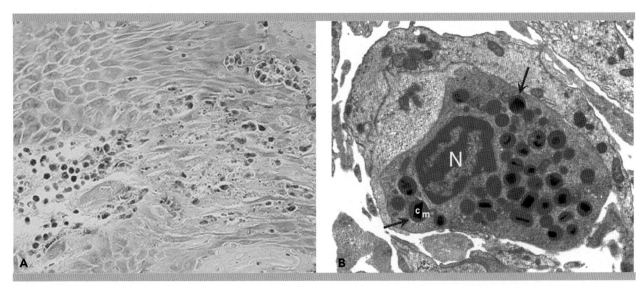

FIGURE 12-12 Eosinophil. *(From Freedberg IM et al: Fitzpatrick's Dermatology in General Medicine, 6th ed. New York: McGraw-Hill, 2003, p. 320.)*

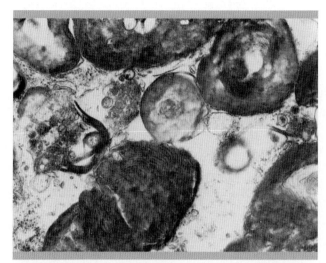

FIGURE 12-13 Mitral valve in Fabry's disease. *(From Freedberg IM et al: Fitzpatrick's Dermatology in General Medicine, 6th ed. New York: McGraw-Hill, 2003, p. 1479.)*

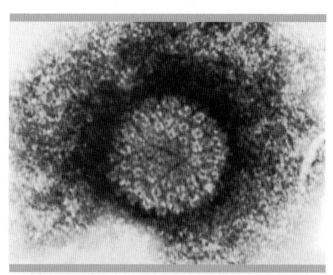

FIGURE 12-15 Herpes virus. *(From Freedberg IM et al: Fitzpatrick's Dermatology in General Medicine, 6th ed. New York: McGraw-Hill, 2003, p. 2037.)*

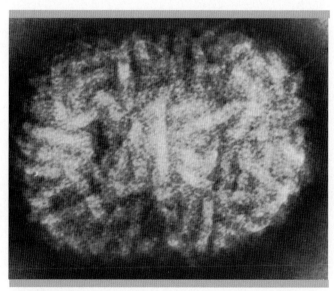

FIGURE 12-14 Pox virus. *(From Freedberg IM et al: Fitzpatrick's Dermatology in General Medicine, 6th ed. New York: McGraw-Hill, 2003, p. 2037.)*

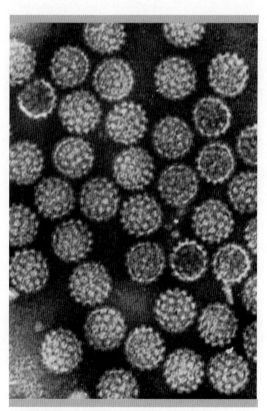

FIGURE 12-16 Papillomavirus. *(From Freedberg IM et al: Fitzpatrick's Dermatology in General Medicine, 6th ed. New York: McGraw-Hill, 2003, p. 2037.)*

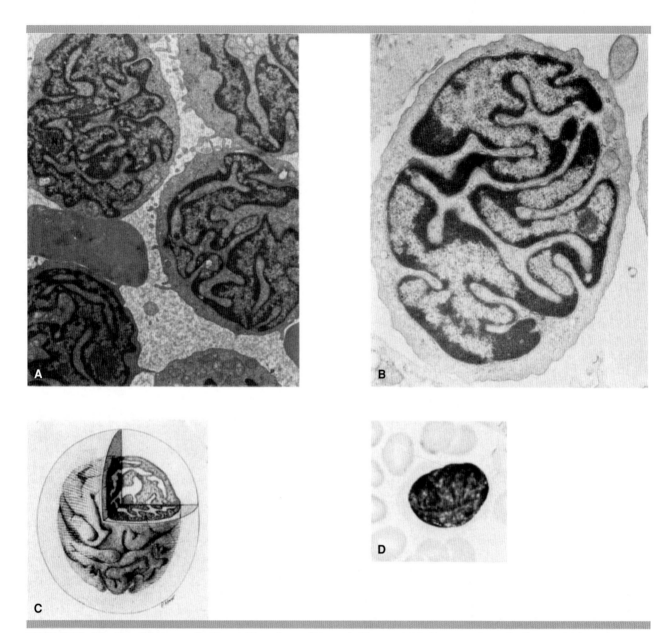

FIGURE 12-17 Sézary cell. *(From Freedberg IM et al: Fitzpatrick's Dermatology in General Medicine, 6th ed. New York: McGraw-Hill, 2003, Figure 108-27.)*

REFERENCES

Daróczy J, Rácz I. *Diagnostic Electron Microscopy in Practical Dermatology.* Budapest: Akadémiai Kiadó; 1987.

Elder DE, Elenitsas R, Johnson BL Jr, Murphy BG, eds. *Lever's Histopathology of the Skin.* Philadelphia: Lippincott Williams & Wilkins; 2005.

Freedberg IM et al. *Fitzpatrick's Dermatology in General Medicine,* 6th Ed. New York: McGraw-Hill; 2003.

Wilborn WH, Hyde BM, Montes LF. *Scanning Electron Microscopy of Normal and Abnormal Human Skin.* Mahwah, New Jersey: Electron Optics Publishing Group; 1985.

Zelickson AS, Mottaz JH. *The Clinical Use of Electron Microscopy in Dermatology,* 4th Ed. Minneapolis: Bolger Publications; 1985.

CHAPTER 13

SURGERY AND ANATOMY

MANUEL DAVILA
TRI H. NGUYEN

1. Anatomic review of arteries, veins, and lymphatics
2. Anatomic review of muscles
3. Anatomic review of nerves
4. Anatomic review of head and neck
5. Electrosurgery
6. Cryosurgery
7. Wound healing
8. Antiseptics
9. Flap review
10. Local anesthesia
11. Sutures

ANATOMIC REVIEW OF ARTERIES AND VEINS AND LYMPHATICS

Arteries of the Head and Neck (Fig. 13-1)

The internal and external carotid arteries and their branches supply the head and neck. In the region of the upper central face (nose, glabella, periorbital, and forehead), vessels from the internal and external carotid systems have intimate anastamoses. These connections are important clinically in that (1) infections in this area may extend intracranially via internal carotid vessels and (2) steroid injections in the periorbital skin may embolize to the retinal artery and cause blindness.

Named arteries give rise to unnamed branches and perforators that nourish overlying muscles, fascia, subcutaneous fat, and skin. Septocutaneous (traveling through septa to skin) and musculocutaneous (perforating muscles to skin) arteries supply the subdermal plexus (arteries at the junction of subcutaneous fat and the deep reticular dermis), which is the main blood supply to the skin. Undermining should be at least below midfat to preserve the subdermal plexus. Immediate subdermal undermining is inappropriate because the subdermal plexus is compromised.

INTERNAL CAROTID ARTERY

Supplies structures inside the skull except for central facial arteries (supraorbital, supratrochlear, infratrochlear, dorsal nasal, and external nasal arteries) that nourish the periorbital skin, forehead, glabella, and nose. The central facial arteries have numerous connections with vessels from the external carotid system.

EXTERNAL CAROTID ARTERY BRANCHES

- Superior thyroid
- Ascending pharyngeal
- Lingual
- Facial
- Occipital
- Posterior auricular
- Maxillary
- Superficial temporal

MAXILLARY ARTERY BRANCHES

- Anterior tympanic
- Middle meningeal
- Inferior alveolar
- Accessory meningeal
- Masseteric
- Pterygoid
- Deep temporal
- Buccal
- Sphenopalatine
- Descending palatine
- Infraorbital
- Posterior superior alveolar
- Middle superior alveolar
- Pharyngeal
- Anterior superior alveolar
- Artery of the pterygoid canal

VI. Vascular system

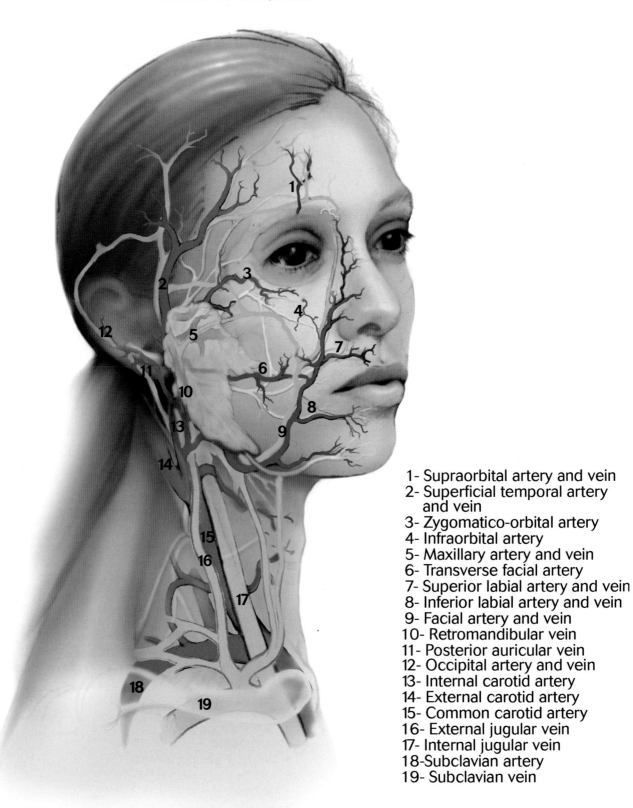

1- Supraorbital artery and vein
2- Superficial temporal artery and vein
3- Zygomatico-orbital artery
4- Infraorbital artery
5- Maxillary artery and vein
6- Transverse facial artery
7- Superior labial artery and vein
8- Inferior labial artery and vein
9- Facial artery and vein
10- Retromandibular vein
11- Posterior auricular vein
12- Occipital artery and vein
13- Internal carotid artery
14- External carotid artery
15- Common carotid artery
16- External jugular vein
17- Internal jugular vein
18-Subclavian artery
19- Subclavian vein

FIGURE 13-1   Arteries and veins of the head and neck.

Venous System of the Lower Extremities (Fig. 13-2)

- Consists of the superficial (above muscular fascia) and deep venous system (below muscular fascia). The superficial and deep systems are connected via perforator veins. Flow is unidirectional and proceeds from the superficial veins, which drain to the deep veins via the perforators, and the deep veins merge to form the common femoral vein
- Venous valves exist only in the lower extremity veins. Greatest density in the calf and progressively fewer valves in the thigh. Venous valves permit only one-way flow (upward) when competent
- Calf muscles act as a muscular pump to drain venous blood. Venous blood is moved only during muscle contraction. Lying still or standing still does not drain the venous system

SUPERFICIAL LEG VEINS

All superficial veins lie above the deep muscular fascia and drain into the deep venous system. Venous thromboses in a superficial vein do not have to be treated with anticoagulation unless the thrombus is progressive or near the junction with a deep vein (proximal thrombus). There are three major networks in the superficial venous system (greater saphenous vein, lesser saphenous vein, and lateral venous system).

- Great saphenous vein (also known as long saphenous vein)
  - Originates from the dorsal arch veins of the foot, runs anterior to medial malleolus, up medial calf, knee, and inner thigh, and empties into the common femoral vein via the saphenofemoral junction (SFJ)
  - The longest superficial vein of the lower leg
  - Most common cause of superficial venous insufficiency
- Small saphenous vein (also known as lesser saphenous vein)
  - Runs behind the lateral malleolus, up the posterior calf, and empties into the popliteal vein (where it empties may vary with individuals) within or near the popliteal fossa
  - Drains skin and superficial fascia of the lateral and posterior side of the foot and leg
- Lateral venous system: series of veins on the lateral thigh that drain this area
- Anterolateral thigh vein: drains the lateral and anterior thigh; empties into the greater saphenous vein; lateral segment is part of the lateral venous system

DEEP LEG VEINS

- All lie below the deep muscular fascia
- Tibial veins: anterior and posterior; drain into popliteal vein
- Popliteal vein: drain into superficial femoral vein

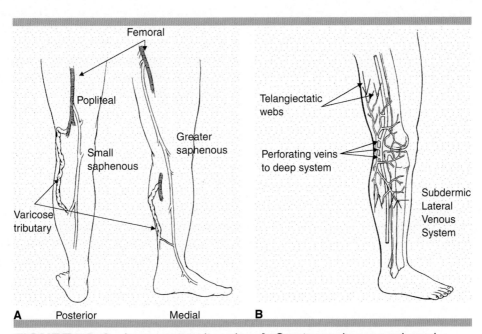

FIGURE 13-2 Lower extremity veins. **A.** Greater saphenous vein and lesser saphenous vein. **B.** Subdermic lateral venous system. *(From Freedberg IM et al: Fitzpatrick's Dermatology in General Medicine, 6th ed. New York: McGraw-Hill, 2003, p. 2551.)*

TABLE 13-1 Lymph Glands of the Head

Occipital	Facial
Posterior auricular	Deep facial
Anterior auricular	Lingual
Parotid	Retropharyngeal

TABLE 13-2 Lymph Glands of the Neck

Submaxillary	Superficial cervical
Submental	Anterior cervical
Deep cervical	

- Femoral vein: joins with deep femoral vein in thigh to form common femoral vein; this is a deep vein despite its name
- Deep femoral vein
- Common femoral vein: at the groin/upper thigh, this is the site of drainage for multiple veins (greater saphenous vein, circumflex-iliac, external pudendal, epigastric)

Lymph Glands of the Upper Extremity (Tables 13-1 and 13-2)

- Divided into two sets: superficial and deep
  - Superficial lymph glands are few and of small size
  - Deep lymph glands are chiefly grouped in the axilla

Lymphatics of the Lower Extremity

- Anterior tibial gland: small and inconstant
- Popliteal glands: small in size and some six or seven in number; imbedded in the fat
- Inguinal glands: situated at the upper part of the femoral triangle

ANATOMIC REVIEW OF MUSCLES

Embryology

- Muscles of mastication
  - Temporalis, masseter, medial pterygoid, lateral pterygoid
  - All derived from first branchial arch mesoderm
  - Innervated by trigeminal nerve [cranial nerve (CN) V]
- Muscles of facial expression (Fig. 13-3 and Table 13-3)
  - Derived from second branchial arch mesoderm
  - Innervated by facial nerve (CN VII)
  - Lower face muscles (risorius, platysma, depressor anguli oris) are derived from an embryonic platysma and tend to not have bony insertions or origins
  - Middle and upper face muscles (muscles of the forehead, scalp, periorbital, upper mouth) of

expression are derived from the embryonic sphincer colli profundus muscle and may have bony insertions

ANATOMIC REVIEW OF NERVES

Motor Nerves to the Face

- Mandibular branch of trigeminal (CN V3): muscles of mastication
- Facial nerve (CN 7): muscles of facial expression
- Oculomotor (CN 3): levator palpebrae superioris
- Sympathetic innervation: superior palpebral muscle of Müller (involuntary elevates upper eyelid in flight or fight situations)

FACIAL NERVE (CN 7) (TABLE 13-4)

- Emerges from cranium through the stylomastoid foramen and runs in the deep body of the parotid in the lateral cheek/jaw. Provides both motor (major function) and sensory innervation (minor role)
- Sensory: contributes to sensory innervation of the external auditory meatus along with auriculotemporal and vagus nerves
- Motor: five branches that innervate the muscles of facial expression—temporal, zygomatic, buccal, marginal mandibular, cervical

Sensory Innervation to the Face (Fig. 13-4 and Table 13-4)

- Supplied by three branches of the trigeminal nerve (CN V): ophthalmic (V1), maxillary (V2), and mandibular (V3) nerves
- Ophthalmic nerve (V1 sensory)
  - Travels through superior orbital fissure and passes through orbit to reach the skin of the forehead, scalp
  - Branches of V1
    - Frontal nerve
      - ▲ Supraorbital nerve
      - ▲ Supratrochlear nerve
    - Nasociliary nerve
      - ▲ Infratrochlear nerve
      - ▲ External nasal branch of anterior ethmoid
    - Lacrimal nerve

IV. Muscles of facial expression and neck muscles

1- Galea aponeurotica
2- Frontalis (frontal belly)
   of epicranius muscle
3- Corrugator supercilii muscle
4- Procerus muscle
5- Orbicularis oculi muscle:
   a.- Orbital part
   b.- Palpebral part
6- Zygomaticus major muscle
7- Zygomaticus minor muscle
8- Levator labii superioris muscle
9- Levator labii superioris
   alaeque nasi muscle
10- Nasalis muscle
11- Risorius muscle
12- Modiolus
13- Masseter muscle
14- Depressor anguli oris muscle
15- Depressor labii inferioris muscle
16- Mentalis muscle
17- Orbicularis oris
18- Depressor septi nasi muscle
19- Sternocleidomastoid muscle
20- Platysma muscle
21- Trapezius muscle

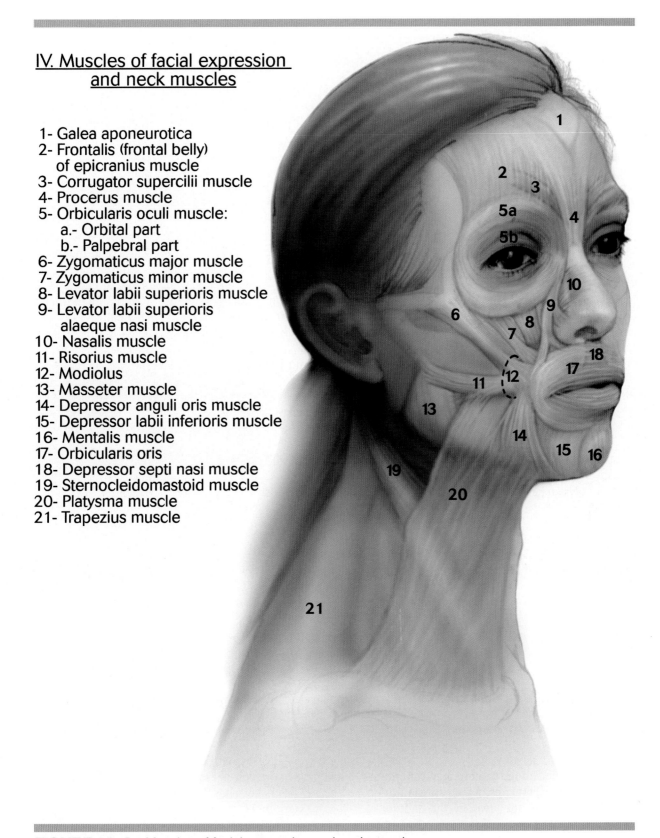

FIGURE 13-3 Muscles of facial expression and neck muscles.

TABLE 13-3 Muscles of Facial Expression with Innervations

Muscle	Action	Branch of Facial Nerve
Mouth-Lip Elevators		
Zygomaticus major and minor	Elevates corner of mouth	Buccal
Levator labii superioris	Elevates upper lip	Buccal
Levator labii superioris alaeque nasi	Lifts upper lip, dilates nares	Buccal
Levator anguli oris	Elevates corner of mouth	Buccal
Risorius	Pulls corner of mouth laterally	Buccal
Mouth-Lip Depressors		
Depressor anguli oris	Depresses corner of mouth (Marionette lines)	Buccal and marginal mandibular
Depressor labii inferioris	Depresses lower lip	Marginal mandibular
Mentalis	Protrudes lower lip (mental crease)	Marginal mandibular
Platysma	Pulls corner of mouth inferiorly (horizontal neck lines), tenses neck	Cervical
Buccinator	Flattens cheek	Buccal
Orbicularis oris	Closes, purses, and protrudes lip (vertical lip lines)	Marginal mandibular
Upper Face Muscles		
Nose Procerus	Pulls skin over glabella inferiorly	Temporal
Nasalis	Dilates nares	Buccal
Depressor septi nasi	Pulls columella inferiorly	Buccal
Periorbital Corrugator supercolli	Pulls eyebrows midially (glabellar lines)	Temporal
Orbicularis oculi	Closes and squeezes eyelids (crow's feet) shut	Temporal and zygomatic
Scalp Occipitalis	Moves scalp posteriorly	Postauricular
Frontalis	Raises eyebrows (horizontal forehead lines)	Temporal

Source: Data from Robinson JK, Anderson Jr R. Skin structure and anatomy, in Robinson JK, Hanke WC, Sengelmann RD, et al. (eds): *Surgery of the Skin: Procedural Dermatology.* London: Elsevier, 2005.

- Maxillary nerve (V2 sensory)
  - Leaves the skull through the foramen rotundum
  - Divides into four branches, which spread out on the side of the nose, the lower eyelid, and the upper lip
  - Branches of V2
    - Zygomaticotemporal
    - Zygomaticofacial
    - Infraorbital
    - Nasopalatine (superior alveolar and palatine nerves: sensation to upper teeth, gingival, palate, nasal mucosa)
- Mandibular nerve (V3 sensory)
  - Exits the cranium through the foramen ovale
  - Five branches of V3 that carry general sensory information from the mucous membranes of the mouth and cheek, anterior two-thirds of the tongue, lower teeth, skin of the lower jaw, side of

TABLE 13-4 Facial Motor Nerve Branches

Nerve	Muscles Innervated	Action
Temporal (frontal)	Frontalis Orbicularis oculi Corrugator supercilii	Wrinkles forehead Closes eye Purses eyebrows
Zygomatic	Orbicularis oculi Procerus	Closes eye Wrinkles nose upwards
Buccal	Lip elevators Orbicularis oris Buccinator	Elevates lip and oral angle Purses lips or pucker Whistling, blowing
Marginal mandibular	Lip depressors	Depress lip and oral angle Protrudes lower lip
Cervical	Platysma	Webs neck, depresses oral angles

the head and scalp, and meninges of the anterior and middle cranial fossae
  - Buccal nerve
  - Lingual nerve
  - Mental nerve
  - Inferior alveolar nerve
  - Auriculotemporal nerve

Facial Nerve Blocks

- The most common facial nerve blocks target the supraorbital (V1), infraorbital (V2), and mental (V3) nerves, which exit into the face through foramina of the same names. These three nerves line up vertically at the midpupillary line, which is 2.5 cm from the facial midline
  - For all nerve blocks, *aspirate* before injecting; use a 30-gauge needle
  - If pain/dysesthesia is elicited during insertion or injection, withdraw the needle slightly to avoid injuring the nerve itself
  - The principle is to *not* inject the nerve directly but to bathe the perineural space with local anesthetic
  - *Wait* at least 10 to 20 minutes for effective anesthesia
  - Intraoral approach to infraorbital and mental nerve is preferred to reduce patient discomfort, which is greater with transcutaneous injections
- Supraorbital nerve block
  - Blocking the supraorbital nerve will anesthetize part of the superior forehead and part of the upper eyelid. If the block is extended medially to include the supratrochlear and infratrochlear nerves, then the medial forehead, glabella, medial canthus, and

upper nasal dorsum and sidewall also will be anesthetized. Extending the block laterally to include the lacrimal nerve will anesthetize the lateral superior forehead and lateral upper eyelid
  - Supraorbital foramen/notch may or may not be palpable. Use the midpupillary line as a guide to the supraorbital nerve
  - Stand behind the patient's head with body in slight reverse Trendelenburg. This position will afford better access to the superior orbital rim and prevent the patient from seeing the needle approach
  - Raise a cutaneous wheal of anesthesia over the superior orbital rim in the midpupillary line. Insert the needle down to the rim until resistance is felt. Aspirate to ensure no blood return, and then inject 1 to 2 ml and massage the site to spread the anesthetic near the nerve
  - If no resistance is felt after inserting the needle 1 cm, then you are likely below the orbital rim or in the foramen itself. Withdraw the needle, and then insert it again, but redirect it to be above the rim
  - To extend the block medially or laterally, a bleb of anesthesia may be injected along the superior orbital rim medially and laterally from the supraorbital starting point
- Infraorbital nerve block
  - Infraorbital nerve block will anesthetize the lower eyelid skin, lower medial cheek, nasofacial sulcus, and part of the nasal sidewall and lateral ala
  - Intraoral (mucosal) approach is preferred. Use a 1-in 30-gauge needle, and when possible, apply viscous lidocaine or EMLA cream to the gingival

1- Frontal region
2- Temporal region
3- Orbital region
4- Zygomatic region
5- Malar/infraorbital region
6- Glabella region
7- Nasal region
8- Nasofacial sulcus
9- Nasolabial fold
   (melolabial fold)
10-Parotid region
11- Buccal region
12- Oral region
   a. upper cutaneous lip
   b. philtrum
   c. mucosal lip
   d. lower cutaneous lip
   e. mental
13- Submandibular triangle
14- Carotid triangle
15- Sternocleidomastoid region
16- Omoclavicular triangle
17- Lateral cervical region
18- Posterior cervical region

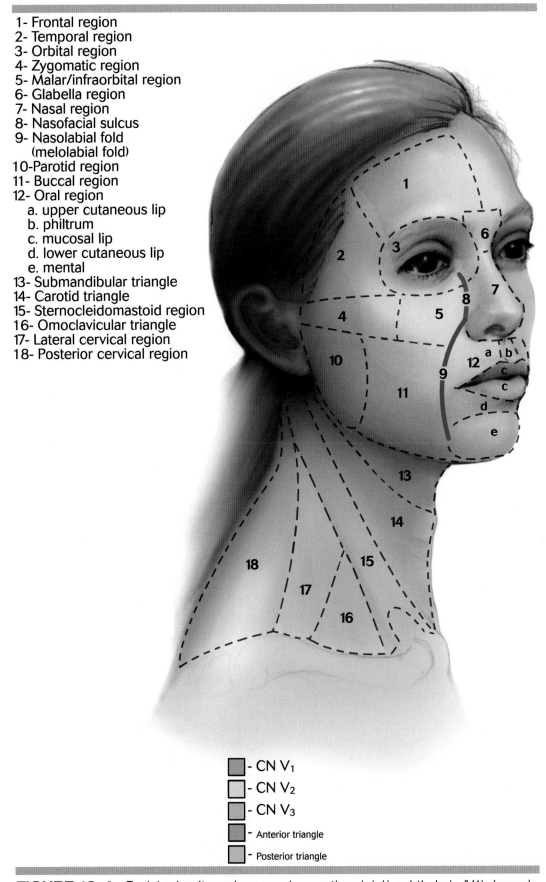

- CN V₁
- CN V₂
- CN V₃
- Anterior triangle
- Posterior triangle

FIGURE 13-4 Facial subunits and sensory innervation: (*pink*) ophthalmic (V1), (*green*) maxillary (V2), (*lavender/blue*) mandibular (V3).

sulcus above the upper canines for 5 minutes prior to injection

- Position yourself on the opposite side of the nerve to be blocked, and have the patient slightly turn his or her head toward you. For example, to block the right infraorbital nerve, stand at the patient's left side. This permits better access to the medially oriented foramen and causes less flexion of the injecting wrist
- Place the third or fourth finger of the noninjecting hand over the infraorbital foramen (1 cm below the palpable infraorbital margin), and peel back the ipsilateral upper lip with the index finger and thumb of the same hand (use a gauze to lift up the lip to avoid slipping)
- Inject a bleb of anesthesia at the gingival-labial sulcus above the apex of the canine fossa. Insert and aim the needle toward the foramen, or just below the overlying finger. Stop when resistance or bone is felt
- Aspirate and confirm that no blood returns, and then inject 2 to 3 ml of local anesthetic. If you are in the proper location, then the finger overlying the infraorbital foramen should feel a bleb of anesthesia rise from underneath. Withdraw slightly, and inject another 1 to 2 ml laterally on each side of the infraorbital foramen. Massage the injected site
- Mental nerve block
  - Mental nerve block will anesthetize the lower lip and chin/jawline and lower gingiva and teeth
  - Intraoral (mucosal) approach is preferred. Use a 1-in 30-gauge needle, and when possible, apply viscous lidocaine or EMLA cream to the gingival-labial sulcus below the second bicuspid for 5 minutes prior to injection
  - Stand behind the patient's head with the body in reverse Trendelenburg. Mark the mental foramen position in the midpupillary line (rarely, the foramen may be palpable; the foramen is approximately midway between the oral commissure and the mandibular rim in the midpupillary line), and place the third or fourth finger of the noninjecting hand over this site. Peel the ipsilateral lower lip outward with the index finger and thumb of the same hand
  - Inject and raise a bleb of local anesthetic at the gingival-labial sulcus below the second bicuspid (second premolar). Insert and aim the needle toward the mental foramen, or below the overlying finger marking the site
  - Aspirate and confirm that no blood returns, and then inject 2 to 3 ml of local anesthetic. If you are in the proper location, the finger overlying the mental foramen should feel a bleb of anesthesia rise from underneath. Withdraw slightly, and

inject another 1 to 2 ml laterally on each side of the infraorbital foramen. Massage the injected site
- Nasal nerve block
  - Sensory innervation to the nose is via the infratrochlear (V1: nasal root, middorsum, and sidewall), external nasal branch of the anterior ethmoid (V1: distal nasal dorsum and tip), infraorbital (V2: lower nasal sidewall and lateral ala), and branches of the nasopalatine (V2: columella, nasal mucosa) nerves
  - *Infratrochlear* nerve: Insert the needle and raise a bleb of anesthesia at the nasal root. Extend the anesthesia on each side of the nasal root and medial canthus
  - *External nasal branch of the anterior ethmoid*: Feel for the junction of the nasal bone and lateral cartilage (palpable hump on the upper to middle nasal dorsum). Inject a bleb of anesthesia (superficial and deep) here, and fan laterally on each side of the nasal sidewall toward the upper alar groove
  - *Infraorbital* nerve: The main trunk may be blocked as above. Alternatively, its peripheral nasal branches may be targeted by continuing the injection from the upper alar groove (from anesthesia of the external nasal branch of the anterior ethmoid) as above and extending it to the lateral ala and then curving underneath to the nasal sill. Repeat on both sides
  - *Nasopalatine* nerve: Extend the nasal sill anesthesia medially to subnasale (junction of columella and upper philtrum
- Auricular nerve block
  - For complete anesthesia of the external auricle, five nerves must be targeted (great auricular, auriculotemporal, lesser occipital, facial, and vagus nerves). Four injection sites are required, and anesthesia is fanned peripherally in a ring-block fashion
    - Great auricular (major sensory nerve to ear sensation to most of the posterior and anterior ear and lower earlobe)
    - Auriculotemporal (preauricular skin and anterosuperior auricle above the inferior crus of the helix; contributes to sensation of external auditory meatus)
    - Lesser occipital (minor role, upper posterior ear)
    - Conchal bowl and external auditory meatus: sensory supply from branches of the facial, vagus, and auriculotemporal nerves (conchal bowl)
  - *Greater auricular* nerve: Inject anesthesia at the midpoint of a line connecting the mastoid process and the mandibular angle. Extend or fan out the

injection both posterior and anterior to the earlobe (where the earlobe joins the jawline)
- *Auriculotemporal* nerve: Insert the needle 0.5 cm anterior to the superior crus of the helix. Aspirate before injecting because the superficial temporal artery pulsation is in proximity. Inject 2 to 3 ml here, and fan out inferiorly (toward the tragus) and posteriorly (behind where the superior helix joins the temporal scalp)
- *Lesser occipital* nerve: Find the midpoint of the postauricular sulcus, inject anesthesia here, and extend it superiorly and inferiorly (toward the lobe)
- *Conchal bowl anesthesia:* Place a bleb of anesthesia at the inferior crus of the helix, and extend it to cover the entire conchal bowl and external auditory meatus

Sensory Nerves of the Neck

- Cervical plexus (three nerves) supplies sensation to the neck. All exit in proximity at the posterior border of the sternocleidomastoid muscle in a region called *Erb's point* (discussed under "Surgical Anatomy: Danger Zone" below)
  - Lesser occipital (sensation to posterior neck, scalp, occiput, and upper posterior ear)
  - Greater auricular (sensation to earlobe and posterior auricle)
  - Transverse cervical (sensation to anterior neck)

Sensory Nerves of the Leg and Foot

- Innervated by five nerves (saphenous, posterior tibial, sural, deep peroneal, superficial peroneal).
- Femoral nerve branches
  - Saphenous nerve
    - Largest cutaneous branch of femoral nerve
    - Enters foot anterior to medial malleolus
    - Provides sensory innervation to the medial aspect of the ankle and the medial-dorsal foot up to the first metatarsal bone
- Sciatic nerve branches (consist of the tibial nerve and common peroneal nerves): Tibial nerve divides into the posterior tibial nerve and sural nerve. Common peroneal divides into the deep peroneal and superficial peroneal nerves
  - Posterior tibial nerve (enters foot posterior to tibial artery at medial malleolus): gives rise to two nerves that supply most of the sensation to the sole of the foot
    - Lateral plantar nerve: lateral sole of foot
    - Medial plantar nerve: medial sole of foot
  - Sural nerve
    - Formed by branches of the common peroneal and tibial nerves
    - Enters the foot posterior to lateral malleolus

- Sensation to lateral and posterior lower third of inferior leg; sensory to small portion of lateral margin of foot and lateral side of fifth toe
- Deep peroneal nerve (underneath flexor retinaculum anteriorly)
  - Branch of the common peroneal nerve
  - At level of the lateral malleolus, it is bounded medially by the tendon of the extensor hallucis longus and laterally by the anterior tibial artery
  - Skin sensation between first and second toes
- Superficial peroneal nerve (above retinaculum): skin sensation of lateral dorsum of foot and toes except for the first interdigital space (deep peroneal nerve) and lateral aspect of the foot (sural nerve)

Nerve Blocks for the Foot

SENSORY INNERVATION TO THE SOLE OF THE FOOT

- Two nerves supply sensation to sole of foot
  - Posterior tibial nerve block (to numb the lateral and medial plantar nerves) will anesthetize most of the plantar surface
  - Sural nerve (if lateral edge of foot and fifth toe are involved)
  - Posterior ankle block
  - Sural nerve
    - Patient is positioned prone with the foot in slight dorsiflexion
    - Needle is inserted lateral to the Achilles tendon and 1 to 2 cm above the level of the distal tip of the lateral malleolus
    - Needle is redirected in a fan-shaped pattern from side to side as anesthetic is infiltrated
  - Posterior tibial nerve
    - Patient is positioned prone with the foot in slight dorsiflexion. Feel for the posterior tibial artery pulsation (the nerve is just behind the artery)
    - Needle is inserted midway between the medial malleolus anteriorly and the Achilles tendon posteriorly. Raise a wheal at this site, and advance the needle toward the posterior tibial artery
    - Tibial nerve lies under the dense flexor retinaculum; advance the needle until a slight give is felt as the needle penetrates the retinaculum
    - Aspirate and confirm no blood return, and inject 5 ml of 1% lidocaine. Another 5 ml is injected as the needle is withdrawn

SENSORY INNERVATION TO THE DORSUM OF THE FOOT

- Three nerves supply sensation to the dorsum of the foot
  - Saphenous nerve for medial dorsum
  - Superficial peroneal nerve for lateral dorsum

- Deep peroneal nerve if plan to work near the first and second toes
- Anterior ankle block
  - Superficial peroneal nerve block
    - Insert needle immediately above and anterior to the lateral malleolus
    - Inject 5 ml anesthetic subcutaneously between the anterior border of the tibia and the superior aspect of the lateral malleolus
  - Deep peroneal nerve block
    - Patient supine and the ankle in slight plantar flexion
    - Needle is inserted at the upper level of the malleoli between the tendons of the tibialis anterior and extensor hallucis longus
    - Tendons can be accentuated by dorsiflexing the ankle and the great toe against resistance
    - If the anterior tibial artery can be palpated, the needle should be inserted just lateral to the artery
    - Needle is advanced deep to the tendons just above the periosteum, and 5 ml of 1% lidocaine is injected after aspiration
  - Saphenous nerve block
    - Insert needle immediately above and anterior to the medial malleolus
    - Inject 3 to 4 ml anesthetic into the subcutaneous tissue around the great saphenous vein

Nerves of the Hand

- The hand is innervated by four nerves
  - Posterior antebrachial cutaneous nerve
  - Radial nerve
  - Ulnar nerve
  - Median nerve
- Fingers are innervated by four digital nerves
  - Two superior or dorsal nerve branches and two inferior or ventral nerve branches
  - On the dorsal surface of the fingers, digital nerves are branches of the radial and ulnar nerves
  - On the ventral or palmar surface of the fingers, digital nerves are branches of the median and ulnar nerves
- Dorsum of the hand
  - Radial nerve: skin of dorsum of thumb and $2\frac{1}{2}$ digits as far as the distal interphalangeal joint
  - Ulnar nerve: ulnar $1\frac{1}{2}$ digits and adjacent part of dorsum of hand
- Palm of hand
  - Ulnar nerve
    - Sensory to skin of ulnar $1\frac{1}{2}$ digits, motor to muscles of hypothenar eminence
    - Motor to ulnar two lumbricals
    - Motor to seven interossei
    - Motor to adductor pollicis muscle

- Median nerve
  - Sensory to skin of the palmar aspect of thumb and $2\frac{1}{2}$ digits, including the skin on the dorsal aspect of the distal phalanges
  - Motor to muscles of thenar eminence
  - Motor to radial two lumbrical muscles

Hand Blocks

MEDIAN NERVE BLOCK

- Provides sensation to the radial aspect of the palm, palmar surface of the thumb, index finger, middle finger, radial half of the ring finger, and the nail beds of the same digits
- Nerve enters the hand between the flexor carpi radialis and palmaris longus tendons beneath the flexor retinaculum
- Both tendons are identified by asking the patient to oppose the thumb and the fifth digit
- Needle is angled at 45 degrees and enters between the tendons at the level of the proximal wrist crease
- Inject 2 to 5 ml local anesthetic
- If the patient has congenital absence of the palmaris longus muscle, the injection can be made on the medial aspect (toward the ulna) of the flexor carpi radialis tendon
- As the needle passes through the flexor retinaculum, a loss of resistance is felt, marking the point at which the injection should be made
- If paresthesias are elicited, the needle should be withdrawn slightly (i.e., approximately 2 mm) to avoid nerve damage or intraneural injection

DIGITAL NERVE BLOCK

- General considerations
  - Avoid circumferential injections, which may lead to digital ischemia
  - Limit injection volumes to 3 ml total
  - Epinephrine may be used cautiously in digital blocks but should be diluted to 1:200,00 or more (see epinephrine discussion in section on local anesthesia below)
  - Block should be as far back as possible from the surgical site
- Two nerves run on each side of the fingers and toes. These may be blocked with injections on each side of the digit
- Needle is inserted perpendicular to the digit, midway between the palmar and dorsal surfaces of the digit, 1 to 2 cm distal to the web space. Once resistance or bone is felt, aspirate to ensure no blood return, then inject 0.5 ml. Withdraw the needle slightly, and redirect the needle to the dorsal surface, and inject 0.5 ml. Repeat 0.5 ml for the palmar surface. The side, palmar, and dorsal injections all may be done

through one insertion point at the side of the finger by redirecting the needle

WEB SPACE BLOCK

- Needle is inserted from the dorsal aspect of the web space and advanced until the tip tents the palmar skin
- Anesthetic is administered along the side of the digit as the needle is withdrawn
- Epinephrine may be used with caution (see epinephrine discussion above and in section local anesthesia below)

SURGICAL ANATOMY: DANGER ZONES (FIG. 13-5)

- The greatest danger is injury to a major motor nerve, especially at its proximal trunk, because permanent paralysis or weakness may result, causing facial asymmetry and atrophy. All motor nerves and major vessels lie below the superficial musculoaponeurotic system (SMAS) plane and muscle. From most superficial to deepest, the facial layers are
  - Epidermis (most superficial)
  - Dermis

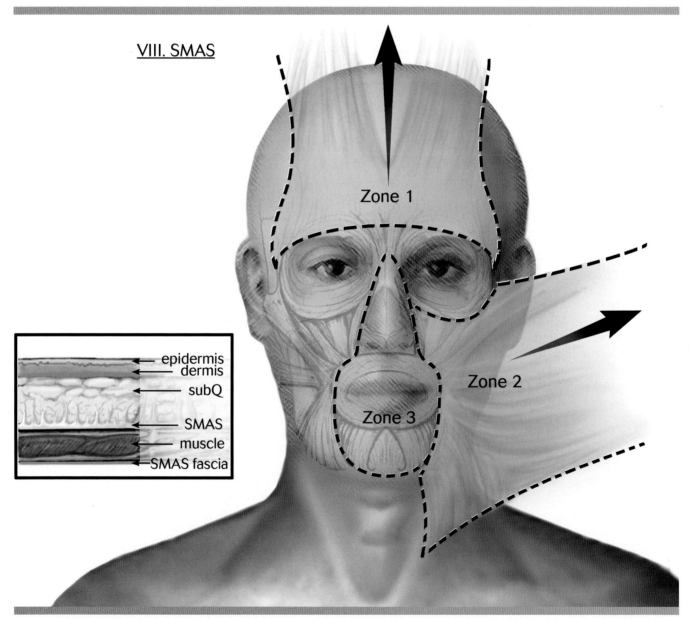

FIGURE 13-5 Superficial musculoaponeurotic system (SMAS).

- Subcutaneous fat
- SMAS
- Muscle
- Deep fat (variable)
- Periosteum
- Bone (deepest)
- Staying above SMAS (when defined) or muscle (when the SMAS is ill-defined) is always safe to avoid motor nerve injury. The SMAS-muscle plane, however, is thin or difficult to identify in three areas, which then are the three *danger zones* in the head and neck for motor nerve injury
  - Temporal nerve (motor to frontalis muscle)
    - Injury will cause drooping of affected eyebrow and flattening of the ipsilateral forehead
    - The nerve is most vulnerable as it exits the superior parotid and crosses the zygomatic arch
    - The nerve is next vulnerable as it travels across the temporal fossa (temple) toward the lateral forehead. Temporal fossa is defined by
      ▲ Superior border: superior temporal line (line palpable from the frontal-temporal hairline to the lateral eyebrow)
      ▲ Inferior border: zygomatic arch
      ▲ Medial border: lateral orbital rim
      ▲ Posterior border: superficial temporal artery and temporal hairline
    - Nerve is protected medial to the superior temporal line because it now lies underneath the frontalis muscle
  - Marginal mandibular nerve (motor to lip depressors)
    - Injury will cause asymmetry of corners of mouth
    - Nerve is relatively superficial as it enters the face where the anterior border of the masseter muscle and mandibular rim intersect. The facial artery also enters the face here. At this region, the marginal mandibular is superifical to the facial artery. The platysma above protects both the artery and the nerve. There is great variation, however, in where the nerve lies relative to the mandibular rim
    - Nerve becomes even more superficial as it travels obliquely up toward the corner of the mouth. As long as one stays above the lip depressor muscles, however, the nerve will not be injured
  - Spinal accessory nerve (motor to trapezius muscle)
    - Injury will cause shoulder drooping and restricted shoulder elevation and abduction
    - Nerve travels in the posterior cervical triangle and may be injured in a region called *Erb's point*. Erb's point is found by drawing a horizontal line connecting the mastoid to the mandibular angle. At the midpoint of this line, a vertical line then is drawn inferiorly to intersect with the posterior border of the sternocleidomastoid muscle (SCM). This intersection is Erb's point, and within a 2- to 4-cm radius of this point, several nerves are at risk: (1) spinal accessory (motor), (2) greater auricular (sensory), and (3) transverse cervical (sensory)
- Other branches of the facial nerve (zygomatic, buccal) are rarely injured because they are well protected by a well-defined layer of SMAS and muscle. Injury to these nerves usually does not cause permanent injury because they have multiple rami and cross-innervate muscles. Nerves medial to a line connecting the lateral canthus to the oral commissure are usually well arborized, and permanent injury is rare medial to this line

Undermining

- Undermining serves to detach or separate vertical and lateral fibrous/fascial attachments that restrict tissue mobility. Undermining usually will increase tissue mobility, decrease wound edge tension, and facilitate wound closure, thereby enhancing postoperative cosmesis
- Disadvantages of undermining include more bleeding and potential injury to deeper structures
- Level of undermining
  - Undermining too deep may be dangerous because vital structures (motor nerves or deep arteries) may be injured
  - Undermining too superficially may compromise tissue viability by thinning the vascular pedicle excessively
  - Undermining should always be above SMAS and muscle with few exceptions. Exceptions include the forehead between the two superior temporal lines laterally and the nose, where undermining should be below the frontalis muscle and nasalis muscle respectively
- Figure 13-6 suggests appropriate planes for undermining in different areas of the face

ANATOMIC REVIEW OF HEAD AND NECK

Superficial Musculoaponeurotic System (SMAS) (Fig. 13-5)

- General definitions
  - Superficial fascia of the face and superficial temporalis fascia (also known as the temporalparietal fascia) are all anatomic extensions

of the SMAS on the face. The superficial fascia of the parotid is also an SMAS extension

- The platysma is the SMAS in the neck
- Superficial fascia of the neck, however, is not SMAS. It is deep to the SMAS/platysma and represents the superficial leaflet of the deep cervical fascia
- The galea on the scalp and its forehead extension (below the frontalis muscle) is also an SMAS equivalent

- SMAS may be thought of as a fascial envelope that encircles the muscles of facial expression in a broad plane across the face. From this fascial plane, fibrous septa extend and insert into the dermis above. Muscles of facial expression, therefore, exert movement of the skin above via the SMAS and its fibrous septal extensions
- The SMAS is a distinct layer in the lateral cheek (zone 2 in Fig. 13-5), temple, and forehead (zone 1 in Fig. 13-5) but becomes wispy or membranous at the medial cheek and around the mouth (zone 3 in Fig. 13-5). At the nose, the SMAS is again distinctive. The SMAS in the scalp and upper face and the SMAS of the lower face fuse at the zygoma
- Importance of SMAS
  - Permits the movement of facial skin in complex expressions
  - Protective anatomic plane: All major motor and sensory nerve trunks and named vessels are deep

(below) to the SMAS. With few exceptions, all motor nerves innervate their respective muscles on the muscle's underside. Staying above the SMAS and muscle, therefore, will prevent motor nerve injury. Peripheral sensory nerves and vessels may perforate the SMAS and travel above it in a superficial plane, but the proximal roots are still sub-SMAS. Example: Supraorbital nerve (sensory) is below SMAS and frontalis muscle at the superior orbital rim where it exits the supraorbital foramen. However, above eyebrow, the nerve penetrates the SMAS and frontalis muscle to travel more superficially, sandwiched between the frontalis muscle below and the fat and forehead skin above

- The SMAS may be plicated and imbricated (done in face lift surgery) to draw tight the facial skin. This is also helpful to decrease wound tension during reconstruction
- Figures 13-6 through 13-8 illustrate anatomy of the eyelid, ear, and nose, respectively

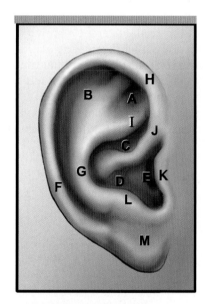

A. Triangular fossa
B. Scaphoid fossa
Concha:
    C. Cymba
    D. Cavum
E. External auditory meatus
F. Helix
G. Antihelix
H. Superior helix
 I. Crura of antihelix
J. Crus of helix
K. Tragus
L. Antitragus
M. Lobule

FIGURE 13-7   Ear anatomy.

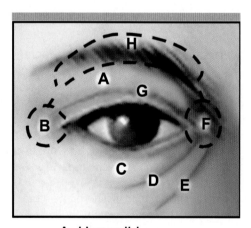

A. Upper lid
B. Lateral canthus
C. Lower lid
D. Infraorbital crease
E. Nasojugal fold
F. Medial canthus
G. Superior palpebral
    sulcus
H. Eyebrow

FIGURE 13-6   Eyelid anatomy.

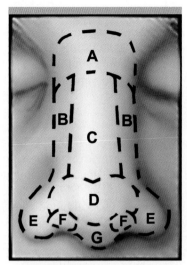

A. Root
B. Lateral side wall
C. Dorsum
D. Tip
E. Ala nasi
F. Soft triangle
G. Columella

FIGURE 13-8 Nasal anatomy.

ELECTROSURGERY (TABLE 13-5)

- Refers to the use of electric current in surgery to produce tissue destruction. Current may be direct current (dc) or alternating current (ac)
  - DC: uses electrons that flow in only one direction. Examples: electrolysis and electrocautery
  - AC: electrons that alternate or regularly reverse direction
    - Ac electrical waveforms may be damped or undamped to produce tissue effects of coagulation, cutting, or fulguration (desiccation)
      - Damped: Waves produced are initially intense and strong and then diminish rapidly. The more rapidly the sine waves return to baseline, the more damped is the current. Damped current coagulates tissue, adding to hemostasis, but causes collateral tissue damage. Examples: electrofulguration, electrodesiccation, electrocoagulation
      - Undamped: Waves produced are pure sine waves. Undamped current cuts tissue without hemostatic effect. Example: electrosection (cutting)
- Complete circuit must exist for electrical energy to flow
- Three basic system components are needed: a power unit, an active electrode, and a dispersive or return electrode
- These three components, along with the patient, form the complete electric circuit
- Monoterminal versus biterminal
  - Monoterminal: delivery of current using only one treatment electrode, without a dispersive electrode. Examples: electrofulguration, electrodesiccation
  - Biterminal: delivery of current via two electrodes, one treatment electrode and one dispersive electrode (usually at a distance from the treatment end). Examples: electrocoagulation and electrosection
    - ▲ Biterminal electrosurgery may be unipolar or bipolar
    - ▲ Unipolar: one treatment electrode and one dispersive electrode (usually a grounding pad at distant site)
    - ▲ Bipolar: A forceps-like device contains both the treatment and the dispersive electrodes

TABLE 13-5 Types of Electrosurgery

Modality	Waveform	Spark Gap Outlet	Voltage	Amperage = Current/Damage
AC				
Electrodessication	Intermittent	Markedly damped	High	Low/moderate
Electrofulguration	Intermittent	Markedly damped	High	Low/moderate
Electrocoagulation	Intermittent	Moderately damped	Moderate	Moderate/high
Electrosection/cutting	Continuous	Undamped	Low	High/high (vaporized)
DC				
Electrolysis			Low	Low
Electocautery			Low	High

△ Current passes from one tine of the forceps to the other tine. Passage of current is restricted between these two tines, which results in substantially less tissue damage than in monopolar devices
△ Bipolar electrosurgery is safest for patients with automatic implantable cardiac defibrillators (AICDs) or pacemakers
△ Dispersive pad is not required because only the tissue grasped between the tines is included in the electric circuit

Properties of Electricity

- Current: flow of electrons during a period of time, measured in amperes (amps)
- Circuit: pathway for the uninterrupted flow of electrons
- Resistance: obstacle to the flow of current, measured in ohms (impedance = resistance)
- Voltage: force pushing current through the resistance, measured in volts
- Direct current (dc): electric current that flows in one direction
- Alternating current (ac): electric current that changes direction during its flow
- Frequency
  - Defined in hertz (Hz)
  - One cycle = the flow of electric current to one direction and back. Hertz is defined as the number of complete cycles per second
  - Usually refers to Ac
- Radiofrequency (rf): an electric current occurring at high frequencies, usually >400,000 cycles per second (Hz)
- Electrode: a physical device; close to or in contact with the patient, through which electrosurgical energy is received or transmitted

Electrocautery

- Refers to a process that uses DC electricity to heat electrodes that are used to produce coagulation
- Tissue effect
  - Results from the application of electrosurgical energy
  - A function of waveform, power setting, electrode size and geometry, activation time, surgical technique (orientation of electrode), and tissue impedance
  - Rate at which heat is produced determines whether a waveform vaporizes tissue or creates a coagulum
  - Hight heat: vaporization
  - Low heat: coagulum

Electrosection (Cutting)

- Undamped waveform; continuous high-frequency ac current causes quick, clean cutting
- Concentrates the energy on a small area
- Causes extreme heating and vaporizing of intracellular fluid that bursts cells

Electrocoagulation

- Biterminal electrosurgery; may be unipolar or bipolar
- A damped waveform that turns on and off several times per second; moderate voltage; moderate/high current
- Excellent for hemostasis of small blood vessels (<2 mm diameter); larger blood vessels (>2 mm) need suture ligation
- Some degree of collateral tissue damage with electrocoagulation
- Average power of a coagulation current is less than that of a cutting current
- Both electrodesiccation and electrofulguration cause superficial coagulation and have hemostatic effects. However, they are technically not electrocoagulation

Electrofulguration (Noncontact Surface Coagulation)

- Monoterminal electrosurgery where treatment electrode is *not* in direct tissue contact. Electric current "sparks" from the electrode tip across the air gap onto the tissue. The electrode is close enough for sparks to bridge the air gap
- Damped waveform; high voltage, low/moderate current
- Intermittent short bursts of high voltage produce superficial coagulation and tissue char

Electrodesiccation

- Monoterminal electrosurgery. Treatment electrode is in contact with tissue
- Damped waveform. Electrofulguration and electrodessication are identical in electrical properties, except that the former is noncontact, and the latter has contact with the treated tissue. Owing to direct tissue contact, charring depth may be slightly deeper in electrodesiccation than in electrofulguration
- No spark is generated

Blended Current

- Blended waveforms are achieved by combining the characteristics of cutting and coagulation waveforms that result in cutting with moderate hemostasis

Ground-Referenced Electrical Surgery Units (ESUs)

- The current is referenced to ground, or rather, the electric circuit is completed through a grounded object

- If there is any interruption or high impedance in the normal return path, the current will seek an alternate path, possibly causing alternate-site burns

Radiofrequency (rf)–Isolated Units

- Most monopolar ESUs are now this type
- The isolation transformer inside the unit isolates the therapeutic current from this ground. Because of this isolation, the therapeutic current is only returned to the ESU and is not connected to earth ground
- This arrangement eliminates the flow of energy if there is no completed pathway to the ESU

Dangers of Electrosurgery

- Burn: A return electrode burn occurs when the heat produced, over time, is not dissipated safely by the size or conductivity of the patient return electrode
- Burn = heat × time/area
- The use of an electrosurgical unit may interfere with the circuitry of an implanted pacemaker
- Patients with an automatic implantable pacemakers and cardioverter/defibrillators (AICDs): The risk of electrosurgery-induced arrhythmia is greater with an AICD than with a pacemaker. Electrosurgery current may mimic the electrical activity of the heart and stimulate the cardiac pacemaker/defibrillator, potentially causing an unnecessary shock (AICD) or an alteration of pacemaker function
- Options for patients with pacemakers or AICDs
  - Electrocautery: safe; no electric current passes into patient
  - Bipolar (biterminal) electrocoagulation: relatively safe in patients with pacemakers and AICDs because the current is restricted between the two forcep tips
  - Unipolar electrocoagulation (biterminal): may be used cautiously in patients with pacemakers and AICD if
    - Bursts of current are short (5 seconds or less)
    - Lowest effective setting is used
    - The dispersive pad/electrode is placed far away from the cardiac device such that the device is not in the path of the current flow
    - The electrosurgery is not directly over the cardiac device
  - Magnet device: placed over a cardiac pacemaker to inhibit it during the procedure. Pacemaker then must be interrogated postoperatively to ensure function
  - AICD deactivation: requires rhythm monitoring and resuscitation abilities during the procedure

CRYOSURGERY (CRYOTHERAPY) (TABLE 13-6)

- Mechanism of action can be divided into three phases: (1) heat transfer, (2) cell injury, and (3) inflammation
- Heat transfer
  - Mechanism by which cryotherapy destroys the targeted cells
  - Quick transfer of heat from the skin to a heat sink
  - Rate of heat transfer depends on the temperature difference between the skin and the liquid nitrogen
  - Liquid nitrogen is applied directly on the skin, and evaporation occurs
  - The heat in the skin is transferred quickly to the liquid nitrogen
  - This process results in the liquid nitrogen evaporating (boiling) almost immediately
- Cell injury
  - Occurs after the cell is frozen, during the thaw
  - Ice crystals do not form until –5 to –10°C
    - Ice crystal formation may be intracellular (more destructive) or extracellular (less tissue damaging)
    - Intracellular ice crystals form with fast freeze; extracellular ice crystals form with slow freeze
  - Greatest destruction seen with
    - Rapid freeze, slow thaw (significant vascular stasis occurs during thaw, contributing to cellular death)
    - Repeat application of rapid freeze and slow thaw
  - Thorough cryotherapy treatment causes basement membrane separation, which may result in blister formation
  - Cell sensitity to cryogen damage
    - Keratinocytes destroyed at –20 to –30°C

TABLE 13-6 Commonly Used Cryogens and Their Temperatures

Cryogen	Boiling Point STP (°C)
Carbon dioxide (solid)	~78.5 (~109.3°F)
Nitrous oxide (liquid)	~89.5 (~129.1°F)
Liquid nitrogen	~195.8 (~320.4°F)

Source: Graham GF, George MN, Patel M: Cryosurgery, in Nouri K, Leal-Khouri S (eds): *Techniques in Dermatologic Surgery.* London: Mosby, 2003.

- Melanocytes are more delicate and only require a temperature of –4 to –7°C for destruction (reason for hypopigmentation with cryotherapy)
  - Dermal fibroblasts: most resistant to freezing, requiring –30 to –35°C
- For malignant tumors, a core tissue temperature of –50°C is required for optimal destruction, whereas benign lesions only require a temperature of –20 to –25°C
- Inflammation
  - Last response to cryotherapy
  - Observed as erythema and edema
  - Inflammation is the response to cell death and helps in local cell destruction

Application of Cryotherapy

- Benign lesions: verruca, xanthelasma, seborrheic keratoses, milia, venous lake, hemangiomas, keloids, lentigines or other epidermal hyperpigmentation, granuloma annulare, prurigo nodularis, myxoid cysts, condyloma
- Malignant lesions: actinic keratosis, basal and squamous cell carcinomas, lentigo maligna, Kaposi's sarcoma

WOUND HEALING

- Wound healing is the restoration of tissue continuity after injury
- Original tissue is replaced with nonspecific connective tissue, which forms a functionally inferior scar
- Epithelialization (sealing of wound) by 48 hours
- Peak collagen formation by 7 days
- Wound tensile strength 20 percent of full by 3 weeks
- Wound tensile strength 60 percent of full by 4 months
- Wound tensile strength never exceeds 80% of full
- Mature scar forms by 6 to 12 months
- Primary healing, delayed primary healing, and healing by secondary intention are the three main categories of wound healing

First-Intention Healing

- Seen in clean, well-perfused, incised surgical wounds and casual wounds inflicted by sharp-edged objects where there is minimum destruction of tissue
- Edges of the wound are closely apposed shortly after injury, and healing occurs without complication
- Epithelial proliferation occurs rapidly (within 24 hours)
- If the wound edges are not reapproximated immediately, delayed primary wound healing transpires

Second-Intention Healing

- When the wound is large, when there has been significant loss or destruction of tissue such that the edges cannot be apposed
- Following tissue injury via an incision, the initial response is usually bleeding followed by vasoconstriction and coagulation
- Wound healing process can be divided into three distinct phases
  - Phase I: Inflammation
    - First 6 to 8 hours
    - Polymorphonuclear leukocytes (PMNs, i.e., neutrophils) flood the wound. Transforming growth factor β (TGF-β) facilitates neutrophil migration (Table 13-7)
    - Monocytes also exude from the vessels and become macrophages once in tissue
    - Macrophages release TGFs, cytokines and interleukin-1 (IL-1), tumor necrosis factor (TNF), and PDGF. Macrophages are the most important cells for wound healing (Table 13-8). Neutropenic or lymphopenic patients do not have impaired wound healing, whereas macrophage-deficient (quantity or function) patients heal poorly
  - Phase II: Granulation
    - Days 5 to 7; can last up to 4 weeks in the clean and uncontaminated wound
    - Fibroblasts have migrated into the wound
    - Wound is suffused with glycosaminoglycans (GAGs) and fibronectin produced by fibroblasts
    - Formation of new vasculature; endothelial cells respond by bud formation
    - Reepithelization occurs with the migration of cells from the periphery of the wound and adnexal structures; reconstitution of the cells of the epidermis into an organized, keratinized, stratified squamous epithelium, which covers the wound defect
  - Phase III: Remodeling
    - Begins after third week; can last for years
    - Dermis responds to injury with a dynamic continuation of collagen synthesis and degradation, and the once highly vascular granulation tissue undergoes a process of devascularization as it matures into less vascular scar tissue

ANTISEPTICS

Infection Control

- Preoperative shaving of hair has been associated with an increase in wound infections. Hairs may be trimmed but not shaved

TABLE 13-7 Growth Factors in Wound Repair

Growth Factor	Effect
Epidermal growth factor and transforming growth factor β (TGF-β)	Reepithelialization
Keratinocyte growth factor (KGF)	Reepithelialization
Heparin-binding epidermal growth factor (HBEGF)	Reepithelialization, fibroblast proliferation
Platelet-derived growth factor (PDGF)	Fibroblast chemotaxis, proliferation, and contraction
Insulin-like growth factor (IGF)	Fibroblast proliferation, extracellular matrix production
Acidic and basic fibroblast growth factors (FGF-1 and FGF-2)	Fibroblast proliferation, angiogenesis
Vascular endothelial growth factor (VEGF)	Angiogenesis
Transforming growth factor β (TGF-β)	Fibroblast chemotaxis and contraction, extracellular matrix production, protease inhibitor production

- Minor procedures such as biopsies: Cleanse with isopropyl alcohol and use nonsterile gloves
- More invasive procedures (excisions with layered closure, flaps, grafts)
  - Skin should be prepared with povidone-iodine (Betadine) or chlorhexidine (Hibiclens) scrub
  - Placement of sterile towels or drapes around the field

Antiseptic

- Agent that kills or inhibits the growth of microorganisms on the external surfaces of the body (Table 13-9)

- Unlike antibiotics that act selectively on a specific target, antiseptics have multiple targets and a broader spectrum of activity, which include bacteria, fungi, viruses, and protozoa

Alcohols

- Alcohol 70% is the optimal strength for killing organisms
- Act by rapid denaturation of biomolecules (DNA, RNA, lipids, etc.) essential to microbial growth and development
- Effective against a broad spectrum of microorganisms

TABLE 13-8 Macrophage Effects

Activity	Effect
Phagocytosis and killing of microorganisms	Wound decontamination
Phagocytosis of tissue debris	Wound debridement
Growth factor release	Formation of new tissue

Source: Bello Y, Falabella A, Eaglstein WH: Wound healing modalities, in Nouri K, Leal-Khouri S (eds): *Techniques in Dermatologic Surgery*. London: Mosby, 2003.

Lie J, Kirsner RS: Wound healing, in Robinson JK, Hanke WC, Sengelmann RD, et al. (eds): *Surgery of the Skin: Procedural Dermatology*. London: Elsevier, 2005.

TABLE 13-9 Topical Antiseptics

	Alcohols	Chlorhexidine Gluconate	Iodine Iodophores	Hexachlorophene	Triclosan
Mode of action	Denaturation of proteins	Disruption of the microbial cell membrane	Oxidation/substitution for elemental form of iodine (free iodine)	Disruption of the microbial cell membrane	Disruption of the microbial cell membrane
Gram-positive bacteria	Excellent	Excellent	Excellent	Excellent	Good
Gram-negative bacteria	Excellent	Good	Good	Fair/Poor	Good (can use for *Pseudomonas*)
Mycobacterium tuberculosis	Good	Fair	Good	Fair	
Virus	Good	Good	Good	Fair	Unknown
Onset of action	Very rapid	Intermediate	Intermediate	Slow/intermediate	Intermediate
Residual activity	None	Excellent	Minimal	Excellent	Excellent
Normal concentration	70–92	4 and 2 (detergent); 0.5 and alcohol; 0.05 water	10, 7.5, 2, 0.5	3	0.3–1.0
Toxicity/side effects	Volatile	Ototoxicity and keratitis	Absorbed through the skin; possible toxicity and irritation	Neurotoxic	Under investigation

- Fastest and greatest reduction in microbial counts on the skin

Chlorhexidine Gluconate (Hibiclens)

- Antiseptic and an antimicrobial agent
- Rapidly acting antiseptic that is effective against both gram-positive and gram-negative bacteria and some fungi
- Antimicrobial action is attributed to disruption of the microbial cell membrane and precipitation of cell contents
- It should not be in contact with eyes, middle ears, and meninges

Triclosan

- Derived from a potent antiseptic called *phenol*
- Effective against gram-positive and most gram-negative bacteria
- Used in soaps, creams, and solutions in concentrations up to 2% for hand and skin disinfection and for skin disinfection prior to surgery
- Avoid contact of this medicine with the eyes

Povidone-Iodine (PVP-I)

- Results from the combination of molecular iodine and polyvinylpyrrolidone

- Combination of iodine with a carrier that decreases iodine availability because molecular iodine can be very toxic for tissues
- Iodine preparations have the added advantage of being sporicidal
- Mechanism of action: Iodine precipitates the proteins of the microorganisms by forming salts via direct halogenation. Approximately 90% of the iodine absorbed by bacterial cells reappears as the iodide, thus confirming oxidative interaction as the major bactericidal activity

Hexachlorophene (Phisohex)

- Chlorinated bisphenol antiseptic with a bacteriostatic action against gram-positive organisms but much less effective against gram-negative organisms
- Antibacterial component in drug and cosmetic products
- Absorbed through intact skin
- Potentially neurotoxic, especially in neonates

Antibiotics and Surgical Procedures (Table 13-10)

- Risk of wound infection after skin surgery is small

TABLE 13-10 Antibiotic Prophylaxis Policy for Prevention of Endocarditis and Prosthesis Infection (MD Anderson Cancer Center, Mohs/Dermatology Surgery Center)

Procedure	Indication	Skin Condition	Prophylaxis
Mohs	High risk	All conditions	Yes
Excision biopsy/cryosurgery/EDC/laser	High risk	Intact	No*
		Inflamed/infected (i.e., inflamed cyst)	Yes

High-Risk Patients (Prophylaxis)	Low-Risk Patients (No Prophylaxis)
<ul><li>Prosthetic valve</li><li>History of bacterial endocarditis</li><li>Mitral valve prolapse with regurgitation</li><li>Mitral valve prolapse without regurgitation in MEN > 45 years</li><li>Any valve dysfunction</li><li>Cardiac malformation</li><li>Hypertrophic cardiomyopathy</li><li>Orthopedic prostheses</li><li>CNS shunts</li><li>Shunt/fistula with nearby inflamed or</li><li>infected tissue</li></ul>	<ul><li>History of rheumatic fever without valve dysfunction</li><li>S/P CABG</li><li>Pacemaker or pacemakers/defibrillator combination</li><li>Physiologic, functional or innocent murmur</li><li>MVP without regurgitation</li><li>Secundum atrial septal defect</li><li>> 6 months postop from repair of ASD (atrial septal defect), VSD (ventricular septal defect), PDA (patent ductus arteriosus)</li><li>Arterial grafts</li><li>Penile prostheses</li><li>Breast implants</li></ul>

Antibiotic Regimens

Non Oral Site (All doses given 30–60 minutes before surgery)	Oral Site (All doses given 30–60 minutes before surgery)
Keflex 2 g PO	Amoxicillin 2 g PO

PCN allergic (type I anaphylaxis reaction)
    Clindamycin 600 mg PO
    Azithromycin or clarithromycin 500 mg PO
	PCN allergic (Type I anaphylaxis reaction)
	    Clindamycin 600 mg PO
	    Azithromycin or clarithromycin 500 mg PO

* Exception: Breach of nasal or oral mucosa, then yes prophylaxis.

- Routine prophylactic antibiotics are usually not indicated except for patients or anatomic sites at greatest risk for infection
- If antibiotics are given, they must be in the bloodstream at time surgery in order to be effective
- Infections are more likely in immunosuppressed, debilitated patients and those with reduced blood flow to the surgical site, e.g., PVD or diabetes mellitus
- Ears, perineum, legs, and feet seem to be the areas at greatest risk for wound infection
- Open wounds almost never become infected, whereas closed wounds with hematomas or a large amount of necrotic tissue are at increased risk for infection
- Prophylactic antiherpesvirus medications are indicated in any lip surgery, including laser procedures
- Risk of bacteremia after skin surgery is slight; risk is similar to control

FLAP AND GRAFT REVIEW

Definition of Terms

- Flap (Table 13-11)
  - Transfer of regional donor tissue (skin and subcutaneous) with its direct vascular supply into a wound defect (recipient site) for closure. Regional tissue may be directly connected to the defect or be nearby but not contiguous. Flaps are usually performed when a primary straight-line closure is not possible (owing to excess tension or potential anatomic/functional distortion)

- Flaps may be categorized by either (1) blood supply (axial versus random pattern) or (2) type of movement (advancement, rotation, transposition)
- *Pedicle:* the vascular supply to a flap (blood vessels are contiguous with the flap)
- *Random-pattern flap:* flap that is nourished by unnamed vessels from underlying arterial perforators. Random flaps rely on a rich vascular plexus of subcutaneous tissue that directly connects with the flap
- *Axial-pattern flap:* flap that has a named vessel for its pedicle. Axial flap examples include (1) paramedian forehead flap (supratrochlear artery), (2) cheek interpolation flap (angular artery), and (3) Abbé (lip-switch) flap (inferior or superior labial arteries). Axial flaps also may be called *interpolation flaps* and typically require at least two separate stages of surgery, usually separated by 3 weeks between stages. Axial-pattern flaps are usually done for larger defects, where either most of the entire subunit is missing
- *Advancement, rotation, transposition flaps:* flaps so named based on their primary type of movement. In reality, flaps may have more than one movement (i.e., advancement and rotation)
- *Tension vector:* the direction of pull or stress on a wound during its closure
- *Primary defect:* the wound that requires closure
- *Secondary defect:* the wound that results from closure of the primary defect
- *Primary movement:* the motion (advancement, rotation, or transposition) and tension vectors required for closure of the primary defect. Rotation and transposition flaps have in common a pivoting

TABLE 13-11 Types of Flaps

Name	Site	Action
Advancement flaps: A-T, O-T, Burrow's triangle wedge	Forehead, eyebrow, helix, preauricular, upper lip	Slides tissue into defect in linear direction; create as single- or double-pedical flap
Rotation Flaps: O-Z, glabellar turn-down, hatchet flap	Scalp, forehead, cheeks nose, lip	Rotates skin (pivots) directly into defect; single or double rotation
Transposition flaps: rhombic, bilobed, nasolabial		Movement (also a rotational or pivoting motion) of donor tissue over an intervening island of normal skin to fill defect

or arclike motion, whereas advancement flaps have a sliding motion in straight lines

- *Secondary movement:* the motion and tension vectors required to close the secondary defect
- *Burow's triangle/dog-ear/standing cutaneous cone:* redundant skin that is removed as wounds are closed
- *Primary Burow's triangle:* The dog-ear directly connected to the primary defect that is removed during closure
- *Secondary Burow's triangle:* the dog-ear directly connected to the secondary defect that is removed during closure
- *Subunit:* a surface area demarcated by either natural or arbitrary lines that has unique textural, cosmetic, or functional characteristics. The upper lip, for example, has four subunits: the bilateral upper cutaneous lip, the philtrum, and the mucosal lip. In general, repairs within a subunit or incisions placed at junctions of subunits yield the best cosmetic results

Advancement Flap

- A random-pattern flap where the primary flap movement is linear. The flap tissue "slides" in a straight line into the recipient site during closure. Advancement flaps typically result in linear, perpendicular lines
- Advancement flaps provide the least mobility among the different flap types
- Types of advancement flaps
  - Unilateral advancement
    - Classic unilateral advancement
    - Burow's wedge advancement flap
    - V-Y advancement flap (an island pedicle flap with advancement as its primary movement)
  - Bilateral advancement
    - Classic H-plasty
    - A-T or O-T advancement (commonly done on chin, ear, and suprabrow) (Fig. 13-9)
- Areas of applications: eyebrow or mustache area, nasal sidewall, temple, upper cutaneous lip, ear (especially helical rim)

Rotation Flap

- Random-pattern flap where the donor tissue pivots directly into the defect in a curved or arclike motion; lines from a rotation flap are typically curved or arciform
- Areas of application: scalp, cheek, nose, upper cutaneous lip. Rotation flaps may close relatively large defects
- *Backcut:* a relaxing incision on the far end of a rotation curve to release lateral flap restraints and facilitate movement
- Rotation flap variations

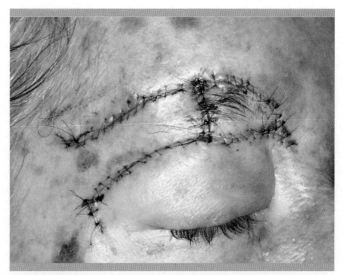

FIGURE 13-9 Bilateral advancement flap. *(From Freedberg IM et al: Fitzpatrick's Dermatology in General Medicine, 6th ed. New York: McGraw-Hill, 2003, p. 2526.)*

- O-Z double rotation flap
- Rieger flap (dorsal nasal rotation flap with backcut at glabella): also known as hatchet flap or glabellar turn-down flap
- Mustarde flap (rotation flap from the lateral canthus/cheek to close lower eyelid or infraorbital defect)

Transposition Flaps

- Donor tissue is nearby but not directly adjacent to defect. The flap, therefore, must move across and over an intervening segment of normal skin to close the defect. Both transposition and rotation flaps have a pivoting and rotational movement. What distinguishes the former is that transpositions must pivot over an intervening area of normal skin to reach the defect, whereas rotation flaps pivot directly into the defect
- Transposition flaps may be random pattern or axial in the pedicle. A common source of confusion is nasolabial (melolabial) transposition (NLTF) versus nasolabial (melolabial) interpolation flap (NLIF). Both flaps are transposition flaps in their movement. NLTF is a one-stage transposition flap, whereas the latter NLIF is a two-stage transposition flap
- Lines from transposition flaps typically are acute (<90 degrees) and Z-shaped or zigzag
- Random-pattern transposition flaps
  - Rhombic flaps
    - Webster: 30-degree transposition (Fig. 13-10)
    - Dufourmental
    - Limberg: 60 degrees

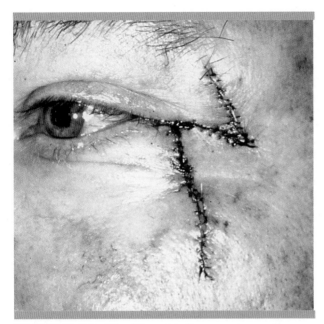

FIGURE 13-10 Rhombic flap, postoperative.
(From Freedberg IM et al: Fitzpatrick's Dermatology in General Medicine, 6th ed. New York: McGraw-Hill, 2003, p. 2583.)

- Nasolabial (melolabial) transposition flap (also known as a banner flap): commonly done for lateral alar defects. Its major disadvantage is that it may blunt the alar groove
- Bilobed transposition: commonly done for distal third nasal tip defects
- Z-plasty: commonly done for scar revision (altering scar length and changing scar orientation)
- Z-plasty: distinct form of transposition often used for scar revision. Z-plasties have two properties: (1) change (redirection) of tension vectors of the original wound/scar and (2) lengthening and breaking up of a scar into multiple zigzag lines. The extent of scar lengthening depends on the degree of transposition of the Z-plasty

Z-plasties and Scar-Lengthening Properties

Degree of Transposition	Extent of Scar Lengthening (percent)
30°	25
45°	50
60°	75

- Axial-pattern transposition flaps (axial flaps are usually done for larger defects, where either most or the entire subunit is missing)

- Paramedian forehead (midline forehead flap): forehead donor flap transposed onto nasal defect based on supratrochlear artery (Fig. 13-11)
- Nasolabial interpolation flap: lower cheek flap at melolabial fold transposed onto nasal ala skin based on angular artery
- Abbé flap (lip-switch flap): lower lip flap (mucosa, muscle, skin, and subcutis) transposed superiorly to repair upper lip defect based on inferior labial artery. The former is most commonly done, but upper lip to lower lip switch based on superior labial artery also may be performed

Island Pedicle Flap (IPF)

- Classically, IPFs are random-pattern flaps. IPFs are unique in that they are completely separated from the surrounding skin (literally an island) and subcutis except for an underlying subcutaneous pedicle directly underneath the flap
- Classically, IPFs are considered advancement flaps, but practically, both advancement and rotation movements are involved. Even transposition movements are possible with IPFs
- IPF suture lines look like a triangle has been moved into the defect
- V-Y advancement is a type of IPF

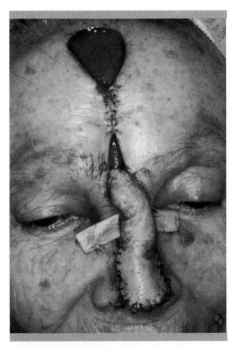

FIGURE 13-11 Paramedian forehead flap, intraoperative.
(From Freedberg IM et al: Fitzpatrick's Dermatology in General Medicine, 6th ed. New York: McGraw-Hill, 2003, p. 2527.)

Autologous Skin Grafts

- Skin that is detached completely from its blood supply, removed from its donor site, and transplanted to a recipient site for wound closure in the same individual
- All grafts require surgery at the donor site for harvesting
- All grafts contract to some degree, but contraction is greatest with split-thickness skin grafts
- Survival of skin grafts depends on the establishment of new vasculature between the wound recipient site and the donor graft. Process of healing occurs in several phases
  - Plasma imbibition (first 48 hours)
    - *Imbibition* means to take in or absorb fluid, causing swelling
    - Ischemic and edematous phase of graft because no blood flow established
    - Grafts survive the first 1 to 2 days by absorbing wound exudate and passive diffusion of nutrients. Graft appears cyanotic and edematous
    - Fibin also forms between the recipient bed and graft, promoting graft adhesion and reducing infection
  - Inosculation (days 2 to 3)
    - Initial establishment of vessels between the recipient bed and graft; new vessels form from the recipient bed and migrate to anastamose with vasculature from the graft
    - Fibrin mesh established during imbibition facilitates vessel migration
  - Capillary ingrowth/revascularization (days 4 to 7)
    - Additional vascular anastamoses occur between wound base and graft
    - Blood flow evident by days 5 to 7
  - Keratinocyte activation (fourth day up to 4 weeks)
    - Epidermal activation and proliferation, greater in split-thickness skin grafts
    - Lymphatic flow reestablished
  - Sensory innervation (begins after 2 to 3 months): starts at edge of graft and moves centrally

Types of Autologous Skin Grafts

- Full-thickness skin graft (FTSG)
  - Entire epidermis and a dermis harvested. Dermis may be of varying thickness depending on donor site
  - Advantages: minimal contraction during healing phase. Potential for good match with recipient site if donor site properly selected. Donor site is usually sutured or closed
  - Disadvantage: Other than donor site morbidity, FTSGs require more metabolic support (thicker) and do not survive as well as STSGs

- Potential FTSG donor sites for facial wounds: upper eyelid, nasolabial fold, pre- and postauricular regions, conchal bowl, and the supraclavicular fossa. Donor sites are selected based on matching qualities for thickness, texture, pigmentation, actinic damage, and morbidity of donor harvesting
- Split-thickness skin graft (STSG)
  - Epidermis and only partial-thickness dermis
  - Thin (0.005 to 0.012 in), intermediate (0.012 to 0.018 in), or thick (0.018 to 0.030 in)
  - Advantages: much thinner, requires less metabolic support, and survives better than FTSGs. Able to cover large wounds, line cavities, resurface mucosal deficits, exposed bone, close donor sites of flaps, and resurface muscle flaps. Harvested from any surface of the body
  - Disadvantages: requires more equipment, significant contraction occurs at recipient site, cosmetically poor compared to FTSGs, and discomfort and appearance of donor site (donor site heals by second intention, a rectangular discolored patch is typical postoperative appearance)

Composite Grafts

- Contains two different tissue layers (i.e., skin and cartilage)
- Advantage: provides structure (cartilage) as well as soft tissue covering. Donor site is usually crus of the helix to include skin and cartilage
- Disadvantage: most metabolically demanding of all graft types. Most composite grafts over 1 cm do not survive completely

LOCAL ANESTHESIA

- Anesthetics block membrane Na^+/K^+ channels, thus preventing effective depolarization and nerve transmission
- Unmyelinated C-type nerve fibers (slow conduction) that conduct temperature and pain are blocked more easily than myelinated A-type fibers (fast conduction) that carry pressure and motor fibers
- Two main groups of local anesthetics: esters and amides. Groups differentiated by their intermediate chain. Cocaine (ester group) is vasoconstricting; all others anesthetics are vasodilating
- Esters: hydrolyzed in plasma and liver by pseudocholinesterases and excreted by kidney
- Amides: *N*-dealkylated and hydrolyzed by microsomal liver enzymes cytochrome P450 3A4
- Lidocaine 1% with 1:100,000 epinephrine
  - Standard local anesthetic for skin surgery

- Very acidic (low pH)
- Addition of $NaHCO_3$ to lidocaine with epinephrine neutralizes solution, reducing burning on injection and facilitating anesthetic diffusion
- Longer-lasting anesthetics (>2 hour duration) are more protein bound and include bupivacaine and etidocaine

Side Effects of Local Anesthetics

- Relative contraindications
  - End-stage liver disease (altered drug metabolism)
  - Severe blood pressure instability
  - Pregnancy (small volumes of lidocaine without epinephrine may be used for essential procedures)
- Absolute contraindications
  - True allergy to the anesthetic (more common with esters than amides)
  - Contraindications for ester anesthetics
    - Severe renal compromise
    - Pseudocholinesterase deficiency
    - Allergy to PABA compounds
- Most frequent side effect encountered
  - Vasovagal reaction with hypotension and bradycardia
  - Rx: Place patient in Trendelenburg position to increase cerebral perfusion; supportive care; atropine for severe reactions

- Local side effects
  - Bruising and edema, especially in periorbital area
  - Transient motor nerve paralysis
  - Prolonged paresthesia: Nerve injury can occur in nerve blocks if needle traumatizes nerve

Lidocaine Toxicity (Table 13-12)

- Maximum dose of lidocaine
  - 5 mg/kg of 1% lidocaine plain
  - 7 mg/kg of 1% lidocaine with 1:100,000 epinephrine
- Starts with circumoral numbness and tingling; can progress to seizures and cardiovascular collapse with severe overdosage; toxic effects are exacerbated by acidosis and hypoxia
- Allergic reactions are usually IgE-mediated type I reactions with urticaria, angioedema, or anaphylaxis with hypotension and tachycardia
- True allergic reactions to ester anesthetics are infrequent, but there is cross-reactivity with PABA, sulfonamides, sulfonylureas, thiazides, and paraphenylene diamine

Prilocaine Toxicity

- Metabolizes to ortho-toluidine, an oxiding agent capable of converting hemoglobin to methemoglobin, potentially causing methemoglgbinemia. Patients at risk of methemoglobinemia include

TABLE 13-12 Systemic Lidocaine Toxicity

Organ system	Signs	Treatment
Central nervous system Early (1–5 μg/ml)	Tinnitus, circumoral pallor, metallic taste in mouth, lightheadedness, talkativeness, nausea, emesis, diplopia	Recognition, observation, hold lidocaine
Middle (8–12 μg/ml)	Nystagmus, slurred speech, hallucinations, muscle twitching, facial, hand tremors, seizures	Diazepam, airway maintenance
Late (20–25 μg/ml)	Apnea, coma	Respiratory support
Cardiovascular system	Myocardial depression, bradycardia, atrioventricular blockade, ventricular arrythmias, vasodilation, hypotension	Oxygen, vasopressors, cardiopulmonary resuscitation
Allergy	Pruritus, urticaria, angioedema, nausea, wheezing, anaphylaxis	Antihistamines; epinephrine 0.3 ml 1:1000 SQ, oxygen, airway
Psychogenic	Pallor, diaphoresis, hyperventilation, lightheadedness, nausea, syncope	Trendelenburg position, cool compresses, observation

- Patients <1 year old
- Patients with G-6-PD deficiency
- Methemoglobinemia-inducing agents: dapsone, nitroglycerin, nitrofurantoin, antimalarials, sulfonamides, phenobarbitol, phenytoin, nitroprusside, acetaminophen
- Application of EMLA to large surface areas and eroded skin (increase absorption)

Bupivacaine Toxicity

- Risk of cardiac toxicity, with ventricular arrhythmias and cardiovascular collapse

Epinephrine

- Epinephrine prolongs duration of anesthesia by 100 to 150 percent and decreases the anesthetic's systemic toxicity by slowing absorption
- Epinephrine is hemostatic in a dilution of up to 1:1,000,000
- Absolutely contraindicated in uncontrolled hyperthyroidism and pheochromocytoma
- Relative contraindications: hypertension, severe cardiovascular disease, pregnancy, and narrow-angle glaucoma, beta blockers, phenothiazines, monoamine oxidase inhibitors, and tricyclic antidepressants
- Epinephrine use in digital anesthesia (fingers/toes): Safe to use in digital blocks and local anesthesia as long as these guidelines are followed:
  - Epinephrine dilution of 1:200,000 or greater
  - Volumes injected are minimal (digital block should not exceed 3 ml—1.5 ml max per side)
  - Circumferential injection (ring block) is avoided
  - Patients with vascular compromise are avoided (smokers, diabetes, peripheral vascular disease, Raynaud's phenomenon)
- In relative contraindications, epinephrine may be used by diluting it to 1:500,000; use sparingly
- Side effects of epinephrine include self-limited palpitations, anxiety, fear, diaphoresis, headache, tremor, weakness, and tachycardia
- Serious side effects include arrhythmias, ventricular tachycardia, ventricular fibrillation, cardiac arrest, and cerebral hemorrhage

Topical Anesthetics (Table 13-13)

- Conjunctiva anesthetized with proparacaine or tetracaine eyedrops
- Superficial mucous membrane anesthesia: Surfacaine, Topicale, Dyclone, Anbesol, viscous lidocaine, and lidocaine jelly
- Intranasal mucosa: 4% to 10% cocaine solution is effective, and hemostatic
- EMLA (eutectic mixture of local anesthetics) cream contains 2.5% lidocaine and 2.5% prilocaine;

applied under occlusion 1 to 2 hours preoperatively depending on location
- Should be applied to intact skin only and in patients older than 1 year of age. Application to denuded skin or to large surface areas may result in substantial prilocaine absorption and risk of systemic methemoglobinemia. Alternative to EMLA is 30% to 40% lidocaine in acid-mantle cream applied under occlusion 1 to 2 hours before the procedure
- ELA-Max (4% lidocaine) liposomal delivery; thus no occlusion necessary; no chance of methemoglobinemia as with EMLA. Available over the counter; comes in 5- and 30-g tubes
- Iontophoresis of lidocaine also can achieve superficial skin anesthesia

Alternatives to Esters and Amides for Local Anesthesia

- Diphenhydramine hydrochloride (Benadryl) 12.5 mg/ml
- Normal saline injected intradermally (transient brief anesthesia)
- Ice or cryogen application; cryoanesthesia with fluoroethyl or frigiderm for superficial procedures; dermabrasion

Tumescent Anesthesia

- *Tumesce* means to swell. *Tumescent anesthesia* (TA) is the use of dilute lidocaine (0.05% to 0.1%) and epinephrine (1:1,000,000) for local anesthesia. Large volumes of TA may be infiltrated subcutaneously to achieve complete anesthesia and effective hemostasis
- Tumescent pharmacology applies only to dilute lidocaine and epinephrine; it cannot be extrapolated to other anesthetics (i.e., lidocaine cannot be substituted for bupivacaine)
- TA applications: originally developed for liposuction. Other uses: face lift surgery, reconstruction, ambulatory phlebectomy, ablative laser resurfacing, hair transplantation, endovenous radiofrequency ablation
- TA advantages
  - Increases maximum safe dose of lidocaine to 55 mg/kg (maximum lidocaine dose for nontumescent formulations is 7 mg.kg of 1% lidocaine and epinephrine)
  - Dilute epinephrine achieves pronounced vasoconstriction of subdermal vessels, thereby limiting systemic absorption while achieving excellent hemostasis
  - Some procedures (liposuction, phlebectomy, endovenous ablation) cannot be done safely in an outpatient setting without TA
- TA disadvantages
  - Requires equipment and understanding of tumescent pharmacology

TABLE 13-13 Local Anesthetics

Generic Name	Trade Name	Primary Use	Relative Potency	Onset	Duration* Plain	Maximum Dose[†] Plain	Maximum Dose with Epinephrine[†]
Amides							
Bupivacaine	Marcaine	Infiltration	8	2–10 min	30–10 h	175mg	250 mg
Dibucaine	Nupercaine	Topical		Rapid	Short		
Etidocaine	Duranest	Infiltration	6	3–5 min	3–10 h	300 mg	400 mg
Lidocaine	Xylocaine	Infiltr./topical	2	Rapid	1–2 h	300 mg	500 mg (3850 mg dilute)
Mepivacaine	Carbocaine	Infiltration	2	3–20 min	2–3 h	300 mg	400 mg
Prilocaine	Citanest	Infiltration	2	Rapid	2–4 h	400 mg	600 mg
Prilocaine/ lidocaine	EMLA	Topical		30–120 min	Short		
Esters							
Benzocaine	Anbersol, etc.	Topical		Rapid	Short		
Chloroprocaine	Nesacaine	Infiltration	1	Rapid	0.5–2 h	600 mg	
Cocaine		Topical		2–10 min	1–3 h	200 mg	
Procaine	Novocaine	Infiltration	1	Slow	1–1.5 h	500 mg	600 mg
Proparacaine	Ophthaine	Topical		Rapid	Short		
Tetracaine	Pontocaine	Infiltration	8	Slow	2–3 h	20 mg	
Tetracaine	Cetacaine	Topical		Rapid	Short		

*Clinically, duration of anesthesia may be less than stated above, especially for head and neck; addition of epinephrine prolongs anesthesia by factor of two.
[†] Maximum doses are for a 70-kg person.

- Swelling of subcutaneous space is typical but may be prolonged in the lower extremities
- Caution warranted with drug interactions (competitors with liver cytochrome P450 enzymes may interfere with lidocaine metabolism and increase toxicity)
- Remember: amides are metabolized by the liver and excreted by the kidney
- Esters are metabolized by tissue pseudocholinesterase and excreted by the kidney; may cross-react with PABA
- Lidocaine is class B in pregnancy; avoid complex procedures in the first trimester

SUTURE REVIEW

Suture Characteristics (Tables 13-14 and 13-15)
- Tensile strength: measure of a material or tissue's ability to resist deformation and breakage
- Knot strength: force required for a knot to slip
- Configuration
  - Monofilament (less risk of infection)
  - Braided multifilament (easier to handle and tie)
- Elasticity: degree suture stretches and returns to original length
- Memory or suture stiffness: inherent capability of suture to return to or maintain its original gross shape

TABLE 13-14 Suture Materials

	Type	Memory	Tissue Reactivity	Tensile Strength Half-Life
Nonabsorbable				
Cotton	Twisted	Low	Very high	—
Nylon (Ethilon, Demalon)	Monofilament	High	Low	—
Nylon (Nurolon, Surgilon)	Braided	Low	Low	—
Polybutester (Novafil)	Monofilament	High	Low	—
Polyester, uncoated (Mersilene)	Bralded	Low	Low	—
Polyester, coated (EthiGoodd)	Bralded	Low	Low	—
Polypropylene (Prolene, Surgilene)	Monofilament	Very high	Very low	—
Silk	Braided/twisted	Very low	High	—
Stainless steel	Monofilament/ braided/twisted	Very high	Very low	—
Absorbable				
Catgut, fast absorbing/mild chromic	Twisted	Very high	High	2 days
Catgut	Twisted	Very high	High	4 days
Catgut, chromic	Twisted	Very high	High	1 week
Polyglactin 910 (Vicryl)	Braided	Very low	Low	2 weeks
Polyglycolic acid (Dexon)	Braided	Very low	Low	2 weeks
Poliglecaprone 25 (Monocryl)	Monofilament	Low	Very low	1 week
Polyglyconate (Maxon)	Monofilament	Low	Very low	1 month
Polydoxanone (PDS)	Monofilament	High	Very low	1 month

Source: Weitzul S, Taylor RS: Suturing techniques and other closure materials, in Robinson JK, Hanke WC, Sengelmann RD, et al. (eds): *Surgery of the Skin: Procedural Dermatology.* London: Elsevier, 2005.

TABLE 13-15 Epidermal Suture Applications

Simple running	Fast epidermal closure May not approximate skin as precisely as simple interrupted May unravel if one segment is severed
Simple interrupted	Time-consuming Best for correcting minor differences in overlapping edge Most accurate for skin approximation
Vertical mattress	Suture line perpendicular to wound edge Time-consuming Best suture for additional wound edge eversion May strangulate wound edge if tied too tightly
Horizontal mattress	Suture line parallel to wound edge Time-consuming Moderate wound edge eversion Helpful in hemostasis for nonspecific wound edge oozing
Running subcuticular	Entire suture is buried in the superficial dermis except for an entry and exit point on either ends of the wound edge Time-consuming Beneficial for closure that requires epidermal support greater than 1 week; running subcuticular suture may be left in place greater than 1 week and removed later without railroad tracks on skin

Note: All epidermal sutures will leave cross-marks of railroad-track lines on skin if not removed within 1 week.

- Plasticity: measure of the ability to deform without breaking and to maintain a new form after relief of the deforming force
- Pliability: ease of handling of suture material; ability to adjust knot tension and to secure knots (related to suture material, filament type, and diameter)

REFERENCES

Baker S, Swanson N: *Local Flaps in Facial Reconstruction.* London: Mosby, 1995.

Bello Y, Falabella A, Eaglstein WH: Wound healing modalities, in Nouri K, Leal-Khouri S (eds): *Techniques in Dermatologic Surgery.* London: Mosby, 2003.

Castro-Ron G, Pasquali P: Cryosurgery, in Robinson JK, Hanke WC, Sengelmann RD, et al. (eds): *Surgery of the Skin: Procedural Dermatology.* London: Elsevier, 2005.

Cook JL, Goldman GD: Random pattern cutaneous flaps, in Robinson JK, Hanke WC, Sengelmann RD, et al. (eds): *Surgery of the Skin: Procedural Dermatology.* London: Elsevier, 2005.

Graham GF, George MN, Patel M: Cryosurgery, in Nouri K, Leal-Khouri S (eds): *Techniques in Dermatologic Surgery.* London: Mosby, 2003.

Larrabee WF, Makielski KH, Henderson JL: *Surgical Anatomy of the Face,* 2nd ed. Baltimore: Lippincott Williams & Wilkins, 2004.

Lie J, Kirsner RS: Wound healing, in Robinson JK, Hanke WC, Sengelmann RD, et al. (eds): *Surgery of the Skin: Procedural Dermatology.* London: Elsevier, 2005.

Nguyen TH: Topical and local anesthesia, in Narins RS (ed): *Cosmetic Surgery.* New York: Marcel Dekker, 2001:411–441.

Nouri K, Trent J, Lodha R: Aseptic techniques, in Nouri K, Leal-Khouri S (eds): *Techniques in Dermatologic Surgery.* London: Mosby, 2003.

Putz R, Pabst R: *Sobotta Atlas of Human Anatomy,* vol 1, 13th ed. Baltimore: Lippincott Williams & Wilkins, 2001.

Robinson JK, Anderson Jr R. Skin structure and anatomy, in Robinson JK, Hanke WC, Sengelmann RD, et al. (eds): *Surgery of the Skin: Procedural Dermatology.* London: Elsevier, 2005.

Soon SL, Washington CV. Electrosurgery, electrocoagulation, electrofulguration, electrodessication, electrosection, electro-cautery, in Robinson JK, Hanke WC, Sengelmann RD, et al. (eds): *Surgery of the Skin: Procedural Dermatology.* London: Elsevier, 2005.

Soriano TT, Lask GP, Dinehart SM: Anesthesia and analgesia, in Robinson JK, Hanke WC, Sengelmann RD, et al. (eds): *Surgery of the Skin: Procedural Dermatology.* London: Elsevier, 2005.

Weiss RA, Feied CF, Weiss MA: *Vein Diagnosis & Treatment: A Comprehensive Approach.* New York: McGraw-Hill, 2001.

Weitzul S, Taylor RS: Suturing techniques and other closure materials, in Robinson JK, Hanke WC, Sengelmann RD, et al. (eds): *Surgery of the Skin: Procedural Dermatology.* London: Elsevier, 2005.

CHAPTER 14

COSMETIC DERMATOLOGY

RAMSEY MARKUS
ASRA ALI

Skin Aging

- Intrinsic: natural aging, genetic process
- Extrinsic: exogenous causes; ultraviolet radiation, smoking
- Photoaging
- Skin is changed or damaged as a result of exposure to ultraviolet radiation in sunlight and other sources
- Long-term effects
  - Wrinkles
  - Discoloration
  - Telangiectasia
  - Susceptibility to cancer
  - Solar elastosis (heliosis): term applied to the chronic inflammatory changes and degradation of elastin and collagen

Ultraviolet B Light (UV-B)

- 290 to 320 nm
- Photons 1000 times more energetic than UV-A
- Absorbed by the epidermis, approximately 10 percent penetrating to deeper layers of the skin
- Causes acute sunburn, skin cancer

Ultraviolet A Light (UV-A)

- UV-A I: 340 to 400 nm
- UV-A II: 320 to 340 nm
- 10-fold greater abundance in terrestrial sunlight compared to UV-B
- Approximately 50 percent of UV-A radiation penetrates the epidermis and reaches the papillary dermis
- Causes delayed tanning

Molecular Mechanism of Photoaging

- UV light activates activator protein 1 (AP-1)
- AP-1 upregulates extracellular matrix–degrading metalloproteinases
- Modules related to aging

- Extracellular signal-regulated kinase (ERK): photoaging
- c-Jun NH_2-terminal kinase (JNK): natural aging
- UV light generates hydroxyl radicals: damages DNA
- Blocks transforming growth factor β (TGF-β) receptor II gene; prevents procollagen promoter with a reduction of collagen formation

Telomeres and Aging Skin

- Telomeres: tandem repeats of the DNA base sequence (TTAGGGG) (T-thymine, G = guanine, A = adenosine), at the end of mammalian chromosomes
- DNA polymerase does not copy the final bases on each chromosome, resulting in telomere shortening after each round of cell division
- When the telomeres become too short, the cell will no longer divide
- 3' telomeric overhang (T-oligos): 3'-guanine-rich single-stranded overhang that is concealed in a protective loop
- Most important: telomeric repeat binding factor 2 (TRF2)
- Exposed during DNA damage or progressive telomere shortening
- T-oligos: taken up into the nucleus and recognized by a sensor; initiates DNA damage signaling

Glogau Photoaging Classification

- Visual grading system used to quantify photodamage
- Type I: no wrinkles
  - Minimal to no discoloration or wrinkling
  - No keratoses (skin overgrowths)
- Type II: wrinkles in motion
  - Wrinkling as skin moves
  - Slight lines near the eyes and mouth
  - No visible keratoses
- Type III: wrinkles at rest
  - Visible wrinkles all the time
  - Noticeable discolorations
  - Visible keratoses

- Type IV: many wrinkles
  - Wrinkles throughout
  - Yellow or gray color to skin
  - Prior skin cancer

Fitzpatrick Skin Types

- Skin type I: very white or freckled, always burns, never tans
- Skin type II: white, usually burns, some ability to tan
- Skin type III: white to olive, sometimes burns, tans easily
- Skin type IV: brown, rarely burns, always tans
- Skin type V: dark brown, very rarely burns
- Skin type VI: black, never burns

BOTULINUM TOXIN (BTX)

- Treatment of hyperfunctional lines that result from the contraction of the underlying facial musculature
- Temporary flaccid paralysis of the injected muscles
- Measured as 1 standard unit (amount injected necessary to kill 50 percent of Swiss-Webster mice)
- Seven serotypes (A–G) bind to different sites on the motor nerve terminal and within the motor neuron
- Botulinum toxin type A and type B are commercially available; A is the most potent
- Botox (Allergan) is approved by the Food and Drug Administration (FDA) for the treatment of blepharospasm, strabismus, cervical dystonia, glabellar rhytides, and hyperhidrosis
  - Currently available in the United States
  - Comes in a vial containing 100 units of Botox A toxin
  - Must be stored frozen and then refrigerated when reconstituted
- Dysport (Ipsen, U.K.)
  - Not currently available in the United States
  - Comes in a vial containing 500 units of Botox A toxin
  - Can be stored at room temperature
  - Myobloc
  - Available in vials containing 2500, 5000, and 10,000 units
  - Does not require constitution and is ready to use at pH 5.6
  - Can be diluted to desired concentration
- Mechanism of action (Fig. 14-1)
  - Blocks neurotransmitter release at peripheral cholinergic nerve terminals
  - Each toxin is made of a light chain and a heavy chain linked by a disulfide bond

- Heavy chain: allows transport of toxin into the cholinergic motor neuron
- Light chain: a Zn^{2+}-containing endopeptidase that blocks acetylcholine-containing vesicles from fusing with the terminal membrane of the motor neuron (SNARE complex)
- Each serotype is composed of three domains: binding, translocation, and enzymatic
- Binding to the motor nerve terminal occurs at the presynaptic membrane and is mediated by the carboxy terminal of botulinum toxin heavy chain
- Neuronal uptake of Botox occurs by endocytosis
- Translocation across cell membrane is mediated by N terminal of botulinum toxin heavy chain (H_N)
- Inhibition of the release of acetycholine from presynaptic motor neurons occurs by cleaving various SNARE proteins using a specific endopeptidase (found on light chains)
- SNARE (synaptosomal-associated protein receptor) proteins are presynaptic proteins involved in exocytosis of acetylcholine
  - Synaptosomal-associated protein (SNAP-25) cleaved by serotypes A and E
  - Vesicle-associated membrane protein (VAMP, Synaptobrevin) cleaved by serotypes B, D, F, and G
  - Syntaxin 1 cleaved by serotype C1
- Events following Botox injection
  - Requires 24 to 72 hours to start to take effect; full effect by 2 weeks
  - Lasts approximately 3 to 5 months
  - Muscle function returns as new neuromuscular junctions form
- Antibodies to Botox
  - Antibody to the binding site on the heavy chain of the Botox molecule
  - Prevents binding of the toxin to its receptor, thereby crippling the actions of the toxin
  - Increased risk of antibody formation at doses of more than 300 units at a time
  - Myobloc binding domain distinct from Botox
  - Antibodies that neutralize Botox A would not neutralize Botox B, and vice versa
- Uses for Botox on the face and neck (Fig. 14-2)
  - Injections under the guidance of EMG monitoring can be performed
  - Numerous injection sites and concentrations published in literature
- Glabellar rhytides are the only FDA-approved use of Botox for wrinkles
- Facial rhytides can be static (gravity or extrinsic causes, e.g., smoke) or dynamic (muscle use)

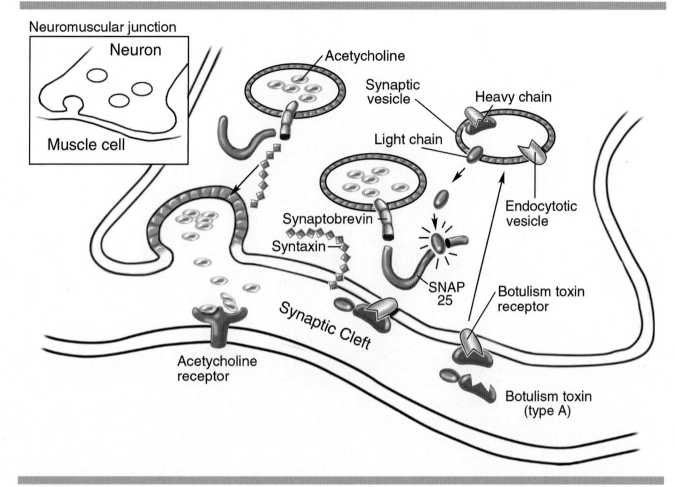

FIGURE 14-1 Botox mechanism of action. *(From Baumann N: Cosmetic Dermatology: Principles and Practice. New York: McGraw-Hill, 2002, p. 140.)*

- Glabellar furrows
  - Muscles involved
  - Procerus: brow depressor
  - Corrugator: brow depressor
  - Orbicularis oculi (medial fibers)
- Complications
  - Eyelid ptosis
  - When Botox affects the levator palpebrae superioris muscle
  - Normally elevates the eyelid
  - May persist for 2 to 4 weeks
  - Risk is minimized by the correct injection volume and site of injection
  - Stay 1 cm above the orbital ridge
  - Have the patient stay vertical for 4 hours
  - Avoid manipulating injection site
  - Aproclonidine 0.5% eye drops (Iopidine)
  - One to three drops three times a day to the affected side
  - Results in 1 to 2 mm of elevation
- Hyperhidrosis (Fig. 14-3)
  - Innervation of the eccrine glands: sympathetic nerves that use acetylcholine as the neurotransmitter
  - Botulinum toxin can temporarily reduce or even abolish sweat production
  - 50 units of Botulinum toxin injected into each axillae
  - Long-term satisfactory median responses lasting 6 to 19 months depending on dose and location
  - Extent of hyperhidrosis: evaluated by performing an iodine starch test of axillae, palms, or soles
- Contraindications to use of Botox
  - History of a neuromuscular disease (Eaton-Lambert syndrome, amyotrophic lateral sclerosis, or myasthenia gravis)
  - Known history of sensitivity to Botox or human albumin
  - Aminoglycosides can interfere with neuromuscular transmission

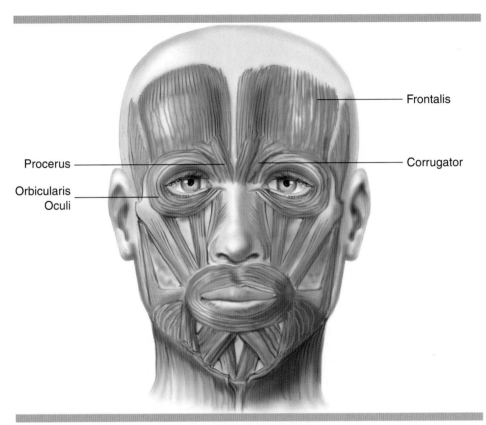

FIGURE 14-2 Muscles of the face treated by Botox. *(From Baumann N: Cosmetic Dermatology: Principles and Practice. New York: McGraw-Hill, 2002, p. 143.)*

- Pregnancy
- Lactation
- Age younger than 12 years

LASER (LIGHT AMPLIFIED BY STIMULATED EMISSION OF RADIATION)

Light Properties

- A quanta of light energy is a photon
- Photons display duality: both particle-like and wavelike behavior
- Electromagnetic radiation (EMR): form of energy, moves through space as a wave and comprised of photons
- Photon energy is proportional to wave frequency and inversely related to wavelength
- Laser characteristics
  - Wavelength λ
  - Power output (watts = joules per second; $P = rate\ of\ energy\ delivery$)
  - Spot size: diameter d and square S
  - Pulse duration (exposition time) T

- Fluence $= PT/S =$ joules/cm^2
  - Energy (joules) delivered per square centimeter of skin during a laser pulse
- Irradiance $= (w/cm^2) =$ concentration of power output per unit area
- Light (infrared, visible, and UV) is a form of electromagnetic radiation (Table 14-1)

Laser Properties

- Monochromaticity
  - Single, discrete wavelength
  - Active medium determines the emission wavelength, which is restricted to a very narrow band
- Coherency
  - Monochromatic light in phase
  - Highly directional
- Collimation: light in parallel fashion to achieve its propagation across long distances without light divergence (constant diameter beam)
- Intensity: amplification process allows the emission of high-energy level laser

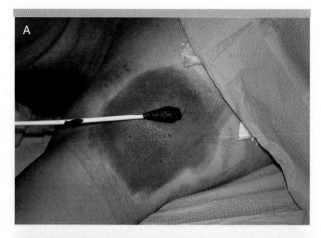

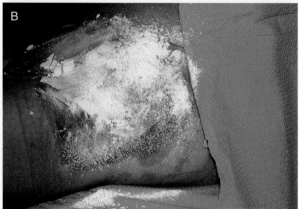

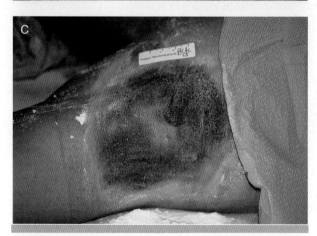

FIGURE 14-3 Hyperhidrosis. In the iodine starch test, A: an iodine solution is applied to the affected area, B: potato starch is then sprinkled over the area, and C: the starch turns black in reaction to sweat, clearly delineating affected areas.

- Chromophores (Fig. 14-4)
  - Skin components that absorb the laser light
  - Lasers effects on tissue components depend on absorption spectra

- Endogenous (water, melanin, protein, and hemoglobin)
  - Exogenous (tattoo ink) (Table 6-5)
- Depth of penetration
  - Depends on absorption and scattering
  - Amount of scattering of laser energy is inversely proportional to the wavelength of incident light
  - Depth of penetration increases with wavelength
- Laser-tissue interactions
  - Photothermal reaction: results directly from the effects of heat
  - Photochemical reaction: reaction of an endogenous or exogenous photosensitizer with UV or visible light
  - Photomechanical reaction: rapid absorption of a laser pulse resulting in a rapid temperature change along with sudden tissue vaporization, shock wave, or pressure wave formation
- Skin optics
  - Reflection: waves encounter a surface or other boundary that does not absorb the energy of the radiation and bounces the waves away from the surface
  - Absorbtion: energy is deposited in a chromophore
  - Scattering: energy is redirected elsewhere in the skin, dermal light scattering varies inversely with wavelength
  - Tyndell effect: short (blue) wavelengths are scattered more long (red) wavelengths
  - Transmission: direction of photon path is unchanged
- Selective photothermolysis
  - Controlled destruction of a targeted lesion without significant thermal damage to surrounding normal tissue
  - Thermal damage can be induced in tissue targets that absorb photons well at the emitted wavelength; pulse duration or exposure time should be shorter than the cooling time or thermal relaxation time (defined as the time required for the targeted site to cool to one-half its peak temperature immediately after laser irradiation) of the target
- Thermal effects on skin cells
  - Increase of 5 to 10°C: cell injury and inflammation
  - Above 60°C: denaturation of protein
  - Above 70°C: denaturation of DNA
  - Over 100°C: vaporization of water

Laser Media (Tables 14-2 through 14-6)

- Solid-state lasers
  - Lasing material distributed in a solid matrix
  - Ruby or neodymium:yttrium-aluminum garnet (Nd:Yag) lasers

TABLE 14-1 Electromagnetic Spectrum

Electromagnetic Spectrum	Wavelengths	Comment
Radio waves	>30 cm	Combines electric and magnetic fields
Microwaves	1 mm–30 cm	Used for radar and cooking (heats water)
Infrared	700 nm–1 mm	Invisible; usually delivers heat
Visible light	400–700 nm	Passes through atmosphere
Ultraviolet	10 nm–350 nm	Majority filtered by ozone layer
X-rays	0.01 nm–10 nm	Ionization of the inner electrons of an atom
Gamma rays	<0.01 nm	From nuclear decay at atom's center

- Gas lasers
  - Helium and helium-neon (HeNe)
  - Primary output of visible red light
- Excimer lasers
  - Name is derived from the terms *excited* and *dimers*
  - Use reactive gases, chlorine and fluorine, mixed with inert gases such as argon, krypton, or xenon
  - When electrically stimulated, a pseudo-molecule (dimer) is produced
  - When lased, the dimer produces light in the ultraviolet range
- Dye lasers: use complex organic dyes
- Semiconductor lasers (diode lasers)

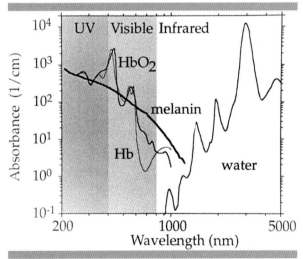

FIGURE 14-4 Chromophores. *(From Freedberg IM et al: Fitzpatrick's Dermatology in General Medicine, 6th ed. New York: McGraw-Hill, 2003, p. 2497.)*

Beam Types (Fig. 14-5)

- Continuous-wave (CW) lasers
  - Continuous beam of light with little or no variation in power output over time
  - Operate with a stable average beam power
  - Long exposure times with low peak power
  - Can result in nonselective tissue injury (scar) as heat spreads from chromophore; examples: CO_2, argon
- Quasi-continuous-mode (QSW)
  - Continuous-wavelength lasers that are mechanically shuttered to deliver pulses of light as short as 20 ms
  - Produce individual pulses of light
  - Energy within the pulse is not constant but rather builds, peaks, and tapers off within a very short time
  - Peak power outputs of pulsed lasers are often up to 100 times the maximum output of CW lasers
  - Argon-pumped tunable dye, potassium-titanyl-phosphate (KTP), copper vapor, krypton
- Pulsed lasers
  - Long pulse (millisecond): 0.5 to 400 ms allows for targeting of most hair and blood vessels (with visible to near infrared lasers)
  - Short pulse (microsecond): modified to produce very short pulses with high peak power in a repetitive fashion; developed to reduce the amount of thermal damage that occurs adjacent to a vaporized area or a laser incision; when applied to CO_2 laser, allows for much safer skin resurfacing
  - Nanosecond (Q-switched)
    - Allows buildup of excessive energy in the laser cavity before discharge
    - Very short (nanosecond) single pulses of extremely high power are released

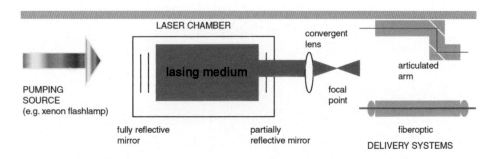

A. Schematic of a typical laser light source. Electrical, chemical, or optical energy input is provided by the pumping source. Note that the initial wavelength of the emitted laser beam is determined by the lasing medium, although this can be altered. Laser energy is delivered to the target via an articulated arm or fiberoptic cable.

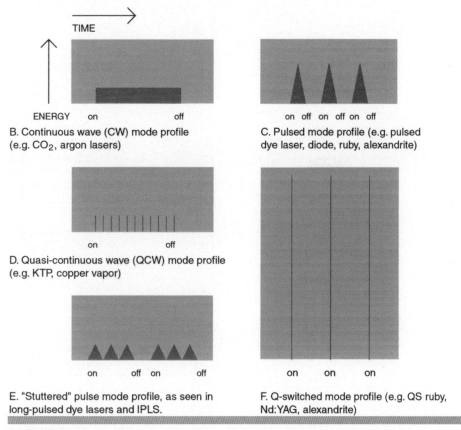

B. Continuous wave (CW) mode profile (e.g. CO_2, argon lasers)

C. Pulsed mode profile (e.g. pulsed dye laser, diode, ruby, alexandrite)

D. Quasi-continuous wave (QCW) mode profile (e.g. KTP, copper vapor)

E. "Stuttered" pulse mode profile, as seen in long-pulsed dye lasers and IPLS.

F. Q-switched mode profile (e.g. QS ruby, Nd:YAG, alexandrite)

FIGURE 14-5 Beam types. *(From Freedberg IM et al: Fitzpatrick's Dermatology in General Medicine, 6th ed. New York: McGraw-Hill, 2003, p. 2494.)*

- Q stands for the quality factor of the laser cavity and represents the rate of discharge of energy of quality-switched lasers

Non-Laser Light Sources
- Intense pulsed light (IPL)
  - Noncoherent light within 500 to 1200 nm
  - Filtered xenon flashlamps are used to eliminate shorter wavelengths

- Single-, double-, or triple-pulse sequences; pulse durations of 2 to 25 ms and delays between pulses ranging from 10 to 500 ms
- Light-emitting diodes (LEDs)
  - Narrow-band light source
  - Emit noncoherent light; restricted range of ±20 nm; pulse signal to stimulate mitochondria in fibroblasts (see Tables 14-2 through 14-6)

TABLE 14-2 Types of Lasers and Light Sources

Laser	Wavelength (nm)	Color	Chromophore	Output
Excimer	308	Ultraviolet	Protein	Quasi-continuous
Narrow-band blue light	407–420	Violet/blue	Endogenous porphyrins	
Argon	488/514	Blue	Vascular and pigmented lesions	CW
Pulsed dye	510	Yellow	Pigmented lesions, vascular lesions	Pulsed
Copper vapor	511/578	Yellow/green	Pigmented lesions, vascular lesions	CW
Krypton	530/568	Yellow/green	Pigmented lesions, vascular lesions	CW
Potassium-titanyl-phosphate (KTP), Nd:YAG, frequency-doubled	532	Green	Pigmented lesions, red tattoos	QS
Argon-pumped tunable dye	577/585	Yellow	Vascular lesions	CW
Pulsed dye	585–595	Yellow	Vascular lesions, hypertrophic/keloid scars, striae, verrucae, nonablative dermal remodeling	Pulsed
Ruby, normal mode	694	Red	Hair removal	Pulsed
QS ruby	694	Red	Pigmented lesions, blue/black/green/ tattoos	QS
Alexandrite, normal mode	755	Red	Hair removal, leg veins	
QS alexandrite	755	Red	Pigmented lesions, blue/black/green Tattoos	QS
Diode	800–810	Red	Hair removal, leg veins	Pulsed
Qs Nd:YAG	1064	Infrared	Pigmented lesions, blue/black tattoos	QS
Normal mode	1064	Infrared	Hair removal, leg veins, nonablative dermal remodeling	Pulsed Pulsed
Nd:YAG	1320	Infrared	Water: nonablative dermal remodeling	Pulsed
Diode	1450	Infrared	Water: nonablative dermal remodeling	Pulsed
Erbium	2940	Infrared	Water	
CO_2	10,600	Infrared	Water (vaporization and coagulation): actinic cheilitis, verrucae, rhinophyma	CW
CO_2	10,600	Infrared	Ablative skin resurfacing, epidermal/dermal lesions	Pulsed

Note: CW, continuous-wave; Nd, neodymium; QS, quality-switched; YAG, yttrium-aluminum-garnet.

TABLE 14-3 Laser Treatment of Tattoo Pigment (Chromophore Is Ink)

Laser Type	Wavelength	Tattoo Pigment
Pigmented pulsed dye	510 nm	Purple, yellow, and orange
Q-switched Nd:YAG, frequency-doubled	532 nm	Red/orange/yellow
Q-switch ruby	694 nm	Blue and blue-black, occasionally green and brown
Q-switch alexandrite	755 nm	Blue, black, and green
Q-switch Nd:YAG	1064 nm	Blue-black

TABLE 14-4 Lasers Used for Vascular Lesions (Chromophore Is Hemoglobin)

Port-wine stain	Pulsed-dye laser, IPL
Hemangiomas	Pulsed-dye laser
Telangiectases	Green-light lasers (532 nm), pulsed-dye laser, diode laser, long-pulsed Nd:YAG (1064 nm)
Pyogenic granuloma	Pulsed-dye laser, carbon dioxide laser, combined continuous-wave/pulsed
Angiofibromas	Carbon dioxide, pulsed-dye laser

TABLE 14-5 Laser Treatment of Pigmented Lesions (Chromophore Is Melanin)

Lentigines	Q-switched ruby, Q-switched alexandrite, Q-switched Nd:YAG (532 nm), IPL
Nevus of Ota	Q-switched ruby, Q-switched alexandrite, Q-switched Nd:YAG (1064 nm)
Congenital melanocytic nevi	Normal ruby, Q-switched ruby, Q-switched Nd:YAG (532 nm)
Café-au-lait macules	Q-switched ruby, Q-switched Nd:YAG (532 nm), copper vapor
Nevus spilus	Normal ruby, normal alexandrite, Q-switched ruby, Q-switched Nd:YAG (532 nm)

TABLE 14-6 Laser and Other Devices for Nonablative Remodeling

Wrinkles or acne scars	Pulsed-dye laser Nd:YAG (1064, 1320 nm) Diode (1450 nm)	Chromophore is hemoglobin Chromophore is water Chromophore is water
Nonsurgical lift	Radiofrequency	Heat from electrical resistance

- Laser safety
  - Fire prevention with CO_2 lasers
    - Saline-soaked drapes or cloths should be used intraoperatively
    - Exposed hair-bearing areas should be kept moist; alcohol-based skin preparations should be strictly avoided
  - Eye protection: permanent visual loss can result
  - Aerosolized particles: smoke evacuator with clean filters and tubing
- Anesthesia
  - Topical anesthetic compounds
    - Can be applied under occlusion for 30 to 90 minutes before laser treatment
    - EMLA cream: lidocaine 2.5% and prilocaine 2.5%
    - LMX: 4% or 5% lidocaine
    - S-Caine peel: lidocaine and tetracaine
      - ▲ Applied to the skin as a cream 30 minutes before treatment
      - ▲ Dries to a thin, flexible film that can be peeled away easily
  - For ablative laser skin resurfacing procedures: consider combination anesthesia: topical, tumescent, nerve blocks, sedation
- Possible laser side effects
  - General: erythema, pain, scar, incomplete removal of target, hyper- and hypopigmentation
  - Laser tattoo or pigmented lesion removal: purpura, eschar
  - Laser treatment of vessels: purpura, vesiculation
  - Laser hair removal: perifollicular edema, vesiculation
  - Ablative laser skin resurfacing
    - Short term: edema, exudation, infection (HSV, *Candida*, or bacterial)
    - Medium term: acne/milia, pruritus, hyperpigmenation, dermatitis
    - Permanent: hypopigmentation, scar, ectropion
  - Nonablative resurfacing: vesiculation
- Skin cooling
  - Decreases risk of vesiculation and pigmentary changes by protecting epidermis
  - Methods of cooling
    - Inert: ice, cold gel, water-cooled glass or sapphire treatment tips
    - Active: air cooling, cryogen spray

CHEMICAL PEELS

- Indications
  - Actinic keratoses
  - Superficial scarring
  - Hyperpigmentation and melasma
  - Mild wrinkles
  - Acne

- Chemical peel strengths
  - Depend on the amount of free acid present
  - Affected by
    - Percentage of acid
    - Type of vehicle used
    - Buffering
    - pK_a of acid preparation
- Free acid availability (pK_a)
  - pK_a = pH at which half is in acid form
  - Lower pK_a = more free acid available
- Defatting
  - Acetone, rubbing alcohol, or Septisol
  - Essential for penetration as most agents are not lipid soluble
- Frost
  - Whitish tint of skin keratin agglutination
  - Dependent on pre-existing degree of photo damage, choice of applicator, adequacy of defatting
  - Level of peel can be correlated with the intensity of the frost
    - Level 0: no frost, stratum corneum
    - Level 1: irregular light frost, superficial epidermis
    - Level 2: uniform white frost with pink showing through, full-thickness epidermal peel
- Depth of peel
  - Superficial: necrosis of all or part of the epidermis
  - Medium: necrosis of the epidermis and part to all of the papillary dermis
  - Deep: wounding extends into the mid-reticular dermis
- Peeling agents
  - Alpha-hydroxyacid (AHA)
    - Glycolic, lactic, citric, and malic acids
    - Dependent on the contact time with the skin
    - Carboxylic acids normally found in many foods
    - Thins the stratum corneum, although the epidermis thickens
    - May increase photosensitivity
  - Glycolic acid
    - Derived from sugar cane
    - Concentrations range from 20% to 70%
    - Decreases corneocyte cohesion by promoting exfoliation of the outer layers of the stratum corneum
    - Neutralize with sodium bicarbonate
    - Dispersal of melanin pigmentation and a return to a more normal rete pattern
  - Lactic acid
    - Derived from sour milk
    - Acts as a humectant (causes the skin to hold onto water), keratolytic
  - Beta-hydroxyacid (BHA)
    - Salicylic acid
    - Derived from willow bark, wintergreen leaves, or sweet birch

- Concentrations of 20% or 30% (OTC preparations contain only 2%)
- Exhibits anti-inflammatory capabilities, producing less irritation
- Lipophilic
- Penetrates the follicular sebaceous material (anticomedogenic effect)
- Does not need to be neutralized, and the frost is visible
- No need to time the peel: After 2 minutes, there is very little absorption of the active agent
- Contraindicated in pregnancy, breast-feeding, and aspirin allergies
- Adverse effect: salicylism (nausea, disorientation, and tinnitus)
- Jessner's solution
  - 14% salicylic acid, 14% lactic acid, 14% resorcinol in alcohol
  - Keratolytic effects
- Carbon dioxide (CO_2)
  - Boiling point: 78°C
  - Physical peeling method
  - Solid block of CO_2 ice dipped in an acetone-alcohol mixture
  - Applied to the skin for 5 to 15 seconds
- Resorcinol
  - 1,3-Dihydroxybenzene
  - 20% to 50%
- Trichloroacetic acid
  - Can be used for superficial, medium, and less often deep peels
  - No need to neutralize
  - No systemic toxicity
  - Causes coagulation of proteins in the skin (results in frost)
- Deep peels
  - Baker Gordon phenol
    - Phenol 88%, 2 ml distilled water, 8 drops Septisol, and 3 drops croton oil
    - Septisol causes deeper penetration of phenol and a deeper peel
    - Croton oil (especially the toxic fraction solubilized in phenol) causes a deeper peel
    - Exfoliation to middle reticular dermis
    - New zone of collagen forms
    - Occluded method uses zinc oxide tape or other artificial barrier product to prevent evaporation of the phenol from the skin, thus enabling the solution to penetrate deeper
    - Litton's formula: replaces Septisol with glycerin
    - Beeson McCollough formula: uses aggressive defatting and heavier application of Baker Gordon solution

- Complications
  - ▲ Arrhythmias (needs ECG and pulse oximeter monitering)
  - ▲ Pigmentary change
  - ▲ Scarring
  - ▲ Infection
  - ▲ Prolonged erythema
  - ▲ Acne
  - ▲ Milia

MICRODERMABRASION

- Produces a superficial ablation, primarily in the epidermis
- Components common to all systems
  - Pump: generates a high-pressure stream of aluminum oxide or salt crystals
  - Connecting tube and handpiece: delivers the crystals to the skin
  - Vacuum: removes the crystals and exfoliated skin
  - Crystals are discarded after use
- Advantages: low risk, rapid recovery
- Contraindications
  - Current or recent use (<1 year) of isotretinoin (Accutane)
  - Active herpes infection
  - Malignant skin tumors
  - Evolving dermatoses
  - Certain keratoses

DERMABRASION

- Manual abrasion, wound healing by second intention allows re-epithelialization to occur from the underlying adnexal structures
- Tattoos, rhinophyma, acne scarring, actinic keratoses, solar elastosis, and discoloration of photoaging
- Helps lesions or defects of epidermis, papillary dermis, and upper reticular dermis
- Abrasive wire or diamond wheel
- Rotational speeds of 12,000 to 15,000 rpm
- High-speed rotary motors are used to drive an abrading end piece
- Depth of procedure: operator-dependent process and depends on coarseness of the dermabrading tip (fraise), number of brush strokes, pressure exerted on the electric handpiece, and tissue contact time
- Contraindications
  - History of hypertrophic scarring

TABLE 14-7 Commonly Used Filler Agents

Type	Ingredient	Comment
Zyderm 1 and 2 Zyplast	Collagen	Bovine origin; FDA approved; 3% allergy; spot test
Cosmoderm 1 and 2 Cosmoplast	Collagen	Human origin; FDA approved; no spot test
Restylane Perlane	Hyaluronic acid	Bruising; injection pain; Resylane is FDA approved for cosmetic use
Radiance	Calcium hydroxyapatite microspheres suspended in polysaccharide gel	Hard texture; calcium scaffold for collagen deposits; *not FDA approved for cosmetic use (off-label)*
Hylaform	Hyaluronic acid	Bruising; injection pain; derived form rooster combs; *not FDA approved (illegal)*
Artecoll	Polymethylmethacrylate microspheres and collagen	Bovine (altered); permanent results; lumpiness; *not FDA approved (illegal)*
Silicone	Synthetic polymer of silica and oxygen	Manufactured at high temperature and pressure; late complications; *not FDA approved (illegal)*
Sculptra	Polygalactic acid	
Captique	Hyaluronic acid	

- Isotretinoin within 6 to 12 months
- Complications
  - Milia formation and a flare-up of acne
  - Transient postoperative hyperpigmentation
  - Postoperative viral infections
  - Hypertrophic scarring

SOFT-TISSUE AUGMENTATION

- Injectable fillers are generally considered soft tissue augmentation materials
- Temporary injectable fillers are the most commonly used soft tissue augmentation products
- Used for wrinkles, scars, and augmentation of the lips and other tissues (Table 14-7)

REFERENCES

Alam M, Dover JS, Arndt KA. Energy delivery devices for cutaneous remodeling: lasers, lights and radio waves. *Arch Dermatol* 2003; 139(10):1351–1360.

Astner S, Anderson RR. Treating vascular lesions. *Dermatol Ther* 2005; 18(3):267–281.

Freedberg IM et al. *Fitzpatrick's Dermatology in General Medicine*, 6th Ed. New York: McGraw-Hill; 2003.

Glogau RG. Aesthetic and anatomic analysis of the aging skin. *Semin Cutan Med Surg* 1996; 15(3):134–138.

Kilmer SL. Cutaneous lasers. *Facial Plast Surg Clin North Am* 2003; 11(2):229–242.

McKee PH. *Pathology of the Skin: With Clinical Correlations.* London: Mosby-Wolfe; 1996.

Matarasso SL, Glogai RG. Chemical face peels. *Dermatol Clin* 1991; 9(1):131–150.

Narins RS, Bowman PH. Injectable skin fillers. *Clin Plast Surg* 2005; 32(2):151–162.

CHAPTER 15

BACTERIAL DISEASES

STEVEN MARCET
ASRA ALI

GRAM-POSITIVE BACTERIAL DISEASES

Impetigo (Fig. 15-1)

* Most often *Staphylococcus aureus* or *group A Streptococcus*
  * Honey-colored crust
  * Treatment: topical mupirocin
* Bullous impetigo (Fig. 15-2)
  * Separation of the epidermis is due to exotoxin produced by staphylococci
  * Toxin binds desmoglein 1
  * Sharply demarcated flaccid bullae without surrounding erythema
  * Seen most frequently in newborns
  * Treatment: dicloxacillin or first-generation cephalosporin, topical mupirocin

Ecthyma

* Deeper, ulcerated impetigo infection
* Often occurring with lymphadenitis
* Thick crusted ulcer mostly on lower legs
* Histology: subcorneal neutrophilic infiltrate
* Treatment: dicloxacillin or first-generation cephalosporin, topical mupirocin

Folliculitis (Fig. 15-3)

* *S. aureus*
* Clinical
  * Red papules/pustules in follicular distribution
  * Perifollicular inflammation
  * Deep: sycosis barbae
  * Lupoid sycosis: chronic form of sycosis barbae associated with scarring
  * Superficial: Bockhart's folliculitis
* Treatment: topical mupirocin

Furuncles/carbuncles (Fig. 15-4)

* *S. aureus*
* Deep-seated nodules around hair follicle

* Multiple furuncles make a carbuncle, evolve from preceding folliculitis
* Treatment: topical mupirocin and dicloxacillin; if large, then also need drainage

Staphylococcal Scalded-Skin Syndrome (Ritter's Disease)

* Seen in children younger than 4 years of age and renal disease patients
* Exotoxins can be classified as A or B: bind directly to the desmosomal protein desmoglein 1
* *S. aureus:* phage group II (types 3A, 3B, and 3C) (types 55 or 71) (exfoliative)
* *S. aureus* originates from a focus of infection other than the skin
* Clinical
  * Superficial blistering owing to disruption of the epidermal granular cell layer [toxic epidermal necrolysis (TEN) shows deeper cleavage below the epidermis]
  * Sparing of mucous membranes
  * Nikolsky's sign present
  * Periorificial and flexural accentuation may be observed
* Laboratory studies
  * Frozen tissue to rule out TEN by level of split
  * If cultures of bullae are negative, culture other sites (blood)
  * Gram's stain and/or culture from the remote infection site
* Treatment: intravenous penicillase-resistant pencillin, fluid therapy, supportive measures
* Prognosis: mortality rate less than 4 percent in children, greater than 50 percent in immunosuppressed patients

Staphylococcal Toxic Shock Syndrome (TSS)

* Toxins produced by *S. aureus* activate production of superantigens as major part of disease

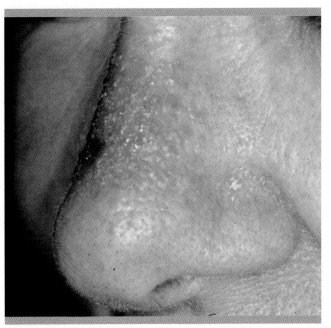

FIGURE 15-1 Impetigo. *(Courtesy of Dr. Steven Mays.)*

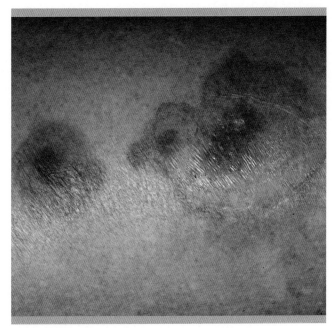

FIGURE 15-2 Bullous impetigo. *(Courtesy of Dr. Steven Mays.)*

process: tumor necrosis factor, interleukin-1, M protein, and interferon-γ
- Toxin-1 (TSST-1) causes most of menstrual-related cases
- Criteria for staph toxic shock syndrome
  - Prodromal period of 2 to 3 days

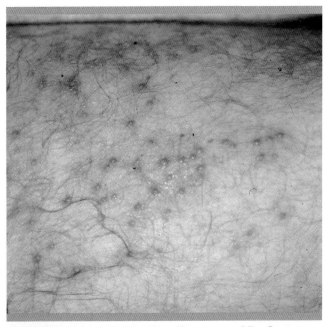

FIGURE 15-3 Folliculitis. *(Courtesy of Dr. Steven Mays.)*

- Criteria for staphylococcal TSS
  - ▲ Fever, hypotension
  - ▲ Skin findings: diffuse rash, occasionally patchy and erythematous, with desquamation occurring approximately 1 to 2 weeks later
  - ▲ Involvement of three or more organ systems (musculoskeletal, renal, hematologic, hepatic, central nervous system)
  - ▲ Absence of serologic evidence of Rocky Mountain spotted fever, leptospirosis, measles, hepatitis B, antinuclear antibody, false-positive Venereal Disease Research Laboratory (VDRL) test results, and antibodies to Monospot testing
- Treatment: Penicillinase resistant penicillin, intravenous gamma globulin, fluid replacement

Streptococcal Toxic Shock Syndrome

- *S. pyogenes* exotoxin A (SPEA) and *S. pyogenes* exotoxin B (SPEB): produced by group A beta-hemolytic streptococci
  - Criteria for streptococcal TSS
    - ▲ Isolation of group A *Streptococcus* from a normally sterile site (e.g., blood, cerebrospinal fluid, surgical wounds) or a non-sterile site (e.g., throat)
    - ▲ Hypotension (as defined earlier)
    - ▲ Involvement of two or more organ systems
    - ▲ Desquamating rash

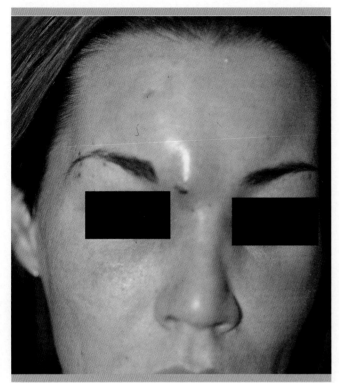

FIGURE 15-4 Furuncules/carbuncles. *(Courtesy of Dr. Steven Mays.)*

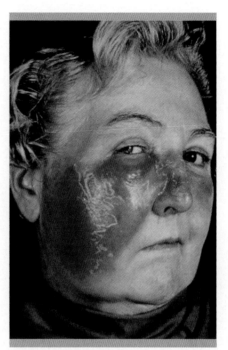

FIGURE 15-5 Erysipelas. *(From Connor DH et al: Pathology of Infectious Diseases. Stamford, CT: Appleton & Lange, 1997, p. 819.)*

- Treatment: intravenous penicillase-resistant pencillin, fluid therapy, and supportive measures

Blistering Distal Dactylitis

- Group A beta-hemolytic *streptococci*
- Tense purulent blister of distal finger or toes, volar pad
- Treatment: dicloxacillin or first-generation cephelasporin

Erysipelas (Fig. 15-5)

- Group A beta-hemolytic *streptococci*
- Febrile illness
- Red, indurated plaque often on face or legs with sharp margins
- Laboratory studies: check antistreptolysin (ASO)
- Treatment: penicllin or erythromycin

Scarlet Fever

- Toxin-producing group A beta-hemolytic streptococci (GABHS)
- Produces erythrogenic exotoxin
- Clinical
  - Fever and pharyngitis
  - Mucous membrane changes: white strawberry tongue turns into red strawberry tongue after 4 days

- Skin changes: 2 to 4 days after initiation of fever, sandpaper-like rash starting on trunk then becomes more generalized; desquamates after 4 to 5 days
- Circumoral pallor
- Pastia's line: linear petchial rash over skin folds (axillary/antecubital)
- Laboratory studies: antistreptolysin O (ASO) titers
- Treatment: penicillin or erythromycin

Erythrasma (Fig. 15-6)

- *Corynebacterium minutissimum* (lipophilic gram-positive aerobic diphtheroid)
- Superficial infection of the intertriginous areas
- White maceration between fourth and fifth webspace
- Inner thighs have reddish brown plaques
- Fluoresce coral red with Wood's lamp owing to coproporphyrin III
- Treatment: erythromycin or benzoyl peroxide wash

Trichomycosis axillaris

- *C. tenuis* (gram-positive diphtheroid)
- White concretions on hair shaft, usually in axillae
- Occasionally affects pubic hair (trichomycosis pubis)
- Often see hyperhidrosis
- Treatment: shave the affected hair; use topical clindamycin or erythromycin

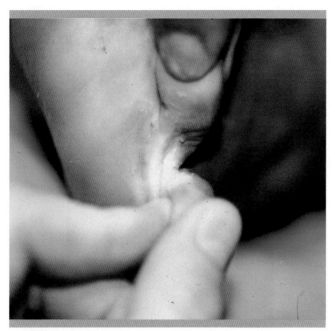

FIGURE 15-6 Erythrasma. *(Courtesy of Dr. Steven Mays.)*

Pitted Keratolysis (Fig. 15-7)

- *Kytococcus sedentarius* (previously *Micrococcus sedentarius*)
- Bacteria proliferate and produce proteinases: destroy the stratum corneum, creating shallow pits on soles
- Seen with sweaty feet

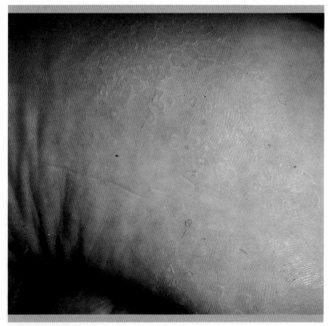

FIGURE 15-7 Pitted keratolysis. *(Courtesy of Dr. Ronald Rapini.)*

- Malodor owing to the production of sulfur-compound by-products
- Treatment: reduce hyperhidrosis, topical clindamycin or erythromycin

Erysipeloid

- *Erysipelothrix rhusiopathiae* (gram-positive bacillus)
- Direct contact with infected meat, fish, or animal products
- Three clinical forms
  - Localized cutaneous form (erysipeloid of Rosenbach): purplish raised plaque, well demarcated on hand
  - Diffuse cutaneous form
  - Generalized or systemic infection associated with endicarditis
- Treatment: penicillin, ciprofloxacin, third-generation cephalosporin

Anthrax

- *Bacillus anthracis* (gram + rod)
- Exposure to sick animals or contaminated wool, hair, or animal hides
- Two virulence factors: (1) D-glutamyl polypeptide capsule; (2) pair of toxins: edema toxin and lethal toxin
  - 1- to 12-day incubation period followed by a low-grade fever and malaise
- Pulmonary anthrax (woolsorter's syndrome)
  - Five percent of anthrax cases
  - Inhalation of anthrax spores
  - Nonspecific symptoms: low-grade fever and a nonproductive cough
  - Hemorrhagic mediastinal infection
  - Can result in septicemic anthrax
  - Chest x-ray: widened mediastinum with hemorrhagic pleural effusions
  - Usually fatal
- Gastrointestinal anthrax
  - Ingestion of infected meat products
  - Mainly affects the cecum
- Cutaneous anthrax
  - Occurs 1 to 7 days after skin exposure
  - "Malignant pustule": central area of coagulation necrosis (ulcer) with edema and vesicles filled with bloody or clear fluid
  - Ruptures with purulent discharge, leaving a black eschar and a permanent scar
- Regional lymphadenopathy may persist
- Anthrax meningitis may occur after bacteremic seeding from any form of anthrax
- Laboratory studies
  - Stain with methylene blue or Giemsa
  - Culture on blood agar: from skin, pleural fluid, cerebrospinal fluid (CSF)

- Serologic diagnosis (ELISA)
- Skin biopsy
- Treatment
  - Pencillin, doxycycline
  - Quinolones if patient is unable to take pencillin, doxycycline
  - Postexposure prophylaxis to prevent inhalation anthrax should be continued for 60 days
- Vaccine exists but is not readily available
- Do not incise and drain secondary to dissemination

Necrotizing Fasciitis (NF)

- Soft tissue infection
- Group A beta-hemolytic *streptococci* or caused by *Clostridium perfringens*
- Type I: polymicrobial
- Type II: group A streptococcal
- Type III: gas gangrene or clostridial myonecrosis
- Can occur as a complication of a number of surgical procedures
- Clinical
  - Begins with erythema progressing to vesiculation or bullae formation
  - Spreads from the subcutaneous tissue along the superficial and deep fascial planes
  - Ischemia and tissue necrosis
  - Crepitus present with gas-forming aerobes
  - Septicemia
  - Fournier's gangrene
    - Localized variant of type I NF involving scrotum and penis
- Diagnosis
  - Standard radiographs or computed tomography (CT) to visualize free air
  - Culture
- Treatment
  - Aerobes (usually gram-negative organisms), ampicillin, and gentamicin
  - Anaerobes, clindamycin, or metronidazole
  - Intravenous immunoglobulin
  - Surgical debridement

GRAM-NEGATIVE BACTERIAL DISEASES

Ecthyma Gangrenosum

- Bacteremia with skin lesions
- *Pseudomonas aeruginosa* (gram-negative rods)
- Clinical
  - Hemorrhagic bullae that develop into black eschars
  - Often in sick hospitalized patients or those with HIV infection
- Treatment: penicillins, aminoglycosides, fluoroquinolones, third-generation cephalosporins, or aztreonam

Green Nail Syndrome

- *P. aeruginosa*
- Greenish discoloration in areas of onycholysis due to pigment production: —pyocyanin: blue, fluorescein: yellow/green, pyomelinin: black
- Seen in people who chronically have their hands in water
- Treatment: acetic acid solution and/or thymol 4% solution

Pseudomonas Folliculitis

- Hot tub folliculitis
- *P. aeruginosa*
- Pustular eruption in follicular distribution on trunk
- Exposure to whirlpools, swimming pools, and hot tubs
- Treatment: acetic acid soaks, quinolones

Gram-Negative Folliculitis

- *Proteus, Klebsiella, Escherichia,* and *Serratia* spp.
- Complication in patients with acne vulgaris and rosacea who have received systemic antibiotics for prolonged periods
- Clinical
- Acne has not been responding to antimicrobial therapy or other therapy: 80 percent of patients
- Patient's acne suddenly flares: 20 percent of patients
  - Superficial pustular lesions without comedones
  - Deep, nodular, and cystic lesions
- Laboratory studies: Gram stain and culture
- Treatment: isotretinoin, systemic antibiotics

Malakoplakia

- Commonly due to *Escherichia coli*
- Immunocompromised patients
- Clinical
  - Yellow to pink papules, nodules, or ulcerations
  - Draining abscesses/sinuses
- Laboratory studies
  - Histology: foamy histiocytes with distinctive basophilic inclusions: Michaelis-Gutmann bodies
  - Culture
- Treatment: quinolone antibiotics (e.g., ciprofloxacin) and sulfonamides (e.g., trimethoprim-sulfamethoxazole)

Rhinoscleroma

- *Klebsiella rhinoscleromatis* (gram-negative coccobacillus)
- Chronic granulomatous condition of the nose and upper respiratory tract
- Inhalation of droplets or contaminated material
- Clinical
  - Three stages: (1) rhinitic, (2) proliferative, (3) fibrotic

- Affects nose most frequently: intranasal rubbery nodules or polyps
- Epistaxis (bloody nose)
- Hebra nose: nasal enlargement, deformity, and destruction of the nasal cartilage
- Histology
  - Mikulicz cells: parasitized histiocytes
  - Russel body: eosinophilic bodies inside and outside plasma cells secondary to increased IgG
- Treatment
  - Surgery combined with antibiotic therapy
  - Tetracycline,ciprofloxacin, and rifampin

Meningococcal Disease (Fig. 15-8)

- *Neisseria meningitides* (obligate nonmotile aerobic encapsulated gram-negative diplococcus)
- Serogroups A, B, C, W135, X, Y, and Z
- Transmitted from person to person via respiratory secretions
- Human upper respiratory tract is the only known reservoir
- Common among individuals with deficiencies of terminal complement components C5 to C9 or properdin, immunoglobulin deficiency, asplenia, and HIV infection
- Direct invasion of endothelial cells and indirect damage from endotoxin release
- Clinical
  - Cutaneous findings
    - Petechiae
    - Pustules, bullae, and hemorrhagic lesions with central necrosis
    - Stellate purpura with a central gunmetal-gray hue
  - Fulminant meningococcemia
    - Can present as purpura fulminans
    - Waterhouse-Friderichsen syndrome: symmetric peripheral gangrene, cyanosis, hypotension, and profound shock
  - Meningitis
    - Headache and a stiff neck
    - Lethargy or drowsiness
  - Chronic meningococcemia: one week to as long as several months with recurrent fever and variable rash usually occurring on pressure areas or around painful joints
- Diagnosis
  - Blood culture on blood agar
  - Lumbar puncture
  - Gram stain of lesional skin biopsy or aspirate specimens
- Treatment: penicillin G, third-generation cephalosporin

Bartonella Species

- Cat-scratch disease, oroya fever, verruga peruana, bacillary angiomatosis, trench fever
- Aerobic gram-negative organisms

CAT-SCRATCH DISEASE (BENIGN LYMPHORETICULOSIS)

- *Bartonella henselae*
- Vector: cat flea (*Ctenocephalides felis*): maintains infection in cats
- Clinical
  - Infection spread by bite or scratch from cat
  - Fever 25 to 75 percent
  - Constitutional symptoms: anorexia, myalgias
  - Red papules appear at the site of scratch (develops over 3 to 10 days)
  - Lymphadenopathy (develops 1 week to 2 months after exposure)
    - Fifty percent have involvement of a single node
    - May last 6 weeks to 2 years
  - Parinaud oculoglandular syndrome: unilateral conjunctivitis and regional lymphadenitis
  - CNS changes 1 to 2 percent: headaches, mental status changes, seizures, encephalitis, cerebro spinal fluid usually normal
- Laboratory studies
  - Indirect fluorescent antibody (IFA) for *Bartonella* (cross-reactivity between *B. henselae* and *B. quintana*)
  - Brown-Hopp tissue Gram stain
  - Warthin-Starry silver staining
  - Fourfold rise in antibody levels
  - Lymph node biopsy: necrotizing granulomas

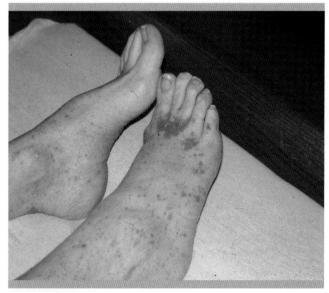

FIGURE 15-8 Meningococcal disease. *(Courtesy of Dr. Asra Ali.)*

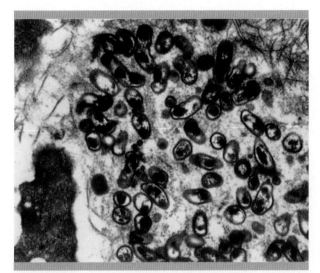

FIGURE 15-9 Bacillary angiomatosis. *(From Connor DH et al: Pathology of Infectious Diseases. Stamford, CT: Appleton & Lange, 1997, p. 408.)*

- Treatment
  - Immunosuppressed patients: erythromycin, doxycycline, septra, rifampin, ciprofloxacin, gentamycin
  - Immunocompetent patients: supportive care

BACILLARY ANGIOMATOSIS (FIG. 15-9)

- *B. henselae, B. quintana*
- Adheres to and invades red blood cells (RBCs)
- Makes an endothelial cell–stimulating factor: proliferation of both endothelial cells and blood vessels
- Clinical
  - Cutaneous patterns
    - Resembles pyogenic granuloma
    - Violaceous nodule (similar to Kaposi's sarcoma)
    - Lichenoid violaceous plaque
    - Subcutaneous nodule
  - *Peliosis* hepatitis
    - Blood-filled cysts in liver of AIDS patients (occasionally are found in spleen)
    - Nausea, vomiting, diarrhea, and fever with hepatosplenomegaly
    - Laboratory studies
  - Histology
    - Bacilli stain with modified Warthin Starry
    - Vascular proliferation with small vessels arranged in clusters; epithelial collarette may be observed
- Treatment
  - Erythromycin, doxycycline
  - May get Jarisch-Herxheimer reaction
    - Self-limited reaction to therapy

- Seen after treatment of syphilis, borreliosis, brucellosis, typhoid fever, trichinellosis, leptospirosis, leprosy, Lyme disease, relapsing fever (epidemic)
- Fever, malaise, nausea/vomiting
- Exacerbation of secondary rash
- Occurs 8 hours after the first injection
- Resolves within 24 hours

TRENCH FEVER

- *B. quintana*
- Incubation period of a few days to a month
- Symptoms begin with chills and fever: relapsing fever every 5 days (also can have single febrile episode occurring for 3 to 5 days or persistent fever lasting 2 to 6 weeks)
- Headaches, neck and back pain
- Groups of erythematous macules or papules measuring 1 cm or less
- Spread by human body louse (*pediculus humanus corporis*)
- Treatment: doxycycline, erythromycin

OROYA FEVER (CARRION'S DISEASE) AND VERRUGA PERUANA

- *B. bacilliformis*
- Vector: sand fly (Lutzomyia verrucarum)
- Clinical
  - Fever begins 3 to 12 weeks after bite
  - Fevers, headache, hemolytic anemia (80 percent of RBCs infected)
  - Skin lesions
    - Small nodules and subsequently become larger
    - Vascular miliary, nodular and mular lesions form (resemble pyogenic granuloma)
    - Can ulcerate, bleed, and heal by fibrosis over several months
    - Various stages may occur together
  - Chronic phase: verruga peruana (Fig. 15-10)
- Laboratory studies
  - Histology: rocha-lima bodies: purple cytoplasmic inclusion bodies in endothelial cells
  - Hemolytic anemia, thrombocytopenia, and elevated liver function studies
- Treatment: chloramphenicol or doxycycline

BRUCELLOSIS (MEDITERRANEAN FEVER, MALTA FEVER, GASTRIC REMITTENT FEVER, AND UNDULENT FEVER)

- *B. abortus, B. melitensis, B. suis,* and *B. canis* (gram-negative rods)
- Seen in meat-packing industry or from unpasteurized dairy products
- Cell wall lipopolysaccharide (LPS): principal virulence factor that enters macrophages

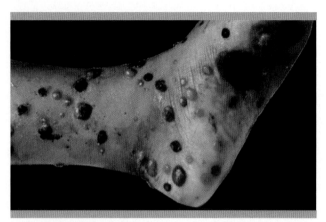

FIGURE 15-10 Verruga peruana. *(From Connor DH et al: Pathology of Infectious Diseases. Stamford, CT: Appleton & Lange, 1997, p. 434.)*

- Infects organs of the reticuloendothelial system (i.e., liver, spleen, bone marrow
- Host response results in tissue granulomas and visceral microabscesses
- Clinical
  - Acute febrile illness
  - Rarely granulomatous disease, erythema nodosum
  - Purpura, erythematous papules/nodules
  - Sacroiliitis, epididymoorchitis in males
  - Meningitis
- Laboratory studies
  - Agglutination titers
  - Culture
  - Immunoglobulin G (IgG) by ELISA
  - Anemia, thrombocytopenia, pancytopenia in 6 percent of patients
  - Elevated liver enzymes
  - Bone marrow: erythrophagocytosis
  - CSF reveals pleocytosis, elevated protein levels
- Treatment
  - Doxycycline and rifampin or trimethoprim-sulfamethoxazole (TMP-SMZ) plus rifampin
  - Drain pyogenic joint effusions or rare paraspinal abscesses

Leptospirosis (Weil Disease or Icteric Leptospirosis)

- *Leptospira interrogans*
- Infects many types of mammals: cats, dogs, cattle, pigs, squirrels
- Transmitted via infected urine and then through contact with contaminated water and soil
- Clinical
  - Two distinct presentations
    - Septicemic: organism may be isolated from blood cultures, CSF, and most tissues
    - Immune: circulating antibodies may be detected or the organism may be isolated from

urine; it may not be recoverable from blood or CSF
- Headaches, fever, petechiae
- Cutaneous lesions: macular or maculopapular eruption with erythematous, urticarial, petechial, or desquamative lesions, jaundice (90 percent of patients manifest a mild anicteric form of the disease)
- Vasculitis of capillaries: petechiae, intraparenchymal bleeding, and bleeding along serosa and mucosa
- Organ involvement: direct hepatic injury, alveolar capillary injury, renal tubular necrosis, myocarditis and coronary arteritis
- CSF: ± encephalitis
- Symptoms: based on species type
- Pretibial fever (Fort Bragg fever)
  - *L. autumnalis*
  - Fevers, pretibial erythema, and ocular symptoms
- Gastrointestinal symptoms: *L. grippotyphosa*
- Aseptic meningitis: *L. pomona* or *L. canicola*
- Jaundice: *L. icterohaemorrhagiae* (83 percent of patients)
- Weil syndrome: profound jaundice, renal dysfunction, hepatic necrosis, pulmonary dysfunction, and hemorrhagic diathesis
- Serologies: microscopic agglutination test (MAT) and the indirect hemagglutination assay (IHA): four-fold increase
- Diagnosis: dark-field microscopy of blood or rising anitbodies
- Treatment: tetracyclines or penicillin (possible Jarisch-Herxheimer reaction)

TICK-BORNE BACTERIAL INFECTIONS

Tularemia (Ohara's Disease, Deer Fly Fever)

- *Francisella tularensis* (gram-negative coccobacillus)
- Vectors: hard tick (*Dermacentor andersoni*) or deer fly (*Chrysops discalis*)
- Clinical
  - Eight forms: depend on mode of transmission: ulceroglandular (most common), glandular, oculoglandular, oropharyngeal, pulmonary, typhoidal, meningeal, chancriform
    - Intracellular parasitism of reticuloendothelial system of humans
    - Infection common in hunters after infected animal exposure via vectors
  - Ulceroglandular
    - Organism enters through a scratch or abrasion.
    - Ulcerates with sporotrichoid spread
    - Regional lymphadenopathy

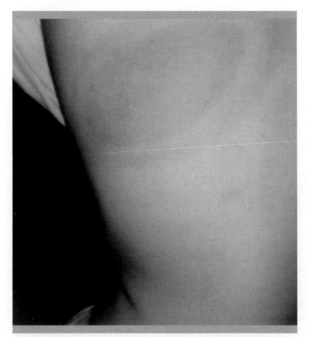

FIGURE 15-11 Lyme disease. *(From Connor DH et al: Pathology of Infectious Diseases. Stamford, CT: Appleton & Lange, 1997, p. 637.)*

- Laboratory studies: serologic testing
- Treatment: streptomycin

Lyme Disease (Fig. 15-11)

- Spirochete *Borrelia burgdorferi*
- Vector: *Ixodes* ticks (hard ticks)
  - Midwestern United States: *I. scapularis, I. dammini*
  - *I. ricinus* and *I. persulcatus* in Europe: Northwestern United States: *I. pacificus*
- Clinical
  - Stage 1: early localized
    - Erythema migrans (EM)
    - Erythematous macule or papule at site of the tick bite, can have central clearing
    - Expands over days to weeks centrifugally
  - Stage 2: early disseminated disease
    - Hematogenous spread
    - Lymphocytic meningitis, cranial neuropathy, carditis (heart block, arrhythmias), and rheumatologic changes (arthralgias, oligoarthritis)
    - Borrelial lymphocytoma: bluish red nodular swelling that is almost always on the lobe of the ear or the areola of the nipple
  - Stage 3: late Lyme disease
    - Acrodermatitis chronica atrophicans (ACA)
    - 20 percent of patients have history of untreated erythema migrans

- Develops 6 months to 10 years later
- Inflammatory phase
- Edema and erythema, usually on the distal extremities
- Loss of subcutaneous fat, with thin, atrophic, and dry skin
- Neurologic changes (meningitis, encephalitis)
- Diagnosis
  - Antibody titer
  - Confirm positive titers with PCR
- Treatment
  - Doxycycline or amoxicillin
  - Pediatric patients: erythromycin

Rickettsioses

- Obligate intracellular gram-negative coccobacilli
- Transmitted to humans by arthropods
- Spotted fever group
  - Rocky Mountain spotted fever (RMSF)
  - Rickettsial pox
  - Boutonneuse fever
- Typhus group
  - Louse-borne (epidemic) typhus
  - Brill-Zinsser disease (i.e., relapsing louse-borne typhus)
  - Murine (endemic or flea-borne) typhus
- Other rickettsial diseases
  - Tsutsugamushi disease (i.e., scrub typhus)
  - Q fever: *Coxiella burnetii*
  - Ehrlichia

ROCKY MOUNTAIN SPOTTED FEVER

- *Rickettsia rickettsii* (obligate intracellular gram - coccobacilli)
- Most common fatal tick-borne disease in the United States
- Vectors
  - Eastern United States: Wood tick *(Dermacentor andersoni)*
  - Western United States: Dog tick *(Dermacentor variabilis)*
- Infects the endothelium
- Clinical
  - Triad: fever, headache, and rash (1 to 2 weeks after tick bite)
  - Multisystem involvement is common
  - Skin lesions
    - Two to four days following fever
    - Blanchable macular rash that starts on extremities and spreads to trunk (centripetal)
    - Face usually spared; involvement of the scrotum or the vulva and palms/soles
    - Macules become petechial over a few days.
    - Desquamation as the rash fades

- Also see hepatosplenomegaly, myocarditis, thrombocytopenia
- Rumple-Leede test
  - Multiple petechiae where sphygmomanometer had been placed
- "Spotless" fever in 10 percent of cases
- Laboratory studies
  - Elevated liver function tests
  - Indirect fluorescent antibody
  - Direct immunofluorescence
  - Immunoperoxidase staining
  - Giemsa stain
  - Weil-Felix assay
- Treatment
  - Tetracycline or chloramphenicol (in pediatric patients)
  - Avoid sulfa treatments; symptoms may worsen

RICKETTSIALPOX

- *R. akari*
- Vector: rodent (mouse) mite (*Allodermanyssus sanguineus*)
- Clinical
  - Papular skin lesions appear at the bite site and then become vesicular with surrounding erythema
  - Dries and forms a black eschar; no scarrring
  - Sudden onset of high-grade fever and chills (3 days after skin lesions), headaches, and myalgias
- Laboratory studies
  - Cultures from blood
  - Direct fluorescent antibody test of biopsies from skin lesions
  - Immunofluorescence antibody (IFA) testing
  - Complement fixation
  - Giemsa stain
- Treatment
  - Self-limited disease
  - Doxycycline or chloramphenicol, quinolones

BOUTONNEUSE FEVER (MEDITERRANEAN FEVER)

- *R. conorii*
- Vector: *Rhipicephalus sanguineus* (brown dog tick)
- Clinical
  - Fever
  - Exanthem: erythematous papules, mainly on the lower limbs
  - Tache noire (eschar, necrotic plaque)
  - Malignant form
    - Criteria: requires two laboratory abnormalities (thrombocytopenia, increased creatinine level, hyponatremia, hypocalcemia, hypoxemia) and two clinical criteria (purpuric rash, stupor, pneumonia, bradycardia, coma, jaundice, gastrointestinal bleeding)

- More common in patients with underlying disease or in elderly persons
- Laboratory studies
  - Immunofluorescent antibody
  - Culture
  - Enzyme-linked immunosorbent assay (ELISA): detects antibodies to lipopolysaccharides (LPS) of *R. conorii*
- Treatment: tetracyclines together with chloramphenicol and quinolones

Typhus Group

- Diagnosis
  - Actual isolation and culture of *rickettsiae* are difficult
  - Serologic tests for antibodies
  - Indirect immunofluorescence assay (IFA)
  - Enzyme-linked immunosorbent assay (ELISA)
  - Indirect immunoperoxidase
  - Weil-Felix test
  - Polymerase chain reaction (PCR): serum or skin biopsy
  - Complement fixation (CF)
- Treatment: doxycycline, chloramphenicol

EPIDEMIC TYPHUS

- *R. prowazekii*
- Vector: human body louse (*Pediculus humanus corporis*)
- Clinical
  - Fever, headache
  - Maculopapular rash occurs on days 4 to 7
  - Begins on the axilla and trunk and spreads peripherally
  - Can become hemorrhagic with necrosis
  - Brill-Zinsser disease: mild reccurence of disease: can occur months, years, or even decades after treatment

MURINE TYPHUS (ENDEMIC TYPHUS)

- *R. typhi*
- Vectors: rat or cat flea (*Xenopsylla cheopis, Ctenocephalides felis*)
- Erythematous macular eruption without becoming hemorrhagic or necrotic following fever

Ehrlichiosis

- Due to gram-negative organisms, resemble *Rickettsia*
- Human monocytic ehrlichioses (HME): *Ehrlichia chaffensis*
- Human granulocytic ehrlichiosis (HGE): *E. phagocytophilia*
- Vector: Lone Star tick (*Amblyoma americanum*) or deer tick (*Ixodes persulcatus*)
- Infects mononuclear cells and granulocytes

- Clinical
  - Rash is rare in ehrlichiosis; however, can develop maculopapular lesions following fever
  - Rare renal failure and encephalopathy
- Laboratory studies
  - Histology: characteristic morulae in the cytoplasm of leukocytes
  - Neutropenia, lymphocytopenia, or thrombocytopenia
- Treatment: tetracyclines; chloramphenicol is not effective in ehrlichiosis

Scrub Typhus (Tsutsugamushi Fever)

- *Orientia tsutsugamushi* (formerly *Rickettsia tsutsugamushi*)
- Vector: trombiculid mite (only the larval stage: chigger): *Leptotrombidium akamushi* and possibly *L. deliense*
- Clinical
  - Headaches, shaking chills, lymphadenopathy, conjunctival injection, fever
  - Painless papule develops at site of bite, and then a central necrosis results with formation of an eschar
  - Five to eight days after infection, dull red rash on trunk and extending to the extremities
  - Pneumonitis or encephalitis can occur
  - Regional lymphadenopathy

SEXUALLY TRANSMITTED BACTERIAL INFECTIONS

Gonorrhea (Fig. 15-12)

- *Neisseria gonorrhoeae* (gram-negative intracellular aerobic diplococcus)

- Clinical
  - Men: urethritis; women: dyspareunia, bleeding or discharge
  - Neonates: bilateral conjunctivitis (ophthalmia neonatorum) after vaginal delivery from an infected mother
  - Acute perihepatitis with hepatic capsular adhesions (Fitz-Hugh-Curtis syndromes)
  - Dissemination: arthritis dermatitis syndrome
    - Septic arthritis: knee is most common site
    - Hemorrhagic vesiculopustular rash, mostly found on the distal extremities
    - Rare gonococcal meningitis and endocarditis
- Laboratory studies
  - Culture on chocalate agar
  - Gram stain
  - Fluorescein-conjugated monoclonal antibodies, enzyme-linked immunoassays
- Treatment: ceftriaxone intramuscular, cefixime, ciprofloxacin

Granuloma Inguinale (Fig. 15-13)

- *Calymmatobacterium granulomatis* (gram-negative rod)
- Clinical
  - Types of skin lesions
    - Ulcerovegetative type (most common)
      - ▲ Beefy red ulcers with clean, friable bases and distinct, raised, rolled margins
      - ▲ Autoinoculation is common
    - Nodular type
      - ▲ Pruritic, soft, red nodules at the site of inoculation
      - ▲ Eventually ulcerate and present a bright red granulating surface

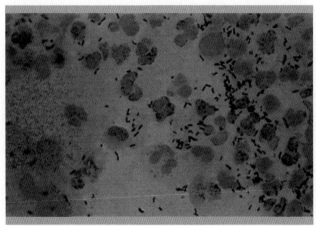

FIGURE 15-12 Gonorrhea. *(From Connor DH et al: Pathology of Infectious Diseases. Stamford, CT: Appleton & Lange, 1997, p. 686.)*

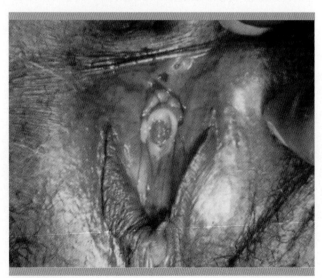

FIGURE 15-13 Granuloma inguinale. *(From Connor DH et al: Pathology of Infectious Diseases. Stamford, CT: Appleton & Lange, 1997, p. 567.)*

▲ Pseudobubo: nodule appears clinically as a lymph node
- Cicatricial type
  ▲ Dry ulcers evolve into cicatricial plaques
  ▲ May be associated with lymphedema
  ▲ Hypertrophic or verrucous type (relatively rare)
  ▲ Vegetating masses may resemble genital warts
- Laboratory studies
  - Culture not possible
  - Smear or biopsy
  - Wright, Giemsa or Warthin-Starry stain
  - Donovan bodies: intracytoplasmic bipolar staining, safety pin–shaped, inclusion bodies seen in histiocytes
- Treatment: doxycycline or bactrim

Lymphogranuloma Venereum (Fig. 15-14)

- *Chlamydia trachomatis* L1, L2, L3 serotypes
- Clinical
  - First stage: small papule usually not seen, lasts 1 week, painless
  - Second stage: buboes (painful lymph nodes) after 2 to 6 weeks; groove sign: enlargement of the inguinal nodes above and the femoral nodes below the inguinal ligament (poupart's)
  - Third stage: fistulas seen more often in women, proctocolitis, results in scarring/chronic lymphatic obstruction (acute rectal syndrome)
- Laboratory studies
  - Complement fixation test with titer of 1:64
  - Culture
  - Immunofluorescent testing with monoclonal antibodies
- Treatment: doxycycline; alternative is erythromycin

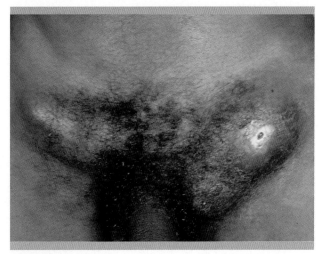

FIGURE 15-14 Lymphogranuloma venereum. *(From Freedberg IM et al: Fitzpatrick's Dermatology in General Medicine, 6th ed. New York: McGraw-Hill, 2003, p. 2199.)*

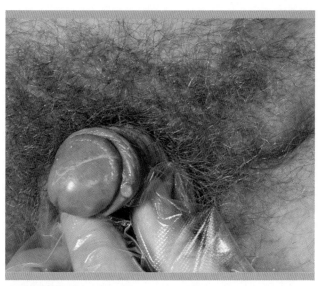

FIGURE 15-15 Chancroid. *(From Freedberg IM et al: Fitzpatrick's Dermatology in General Medicine, 6th ed. New York: McGraw-Hill, 2003, p. 2195.)*

Chancroid (Fig. 15-15)

- *Haemophilus ducreyi* (gram-negative bacillus)
- Clinical
  - Painful ulcers
  - Soft chancre, multiple painful ragged punched-out ulcers, with ragged undermined borders
  - Grayish fibrinous membrane covers the base of the ulcer
  - Lymph node involvement mostly unilateral and can rupture
  - Bubo: tender, fixed, inguinal lymphadenopathy
- Diagnosis
  - Gram staining: organisms in a school-of-fish pattern
  - Culture
- Treatment
  - Penicillin and tetracycline
  - Buboes should be drained

Syphilis

- *Treponema pallidum* (microaerophilic spirochete)
- Primary
  - Within 3 weeks
  - Highly infectious painless chancre (ulcerated lesion with a surrounding red areola)
  - Lasts 10 to 14 days
  - Buboes
    - Enlarged, nontender lymph nodes
- Secondary
  - Month after chancre
  - Hair (moth eaten): caused by papular follicular syphilids
  - Mucous membrane
    - Condyloma lata: Infectious papules develop at the mucocutaneous junctions
    - pharyngitis

- Mucous patches: silver-gray erosions with a red areola
- Skin: bilaterally symmetric discrete round macules on the trunk and proximal extremities (often affecting palms and soles); can become necrotic
- Ocular: anterior uveitis
- Latent syphilis
  - No clinical manifestations
  - Only evidence is positive serologic test for syphilis
    - Follows secondary stage
  - Categories
    - Early latent: <1 year's duration
    - Late latent: ≥1 year's duration or of unknown duration
- Tertiary
  - Within 3 to 10 years of infection
  - Gummas: granulomas of skin and bone
  - Neurologic: subacute meningitis
    - Tabes dorsalis: demyelination of the posterior columns, dorsal roots, and dorsal root ganglia (e.g., ataxic wide-based gait and foot slap)
    - Argyll Robertson pupil: small, irregular pupil that reacts normally to accommodation but not to light (Romberg sign)
  - Cardiovascular (aortic aneursym)
- Congenital syphilis
  - Early (<2 years of age)
    - Mucocutaneous
      ▲ Snuffles: rhinitis
      ▲ Rhagades (Parrot lines): depressed linear scars radiating from the orifice of the mouth
      ▲ Condyloma lata and mucous patches
    - Bone changes
      ▲ Cranio tabes: reduction in mineralization of the skull, with abnormal softness of the bone
      ▲ Pseudoparalysis of Parrot: child keeps limb still secondary to pain from osteochondritis
      ▲ Osteochondritis: sawtooth x-ray lesion
    - Skin
      ▲ Copper-colored papulosquamous eruption
      ▲ Hematologic: jaundice, thrombocytopenia
  - Late (>2 years of age)
    - Mucocutaneous
    - Interstitial keratitis
    - Corneal opacities
    - Hutchinson teeth: peg-shaped incisors
    - Mulberry molars: poorly developed cusps
    - Saddle nose: owing to gummatous periostitis
    - Syphilitic pemphigus: congenital bullae with purulent fluid on palm
    - Bone changes
      ▲ Saber shin: anterior bowing of tibia
      ▲ Frontal bossing

      ▲ Higomenaki's sign: unilateral sternoclavicular enlargement
      ▲ Bulldog jaw
    - Recurrent arthropathy
    - Cranial nerve VIII deafness
- Diagnosis
  - Histology: perivascular infiltration, chiefly by lymphocytes, plasma cells, and macrophages with warthin starry stain
  - Identification of *T. pallidum* in lesions on tissue
    - Dark-field microscopy: immediate result
    - DFA-TP (direct fluoresence antibody test): direct fluorescent antibody *T. pallidum*, 1 to 2 days
  - Nontreponemal serology screening
    - Venereal Disease Research Laboratory (VDRL): Measure IgM and IgG antibody directed against a cardiolipin lecithin-cholesterol antigen; not specific for *T. pallidum;* used to follow response to therapy
  - Prozone effect
    - May cause a false-negative reaction
    - Occurs when the reaction is overwhelmed by antibody excess and may happen in late primary or secondary syphilis
    - Should dilute the serum to at least a 1/16 dilution
  - Rapid plasma reagin (RPR)
    - Develops 1 to 4 weeks after chancre
    - Fourfold decline in titer by 3 months following treatment
    - False-positive RPR results occur in 1 to 2 percent of the normal population.
  - Treponemal tests
    - FTA-ABS: fluorescent treponemal antibody absorption
      ▲ Reactive 4 to 6 weeks after infection
      ▲ Remains reactive for many years
      ▲ Does not indicate response to therapy
      ▲ Does not distinguish between syphilis and other treponematoses
      ▲ Antibody (IgM and IgG) directed against *T. pallidum*
    - MHA-TP: microhemagglutination assay *T. pallidum* test
      ▲ Remains reactive for life
      ▲ Not recommended for monitoring reinfection or the efficacy of treatment
- Treatment
  - Penicillin 2.4 million units IM
  - Jarisch-Herxheimer reaction

MYCOBACTERIA

Leprosy (Hansen's Disease)

- Chronic granulomatous infection that affects skin and nerves

- *Mycobacterium leprae*
- Transmitted: respiratory, human to human, armadillos, and sphagnum moss
- Pregnancy is a precipitating factor for leprosy in 10 to 25 percent
- Incubation: up to 5 years and may be 20 years or longer
- Clinical
  - Neurological
    - Acral distal symmetric anesthesia
    - Palsies of cranial nerves V and VII
    - Nerve enlargement
    - Predilection for superficial nerves (temperature is cooler)
    - Great auricular, ulnar, median, superficial peroneal, sural, and posterior tibial nerves
    - Anesthetic skin lesions
  - Cutaneous: varies based on type of infection
  - Classification
    - Depends on the level of host cell-mediated immunity
    - TT (polar tuberculoid) ↔ BT (borderline tuberculoid) ↔ BB (borderline) ↔ BL (borderline lepromatous) ↔ LLs (subpolar lepromatous), LLp (polar lepromatous)
    - Levels are not static: patients can move through spectrum of disease through upgrading or downgrading reactions
- Indeterminate leprosy (IL)
  - Early form
  - One to a few hypopigmented, macules
- Tuberculoid leprosy (TT)
  - Paucibacillary
  - Predominance of CD4$^+$ cells: cell-mediated immunity can localize infection
  - T$_H$1 (proinflammatory) profile: interleukin 2 (IL-2), interferon-δ (IFN-δ), and IL-12
  - Clinical
    - Erythematous large plaque with well-defined borders and atrophic center
    - Tender, thickened nerves
    - Lesions are anesthetic and anhidrotic
  - Histology
    - Resembles tuberculosis
    - Two histologic patterns
      ▲ Mature epithelioid tubercles surrounded by lymphoid mantles
      ▲ Abundant large Langhans' giant cells, fibrinoid necrosis, occasional foci of caseation necrosis, and heavy exocytosis (associated with TT upgraded from BT)
    - Tissue may be negative for AFB owing to paucibacillary nature
  - Prognosis: spontaneous resolution or progression
- Borderline tuberculoid leprosy (BT)

- Host response is insufficient for self-cure
- Annular plaques but with satellite papules
- Multiple (occasionally solitary) anesthetic large (>10 cm) asymmetric lesions
- Symmetric nerve enlargement or palsy
- Histology: epithelioid tubercules, fewer lymphocytes than in TT; usually negative for AFB
- Borderline leprosy (BB)
  - Most unstable type
  - Patients quickly up- or downgrade to a more stable disease
  - Multiple annular plaques with indistinct borders compared with TT lesions; can have classic dimorphic lesions
  - Mild anesthesia
  - Histology
    - Granulomas have epithelioid differentiation; no giant cells or lymphoid mantle
    - AFB are found easily
- Borderline lepromatous leprosy (BL)
  - Host resistance too low to restrain bacillary proliferation
  - Destructive inflammation in nerves still occurs
  - Dimorphic lesions: hypesthetic annular patches with poorly marginated borders (lepromatous-like) and sharply marginated inner ones (tuberculoid-like)
  - Annular punched-out-appearing lesions also occur
  - Histology
    - Granulomas with lymphocytes and foamy macrophages
    - Nerves with lamination of the perineurium with inflammatory cell infiltration; bacilli and globi (*M. leprae* within multinucleate Virchow giant cells derived from histiocytes)
  - Patients remain in this stage, improve, or regress
- Lepromatous leprosy (LL)
  - Multibacillary
  - Predominance of CD8$^+$ cells
  - T$_H$2 (anti-inflammatory) profile: IL-4 and IL-10
  - Lack of cell-mediated immunity permits progression of the infection
  - Clinical (Fig. 15-16)
    - Poorly defined symmetric skin-colored plaques and nodules
    - Anhidrosis
    - Diffuse dermal infiltration
    - Leonine facies: widening of the nasal root
    - Madarosis: lateral alopecia of the eyebrows and lashes
    - Acral distal symmetric anesthesia
    - Testicular infection: invasion of the seminiferous tubules causing sterility
  - Subpolar lepromatous (LLs): can develop reversal reactions and erythema nodosum leprosum

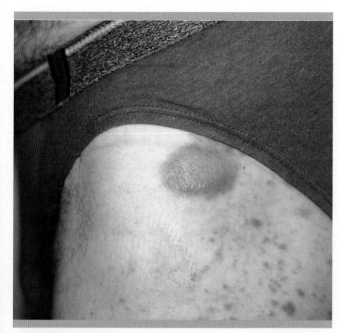

FIGURE 15-16 Lepromatous leprosy. *(Courtesy of Dr. Steven Mays.)*

- Polar lepromatous (LLp): develops erythema nodosum leprosum
- Histology: Grenz zone (superior area of spared dermis), foamy macrophages with globi
- Untreated LL is progressive
- Relapsing Leprosy
- Multibacillary patients who are noncompliant or develop drug resistance
- Clinical
  - Recurrence of initial presentation
  - Florid dermatofibroma-like lesions (histioid leprosy)
  - Develop a reactional state
- Reactional states: destructive inflammatory processes
- Jopling's type 1 reversal reaction
  - Delayed-type hypersensitivity reaction
  - Common in BL patients
  - Patients either upgrade to a more resistant state, remain unchanged, or downgrade to a less resistant state
  - Clinical
    - Abrupt conversion of previously quiescent plaques to tumid lesions and/or develop new tumid lesions in clinically normal skin
    - Dusky purple erythematous plaques
    - Iritis and lymphedema (elephantiasis graecorum)
    - Neuritis
- Jopling's type 2 reaction
  - Erythema nodosum leprosum

- Often in LL but also in BL before, during, or after therapy
- Clinical
  - Crops of tender bright pink nodules in clinically normal skin
  - Fever, anorexia, and malaise
  - Upper and lower extremities, facial lesions in 50 percent
  - Arthralgias
  - Neutrophilic leukocytosis
  - Abrupt fall in hematocrit
- Lucio reaction
  - Mexico and the Caribbean
  - Seen in Latapi's lepromatosis (diffuse nonnodular lepromatous leprosy with hemorrhagic infarcts)
  - Purplish suffusion of the hands and feet
  - Telangiectases
  - Nasal septum perforation
  - Total alopecia of the eyebrows and lashes
  - Acral distal symmetric anesthesia
  - Crops of necrotic lesions
  - Ulceration
  - Histology: ischemic necrosis secondary to endothelial parasitization by AFB; thrombosis in deep vessels
  - Rifampin is the treatment of choice
- Laboratory changes
  - Hyperglobulinemia
  - False-positive serologic test for syphilis
  - Anemia of chronic disease
  - Mild lymphopenia
  - Elevated serum lysozyme and angiotensin-converting enzyme
  - Proteinuria due to focal glomerulonephritis in ENL
  - Testicular involvement in LL males manifests as high serum follicle-stimulating hormone (FSH) and luteinizing hormone (LH) but low testosterone
  - Lepromin skin testing
    - Not useful in diagnosis
    - Helps in classification
  - All TT and most BT are positive and BB through LLp are negative
- Treatment
  - Paucibacillary (tuberculoid) disease
    - Dapsone (bacteriostatic) 100 mg daily
    - Supervised rifampin (bactericidal) 600 mg monthly for 6 months
  - Multibacillary (lepromatous) disease
    - Dapsone 100 mg daily + supervised rifampin 600 mg monthly + clofazimine (bacteriostatic) 50 mg daily (unsupervised) and 300 mg monthly (supervised) for 2 years
    - Alternative combination of minocycline (bactericidal) 100 mg daily + rifampin 600 mg daily for 2 to 3 years, followed by monotherapy

- Reversal reactions
  - Prednisone (0.5 to 1.0 mg/kg per day)
  - Prevents permanent nerve damage
  - Minimum of 6 months
- ENL
  - Thalidomide is the treatment of choice
  - Prednisone + clofazimine 200 mg daily

TUBERCULOSIS

- *Mycobacterium tuberculosis*
- Aerobic, intracellular, curved rods, acid fast
- Transmitted by airborne droplet nuclei
- Causes epithelioid granulomas with central caseation necrosis
- Clinical
  - Multiorgan infection
    - Pulmonary: productive cough, fever, and weight loss, hemoptysis or chest pain
    - Meningitis: headache that is either intermittent or persistent, mental status changes
    - Skeletal: spine (Pott disease), arthritis: hip or knee
    - Genitourinary: flank pain, dysuria, or frequency
    - Gastrointestinal TB: nonhealing ulcers
  - Cutaneous TB
    - Verrucosa cutis
      - ▲ Direct inoculation
      - ▲ Prior infection
      - ▲ Purplish or brownish-red warty growth
    - Lupus vulgaris
      - ▲ Hematogenous spread
      - ▲ Persistent and progressive
      - ▲ Sharply defined reddish brown papule, plaques with a gelatinous consistency (apple-jelly color)
    - Cutis orificialis
      - ▲ Autoinoculation into the periorificial skin and mucous membranes
      - ▲ Yellow/red nodule on mucosa that results in ulceration
      - ▲ Patients with advanced TB
      - ▲ Tuberculin sensitivity is strong
    - Scrofuloderma
      - ▲ Direct extension of underlying TB infection of lymph nodes, bone, or joints
      - ▲ Associated with TB of the lungs
      - ▲ Firm, painless lesions that eventually ulcerate with a granular base
      - ▲ Tuberculin sensitivity is strong
    - Metastatic tuberculous abscess (tuberculous gumma)
      - ▲ Occurs following hematogenous spread of mycobacteria to skin in tuberculin-sensitive individuals
      - ▲ Painless, fluctuant, subcutaneous abscesses form singly or at multiple sites
  - Miliary TB
    - ▲ Chronic infection
    - ▲ Hematogenous spread from the primary infection (usually in the lungs) to other tissues
    - ▲ Small red spots that develop into ulcers and abscesses
    - ▲ Immunocompromised patients, e.g., HIV, AIDS, cancer
  - Tuberculid: hypersensitivity reactions to tubercle bacillus
    - ▲ Erythema induratum (Bazin disease): Recurring subcutaneous nodules that may ulcerate and scar are seen in the posterior calves of women's legs; tubercle bacilli are not seen; mycobacterial cultures usually are negative
    - ▲ Papulonecrotic tuberculid: crops of recurrent necrotic skin papules on knees, elbows, buttocks or lower trunk that heal with scarring after about 6 weeks
    - ▲ Lichen scrofulosorum: lichenoid eruption of small follicular papules in young persons with underlying TB
- Laboratory studies
  - Tuberculin skin test
  - Chest radiograph
  - Culture of sputum specimens
  - Skin biopsy
- Treatment
  - Drug treatment is for 2 months
  - Isoniazid
  - Rifampin
  - Pyrazinamide
  - Ethambutol or streptomycin

Atypical Acid-Fast Mycobacterium (AFB)

- Facultative saprophytes and entities that are acid-fast: do not cause tuberculosis or leprosy
- Categorized based to their association with human disease according to their production of yellow or orange pigment and their rate of growth
- Group 1
  - Photochromogens (pigmentation on exposure to light)
  - *M. kansasii, M. marinum, M. simiae*
- Group 2
  - Scotochromogens (pigmentation formed in the dark)
  - *M. scrofulaceum, M. szulgai, M. gordonae*
- Group 3: nonchromogens (no pigmentation)
  - *M. malmoense, M. xenopi, M. avium-intracellulare*
- Group 4
  - Fast growers (groups 1,2, and 3 grow slowly)

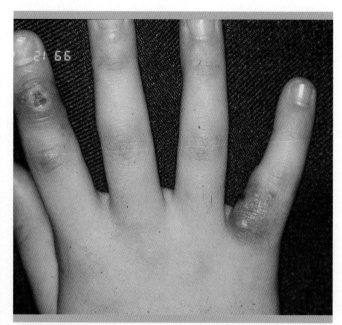

FIGURE 15-17 *M. marinum. (Courtesy of Dr. Asra Ali.)*

- Three to five days (e.g., *M. fortuitum*, *M. chelonae*, *M. abscessus*)
- *M. marinum* (Fig. 15-17)
  - Fish tank granuloma
  - Occurs when contaminated water is exposed to skin that has experienced open trauma
  - Isolated nodule typically on the upper extremity
  - Lymphangitic spread with several nodules
- *M. avium-intracellulare* complex (MAC)
  - May cause lung disease in humans
  - Usually requires an immunocompromised host (such as in humans with AIDS)
  - Skin disease rare: plaques, nodules, ulcers
- *M. ulcerans*
  - An emerging pathogen that causes Buruli ulcer in humans, deeply undermined, with scarring; lymphedema may result
  - Strict temperature requirements for growth (33°C)
  - Strict growth limited to fatty tissue beneath the dermis

- *M. kansasii*
  - Pulmonary and extrapulmonary disease in humans similar to tuberculosis, cellulitis, and abscesses
  - Difficult to treat; does not respond well to drugs
  - Grows well at 37°C
  - Most often recognized in immunocompromised host
- *M. scrofulaceum*
  - Causes scrofula (cervical adenitis)
  - Does not respond well to drugs
- *M. fortuitum* (rapidly growing mycobacteria) (also *M. chelonae* and variety *abscessus*): causes chronic abscesses in humans
  - Primary cutaneous oculation
  - May be resistant to treatment
- Diagnosis: stain with carbolfuchsin (basic dye, red in color)
- Treatment
  - Rifampin
  - Ethambutol
  - Minocycline
  - Trimethoprim and sulfamethoxazole
  - Clarithromycin

REFERENCES

Blume JE, Levine EG, Heymann WR. Bacterial Diseases, in: Bolognia JL et al. *Dermatology*. London: Mosby; 2003.

Chian CA, Arrese JE, Pierard GE. Skin manifestations of Bartonella infections. *Int J Dermatol*. 2002; 41(8):461–466.

Czelusta AJ, Yen-Moore A, Evans TY, Tyring SK. Sexually transmitted diseases. *J Am Acad Dermatol* 1999; 41(4): 614–623.

Freedberg IM et al. *Fitzpatrick's Dermatology in General Medicine*, 6th Ed. New York: McGraw-Hill; 2003.

McKee PH. *Pathology of the Skin: With Clinical Correlations*. London: Mosby-Wolfe; 1996.

McGinley-Smith DE, Tsao SS. Dermatoses from ticks. *J Am Acad Dermatol* 2002; 49(3):363–392.

Myers SA, Sexton DJ. Dermatologic manifestations of arthropod-borne diseases. *Infect Dis Clin North Am* 1994; 8(3):689–712.

Sadick NS. Current aspects of bacterial infections of the skin. *Dermatol Clin* 1997; 15(2):341–349.

CHAPTER 16

IMMUNOLOGY REVIEW

GENEVIEVE WALLACE
JENNIFER CLAY CATHER

CELLS OF THE IMMUNE SYSTEM

- The pluripotent hematopoietic stem cell gives rise to the common lymphoid progenitor and a common myeloid progenitor
- Three types of lymphocytes differentiate from a common lymphoid stem cell in the bone marrow and are identified based on their particular surface molecules: T-lymphocytes, B-lymphocytes, and natural killer cells (NK cells)
  - T-cell development starts when progenitor cells exit the bone marrow and undergo further maturation and selection in the thymus for the expression of antigen receptors useful in self/nonself discrimination (Fig. 16-1)
    - In the thymus, T cells rearrange their specific T-cell antigen receptors (TCRs) and then express CD3 along with the TCRs on their surface
    - The TCR for antigen is a heterodimeric integral membrane molecule expressed exclusively by T-lymphocytes
    - Positive and negative selection during thymocyte differentiation allows for the capacity for self/nonself discrimination
    - Different subpopulations exist based on surface expression of CD4 and CD8, as well as by their function in the immune response
    - Helper T-cells (T_H cells) express CD4 surface molecules and recognize antigen bound to class II major histocompatablilty complex (MHC) molecules
      - ▲ Play a central role in the initiation and regulation of immune responses through the secretion of cytokines and activation of macrophages
      - ▲ Important effectors of cell-mediated immunity

- ▲ Essential contributers to the generation of chronic inflammatory responses
- ▲ Cytotoxic activity either through the elaboration of cytotoxic cytokines (i.e., lymphotoxin, tumor necrosis factor α) or directly through interaction with antigen bound to MHC class II molecules
- ▲ Function depends on the cytokine profile produced, which characterizes them as T_H type 1 (T_H1) or T_H type 2 (T_H2)
- ▲ Three types of T cells based on their function: T_H0, T_H1, T_H2
  - △ Precursor T_H cell first differentiates into a T_H0 cell, producing interferon-α, (IFN-α), IFN-γ, and interleukin 4 (IL-4)
  - △ Cytokine environment determines whether the T_H0 cell will differentiate toward T_H1 or T_H2 profile
  - △ T_H1 cells produce primarily IFN-α, IL-2, and tumor necrosis factor α (TNF-α); important in cell-mediated immunity to intracellular pathogens (i.e., tubercle bacillus)
  - △ T_H2 cells produce predominantly IL-4, IL-5, IL-6, IL-10, IL-13, and IL-2 ; predominate in immediate or allergic type I hypersensitivity
- Cytotoxic T cells (Tc cells): cytotoxic effectors
  - ▲ Express CD8 surface molecules and recognize antigen bound to class I MHC molecules
  - ▲ Capable of direct killing of target cells expressing an appropriate viral peptide bound to a self-MHC class I molecule
  - ▲ Highly specific process that requires direct apposition of Tc cell and target cell membrane

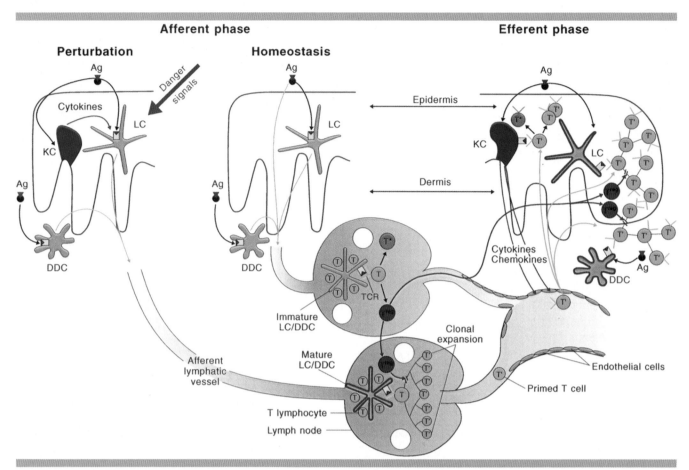

FIGURE 16-1 T-cell development. *(From Freedberg IM et al: Fitzpatrick's Dermatology in General Medicine, 6th ed. New York: McGraw-Hill, 2003, p. 270.)*

- ▲ Following killing, Tc cell is capable of detaching from target and seeking another target cell
- ▲ Destruction of target cells requires the insertion of perforins from the Tc cell into the target cell membrane that results in fragmentation of target cell nuclear DNA (apoptotic)
- – Suppressor T cells
  - ▲ Express CD8 surface molecules
  - ▲ Function as suppressors or downregulators of immune responses
  - ▲ Difficulty in defining the molecular basis of this activity
  - ▲ Thought to involve the production of non-specific inhibitory cytokines
- • Natural killer (NK) cells (large granular lymphocytes): ~2 percent of the circulating lymphocytes
  - – Reside in blood, spleen, lung, liver, gastrointestinal (GI) tract, and uterine deciduas

- – Main function is to provide cytotoxic activity toward virally infected cells and neoplastic cells—both antibody-independent and -dependent pathways exist
- – Respond early to microbial assault and interact with other cells of the innate immune system; able to nonspecifically kill target cells without prior sensitization
- – An important component of the innate (nonspecific) immune system
- – While they express neither a T-cell receptor nor a B-cell receptor, NK cells demonstrate specificity in their ability to recognize targets
- – Express distinct surface molecules
  - ▲ CD16 is a receptor for the Fc portion of Ig (used in antibody-dependent cellular cytotoxicity)
  - ▲ CD56 is a neural adhesion molecule that can bind to CD56 on other cells
- – Activated by IL-2, IL-7, and IL-12

▲ NK cells express the beta chain of the IL-2 receptor; therefore, resting NK cells can respond directly to IL-2

▲ Capable of producing cytokines following activation, such as IFN-γ and TNF-α, which can affect the proliferation and differentiation of other cell types

   – Mechanisms of cytotoxicity

     ▲ NK cells lyse targets through calcium-dependent release of preformed granules that contain perforin and granulysin

       △ Perforin, like complement, intercalates into the target cell membrane, forming pores

       △ Granulysin is a cationic protein that can induce apoptosis by initiating DNA fragmentation; may potentiate the activity of perforin in the lysis of target cells

     ▲ Receptor-induced apoptosis

       △ Activated NK cells will induce apoptosis or lysis of target cells expressing certain receptors such as FAS and TRAIL ligands death receptor-4 and death receptor-5

       △ NK cells are also capable of killing specifically when they are provided with an antibody [antibody-dependent cellular cytotoxicity (ADCC)]; ADCC occurs via binding of the antibody to the Fcγ receptor (CD16) located on the NK cell, leading to apoptosis of the target cell

• B-lymphocytes (B cells): antibody-producing cells

   – Represent 5 to 10 percent of the lymphocytes found in the blood

   – Express cell membrane immunoglobulin (Ig): Majority expresses both IgM and IgD

   – A small minority of B cells expresses surface IgG or IgA

   – Possess a variety of receptors on their surface (complement receptors, class I and II MHC molecule receptors)

   – Analogous to T cells, B cells have specific antigen receptors, which are immunoglobulins (Ig)

   – On activation and cross-linking of surface Ig by specific antigen, B cells undergo proliferation and differentiation to produce plasma cells

   – Plasma cells are nondividing, specialized cells whose only function is to secrete Ig

   – Immunoglobulins (Igs) (Fig. 16-2)

     ▲ Exquisite specificity for antigen is achieved by a mechanism of genetic recombination that is unique to Ig and T-cell receptor genes

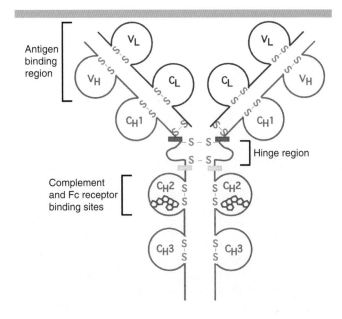

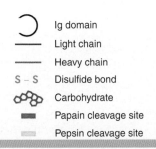

- Ig domain
- Light chain
- Heavy chain
- S – S Disulfide bond
- Carbohydrate
- Papain cleavage site
- Pepsin cleavage site

FIGURE 16-2 Immunoglobulin (Ig) molecule. *(From Freedberg IM et al: Fitzpatrick's Dermatology in General Medicine, 6th ed. New York: McGraw-Hill, 2003, p. 281.)*

     ▲ The antigen-binding site consists of a highly variable sequence created by the juxtaposition of two constituent polypeptides

     ▲ Heavy (H) chain: one of two alternative light (L) chains, κ or λ

     ▲ These polypeptides can be divided into two segments

       △ An antigen-binding amino-terminal variable domain

       △ One or more carboxy-terminal constant (nonvariable) domains that are generally responsible for biologic functions and activities of the molecule

   – Ig antigen receptor

     ▲ A virtually limitless array of specific-antigen receptors is possible

     ▲ The great variability is accomplished by recombination of genomic segments that encode the variable portions of Ig

▲ The products of these rearranged genes provide the B cell with its own unique receptor

▲ The mature receptor consists of the products of two or three such rearranged segments
  △ V (variable) and J (joining) for IgL chains
  △ V, D (diversity), and J for IgH

▲ DNA rearrangement
  △ Controlled by recombinases
  △ Sequential and carefully regulated process
  △ Leads to translation of one receptor of unique specificity for any given B-lymphocyte
  △ Unique specificity is achieved through a process termed *allelic exclusion* (only one member of a pair of allelic genes potentially contributing to an Ig is rearranged at a time)

▲ Somatic hypermutation
  △ A feature of the V-region construction that is unique to B cells
  △ As antigen is introduced into the system, and mature B cells remain genetically responsive to the antigenic environment
  △ As a result, a few B cells increase their affinity for the antigen
  △ Higher-affinity B cells are preferentially activated at exposure to the antigen
  △ As a result, the average affinity of antibodies produced during the course of an immune response increases (termed *affinity maturation*)

– Secretion of Ig molecules

▲ The cell-surface antigen receptors can be secreted in large quantities as antibody molecules

▲ The effector functions of antibodies can be carried out in solution or at the surface of other cells

▲ Secretion is accomplished by alternative splicing of Ig transcripts to include or exclude a transmembrane segment of the Ig heavy chains

– Ig classes (isotypes)(Table 16–1)

▲ Five major classes in order of abundance: IgG, IgM, IgA, IgD, and IgE

▲ Determined by the sequence of the constant region of its heavy chain (Ch)

▲ Isotype or class switching: B cell can change the class of antibody molecule that it synthesizes by using different Ch genes without changing its unique antibody specificity

• Common myeloid progenitor gives rise to the granulocytes (neutrophils, eosinophils, basophils), macrophages, dendritic cells, and mast cells

• Phagocytic cells (macrophage, neutrophils) recognize pathogens via cell-surface pattern-recognition receptors (PRRs)

• Macrophage mannose receptor: only on macrophages

  ▲ Recognize certain sugar molecules found on bacteria and some viruses (HIV)

  ▲ A direct phagocytic receptor (transmembrane bound)

– Scavenger receptors: recognize anionic polymers and also acetylated low-density lipoproteins

  ▲ Involved in the removal of old red blood cells

TABLE 16-1 Classes of Immunoglobulin

Characteristic	IgG	IgA	IgM	IgD	IgE
Heavy chain	γ	α	μ	δ	ε
Light chain	κ, λ	κ, λ	κ, λ	κ, λ	κ, λ
J chain	−	+	+	−	−
Molecular weight	150,000	160,000– 400,000	900,000	180,000	190,000
Serum half-life (days)	23	6	5	3	2
Serum concentration	1200	140–400	20–50	4	0.02
Complement fixation	+	±	+	−	−
Placental transfer	+	−	−	−	−

Used with permission from Freedberg IM et al: *Fitzpatrick's Dermatology in General Medicine,* 5th ed. New York: McGraw-Hill, 1999, p. 380.

▲ Also involved in the removal of pathogens
- CD14: on monocytes and macrophages
  ▲ Lipopolysaccharide (LPS) binds to LPS-binding protein, and this complex interacts with CD14
  ▲ CD14 interacts with toll-like receptor 4, which then activates the NFκB in the nucleus
- Mannan-binding lectin: initiates complement cascade (see complement below)
- Secreted soluble pattern-recognition receptors circulate in blood and lymph and facilitate phagocytosis and killing of the bound pathogen
- PRRs detect pathogen-associated molecular patterns (PAMPs), which are highly conserved amino acid sequences that are not shared with their host
- Ligation of PRRs leads to phagocytosis, destruction of pathogen, and cytokine release
• Dendritic cells express costimulatory molecules and cytokines in response to pathogen antigens
- Proteoglycans first recognized by PRRs
- Then costimulatory molecules and cytokines are upregulated via toll-like receptor-2

THE IMMUNE RESPONSE (FIG. 16-3)

• The human body can respond to antigen via innate and/or adaptive immunity
• Innate immunity (nonspecific, nonclonal, no anamnestic characteristics)
  • Characteristics
    - Immediate first line defense against pathogens composed three major components

▲ Nonspecific physical and chemical barriers
▲ Recruitment and activation of leukocytes [toll-like receptors (TLRs) → phagocytic granulocytes, monocytes-macrophages, etc.)
▲ Release and/or activation of extracellular humoral mediators (i.e., cytokines, complement)
- Exists prior to exposure to a given microbe or antigen (requires no previous exposure) and is rapidly available on pathogen encounter (minutes)
- Immune response is independent of specific antigen receptors and instead uses PRRs for carbohydrate and lipid structures that are germline-encoded with limited ligand diversity
• Key components
  - Physical and chemical barriers to pathogen invasion
    ▲ Skin, mucous membranes, cilia, and secretions (mucous and sweat) cover body surfaces and prevent microorganisms and other potentially injurious agents from entering the tissues beneath
      △ Mucous traps, dissolves, and sweeps away foreign substances
      △ Sweat contains lactic acid and other other substances that maintain the surface of the epidermis at an acidic pH, thereby decreasing colonization by bacteria and other organisms
    ▲ Chemical barrier antimicrobial substances include enzymes that can directly injure or kill microbial pathogens

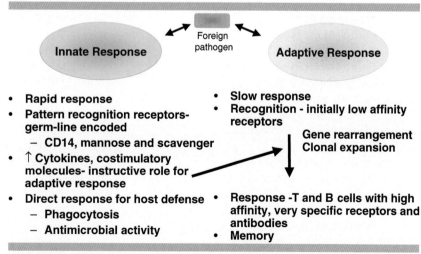

FIGURE 16-3 The immune response. *(From Freedberg IM et al: Fitzpatrick's Dermatology in General Medicine, 6th ed. New York: McGraw-Hill, 2003, p. 247.)*

△ Defensins (alpha or beta) and catheli-cidins have multiple receptor-mediated effects on the immune cells

△ Defensins secreted by resident epithelial cells or by transient leukocytes coat and destabilize the cell membrane of pathogens

♦ β-Defensins interact with CCR6

♦ Defensins are direct chemoattrac-tants for immature dendritic cells

♦ Defensins may facilitate microbial antigen delivery to dendritic cells

△ Cathelicidins are secreted by neu-trophils, keratinocytes, epithelial cells, mast cells, and monocytes-macrophages

- Activation of immune cells

▲ Phagocytic cell PRRs recognize highly con-served pathogen amino acid sequences and result in a variety of signals described pre-viously

▲ Natural killer (NK): activated by INF-γ, INF-β, and macrophage-derived cytokines (TNF-α, IL-12)

▲ Dendritic cells are stimulated to move from the periphery to the lymph node by TNF-α, where they mature from phagocytes into nonphagocytic efficient antigen-presenting cells

▲ Common stem cell precursor for eosinophils and basophils; therefore, many similarities

△ Eosinophils

♦ IL-5 (released by T_H2 cells) increases the production of mast cells in the bone marrow

♦ Possess chemokine receptors that, when bound, activate, degranulate, and coordinate chemotaxis

◇ CCR3 binds to eotaxin 1 and 2, MCP-3, MCP-4, and RANTES

◇ CCR2 binds to MCP-1

♦ After cytokine and chemokine acti-vation, the high affinity IgE recep-tors (FcεRI) are expressed along with an increase in complement receptors

♦ Degranulation releases major basic protein, which causes degranulation of mast and basophils

△ Basophils

♦ Growth factors include IL3, IL-5, and GM-CSF

♦ TGF-β + IL3 suppress eosinophil dif-ferentiation and promote basophil differentiation

♦ Eotaxins attract and degranulate (release histamine and IL-4)

- Toll-like receptors (TLRs)

▲ Found on macrophages, dendritic cells, and epithelial cells

▲ Innate transmembrane receptors that recog-nize different types of pathogen-associated molecular patterns (PAMPs), which are molecular patterns unique to pathogens

▲ Ligands include lipopolysaccharide, pepti-doglycan, CpG DNA

▲ Humans have at least 10 different TLRs

▲ TLRs identify the nature of the pathogen and result in NFκB activation, which results in appropriate cytokine and chemokine expression, along with increased expression of additional immune system receptors

- Bridging innate immunity to adaptive immunity

▲ Macrophages and dendritic cells present antigens to T cells

▲ Interaction of PAMPs and TLRs on the sur-face of dendritic cells triggers secretion of innate immune cytokines (INF-α, INF-β, IL-12, TNF-α) and chemokines, which may affect both T and B cells

▲ Pathogens coated with fragments of the complement protein C3 bind strongly to B cells

• Adaptive immunity (inducible and antigen-specific) refers to antigen-specific immune response (humoral and cell-mediated immunity, mediated by specific antibodies)

• Humoral immunity

- Antibodies, dissolved in blood, lymph, and other body fluids, bind the antigen and trigger a response to it (release cytokines)

- Viruses and intracellular parasite antigens

▲ Processed into peptides within antigen-pre-senting cells (APCs) and are bound to the heavy chain of an MHC class I and pre-sented to a CD8+ or CD4+ (cytotoxic) T cell

▲ If a specific antigen encounters its specific T-cell receptor, IL-2 is released, and T-cell activation, along with expansion of the antigen-specific cytotoxic T-cell (Tc) line, follows

▲ If an antigen-specific Tc cell encounters a cell expressing its specific antigen, the acti-vation signal that ensues results in exocyto-sis of granzymes (granules containing enzymes), perforins, cytolysins, lymphotox-ins, and serine esterases, which kill the APC

- Extracellular antigens
  - ▲ Taken up by APCs by pinocytosis and then processed into peptides
  - ▲ Peptides are presented in the context of an MHC class II molecule to a CD4+ T cell
- After activation, CD4 and CD8 cells may differentiate toward T_H1 or T_H2 cytokine profiles depending on cytokine milieu
  - ▲ T_H1 cell activation
    - △ Goal: macrophage activation and increased cell-mediated immunity
    - △ T_H1 cytokine profile: IL-2, IFN-γ, TNF-α, and IL-12
      - ◆ IL-2: T- and B-cell activation
      - ◆ IFN-γ: activator of macrophages and NK cells
      - ◆ TNF-α: activates macrophages and stimulates the acute-phase response along with IL-1
  - ▲ T_H2 cell activation
    - △ Goal: B-cell activation
    - △ IL-2 production by TH1 cells induces the CD4+ T_H2 cells to transform, differentiate, and divide
    - △ T_H2 cytokine profile: IL-4, IL-5, IL-10, and IL-13
      - ◆ IL-4: promotes the synthesis of antibodies by stimulating B-cell differentiation
      - ◆ Downregulates IFN-γ; therefore, can suppress cell-mediated immunity
      - ◆ Can cause production of IgE
      - ◆ IL-5: helps with B-cell differentiation
      - ◆ Facilitates IgA synthesis
      - ◆ Stimulates growth of eosinophils
      - ◆ IL-4, IL-10, and IL-13 can inhibit T_H1 cell release of IFN-γ and IL-2; thus capable of suppressing cell-mediated immunity
- B-cell response
  - ▲ Like T cells, B cells contain membrane-bound IgM antibody specific for the antigen epitope
  - ▲ Primary immune response: initial encounter
    - △ Antigen bound to the APC receptor along with cytokines IL-2 and IL-4 (stimuli for T cells) triggers the antigen-specific B cell to differentiate and divide
    - △ IgM is secreted initially, and subsequent gene arrangements result in a switch to IgG, IgA, and IgE
    - △ B memory cells of all classes are generated and migrate to various lymphoid tissues, where they have extended survival

- △ Plasma cell: B cell that secretes antibodies
- ▲ Secondary immune response: subsequent exposure to the same antigen
  - △ Activation of antigen-specific B cell results in more efficient antibody synthesis and faster isotype switching from IgM to IgG
  - △ A greater amount of IgG with higher affinity for the antigen during subsequent encounters
  - △ Predominance of IgA secretion in mucosal tissues
- • Cell-mediated immunity (CMI)
  - Mediated by T cells, macrophages, and NK cells
  - Directed toward intracellular microorganisms and neoplastic cells
  - Mechanism of action
    - ▲ T_H1 cells become sensitized to the antigen and release TNF-α and IFN-γ
    - ▲ TNF-α and IFN-γ activate macrophages that subsequently release IL-12
    - ▲ Activated macrophages kill target cells through phagocytosis and release of microbicidal agents (reactive oxygen species, IL-1, thrombin, TGF-β, TNF-α)
    - ▲ CD8+ Tc cells
      - △ IL-12 activates CD8+ (Tc) cell proliferation
      - △ Antigen binding to receptors results in release lytic agents (perforins, cytolysins, lymphotoxins)
  - Antibody-dependent cellular cytotoxic (ADCC) reactions
    - ▲ Target cell is linked to the T cell by an antibody bridge
    - ▲ Fab portion of the antibody binds to a specific membrane antigen on the target cell
    - ▲ Fc portion of the antibody binds to the Fc receptor on the T cell

HYPERSENSITIVITY REACTIONS

- • Resulting from humoral immunity or cell-mediated immunity
- • Type I: anaphylaxis reactions (IgE-mediated)
  - • Immediate hypersensitivity reactions: Symptoms begin within 30 minutes of the exposure
  - • Clinical classification: Type I reactions are categorized as local or systemic
    - Local: allergic rhinitis, allergic asthma, atopic (familial predisposed) dermatitis
    - Anaphylaxis: hypersensitive response in genetically susceptible individuals to small

amounts of antigen to which they have been sensititized previously

- ▲ Generalized vasodilation and increased vascular permeability can lead to hypotension, shock, and ultimately death
- ▲ Early signs and symptoms include angioedema, urticaria, dyspnea, vomiting, and abdominal cramping
- Common triggers are foods (peanuts, eggs, shellfish), drugs (aspirin, radiocontrast media, penicillin and other beta-lactam antibiotics), *Hymenoptera* venom, and pollens
- Mechanism
  - Sensitization to a particular antigen occurs after an initial exposure by injection, ingestion, inhalation, or insect sting
  - IgE antibody is produced, which then binds to its receptor on the surface of mast cells and basophils
  - After reintroduction of antigen to the sensitized host, the antigen binds to several cell-bound IgE antibody molecules, resulting in cross-link and signal transduction
  - Mast cells degranulate and release histamine, leukotriene, serotonin, and bradykinin, resulting in vasodilation, increased vascular permeability, contraction of smooth muscle in brochi, and increased secretions
  - Primary mediators include TNF-α, IL-1, IL-6, prostaglandins, leukotrienes, and histamine
- Treatment: epinephrine, diphenhydramine, aminophylline, and corticosteroids
- Type II reactions: cell surface antigen-antibody cytotoxicity reactions (antibody-mediated)
  - Antibody is directed against an antigen that may be intrinsic (innately part of the host tissues) or extrinsic (absorbed onto host tissue surfaces during exposure)
  - IgG and IgM antibodies bound to these antigens form in situ complexes that activate the classical pathway of complement and generate mediators of acute inflammation at the site
  - Antibody-dependent cell-mediated cytotoxicity (ADCC): NK cells destroy antibody-coated target cells via perforins and serine proteases, which results in pore formation and cell lysis
  - In some cases, formation of the antigen-antibody complexes does not lead to activation of the complement system but still can lead to cell injury
  - Examples of cytotoxic reactions: transfusion reactions, reactions to certain drugs (penicillin, quinidine, methyldopa), and autoimmune hemolytic anemia or thrombocytopenia
- Type III reactions: antigen-antibody complex reactions
  - Circulating antibodies bind to antigen and form complexes that, in the presence of excess antigen, escape phagocytosis and deposit on the surface of blood vessels or tissues
  - Antigen-antibody complexes activate complement and release C5a that acts as a potent neutrophil chemotactic factor and anaphylatoxin; clotting factors are also activated
  - Neutrophils are attracted to the area of complex deposition and release lysosomal enzymes, causing tissue destruction
  - Examples of antigen-antibody complex reactions
    - Arthus reaction: local type III reaction usually seen when antigen is injected into the skin
      - ▲ An IgG antibody directed against the antigen forms immune complexes that bind Fc receptors on leukocytes and mast cells
      - ▲ The immune complexes also activate complement and release of chemotactic factors (C3a, C5a), leading to neutrophil infiltration and activation
    - Serum sickness is an allergic vasculitis characterized by joint pain, fever, pruritic rash, and lymphadenopathy that leads to a complement-mediated systemic immune complex reaction
      - ▲ Occurs by the injection of foreign serum or its products into the blood
      - ▲ Antibody-antigen complexes activate the complement cascade and also trigger ligation of the FcγRIII mast cell receptor, resulting in histamine release
      - ▲ Associated medications include sulfonamides, penicillin, cephalosporins, phenytoin, thiourea, and more recently, Lamictel and streptokinase
- Type IV reactions: delayed-type hypersensitivity (DTH) reactions
  - Consequence of cell-mediated immunity (antigen-specific T cells): appears in 24 to 48 hours
  - Three clinical examples exist
    - Delayed-type hypersensitivity: antigen introduced by sting (venom) or iatrogenically (PPD)
    - Contact hypersensitivity: antigen in the form of haptens from a topical exposure (i.e., Rhus dermatitis, nickel)
    - Gluten-sensitive enteropathy: antigen introduced parenterally
  - Common pathway
    - An antigen to which a person has been exposed previously is introduced to the skin or gut
    - APCs process antigen and present to specific memory $T_H 1$ cells

- T_H1 cells release proinflammatory cytokines (i.e., IFN-γ and TNF-β), which results in activation of macrophages and increased vascular permeability

CYTOKINES

- Polypeptides serve as intercellular messengers in order to mediate immune responses
  - Autocrine in nature: affect the cell that releases the cytokine
  - Paracrine in nature: affect the adjacent cells
  - Endocrine in nature: affect distant cells
- Produced by inflammatory cells (lymphocytes, monocytes) as well as resident cells in the skin (keratinocytes, Langerhans cells, and endothelial cells)
- Variable effects: see Table 16-2 on specific cytokines and their actions
- Involved in innate immunity (occurs without the activation of B or T cells) or adaptive immunity (depends on a B or T cell reacting to a specific antigen)
- T_H1 versus T_H2 T-cell cytokines
  - T_H1: produce IFN-α and IL-2
    - Result in activation of macrophages

- Predominate in psoriasis and allergic contact dermatitis
- T_H2: produce IL-4, IL-5, IL-6, and IL-10
  - Result in activation of mast cells, eosinophils, and B cells
  - Predominate in advanced CTCL, parasitic infections, and atopic dermatitis
- Medications that target cytokines include receptor fusion proteins (etanercept), monoclonal antibodies (infliximab and adalimumab), and receptor antagonists that neutralize or inhibit various cytokines

CHEMOKINES

- Class of cytokines that express both chemoattractant and cytokinetic properties
  - Leukocytes can respond to a panel of different chemokines
  - Neutrophils are recruited first
  - Monocytes and immature dendritic cells are recruited later
- Structures contain a four-cysteine motif with a disulfide bond between cysteines 1,3 and 2,4 along with an N-terminus critical for receptor recognition and activation
- Four subfamilies, based on the position of the first two of four conserved cysteines (α, β, γ, and κ)

TABLE 16-2 Major Families of Cytokine Receptors

Receptor Family	Example	Major Signal Transduction Pathways(s) Leading to Biologic Effects
IL-1 receptor family	IL-1R, type 1	NF-κB activation via TRAF6
TNF receptor family	TNFR1	NF-κB activation involving TRAF2 and TRAF5
		Apoptosis induction via "death domain" proteins
Hematopoietin receptor family (class I receptors)	IL-2R	Activation of Jak-STAT pathway
Interferon/IL-10 receptor family (class II receptors)	IFN-γR	Activation of Jak-STAT pathway
Immunoglobulin superfamily	M-CSFR	Activation of intrinsic tyrosine kinase
TGF-β receptor family	TGF-βR, type I and II	Activation of intrinsic serine/threonine kinase coupled to SMADs
Chemokine receptor family	CCR5	Seven transmembrane receptors coupled to G-proteins

M-CSF, macrophage colony-stimulating factor; SMAD Sma- and Mad-related protein.

Used with permission from Freedberg IM et al: *Fitzpatrick's Dermatology in General Medicine*, 6th ed. New York: McGraw-Hill, 2003, p. 286.

- Multiple cell types can produce the same chemokine, and a cell can produce many different chemokines in response to a single stimulus
- Chemokine receptors
  - Members of the large family of G protein–coupled receptors possessing seven transmembrane-spanning domains
  - One receptor is capable of binding to various chemokines
  - Binding of the ligand to the chemokine receptor induces conformational changes in the receptor and leads to activation of G proteins
  - The G protein causes exchange of GDP for GTP and begins a chain of events resulting in intracellular signaling responses
- Biologic effects of chemokines
  - Influences leukocyte trafficking at all stages of maturation
  - Regulates cells trafficking within primary and secondary lymphoid organs (i.e., from bone marrow to the spleen, lymph node, or thymus)
  - Controls the type of inflammatory infiltrate at a site of inflammation
  - Regulates the expression and activity of adhesion molecules on the leukocyte surface to increase the adhesion of leukocytes to activated endothelium
  - Recruitment and activation of neutrophils and mononuclear cells to sites of inflammation
  - Regulates proliferation of subsets of mature stem cells and immature progenitor cells
- Secretion of chemokines
  - Released by endothelial cells, leukocytes, and tissue cells at the sites of inflammation
  - Locally retained on cell surface proteoglycans, establishing a chemokine chemical gradient that begins at the endothelium surface and increases as the cell approaches the focus of inflammation
  - Thought to be upregulated in inflammatory foci and certain inflammatory diseases (i.e., glomerulonephritis, rheumatoid arthritis, ulcerative colitis, and Crohn's disease)

EICOSANOIDS

- Large, complex family of immunomodulatory and vasoactive compounds derived from arachadonic acid (AA) generated by mast cells, basophils, eosinophils, and mononuclear leukocytes
- General
  - Peroxidation of AA by phospholipases generates prostaglandins [via the cyclooxygenase (COX) pathway] or thromboxanes and leukotrienes [via the lipooxygenase (LO) pathway]
  - Play a key role in inflammatory and anaphylactoid responses

- Arachadonic acid
  - Polyunsaturated fatty acid with 20 carbon atoms and four double bonds
  - Resides in cell membrane lipids
  - Derived from dietary sources or synthesized by desaturation and elongation of linoleic acid
- Cyclooxygenase (COX) pathway
  - Key enzyme in the pathway, cyclooxygenase (COX), has two different isoforms
    - COX-1: constitutively expressed in cells and associated with cellular homeostasis
    - COX-2: requires specific induction, upregulated in inflammatory conditions, and associated with synthesis of proinflammatory prostaglandins
    - COX-1 and COX-2 are inhibited by nonsteroidal anti-inflammatory drugs
  - Derivatives of the cyclooxygenase pathway
    - Prostaglandins (PGs)
      ▲ PGD2 released by activated mast cells
        △ Generated very rapidly after IgE-dependent activation
        △ Enhances venular permeability
        △ Promotes leukocyte adherence to vascular endothelial cells
        △ Coronary and pulmonary vasoconstrictor
        △ Peripheral vasodilator
        △ Potent inhibitor of platelet aggregation
        △ Chemokinetic for neutrophils and in conjunction with LTD4 can induce the accumulation of neutrophils in the skin
        △ Important hypotensive effects, particularly in mastocytosis, suggesting that it is probably an important contributor to the anaphylactic response
        △ Metabolite of PGD2 is elevated in patients with systemic mastocytosis
      ▲ PGE2
        △ Proinflammatory effects
        △ Released in response to infection with ameba (specifically *Entamoeba histolytica*) and parasites
        △ Released by endothelial cells following trauma, leading to tissue inflammation
        △ Plays an important role in the secondary immunosuppression following surgical stress
        △ Synthesized by the synovial lining in rheumatoid arthritis
      ▲ PGI2 and PGE2
        △ Potent vasodilators
        △ Enhance capillary permeability and edema formation
  - Derivatives of lipoxygenase (LO) pathway
    - Thromboxanes/thromboxane A2

- Promotes platelet aggregation, bronchoconstriction, and vasoconstriction
- Contributes to the pulmonary hypertension and acute tubular necrosis that occurs in shock
- Predominately found in platelets and monocytes
- Leukotrienes
  - Mediate wheal and flare reactions, edema formation, and bronchial constriction
  - Combined with histamine can result in hypotension
  - One of the major inflammatory mediators involved in asthma pathogenesis
  - Enhances airway hyperresponsiveness and smooth muscle hypertrophy
  - Causes mucus hypersecretion and mucosal edema
  - Induces influx of eosinophils into the airway tissue key players in anaphylactic reactions and IgE-mediated syndromes
  - Mediators of the vascular sequelae of anaphylaxis as well as of shock states resulting from sepsis or tissue injury
- LTB4
  - Predominantly formed and released by neutrophils
  - Neutrophil chemoattractant
- LTC4
  - Derived from activated mast cells, basophils, and eosinophils
  - Potent vasodilator

COMPLEMENT

- General
  - Group of plasma and cell membrane proteins that play a role in inflammation, tissue injury, hemostasis, and immune response to antigens
  - Some of the proteins exists as precursor (inactive) enzymes that are cleaved by proteolysis; products then act as a catalyst for the next step in the cascade
  - The central step of the complement pathway is the generation of C3b cleavage by C3 convertases and subsequent assembly of C5b-9, the membrane attack complex (MAC)
- Main functions
  - Lysis of cells: examples: *Neisseria,* allografts
  - Generate inflammatory mediators and chemotactic fragments
  - Opsonization for enhanced phagocytosis
- Three pathways for complement activation
  - Classical pathway
    - Activated primarily by antibody-antigen complexes

- Also activated by oligosaccharides, porins from gram-negative bacteria, ligand-bound C-reactive protein
- The starting point of the classical pathway is C1
- Steps of classical pathway
  - Aggregation of IgG or IgM activates C1
  - C1 is a calcium-dependent complex of three subunits: C1q, C1r, and C1s
  - Activated C1 then cleaves C4 to C4a and C4b
  - C4a is a weak anaphylatoxin
  - C4b binds C2 in the presence of Mg^{2+}
  - C1 cleaves the attached C2 into C2b and C2a
  - C2b is released, cleaved by plasmin, and has kinin-like activity
  - C2a stays bound to C4 to form C4b2a—the classical pathway C3 convertase that generates C3
- Alternative pathway
  - Activation usually occurs independent of antibody
  - May be activated by bacterial surfaces, virus-infected cells, certain viruses, abnormal erythrocytes, and lymphoblastoid cell lines
  - The starting point of the alternative pathway is C3b
  - Steps of the alternative pathway
    - Starts with internal hydrolysis of C3 on interaction with water to form C3 (H_2O)
    - C3 (H_2O) then binds factor B and magnesium
    - Factor D then cleaves the bound factor B into Ba and Bb
    - Ba is released
    - Bb stays bound to C3(H_2O) to form C3 (H_2O), which is the initial C3 convertase of the alternative pathway that cleaves C3
    - C3 is cleaved to C3a and C3b
    - C3a is released and becomes a potent anaphylatoxin
    - C3b binds factor B in the presence of magnesium, and factor B is cleaved by factor D into Bb and Ba
    - Ba is released
    - Bb stays bound to form C3bBb, the C3 convertase of the alternative pathway
- Lectin pathway
  - C4 activation can be achieved without antibody and C1 participation
  - Pathway is initiated by three proteins: a mannan-binding lectin (MBL) [mannan-binding protein (MBP)], which interacts with two mannan-binding lectin–associated serine proteases (MASP and MADSP2), analogous to C1r and C1s

- This interaction generates a complex analogous to C1qrs and leads to antibody-independent activation of the classical pathway
- Common portion of pathway
  - At this point, the classical, alternative, and lectin pathways all have generated C3b using their respective C3 convertases, C4b2a, and C3bBb
  - The two convertases assist in the cleavage of C3 to C3a (an anaphylatoxin) and C3b
  - C3b binds to the next protein, C5
  - C5 is also cleaved by the C3 convertases into C5a and C5b
  - C5a is released and becomes the most potent anaphylatoxin
  - C5b becomes the point of assembly for MAC (membrane attack complex)
  - C5b associates with target cell membrane and C6
  - C5b6 then associates with the assembly of C7, C8, and C9
  - C5b6789 is the MAC that forms transmembrane channels (holes) in the cell membrane that allow an influx of water and ions to cause cell swelling and lysis
- Points of regulation
  - Classical pathway
    - C1 is inhibited by C1 inhibitor (C1INH)
    - C1 esterase inhibitor (C1INH) deficiency causes angioedema
    - Factor I inhibits formation of C3 convertase
    - C4-binding protein inhibits formation of C3 convertase
    - Decay accelerating factor (DAF) inhibits formation of C3 convertase
  - Alternative pathway
    - Factor H inhibits formation of C3 convertase
    - Factor P (properdin) protects C3 convertase
- Anaphylatoxins
  - C3a, C5a, C4a
  - Cause release of histamine from mast cells, degranulation of basophils, increase in vascular permeability
  - Anaphylatoxins are regulated by a carboxipeptidase present in plasma

COMMON DERMATOLOGIC DISEASES WITH IMMUNOLOGIC PATHOGENESES

Vitiligo

- Clinical: depigmentation patches of skin in various distributions on the body
- Etiology: loss of melanocytes from the epidermis
- Considered by most to be an autoimmune phenomenon

- Both melanocyte autoantibodies and T cells are involved in the pathogenesis
- Associated with other autoimmune diseases as well as organ-specific autoantibodies: diabetes mellitus, pernicious anemia, systemic lupus erythematosus, thyroid disease (Graves' disease)
- Treatment: steroids, immune modulators: calcinuerin inhibitors, phototherapy, punch grafts

Psoriasis

- Clinical: a systemic inflammatory disorder that manifests as sharply dermarcated red plaques with silvery-white scales on the extensor surfaces and scalp
- Types
  - Plaque psoriasis: raised lesions most common on the extensor surfaces of the knees, elbows, scalp, and trunk (Fig. 16-4)
  - Guttate psoriasis: droplike lesions; may follow streptococcal pharyngitis
  - Inverse psoriasis: flexural surfaces, intertrigenous areas
  - Pustular psoriasis: can occur with fever
  - Erythrodermic psoriasis: nail changes: nail pitting, oil spots, and onycholysis
  - Scalp psoriasis
  - Inflammatory progessive arthritis: Approximately 10–30 percent of patients with psoriasis develop psoriatic arthritis; asymmetric oligoarthritis occurs in as many as 70 percent of patients
- Pathogenesis
  - Activated memory T-lymphocytes release proinflammatory cytokines, which results in proliferation of keratinocytes and leukocyte recruitment
  - CD4+ and CD8+ T cells are both present
  - T_H1 cytokines (IL-2, INF-α, IL-12, and TNF-α) are produced by the T cells, keratinocytes, and antigen-presenting cells
  - Elevated TNF-α levels lead to increased production of proinflammatory cytokines by T cells and macrophages
- Treatments target T cells or their cytokines
- Ultraviolet A (UV-A) light; etanercept, efalizumab, psoralen plus UV-A light (PUVA); UV-B light; Goeckerman regimen uses coal tar followed by UV-B exposure; in the Ingram method, the drug anthralin is applied to the skin after a tar bath and UV-B treatment; oral retinoids; methotrexate; cyclosporine; alefacept; infliximab; adalimumab; topical steroids; topical calcipotriene; coal tar; topical tazarotene; laser treatment; and combinations of the preceding treatments; patients should avoid oral steroids owing to rebound effect

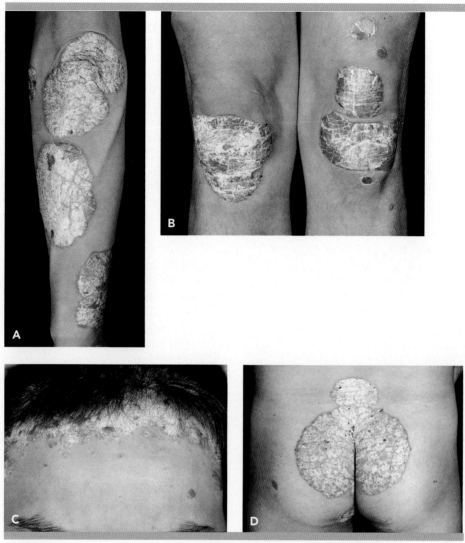

FIGURE 16-4 Psoriasis. *(From Freedberg IM et al: Fitzpatrick's Dermatology in General Medicine, 6th ed. New York: McGraw-Hill, 2003, p. 408.)*

Alopecia Areata (AA)

- Clinical: an autoimmune nonscarring alopecia; usually localized; however, more severe forms may affect the entire scalp (alopecia totalis) or body (alopecia universalis)
- Pathogenesis
  - Associated with certain HLA alleles (HLA-DR4, -DR6, -B12, -B18, -B13, and -B27)
  - CLA+ CD4 and CD8 T-lymphocytes are thought to be involved in the pathogenesis
  - Associated autoimmune diseases: diabetes mellitus, systemic lupus erythematosus, Graves', and vitiligo

Sarcoid

- Clinical: A multisystemic disorder of unknown etiology with a myriad of clinical presentations;

cutaneous lesions, seen in 25 percent of patients, are categorized as specific or nonspecific based on the histologic presence or absence of noncaseating epithelioid granulomas, respectively; systemic involvement is seen in 70 percent of cutaneously involved patients

- Nonspecific (biopsy does not show granulomas)
  - Erythema nodosum: most common nonspecific lesion; tender, erythematous nodules most commonly on legs; associated with a better prognosis
  - May be self-limited and asymptomatic; better prognosis
- Specific
  - Lupus pernio: violaceous patches and plaques on nose more common in women and

associated with pulmonary involvement; resolution with scarring is possible; marker for insidious disease; progresses over many months; worse prognosis
- Papules/plaques/nodules
- Head and neck more common for papules
- Legs: plaques; angiolupoid sarcoid (plaques with telangectasias); marker for pulmonary fibrosis
- Subcutaneous nodules (Darier-Roussy): firm, painless subcutaneous nodules that represent sarcoidosis; limited to the subcutaneous tissue
- Scar sarcoidosis (i.e., vaccination site, tattoos)
- Unique variants: ulcerative (legs), icthyosiform lesions, scarring/nonscarring alopecia
- Syndromes
  - Lofgren's syndrome: hilar adenopathy, EN, fever, migrating polyathritis, and acute iritis
  - Heerenfort-Waldenstrome syndrome (uveoparotid fever): parotid gland enlargement, fever, cranial nerve palsy, anterior uveitis
- Systemic disease manifestations
  - Pulmonary
    - Interstitial lung disease may be subclinical.
    - Symptoms: dyspnea, dry cough
    - Fifty percent clear spontaneously
  - Lymphadenopathy: hilar, cervical, axillary, inguinal
  - Ophthalmic: anterior uveitis
  - Cardiac: ECG rhythm disorders owing to conduction abnormalities
  - Gastrointestinal: hematemesis, 10 percent with granulomas
  - Neurologic: facial palsy
  - Renal: overproduction of 1-25 hydroxy, increased Ca^{2+}
  - Muscle: biopsy: granulomas, no symptoms
  - Bone: If hands involved, check for bone cysts; joint pain in 25 to 40 percent
- Diagnosis
  - Histology
    - Naked (no inflammation at periphery), noncaseating granulomas, Schaumann bodies (round, laminated, calcified body), asteroid bodies (star-shaped eosinophilic structure)
    - Must exclude infection, foreign-body reaction (zirconium, beryllium, silica, etc.), other inflammatory disorders (rosacea, cutaneous Crohn's, etc.), and neoplastic disorders (granulomatous MF and sarcoidal response to underlying lymphoma)
  - Chest x-ray:
    - Stage I: hilar adenopathy
    - Stage II: hilar adenopathy with infiltrates
    - Stage III: pulmonary infiltrates with adenopathy
    - Stage IV: end-stage fibrosis
- Kveim-Siltzbach test: Injection of sarcoidal spleen extract into a patient with sarcoid results in typical granulomatous reaction 4 to 6 weeks later; false-positive results are possible
- Laboratory studies
  - Polymorphisms in the gene encoding angiotensin-converting enzyme (ACE); ACE levels may be elevated in two-thirds of patients; false-egative rate is 40 percent, whereas the false-positive rate is 10 percent; not used for diagnosis as much as for predicting disease progression with serial measurements
  - Increased erythrocyte sedimentation rate (ESR) in two-thirds of patients
  - Lymphopenia with a reduced CD4:CD8 ratio
  - 24-hour urine serum: Ca^{2+} elevated
- Treatments are numerous
  - Steroids suppress T-helper cells
  - Antimalarials [hydroxychloroquine (Plaquenil) and chloroquine (Aralen)]
  - Antimetabolites: methotrexate, chlorambucil, imuran
  - Minocycline
  - Retinoids
  - Thalidomide
  - Biologics that target T cells or TNF may be useful

Urticaria/Angioedema

- Edema formation in specific layers of the skin
- Clinical
  - Urticaria involves only the superficial portion of the dermis; presents as well-circumscribed wheals with erythematous, raised, serpiginous borders and blanched centers; may coalesce to become giant wheals; usually pruritic
    - Can involve any area of the body from the scalp to the soles of the feet
    - Appears in crops, with old lesions fading within 24 hours as new ones appear
  - Angioedema presents as well-demarcated, localized edema involving the deeper layers of the skin, including the subcutaneous tissue
    - Angioedema often occurs in the periorbital region involving the lips
    - Although self-limited in duration, angioedema involvement of the upper respiratory tract may be life-threatening owing to laryngeal obstruction
  - Recurrent episodes of urticaria and/or angioedema of less than 6 weeks' duration are considered acute; >6 weeks' duration is designated as chronic
- Pathology
  - Dermal edema characterizes urticaria

- Edema of both the dermis and subcutaneous tissue characterizes angioedema
- Collagen bundles are widely separated
- Venules are often dilated
- Perivenular infiltrate may include lymphocytes, eosinophils, and neutrophils
- Classification based on etiology
  - Ig-E dependent: due to specific antigen sensitivity (pollens, foods, drugs, fungi, molds, *Hymenoptera* venom, helminthes)
    - Mechanism
      - ▲ A sensitized individual possesses IgE antibodies against a specific antigen
      - ▲ IgE antibodies are attached to the surfaces of mast cells
      - ▲ When rechallenged with the same antigen, the result is release of biologically active products from the mast cells, the most important being histamine
    - Physical urticaria: numerous types
    - Dermographism: linear wheals following minor pressure or scratching of the skin
    - Solar urticaria: characteristically occurs within minutes of sun exposure and often is a sign of erythropoietic protoporphyria
    - Cold urticaria: precipitated by exposure to the cold, and therefore, exposed areas usually are affected
      - ▲ In some cases, the disease is associated with abnormal circulating proteins, more commonly cryoglobulins and less commonly cryofibrinogens and cold agglutinins
      - ▲ Additional systemic symptoms include wheezing and syncope, thus explaining the need for these patients to avoid swimming in cold water
  - Cholinergic urticaria: precipitated by heat, exercise, or emotion; characterized by small wheals with relatively large flares; occasionally associated with wheezing
  - Complement-mediated
    - Hereditary/acquired angioedema
      - ▲ Caused by C1 inhibitor deficiency
      - ▲ Occurs without accompanying urticaria
      - ▲ May be inborn as an autosomal dominant trait (hereditary) or may be acquired
      - ▲ Trauma often precipitates attacks
      - ▲ Results in massive local swelling and occasionally fatal laryngeal edema
    - Serum sickness
      - ▲ Due to deposition of immune complexes in blood vessel walls
      - ▲ Leads to fixation of complement and inflammation
  - Nonimmunologic

- Direct mast cell–releasing agents: opiates, antibiotics, curare, D-tubocurarine, radiocontrast media
- Agents that alter arachidonic acid metabolism: aspirin and other NSAIDs, azo dyes, benzoates
- Blocks the production of prostaglandins from arachidonic acid
- The pathway is then shifted to the production of other metabolites, including leukotrienes
- Leukotriene release ultimately results in release of vasoactive substances (histamine) that alter vascular permeability and produce dermal edema (urticaria)
  - Idiopathic
    - Chronic idiopathic urticaria
      - ▲ Autoantibodies to the high-infinity IgE receptor or to IgE itself have been identified in these patients
      - ▲ Autoantibodies possess histamine-releasing activity
- Systemic diseases associated with urticaria
  - Urticarial vasculitis (immune complex–mediated)
    - Individual lesions tend to last longer than 24 hours and usually develop central petechiae that can be observed even after the urticarial phase has resolved
    - On biopsy, there is a leukocytoclastic vasculitis of the small blood vessels
    - Sometimes a reflection of an underlying systemic illness such as lupus erythematosus, Sjögren's syndrome, hereditary complement deficiency, serum sickness (drug induced?), or infections such as hepatitis B or C infection
    - Treatment
      - ▲ Any suspected medication should be discontinued
      - ▲ Avoidance of precipitating factors may be helpful for some of the physical urticarias, such as solar and cold urticaria
      - ▲ Symptomatic therapy usually includes H_1 antihistamines given on a regular rather than an intermittent, as-needed basis
      - ▲ The tricyclic antidepressant doxepin (Sinequan) is also effective and has been shown to have both H_1 and H_2 antihistamine activity

Graft-Versus-Host Disease (GVHD)

- Occurs when immunologically competent cells are introduced into an immunoincompetent host
- Most commonly seen in hematopoietic cell transplantation (HCT), both allogeneic (between two individuals) and autologous (from the same individual)

- Solid-organ transplants, blood transfusions, and maternal-fetal transfusions also have been reported to cause GVHD
- The skin often is the earliest organ affected
- GVHD remains a primary cause of morbidity and mortality after HCT
- Classifications: arbitrarily defined based on days from transplant
  - Acute GVHD
    - Occurs within the first 100 days of a transplant
    - Consists of a triad of dermatitis, enteritis, and hepatitis
    - Usually begins as scattered erythematous macules and papules that may evolve into a generalized erythroderma or bullous eruption (Fig. 16-5)

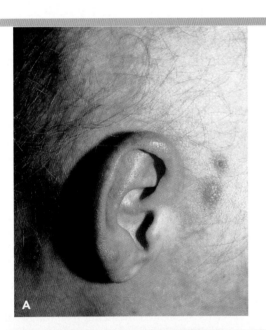

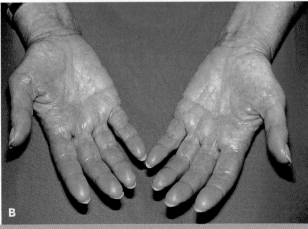

FIGURE 16-5 Erythematous macules. *(From Freedberg IM et al: Fitzpatrick's Dermatology in General Medicine, 6th ed. New York: McGraw-Hill, 2003, p. 1146.)*

- Mediated by T_H1 cells
- Graded in five steps (0–IV)
- Grade 0: no clinical evidence of disease
- Grade I: rash on less than 50 percent of skin and no gut or liver involvement
- Grade II: rash covering more than 50 percent of skin, bilirubin 2 to 3 mg/dl, diarrhea 10 to 15 ml/kg per day, or persistent nausea
- Grade III or IV: generalized erythroderma with bullous formation, bilirubin greater than 3 mg/dL, or diarrhea more than 16 ml/kg per day
  - Chronic GVHD
    - Develops after 100 days
    - Consists of an autoimmune syndrome directed toward multiple organs
    - May occur as a late phase of acute GVHD or as a distinct entity
    - The skin is the primary organ involved and may be characterized as localized or generalized with lichen planus–like or sclerodermoid lesions commonly encountered
    - Mediated by T_H2 cells
- Pathophysiology
  - Three components are required for the development of GVHD
    - The graft must contain immunologically competent cells
    - The host must appear foreign to the graft
    - The host must be incapable of reacting sufficiently against the graft
  - Disease is caused by recognition of epithelial target tissues as foreign by the immunocompetent cells and subsequent induction of an inflammatory response and eventual apoptotic death of the target tissue (regardless of whether the immunoreactive T cells are derived from a nonidentical donor or from the recipient)
  - While T cells may orchestrate the initial inflammatory response, many cell types (e.g., CD4+, CD8+ T-cell subsets, natural killer cells) are found at sites of epithelial injury
- Histology
  - Acute: epidermal basal vacuolization, followed by epidermal basal cell apoptotic death with lymphoid infiltration; satellite cell necrosis (direct apposition of a lymphocyte to a necrotic keratinocyte)
  - Chronic: basal cell degeneration and necrosis, epidermal atrophy, and dermal fibrosis; lichenoid changes with mononuclear infiltrates, epithelial cell necrosis
- Treatment
  - Immunosuppression is the mainstay of therapy: Limiting the graft-versus-host tissue response while maintaining the graft-versus-tumor effect is crucial

- T-cell depletion with Campath 1H or thymoglobulin during transplant is useful
- Prophylaxis with cyclosporine, mycophenolate mofetil, and tacrolimus is common; however, exacerbations of GVHD frequently require prednisone
- Newer biologicals (CTLA-4-Ig, infliximab, etanercept, and anti-CD25 agents such as daclizumab) appear interesting and may prove useful
- Immune modulation with photopheresis or phototherapy also has been helpful

Atopic Eczema (Atopic Dermatitis)

- Clinical: pruritic poorly demarcated, erythematous scaly patches, small vesicles, excoriations, crusting, and frequent impetiginization that have a predilection for the skin flexures (neck, antecubital fossa, and popliteal fossa) in children and extensors in adults; chronic scratching and rubbing can lead to hyperpigmentation and lichenification; periorbital fold (Denny Morgan sign) may be present
- Pathogenesis
  - Believed to be multifactorial
  - Allergens (house dust mites, pollen, animal dander), outdoor pollution, climate, diet, and prenatal or early-life factors such as infections
  - Patients appear to have a genetic predisposition that can then be exacerbated by these numerous factors
- Histology: edema within the epidermis (spongiosis) and infiltration with lymphocytes and macrophages in the superficial dermis
- Diagnosis
  - Made by the typical morphology and distribution of the lesions
  - Family and personal history of atopy (asthma, allergic rhinitis, or atopic dermatitis) also can help with the diagnosis
- Prognosis
  - There is currently no cure; however, various interventions exist to control symptoms
  - Can be expected to clear in 60 to 70 percent of children by their early teens, although relapses may occur
- Treatment
  - Includes emollients, oral antihistamines, topical corticosteroid ointments, topical tacrolimus, topical pimecrolimus
  - More severe cases sometimes use UV-B phototherapy or PUVA
  - Occasionally, a short course of systemic steroids is necessary to bring the disease under control
  - Steroid wet wraps and baths are helpful in treating acute atopic dermatis

- Avoidance of environmental factors that enhance itching is important
- Moisturizers reduce dry skin and itching
- Calcinuerin inhibitors

Nummular Eczema (Nummular Dermatitis)

- Occurs most frequently in patients who are in their fifties and sixties
- In temperate climates, this condition is seen most frequently in the winter
- More frequently encountered in patients of Asian descent
- The etiology is unclear, although xerosis plays a significant role in the pathogenesis
- Clinical
  - Pruritic, coin-shaped, erythematous patches that exhibit scale (hyperkeratosis) and occasionally pin-head sized vesicles on the legs, arms, and legs (in decreasing order of frequency)
  - Lesions may become excoriated and lichenified
- Treatment
  - Liberal use of emollients, avoidance of long hot showers, topical use of corticosteroids or immune modulators, and oral antihistamines
  - Severe cases may require UV-B phototherapy, PUVA, or oral corticosteroids

Seborrheic Eczema (Seborrheic Dermatitis)

- Clinical: erythematous patches and plaques with indistinct margins and yellowish, greasy-appearing scales affecting sebaceous hairy regions of the body (scalp, eyebrows, nasolabial creases, ears, chest, intertriginous areas, axilla, groin, buttocks and inframammary folds)
  - A common problem affecting 3 to 5 percent of the healthy population
  - Waxing and waning course that parallels the increased sebaceous gland activity occurring in infancy and after puberty
  - A variable amount of pruritus
  - The mildest form, dandruff, has white scale without erythema
  - Refractory or more widespread disease may be associated with underlying HIV infection (approximately one-third of patients with AIDS and AIDS-related complex) or neurologic disorder (i.e., Parkinson's disease)
- Pathogenesis
  - Thought to be an inflammatory reaction to the resident skin yeast, *Pityrosporum ovale*
  - *P. ovale* is a lipophilic yeast that is normally found on the seborrheic regions of the skin
  - The most effective antiseborrheic shampoos have antifungal activity against the yeast organisms

- Diagnosis: usually made on clinical grounds alone
- Treatment
  - Antiseborrheic shampoos containing zinc pyrithione, selenium sulfide, or ketoconazole are the mainstay of treatment
  - Topical steroid lotion or gel (hairy areas) and hydrocortisone cream or ketoconazole cream (nonhairy areas)

REFERENCES

Asadullag K, Sterry W: Analysis of cytokine expression in dermatology. *Arch Dermatol* 2002; 138(9).

Assmann T, Ruzicka T: New immunosuppressive drugs in dermatology (mycophenolate mofetil, tacrolimus): Unapproved uses, dosages, or indications. *Clin Dermatol* 2002;20: 505–514.

Athman R, Philpott D: Innate immunity via toll-like receptors and Nod proteins. *Curr Opin Microbiol* 2004; 7(1):25–32.

Craze M, Young M: Integrating biologic therapies in to a dermatology practice: practical and economic considerations. *J Am Acad Dermatol* 2003; 49:S139–142.

Dempsey PW, Vaidya SA, Cheng G: The art of war: Innate and adaptive immune responses. *Cell Mol Life Sci* 2003; 60(12): 2604, 2621.

Gilhar A, Landau M, Assy B, Shalaginov R, Serafimovich S, Kalish RS. Mediation of alopecia areata by cooperartion between CD4+ and CD8+ T lymphocytes: transfer to human scalp explants on Prkdc(scid) mice. *Arch Dermatol* 2002; 138(7): 916–922.

Greaves MW: The immunopharmacology of skin inflammation: The future is already here! *Br J Dermatol* 2000; 143(1):47–52.

Janeway CA Jr, Medzhitov R: Innate immune recognition. *Annu Rev Immunol* 2002; 20:197–216.

Mackel SE, Jordan RE. Leukocytoclasitc vasculitis. A cutaneous expression of immune complex disease. *Arch Dermatol* 1982; 118(5): 296–301.

Stanley MA: Imiquimod and the imidazoquinolones: Mechanism of action and therapeutic potential. *Clin Exp Dermatol* 2002; 27(7):571–577.

Victor FC, Gottlieb AB, Menter A. Changing paradigms in dermatology: tumor necrosis factor alpha blockade in psoriasis and psoriatic arthritis. *Clin Dermatol* 2003: 21(5):392–397.

Williams JDL, Griffiths CEM: Cytokine blocking agents in dermatology. *Clin Exp Dermatol* 2002; 27(7):585.

CHAPTER 17

VIRAL DISEASES

HOLLY BARTELL
STEPHEN K. TYRING

DNA VIRUSES

1. Pox viruses (these viruses replicate in the cytoplasm)
   - Molluscipox: molluscum
   - Orthopox: vaccinia, smallpox, cowpox
   - Parapox: Orf, milker's nodules
2. Papillomaviruses
3. Herpes viruses
4. Hepadnavirus
5. Adenoviruses (these viruses replicate in the nucleus)

Pox Viruses

Molluscipox (Molluscum Contagiosum; MCV)

- Clinical
  - Mainly pediatric age group; dome-shaped umbilical papules
  - Children commonly acquire virus by close contact.
  - Genital papules: usually sexually transmitted
  - In immunocompromised patients, especially HIV infection, thousands of papules
  - Positive Koebner reaction
- Two main subtypes: MCV I and MCV II; both are genital/nongenital; MCV I more prevalent than MCV II (except in HIV patients)
- Incubation 1 week to months
- Free virus cores found in all layers of epidermis
- Molluscum bodies have large numbers of maturing virions; sealed off by collagen and lipid-rich saclike structure protecting the virus from host defenses
- Histology: Henderson-Paterson bodies (molluscum bodies) = viral particles in infected keratinocytes, eosinophils
- Treatment: curettage, liquid nitrogen, cantharidin, lactic acid, CO_2, imiquimod, trichloroacetic acid, cidofovir in immunocompromised patients

Orthopox

1. Smallpox
2. Vaccinia
3. Monkeypox
4. Cowpox

Smallpox

- Caused by variola virus; variola minor also known as alastrim
- Clinical
  - Incubation 12 to 13 days, fever, malaise, backache, exanthema that appears after 2 to 4 days; macules $\rightarrow$ papules $\rightarrow$ vesicles $\rightarrow$ pustules
    - Four clinical types: ordinary, modified (by previous vaccination), flat, and hemorrhagic
    - Latter two have highest mortality rate: 30 percent fatal
  - Discrete pox eruption; firm, deep-seated papules: vesiculated and umbilicated lesions; later crust forms; lesions all in same stage
  - Complications: corneal ulceration, laryngeal lesions, encephalitis, hemorrhage
  - Variola major: fatal secondary to pulmonary edema from heart failure
- Progressive vaccinia related to immunosuppression, malignancy, radiation therapy, or AIDS
- Vaccination: postvaccinal encephalitis and progressive vaccinia; high level immunity for 3 to 5 years and decreasing immunity thereafter
- Histology: balloon and reticular degeneration with hemorrhage inclusion bodies, polymorphonuclear cells
- Treatment: no antiviral treatment for smallpox; cidofovir suggested

Vaccinia (Figs. 17-1 and 17-2)

- Laboratory virus used to vaccinate against smallpox and monkeypox
- Infection occurs primarily in laboratory workers

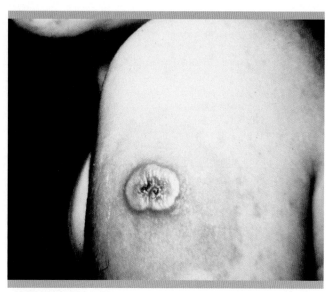

FIGURE 17-1 Vaccinia. *(Courtesy of Dr. Stephen Tyring.)*

- Clinical
  - Papule appears in 2 to 3 days, followed by umbilicated Jennerian vesicle; scab ensues; pitted scar results
  - Pustule at day 7 confirms successful vaccination
  - Generalized vaccinia
    - Secondary to viremia
    - Can occur 6 to 9 days after vaccination
    - Can get eczema vaccinatum (usually only in immunocompromised patients or patients with nonintact skin barrier)
- Treatment: Cidofovir suggested

Monkeypox

- Occasionally infects humans; predominantly residents of western and central Africa; can get protection from vaccinia

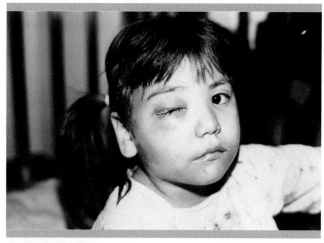

FIGURE 17-2 Vaccinia eye. *(Courtesy of Dr. Stephen Tyring.)*

Cowpox

- Infects cows, but more common in cats
- Cow/cat teats: sites of injury
- Lymphadenopathy, fever

PARAPOX

1. Orf
2. Paravaccinia (milker's nodule)

Orf (Ecthyma Contagiosum, Scabby Mouth)

- Large ovoid virus, 250 × 160 nm with surface tubules, resistant to drying, lipid solvent (ether and chloroform)
- Endemic among sheep and goats, oxen; infection from animals or fomites: barn door, troughs
- Sheep farmers, veterinarians mainly affected
- 4 to 7 days incubation
- Clinical
  - Nodules around mouth, nose of animals; heal in 1 month
  - Lymphadenopathy, malaise, fever
  - Painful lesions: fingers; flat, dome-shaped bullae with minimal fluid, central crust; bleed easily with scarring
  - 36-day period with six clinical stages: Each lasts 6 days
    - Papular: red elevated lesion
    - Target: nodule with red center, white ring, red halo
    - Acute stage: weeping surface
    - Regenerative stage: thin, dry crust with black dots
    - Papillomatous stage: small papillomas over surface of lesion
    - Regressive: thick crusts heal with scarring
- Histology
  - Vacuolization of cells in the upper third of stratum spinosum: multilocular vesicles, acanthosis, eosinophilic inclusion bodies in cytoplasm and nucleus of infected cells
  - Mixed infiltrate, loss of epidermis over central part of lesion
  - Weeping stage: necrosis with massive infiltrate of mononuclear cells
- Diagnosis: history and physical, confirmed by cell culture, fluorescent antibody, complement fixation, electron microscopy, or histologic study
- Treatment: spontaneous remission

Milker's Nodules (Paravaccinia)

- Endemic to cattle, on cow teats
- 150 × 300 nm, brick-shaped
- Clinical
  - Solitary nodule on finger
  - Increases slowly in size over a period of 1 to 2 weeks

TABLE 17-1 Nongenital Cutaneous Disease

	HPV Type
Common warts (verrucae vulgaris)	1, 2, 4, 26, 27, 29, 41, 57, 65
Plantar warts (myrmecia)	1, 2, 4, 63
Flat warts (verrucae plana)	3, 10, 27, 28, 38, 41, 49
Butcher's warts (common warts of people who handle meat, poultry, and fish)	7
Mosaic warts	2, 27, 57
Ungual squamous cell carcinoma	16
Epidermodysplasia verruciformis (benign)	2, 3, 10, 12, 15, 19, 36, 46, 47, 50
Epidermodysplasia verruciformis (malignant or benign)	5, 8, 9, 10, 14, 17, 20, 21, 22, 23, 24, 25, 37, 38

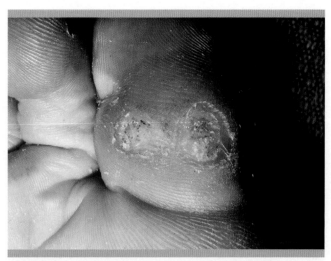

FIGURE 17-3 Plantar warts. *(Courtesy of Dr. Stephen Tyring.)*

- Nodules are painless and bluish red in color
- Lesions heal without scarring
- Usually no fever
- Histology: similar to Orf

Human Papillomavirus (HPV)

- Three categories used to describe HPV clinically
  - Anogenital and/or mucosal
  - Nongenital cutaneous (Table 17-1)
  - Epidermodysplasia verruciformis (EV)

DISEASES AND ASSOCIATED HPV SUBTYPES
Nongenital Cutaneous Diseases

1. Palmoplantar warts (myrmecia) (Fig. 17-3)
   - "Anthill": HPV1
   - Volar aspects of palms/soles, tips of fingers/toes
   - Covered with thick callus
   - Histology: increased keratohyaline granules; cytoplasm of cells with eosinophilic granules coalesces to form irregularly shaped inclusion bodies
   - Treatment: cryotherapy, CO_2 laser, cantharidin, combination therapy using cryodestruction or surgery and imiquimod
2. Common warts (verruca vulgaris)
   - HPV2, HPV4
   - Verrucous papules on glaberous skin
   - Can koebnerize
   - Treatment: salicylic acid, 50% tricholoacetic acid, cantharidin, cryotherapy with liquid nitrogen, electrodesiccation, combination therapy using cryodestruction or surgery and imiquimod
3. Flat warts (verrucae plana) (Fig. 17-4)
   - HPV3, HPV10
   - Slightly elevated flesh-colored papules that may be smooth or slightly hyperkeratotic
   - Can koebnerize, so can increase
   - Treatment: retinoic acid 0.05% applied daily until desquamation occurs; mild irritation may occur
4. Epidermodysplasia verrucifomis (EV)
   - HPV5 and HPV8 are the most common cause of cancer
   - Approximately 15 others are less oncogenic
   - Autosomal recessive, lesions: polymorphic, verruca plana–like, red-brown plaques
   - Malignant transformation = 50 percent; age forties and fifties, especially in immunocompromised patients
   - Onset 6 to 8 years, locally destructive, mucosal involvement
   - Histology: uneven keratohyaline granules; large, course granules in the epidermis; koilocytes; gray cytoplasm; increase in amount of cytoplasm
   - Treatment
     - No effective treatment

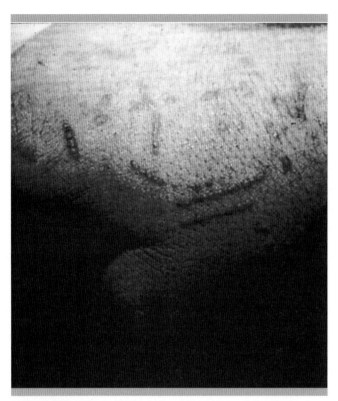

FIGURE 17-4 Flat warts. *(Courtesy of Dr. Robert Jordan.)*

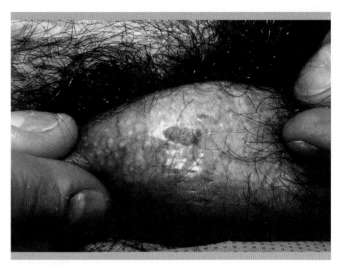

FIGURE 17-5 Anogenital disease. *(Courtesy of Dr. Stephen Tyring.)*

- Counsel patients to protect the skin from ultraviolet radiation exposure; radiation therapy is contraindicated in EV
- Retinoids: For example, long-term isotretinoin has been shown to decrease number of benign lesions and slow appearance of premalignant and malignant lesions

5. Butcher's warts
   - HPV7
   - Proliferative hand warts
   - Histology: verrucae, acanthotic epidermis, papillomatosis, hyperkeratosis, parakeratosis, elongated rete ridges; dermal vessels are prominent; koilocytotic cells (large keratinocytes with eccentric, pylenotic nucleus, surrounded by a perinuclear halo)

Anogenital Disease (Fig. 17-5 and Table 17-2)

1. Bowenoid papulosis
   - HPV16, -18, and -33 (oncogenic)
     - Intraepithelial neoplasia of the genitalia with bowenoid histologic features, papules/plaques on genitalia
     - Young, sexually active adults; cervix in females
   - Histology: full-thickness dysplasia, dysplastic keratinocytes

- Treatment: cryotherapy, laser, excision, topical retinoids, 5-fluorouracil 5% solution, imiquimod 5% cream (low recurrence rates)

2. Condyloma acuminatum
   - HPV6 and HPV11
   - Less commonly HPV16, -18, -21, -22, and -55
   - Clinical
     - Exophytic cauliflower-like lesions that usually are found near moist surfaces
     - Perianal area, vaginal introitus, vagina, labia, and vulva
   - Histology
     - Parakeratosis (mucosa), papillomatosis, acanthosis, elongated rete ridges, mitotic figures occasionally
     - Koilocytes: dark nuclei with dyskeratosis

TABLE 17-2 Anogenital Disease

	HPV Type
Condylomata acuminata	6, 11, 30, 42, 43, 44, 45, 51, 52, 54
Bowenoid papulosis	16, 18, 34, 39, 42, 45
Bowen disease	16, 18, 31, 34
Giant condylomata (Buschke-Löwenstein tumors)	6, 11

3. Verrucous carcinoma
   - Epithelioma cuniculatum: plaque on sole of foot, like a nonhealing wart; associated with HPV2 (rarely) and HPV16/low-grade squamous cell carcinoma (SCC)
   - Giant condyloma of Buschke and Lowenstein
     - HPV6, HPV11, hypergranulosis (usually no granular layer)
     - Slow-growing, locally destructive verrucous lesion that typically appears on the penis but may occur elsewhere in the anogenital region
   - Oral florid papillomatosis: mucosa, usually no granular layer

Nongenital Mucosal Disease (Table 17-3)

1. Oral focal epithelial hyperplasia (Heck disease)
   - Focal epithelial hyperplasia
   - Lower labial mucosa
   - Multiple flat-topped or dome-shaped pink-white papules, 1 to 5 mm, some lesions coalescing into plaques
   - Histology
     - Hyperplastic mucosa with thin parakeratotic stratum corneum
     - Acanthosis, blunting and anastomosis of rete ridges
     - Pallor of epidermal cells as a result of intracellular edema

TREATMENTS FOR HPV

- Topical agents
  - Salicylic acid
    - Over-the-counter treatment
    - Removes surface keratin
    - Cure rates from 70 to 80 percent are reported
  - Cantharidin
    - Dried extract of the blister beetle
    - Causes epidermal necrosis and blistering
    - Treatment may require weekly repetition
  - Dinitrochlorobenzene (DNCB)
    - Powerful sensitizing agent
    - Induces an allergic contact dermatitis
    - Causes local inflammation and an immune response
    - Cure rates from 65 to 90 percent
    - Reported mutagen
  - Dibutyl squaric acid
    - Contact sensitizer
    - Unlike DNCB, it is not a mutagen and therefore may be a safer alternative
  - Trichloroacetic acid
    - Caustic compound
    - Causes immediate superficial tissue necrosis
    - Concentrations up to 80%
    - May require weekly applications
  - Podophyllotoxin
    - Derived from the roots of the Indian podophyllum plant
    - Binds to tubulin and prevents microtubule assembly
    - Genital wart treatment: application twice daily for three consecutive days per week for up to 4 weeks
  - Fluorouracil (5FU)
    - Used primarily to treat actinic keratoses
    - Antimetabolite: fluorinated pyrimidine
    - Active form inhibits DNA synthesis by inhibiting the normal production of thymidine
    - Effective in treating warts when used under occlusion daily for up to 1 month
  - Imiquimod 5% cream
    - Topical cream approved for treating genital warts; used for other HPV infections
    - Anogenital warts: treat at night, three times a week
    - Common warts: treat nightly under occlusion
    - Palmoplantar warts: treat nightly under occlusion, alternate with a keratolytic
    - Potent stimulator of proinflammatory cytokine release
    - Works best as part of combination therapy for nonanogenital warts
  - Cidofovir
    - Nucleotide analogue of deoxycytidine monophosphate
    - Used for refractory condyloma acuminata and recurrent genital herpes
    - Cidofovir gel applied once or twice daily
    - Must be compounded
  - Tretinoin: disrupts epidermal growth and differentiation, thereby reducing the bulk of the wart
- Systemic agents
  - Cimetidine
    - Type 2 histamine receptor antagonist
    - Immunomodulatory effects
    - Results have varied
    - Oral, 25 to 40 mg/kg tid × 3 months

TABLE 17-3 Nongenital Mucosal Disease

	HPV Type
Oral focal epithelial hyperplasia (Heck disease)	13, 32
Oral carcinoma	16, 18
Oral leukoplakia	16, 18

- Intralesional injections
  - Bleomycin
    - Cytotoxic polypeptide that inhibits DNA synthesis in cells and viruses
    - Side effects of bleomycin include pain with injection, local urticaria, Raynaud phenomenon, and possible tissue necrosis
    - If used periungually, bleomycin may cause nail dystrophy or loss
  - Interferon-α
    - Naturally occurring cytokine with antiviral, anticancer, and immunomodulatory effects
    - Intralesional administration is more effective than systemic administration and is associated only with mild flulike symptoms
    - Treatments may be required for several weeks to months before beneficial results are seen
    - Use for warts that are resistant to standard treatments
- Surgical care
  - Cryosurgery: Liquid nitrogen (–196°C) is the most effective method of cryosurgery
  - Lasers
    - Carbon dioxide lasers
      - ▲ Procedure can be painful and leave scarring.
      - ▲ Risk of nosocomial infection also exists in health care workers because HPV can be isolated in the plume
    - Flashlamp-pumped pulse dye laser
      - ▲ Mixed results in treating warts
      - ▲ Decreased risk of scarring and transmission of HPV in the smoke plume
  - Electrodesiccation and curettage
    - May be more effective than cryosurgery
    - Painful
    - More likely to scar
    - HPV can be isolated from the plume
  - Surgical excision: Avoid using because of the risks of scarring and recurrence.

Human Herpes Viruses (HHV)

- dsDNA
- Eight main types
  - HHV 1: herpes simplex 1 (HSV-1): herpes labialis > genitalis
  - HHV 2: herpes simplex 2 (HSV-2): herpes genitalis > labialis
  - HHV 3: varicella-zoster virus (VZV): chickenpox/herpes zoster
  - HHV 4: Epstein-Barr virus (EBV): mononucleosis, Gianotti Crosti, Burkitt's lymphoma, oral hairy leukoplakia
  - HHV 5: cytomegalovirus (CMV): retinitis in AIDS patients
  - HHV 6: roseola infantum (exanthema subitum)
  - HHV 7: possible pityriasis rosea
  - HHV 8: Kaposi's sarcoma

HERPES SIMPLEX VIRUS (HSV)

Herpes Simplex 1 (HSV-1)

- Belongs to the family Herpesviridae
- Humans are the only natural reservoirs, and no vectors are involved in transmission.
- Eighty percent of U.S. adults infected, 85 percent of adults infected worldwide
- Ninety percent orofacial, 10 percent genital
- Mode of transmission is by close personal contact
- Viral properities
  - Neurovirulence: capacity to invade and replicate in the nervous system
  - Latency
    - Establishment and maintenance of latent infection in nerve cell ganglia
    - HSV-1 infection: Trigeminal ganglia are involved most commonly
  - Reactivation
    - Induced by a variety of stimuli: fever, trauma, emotional stress, sunlight, menstruation
    - Recurrent infection and peripheral shedding of HSV
    - Occurs more frequently in the oral rather than the genital region
    - More frequent and severe in immunocompromised patients
  - Primary infection is subclinical (90 percent), gingivostomatitis (10 percent)
  - Forty percent recur, three to four times per year
  - Thirty percent of primary but less than 5 percent of recurrent genital HSV
- Clinical
  - Gingival stomatitis
    - Abrupt onset
    - Children aged 6 months to 5 years
    - High fever (102 to 104°F)
    - Anorexia and listlessness
    - Gingivitis is the most striking feature.
    - Vesicular lesions develop on the oral mucosa, tongue, and lips and later rupture and coalesce, leaving ulcerated plaques
    - Regional lymphadenopathy
    - Acute herpetic pharyngotonsillitis
    - Pharyngitis and tonsillitis
    - Acute disease lasts 5 to 7 days
    - Viral shedding may continue for 3 weeks
  - Herpes labialis
    - Most common manifestation of recurrent HSV-1
    - Prodrome of pain, burning, and tingling often occurs at the site

- Erythematous papules that develop rapidly into tiny, thin-walled, intraepidermal vesicles that become pustular and ulcerate
- Maximum viral shedding is in the first 24 hours of the acute illness but may last 5 days
- Diagnosis
  - Histology: acantholysis, intraepidermal vesicle, balloon and reticular degeneration, intranuclear eosinophilic inclusion bodies, multinucleated keratinocytes (not specific)
  - Viral culture
  - Polymerase chain reaction (PCR) techniques: detection of HSV DNA
  - Immunofluorescent staining of the tissue culture cells or of smear can quickly identify HSV and can distinguish between types 1 and 2
  - Antibody testing
  - Tzanck smear: multinucleated giant cells → nucleus divides but not cell; nuclear molding
- Treatment: See HSV-2 below

Herpes Simplex 2 (HSV-2) (Fig. 17-6)

- Primary genital herpes; asymptomatic in most patients
- Seventy percent of primary, >95 percent of recurrent genital herpes
- Women 45 percent more chance of infection compared with men
- Primary infection asymptomatic: 75 percent
- Ninety-five percent of asymptomatic females and males actively shed virus at some point in time
- Eighty percent transmission secondary to asymptomatic shedding
- Ninety percent recur
- Clinical
  - Incubation period is 3 to 7 days
  - Cervical vesicles resulting in ulcers; can recur with or without external lesions
  - Ulcerative lesions persist from 4 to 15 days

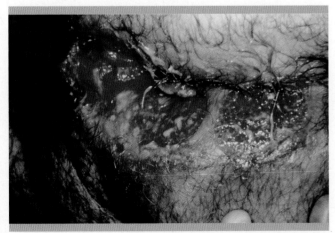

FIGURE 17-6 Herpes simplex type 2 (HSV-2). *(Courtesy of Dr. Stephen Tyring.)*

- Viral shedding is about 12 days.
- Primary HSV systemic complaints > 70 percent: fever, dysuria, malaise, lymphadenopathy, females greater than males
- Spread by sexual contact (1 to 2 percent days/year male, 6 to 8 percent female: asymptomatic transmission)
- Treatment
  - Acyclovir
    - First episode: 200 mg five times daily or 400 mg tid for 7 to 10 days
    - Recurrent genital herpes: 200 mg PO five times daily or 400 mg tid for 5 days
    - Chronic suppressive therapy: 400 mg bid or 200 mg three to five times daily
  - Valacyclovir (Valtrex)
    - First episode 1 g bid for 10 days
    - Recurrent attacks: 500 mg twice daily for 3 days or 2 g bid for one day
    - Suppressive dosing for HSV: 500 mg to 1 g/d
  - Famciclovir (Famvir)
    - First episode: 250 mg tid for 10 days
    - Recurrent outbreaks: 125 mg twice daily for 5 days
    - Suppression: 250 mg bid

Herpes Simplex Virus in Immunosuppressed Patients

- HIV: 95 percent coinfected with HSV-1/HSV-2 or both
- Fifty-two percent of HIV infections among people who also have herpes simplex virus type 2 can be associated with infection with the herpes virus
- Recurrent HSV may last much longer compared with immunocompetent hosts (>30 days)
- Chronic ulcerative HSV: persistent ulcers and erosions starting on the face or perineal region
- Generalized acute mucocutaneous HSV: dissemination and fever after localized vesicular eruption
- Systemic HSV: follows oral or genital lesions; areas of necrosis in liver, adrenals, pancreas
- HIV: 5 to 8 percent resistant to acyclovir.
- Treatment of genital ulcers caused by HSV-2 with specific antivirals has been shown previously to reduce HSV-2 and HIV shedding.
- Acyclovir-resistant HSV in HIV patients
  - 1% Cidofovir (compounded)
  - Foscarnet
    - Reversibly inhibits viral DNA polymerase
    - Does not need thymidine kinase
    - Side effects: penile ulcer, nephrotoxicity

Various Herpes Presentations

- Herpetic whitlow
  - HSV of the fingers of the hand occurs at or near the cuticle or at other sites associated with trauma
- HSV-2 > HSV-1

- Herpes gladiatorum
  - Direct skin-to-skin contact among wrestlers
  - Scattered cutaneous HSV-1 lesions
- Herpetic keratoconjunctivitis: recurrent erosions of the conjunctiva and cornea that can lead to blindness
- Lumbosacral herpes simplex virus: infection is typically asymptomatic
- Herpes-associated EM (HAEM)
  - Consistent with delayed-type hypersensitivity (DTH) reactions
  - Targetoid lesions not always limited to palms and soles
- Eczema herpeticum: widespread HSV infection in patients with skin disorders such as atopic dermatitis, Darier's disease, pemphigus, or Sézary syndrome
- HSV encephalitis
  - Most common cause of sporadic encephalitis
  - Sudden onset of fever, HA, confusion, temporal lobe sign
  - Seventy percent mortality if not treated
- Ramsey Hunt (usually VZV or HSV-1)
  - Infection of the facial nerve
  - Symptoms on the affected side typically include facial weakness and a painful herpes-type skin eruption on the pinna of the ear, and there is frequently vestibulocochlear disturbance
  - Recovery of facial movement occurs in about 50 percent of treated patients

Congenital Herpes Simplex Virus

- One in 3500 vaginal births
- Transmission
  - Perinatally: 90 percent; congenitally: 5 to 8 percent; few postnatally
  - Risk of transmission: 50 percent if mother has primary infection, 3 to 5 percent if mother has recurrent disease
- If lesions on infant in first 10 days, mortality is 20 percent
- If transmission in first 8 weeks, severe defects result
- Mortality rate (if no treatment) is 65 percent transplacental, 80 percent HSV-2, 20 percent HSV-1
- Birth canal transmission: lesions usually on scalp, face; associated encephalitis, hepatoadrenal necrosis, pneumonia, death
- Treatment
  - Pregnancy
    - Give treatment from week 36 until delivery in infected females
    - Valacyclovir 1 g qd
    - Famciclovir 250 mg bid
    - Acyclovir 400 mg bid or 200 mg three to five times daily
  - IV acyclovir for neonates: 30 mg/kg per day

VARICELLA-ZOSTER VIRUS [HUMAN HERPES VIRUS 3 (HHV 3)]

- Causes chickenpox and herpes zoster
- Chickenpox
  - Transmitted to others from the skin and respiratory tract
  - VZV remains dormant in sensory nerve roots after primary infection
  - Low-grade fever precedes skin manifestations by 1 to 2 days
  - incubation period of about 2 weeks
  - Lesions: "dewdrops on a rose petal"; begin on face, scalp, trunk, with relative sparing of the extremities
  - Lesion starts as a red macule and passes through stages of papule, vesicle, pustule, and crust with pruritus
  - Simultaneous presence of different stages of the rash
  - Congenital varicella syndrome
    - First 20 weeks of pregnancy: 2 percent risk of complications
    - Perinatal infection occurs within 10 days of birth
    - If female gets VZV 5 days before or 2 days after delivery, mortality is 30 percent
    - Intrauterine growth retardation, microcephaly, cortical atrophy, limb hypoplasia, microphthalmia, cataracts, chorioretinitis, and cutaneous scarring
  - Infantile zoster
    - Manifests within the first year
    - Maternal varicella infection after the twentieth week of gestation
  - Neonatal varicella
    - Any infant with clinical or laboratory-confirmed varicella
    - Onset in the first month of life
    - Without features of varicella embryopathy
    - Infection may result from peripartum maternal infection or postnatal exposure
- Treatment
  - Healthy children may not need acyclovir, but it allows them to return to school sooner
  - Acyclovir: 20 mg/kg; given orally four times daily for 5 to 7 days
  - Avoid aspirin to prevent Reye's syndrome
  - Symptomatic care
  - Adults
    - Acyclovir, famciclovir, valacyclovir at shingles doses
    - Most effective if it is started within the first 24 to 72 hours after development of vesicles
  - Varicella vaccine
    - Two doses 4 to 8 weeks apart if older than 12 years of age
    - One dose if 1 to 12 years of age

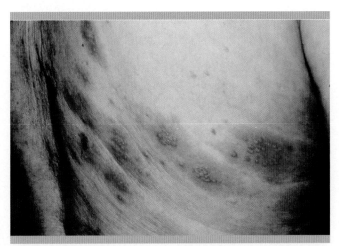

FIGURE 17-7 Zoster (shingles). *(Courtesy of Dr. Stephen Tyring.)*

- Seroconvertion: adolescents and adults: 78 percent after the first dose and 99 percent after the second dose
- Zoster (shingles) (Fig. 17-7)
  - Due to reactivation of latent VZV in sensory ganglion (20 percent incidence unless immunocompromised)
  - Rash preceded by prodrome: fever, malaise, headache, localized pain in the involved dermatome
  - Constitutional symptoms develop initially
  - Rash in a unilateral dermatomal distribution with erythema, vesicles, pustules, or crusting
  - Contagious until crusted
  - Incidence: 66 percent in patients older than 50 years
  - Hutchinson sign: zoster on tip of nose (ophthalmic nerve, nasociliary division), could result in herpetic keratitis
  - Zoster sine herpete: segmental pain without lesions
  - Ophthalmic zoster: ocular disease (20 to 70 percent), cicatricial lid retraction, ptosis, keratitis, scleritis, uveitis, secondary glaucoma, oculomotor palsies, chorioretinitis, optic neuritis, panophthalmitis
  - CNS zoster: has asymptomatic cerebrospinal fluid (CSF) changes
  - Primary varicella pneumonia: 14 percent, higher in adults and immunocompromised patients
  - Reye's syndrome: acute fetal encephalopathy associated with fatty degeneration of the liver, associated with aspirin treatment
  - Bacterial superinfections: usually due to *Staphylococcus aureus*
  - Acute cerebellar ataxia: unsteady gait 11 to 20 days following rash
  - Guillian-Barré syndrome: acute idiopathic polyneuritis
  - Encephalitis with headache, fever, photophobia, nausea, vomiting, nerve palsies

- Motor paralysis (1 to 5 percent), extension from sensory ganglion to anterior horn, first 2 to 3 weeks
- Ramsey Hunt: facial palsy secondary to herpes-zoster infection of facial (VII) and auditory (VIII) nerves; affects external ear, tympanic membrane; causes tinnitus, vertigo, deafness, otalgia, loss of taste
- Postherpetic neuralgia (PHN)
- Pain greater than 1 month after vesicles; occurs in 10 to 15 percent of patients; resolves: 50 percent by 3 months, 75 percent by 1 year
- Occurs in 60 percent of patients over age 60
- Diagnosis
  - Nonspecific tests
    - Tzanck smear: multinucleated giant cells, nuclear molding
    - Histology: intraepidermal vesicle, ballooning degeneration, reticular degeneration, inclusion bodies, margination of chromatin, vascular involvement (75 percent VZV)
  - Specific tests
    - Culture of viruses
    - PCR
- Treatment
  - Acyclovir: 800 mg five times daily for 7 days
  - Valacyclovir: 1 g three times daily for 7 days
  - Famciclovir: 500 mg three times daily for 7 days
  - Pain and pruritus: analgesics, oral antipruritics, calamine lotion, cool compresses
- Treatment of PHN
  - Nonnarcotic or narcotic analgesic
  - Capsaicin cream
  - Topical every 4 hours for pain relief; enhances release of substance P, burning sensation
  - Topical lidocaine gel or patch: for pain relief
  - Tricyclic antidepressant: dosages much less than needed for treatment of depression: amitryptyline, maprotiline, desipramine
  - Anticonvulsants: carbamazepine, gabapentin
  - Sympathetic nerve blockade
  - Steroids: methylprednisolone
  - Transcutaneous electrical stimulation
- Vaccine: to increase immunity in persons with a history of primary VZV in order to decrease zoster

EPSTEIN-BARR VIRUS [HUMAN HERPES VIRUS 4 (HHV 4)]

- dsDNA; replicates in the nucleus
- Infects mainly B-lymphocytes
- After acute infection, EBV persists for life as a latent infection
- Clinical
  - Mononucleosis
    - Triad: fever, sore throat, lymphadenopathy (5 to 15 percent)

- Rash: maculopapular (3 to 15 percent of patients)
- Eighty percent of patients have rash if treated with amoxicillin or ampicillin
- Treatment of infectious mononucleosis is supportive care
- Antipyretics, analgesics, topical steroid for cutaneous manifestations
- Prednisone for complications such as hemolytic anemia, thrombocytopenia, or lymphadenopathy that compromises the airway
  - Oral hairy leukoplakia
    - Usually associated with HIV patients
    - Secondary nonmalignant hyperplasia of epithelial cells
    - Accentuated vertical folds laterally on tongue
    - Mucosa appears white and thick: does not scrape off
    - Pathology: papillomatosis
  - Kikuchi's syndrome: hyperimmune reaction to an infectious agent causing regional lymph node enlargement
  - Mucocutaneous lymphoma: B-cell lymphoma
  - Burkitt's lymphoma
    - High-grade B-cell lymphoma
    - EBV genome can be detected in tumor cells
  - Nasopharyngeal carcinoma
    - Malignant tumor of the squamous epithelium of the nasopharynx
    - Patients have high levels of antibodies to EBV antigens
    - EBV genome is present in nasopharyngeal carcinoma cells
  - Gianotti-Crosti (infantile papular acrodermatitis)
    - Symmetric lichenoid papules that spare the trunk
    - Also associated with hepatitis B, adenovirus, CMV
- Diagnosis of EBV
  - Leukocytosis
  - Lymphocytosis
  - Elevated liver function test results
  - Heterophile antibody test
    - Polyclonal secretion of antibodies by infected B cells
    - (Heterophile test) nonspecific antibodies that agglutinate horse or sheep erythrocytes;heterophile antibodies may persists for 3 months after onset of illness
  - Monospot test: measure acute infectious mononucleosis heterophile antibodies in a rapid qualitative fashion
  - EBV serology
    - Major viral antigens:
    - Latent = EBNA → EBV nuclear antigens
    - LDMA (lymphocyte-defected mem. antigen)
    - Early = EADR → early antigen, diffuse restricted

- Late = VCA → viral capsid antigen, MA → membrane antigen
- Treatment
  - Most are self-limited; treat symptomatically
  - Oral hairy leukoplakia: acyclovir 400 mg five times daily

CYTOMEGALOVIRUS (CMV) [HUMAN HERPES VIRUS 5 (HSV-5)]

- Enveloped dsDNA
- Latent infection in the host occurs after infection; may reactivate during a period of immunosuppression
- Primary infection
  - Usually asymptomatic
  - Maculopapular rashes and ulcers
  - Can cause fever of unknown origin
  - Enlargement of the lymph nodes and spleen
- Complications
  - CMV pneumonia (19 percent)
  - Mononucleosis-like syndrome after treatment with ampicillin or amoxicillin
  - Guillain-Barré syndrome
  - Bone marrow transplant patients have highest mortality (85 percent) secondary to pneumonia
  - Four times increase mortality for solid-organ transplant
  - Gianotti-Crosti associated with CMV, hepatitis B, adenovirus, EBV
- Congenital cytomegalovirus
  - Pregnancy: 2 percent of seronegative patients develop asymptomatic CMV
  - Fifty-five percent have intrauterine infection
  - Most common congenital viral infection (1 percent of U.S. infants)
  - First trimester: intrauterine growth retardation, retinitis, optic nerve malformations
  - "After first trimester" hepatitis, pneumonia, purpura, DIC
- HIV and CMV: Retinitis is the most common symptom
- Diagnosis
  - Histology: vasculitis, "owl's eyes"; basophilic intranuclear inclusions
  - CMV antibodies
  - Antigenemia
  - Shell vial assay
- Treatment
  - Foscarnet: treats virus that is resistant to ganciclovir
  - Cidofovir: treatment of refractory CMV retinitis
  - Ganciclovir: drug of choice for treatment of CMV disease
  - Valganciclovir
  - Fomivirsen

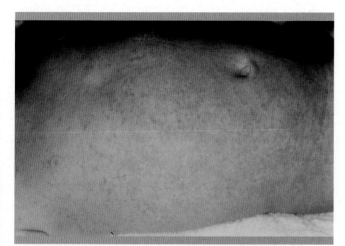

FIGURE 17-8 Roseola infantum. *(Courtesy of Dr. Stephen Tyring.)*

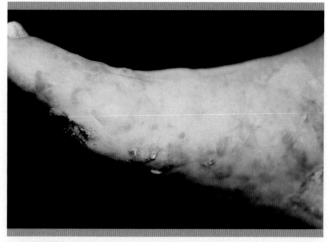

FIGURE 17-9 Kaposi sarcoma (classic). *(Courtesy of Dr. Stephen Tyring.)*

HUMAN HERPES VIRUS 6 (HHV 6): ROSEOLA INFANTUM (EXANTHEMA SUBITUM/SIXTH DISEASE) (FIG. 17-8)

- Enveloped DNA viruses; spread by oropharyngeal secretions
- Most common childhood exanthem
- Clinical
  - Six months to 2 years: 95 percent; incubation: 5 to 15 days; lasts 1 to 2 days
  - Spread of infection during the febrile and viremic phase of the illness
  - Abrupt onset with high fever (102.2 to 105.8°F)
  - Child generally in no distress
  - Bulging anterior fontanelle, tonsillar and pharyngeal inflammation, tympanic injection, and lymph node enlargement
  - Fever drops on the fourth day, coinciding with onset of a rash
  - Rash: starts on trunk and may spread to neck and upper and lower extremities
  - Pink macules: 2 to 5 mm
  - Upper respiratory infection, adenopathy, central nervous system, intussusception, thrombocytic purpura, mononucleosis (as in adults)
  - Palpebral edema (Berliner's sign, "heavy eyelids") and periorbital edema
  - Seizures (6 to 15 percent) during the febrile phase
- HIV + HHV 6: tropism for CD4+ cells; upregulation of CD4 expression, which is needed by the gp120 unit of HIV to infect cells
- Bone marrow transplant patients: idiopathic bone marrow suppression secondary to virus
- Diagnosis: PCR
- Treatment: symptomatic; a few case reports describe foscarnet and/or ganciclovir to be successful, but dosages are not known
- Course: no sequelae generally observed

HUMAN HERPES VIRUS 7 (HHV 7)

- Significant homology with HHV 6
- No clinical disease has been definitely linked to HHV 7; with questionable relationship to pityriasis rosea
- Eighty-five percent of adults are seropositive, and most infections develop within first 5 years of life
- Transmitted through saliva
- Diagnosis: serology
- Treatment: symptomatic

HUMAN HERPES VIRUS 8 (HHV 8): KAPOSI SARCOMA (FIGS. 17-9 AND 17-10)

- Proliferation of spindle cells thought to have an endothelial cell origin
- Four types
  - Endemic African KS: usually aggressive course
  - Epidemic AIDS-related KS: patients with advanced HIV infection
  - Immunocompromised (iatrogenic) KS: patients receiving immunosuppressive therapy; visceral involvement
  - Classic KS: elderly men of Mediterranean and eastern European background; protracted and indolent course
- Clinical
  - Cutaneous and visceral lesions
  - Brown, pink, red, or violaceous papules or nodules
  - Mucous membrane involvement is common
- Diagnosis: histology: spindle cells, prominent slitlike vascular spaces, and extravasated red blood cells
- Treatment
  - Antiretroviral therapy
  - Solitary KS lesions may be excised surgically or removed using laser surgery

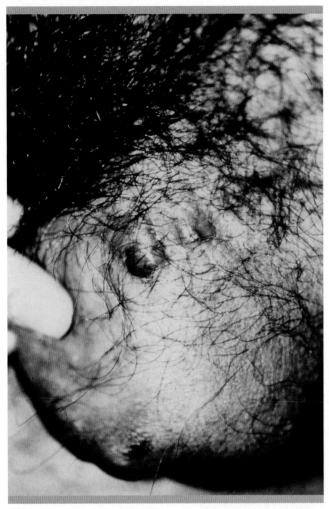

FIGURE 17-10 Kaposi sarcoma (scrotal in patient with AIDS). *(Courtesy of Dr. Stephen Tyring.)*

- Radiation
- Topical retinoids
- Intralesional vinblastine
- Interferon-α
- Chemotherapy: liposomal doxorubicin, liposomal daunorubicin, vincristine, vinblastine, bleomycin, and paclitaxel

HERPES VIRUS B: HERPES SIMIAE

- Transmitted to humans through primates of the *Macaca* species from a bite, scratch, or open wound
- Neurotropic: remains latent in ganglia
- In humans: initial local erythema, vesicular eruption with constitutional symptoms
- Vesicular eruption at site of injury
- Death secondary to encephalitis; very high mortality rate
- Treatment: nucleoside analogues (e.g., intravenous acyclovir)

Parviviruses

PARVOVIRUS B19: "SLAPPED CHEEKS," FIFTH DISEASE, ERYTHEMA INFECTIOSUM

- ssDNA
- Tropism for rapidly dividing erythrocyte precursors
- Clinical
  - Twenty percent are asymptomatic.
  - Headache, coryza, and low-grade fever about 2 days prior to the onset of the rash
  - Characterized by a "slapped cheek" appearance of the face on the first day
  - Erythematous, lacy eruption on the trunk and extremities
  - Red round macules appear on the arms and legs
  - After rash fades, a lacy marble-like pattern to the skin appears: not contagious at this stage
  - Eruption can last 5 to 9 days and can recur for weeks or months with triggers such as sunlight, exercise, temperature change, bathing, and emotional stress
  - Headache, pharyngitis, fever, malaise, myalgias, coryza, diarrhea, nausea, cough, and conjunctivitis
  - Papular-pruritic "gloves-and-socks" syndrome: Erythematous exanthem of the hands and feet with a distinct margin at the wrist and ankle joints is present along with pain and edema
  - Arthralgias or arthritis: 10 percent of children
- Complications: aplastic crisis in patients with increased red blood cell turnover, chronic anemia in immunocompromised persons, patients with chronic hemolytic anemia, fetal hydrops, sickle cell anemia, G6PD deficiency, and β-thalassemia
- Diagnosis
  - Parvovirus serology (IgM and IgG) can be determined.
  - Complete blood count (CBC): low reticulocyte count (0 to 1 percent)
- Treatment
  - Ibuprofen or acetaminophen for fever (to prevent Reye's syndrome: aspirin use is contraindicated)
  - Red blood cell (RBC) transfusions for aplastic crisis

HEPATITIS B

- Hepadna virus
- Partially double-stranded circular DNA
- Encodes four overlapping open reading frames as follows:
  - S for the surface or envelope gene encoding the pre-S1, pre-S2, and S protein
  - C for the core gene, encoding for the core nucleocapsid protein and the e antigen
  - X for the X gene encoding the X protein

- P for the polymerase gene, encoding a large protein promoting priming, RNA-dependent and DNA-dependent DNA polymerase and RNase H activities
- Transmitted sexually and perinatally
- Incubation approximately 75 days
- Clinical
  - Prodromal or preicteric phase: serum sickness–like; develops in 20 to 30 percent of patients: arthropathy, proteinuria, hematuria
  - Icteric phase: jaundice (10 days after the appearance of constitutional symptomatology and lasting for 1 to 3 months), nausea, vomiting, and pruritus
  - Skin: urticaria/vasculitis secondary to perivascular deposition of immune complexes, hepatitis B + C3, IgM, or IgG
- Associated conditions
  - Transient hypocomplementemia associated with urticaria
  - Polyarthritis nodosa: associated with arthralgias, fever, malaise, renal disease, nodules
  - Globulinemia: associated with chronic HBV, purpura, arthropathy, renal disease, necrotizing vasculitis, with mixed IgG and IgM
  - Others: erythema nodosum, urticaria, lichen planus, leukocytoclastic vasculitis, Gianotti-Crosti
- Diagnosis
  - Active hepatitis B: high levels of alanine aminotransferase (ALT) and aspartate aminotransferase (AST); HBsAg (Australian antigen) and HBeAg (marker of infectivity) identified in the serum; HBcAb (IgM)
  - Chronic inactive hepatitis B: HBsAg, HBcAb of IgG type, and HBeAb also are present in the serum.
  - Chronic active hepatitis B: mild to moderate elevation of the aminotransferases
- Treatment: interferon-α, lamivudine, adefovir dipivoxil
- Hepatitis B vaccine

RNA VIRUSES

1. Picornaviruses
   - Nonenveloped (naked) virions
   - Size range of 20 to 25 nm
   - Capsids composed of four different proteins
   - Genome is single-stranded (ss) RNA
   - Size range of 7500 to 8500 nucleotides
   - Three major human genera
     - Rhinoviruses
     - Hepatovirus: hepatitis A virus (HAV)
     - Enteroviruses
       ▲ Poliovirus
       ▲ Enterovirus
       ▲ Coxsackievirus
       ▲ Echovirus
2. Togaviruses
   - Enveloped
   - ssRNA
   - Rubella
3. Flaviviruses
   - Enveloped
   - ssRNA
   - Hepatitis C, yellow fever, dengue fever, West Nile virus
4. Retroviruses
   - ssRNA
   - Enveloped
   - Contain reverse transcriptase
   - HIV
5. Paramyxoviruses
   - Spherical
   - Enveloped virus
   - ssRNA
   - Measles
6. Arenaviruses: Lassa fever, Argentine hemorrhagic fever, and related viruses
7. Bunyaviruses
   - ssRNA
   - Enveloped
   - Helical symmetry
   - Sandfly fever virus and Hantaan virus

Picornaviruses

ENTEROVIRUSES

Hand, Foot, and Mouth Disease (Fig. 17-11)

- Coxsackie A-16, enterovirus 71 (CNS involvement)
- Oral-oral/oral-fecal, highly contagious
- Clinical
  - Incubation: 3 to 6 days
  - Prodrome enanthem: fever, malaise, abdominal pain
  - Oral ulcerative lesions: hard palate, tongue, buccal mucosa, 2 to 10 lesions develop over 5 to 10 days; vesicles on an erythematous base
  - Cutaneous
    - Hands, feet, and buttocks
    - Few hundred lesions
    - Hands > feet, erythematous macules, gray center, run parallel to skin lines, vesicles surrounded by red areola, elliptical
    - Resolves spontaneously after 1 week
- Diagnosis
  - Histology: intraepidermal blister: neutrophils, monocytes, necrotic roof, intercellular edema (reticular edema/balloon degeneration), edematous dermis, intracytoplasmic particles in a crystalline array

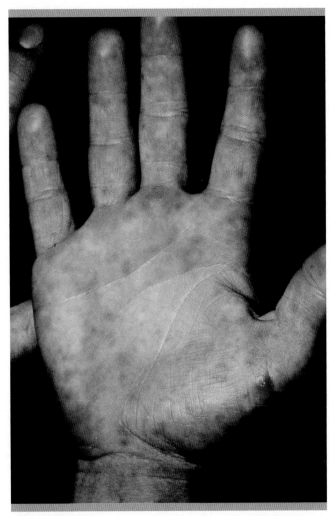

FIGURE 17-11 Hand, foot, and mouth disease. *(Courtesy of Dr. Stephen Tyring.)*

- Cell culture
- PCR of blood, stool, pharyngeal, vesicle (fecal least specific)
- Treatment: symptomatic

Herpangina

- Spread via the fecal-oral route
- Etiology
  - Coxsackieviruses A 1–10, 16, or 22
  - Echovirus 6, 9, 11, 16, 17, 22, and 25
  - Enterovirus 71
- Clinical
  - Sudden onset of fever, headache, back/extremity pain
  - Incubation period typically is 7 to 14 days
  - Lesions on mucous membranes: soft palate tonsillar pillars, fauces, uvula
  - Gray/white papulovesicular lesions, 1 to 2 mm, erythema surrounding

- Exanthem: Characteristics vary
- Treatment: self-limited

HEPATOVIRUS

Hepatitis A

- Picornavirus
- Transmission: fecal-oral route
- Incubation: 2 to 7 weeks
- Fourteen percent of cases manifest as a transient, discrete, maculopapular, urticarial, or petechial rash
- Rarely, persistent hepatitis A develops into a globulinemia with cutaneous vasculitis
- Treatment: mild self-limited disease
- Combination vaccine for the prevention of hepatitis A and hepatitis B virus has been approved

Paramyxovirus

RUBEOLA/MEASLES

- Paramyxovirus, RNA virus
- Most infectious virus known
- Responsible for more than 1 million deaths worldwide
- Three types
  - Typical
  - Modified: partial immune host
  - Atypical: previously immunized
- Four phases
  - Incubation: 10 to 12 days
  - Prodrome: three Cs of measles: cough, coryza, and conjunctivitis
  - Enanthem: Koplik spots (24 hours before rash): red spots on buccal mucosa with white center (gray)
  - Exanthem: fourth day (lasts 5 days); not pruritic, red macules, papules that begin on the face and behind the ears and then spread to trunk, limbs
- Complications: encephalitis (1 in 800), purpura = secondary to thrombocytopenia, otitis media and pneumonia from the secondary bacterial infection, tuberculosis, subacute sclerosing panencephalitis (SSPE)
- Diagnosis
  - Serology: (hemagglutination inhibiting Ab) ELISA
  - Histology: hyaline necrosis, necrotic epithelium, intranuclear inclusions, multinucleated giant cells (Warthin-Finkelday cells)
- Treatment: vitamin A
- Vaccine: Protective titers can last greater than 16 years

Togaviruses

RUBELLA: GERMAN MEASLES (FIG. 17-12)

- ssRNA togavirus
- Clinical
  - Incubates 2 to 3 weeks; spread by nasal droplet infection

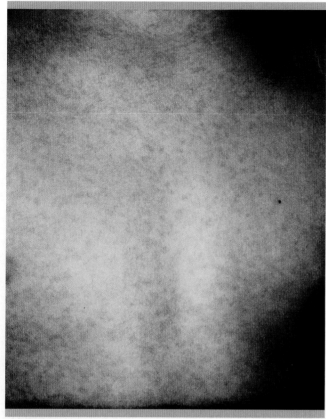

FIGURE 17-12 Rubella. *(Courtesy of Dr. Stephen Tyring.)*

- Known as "3-day measles"
- Generalized tender lymphadenopathy: involves all nodes, most striking in the suboccipital, postauricular, and anterior and posterior cervical nodes
- Exanthem lasts 1 to 3 days, first leaving the face and may be followed by desquamation
- Forscheimer's spots: nonspecific enanthem of pinpoint red macules and petechiae that can be seen over the soft palate and uvula just before or with the exanthem
- Syndrome of low-grade fever, chronic fatigue, and myalgias can persist for months or years but rare
- Congenital rubella syndrome
  - Fetus of a pregnant woman without immunity to the virus
  - Fifty percent with complications if infant infected in the first trimester
  - Ophthalmologic: cataracts, retinopathy
  - Cardiac abnormalities: patent ductus arteriosus, pulmonary stenosis
  - Sensineural deafness
  - Neurologic: meningoencephalitis, mental retardation with behavioral disorders
  - "Blueberry muffin" baby: dermal extramedullary hematopoiesis
  - Thrombocytopenia with purpura and petechiae

- Diagnosis: culture from nose, urine
- Treatment
  - No adequate treatment is available for pregnant women exposed to rubella
  - No specific treatment for rubella exists; the disease usually is self-limited
  - Preventative measures include vaccine—as part of the combined MMR usually given between 12 and 15 months of age—and some experts recommend a second vaccination at 4 to 6 years of age

Flaviviruses

HEPATITIS C

- Acute
  - ssRNA
  - Parenteral transmission, tatoos
  - Incubation: 6 to 7 weeks
  - Thirty to forty percent have symptoms (jaundice)
  - Symptoms indistinguishable from other types of acute viral hepatitis
  - Fluctuating serum aminotransferase levels
- Chronic
  - Most common cause of chronic viral hepatitis (70 to 85 percent patients will develop)
  - Defined as elevated ALT enzyme levels for a period of at least 6 months
  - Cirrhosis: 8 to 46 percent of patients
  - Diseases associated with chronic hepatitis C
    - Immune complexes: skin, kidney (glomerulonephritis)
    - Sialadentitis
    - Autoimmune thrombocytopenic purpura
    - Lymphoma: increased antibodies to HCV in patients with non-Hodgkin's B-cell lymphoma (20 to 40 percent)
    - Mixed cryoglobulinemia (types II and III)
    - Porphyria cutanea tarda
    - Lichen planus
    - Polyarteritis nodosa (5 percent)
    - Pruritus (39 percent)
- Treatment: Peginterferon-α, pegylated interferon plus ribavirin

Retroviruses

HUMAN IMMUNODEFICIENCY VIRUS

- ssRNA retrovirus
- p24 nucleocapsid protein; gp41 and gp120 are envelope proteins
- Reverse transcriptase
- DNA polymerase
  - Transcribes single-stranded RNA into double-stranded DNA
  - Integrated into host DNA

- Primary symptoms: headache, retroorbital pain, muscle aches, fever, pharyngitis, fatigue, lymphadenopathy, and a fine morbilliform rash
- Cutaneous manifestations seen in HIV-infected individuals
  - Acute exanthem of HIV disease
  - Herpes simplex virus
  - Cytomegalovirus
  - Oral hairy leukoplakia
  - Human papillomavirus
  - Molluscum contagiosum
- Diagnosis
  - ELISA
  - Western blot assay
  - Viral load measured by PCR
- Treatment
  - Nucleoside reverse transcriptase inhibitors (NRTI's)
    - Zidovudine: 200 mg three times daily
    - Lamivudine: 150 mg twice daily
    - Stavudine: 40 mg twice daily
    - Didanosine: 200 mg twice daily
    - Zalcitabine: 0.75 mg three times daily
    - Abacavir: 300 mg twice daily
    - Emtricitabine: 200 mg daily
    - Combivir: combination of 300 mg zidovudine + 300 mg abacavir taken twice daily
    - Trizivir: 300 mg zidovudine + 150 mg lamivudine + 300 mg abacavir taken twice daily
  - Nonnucleoside reverse transcriptase inhibitors (NNRTI's)
    - Nevirapine: 200 mg for 14 days and then 200 mg twice daily
    - Delavirdine: 400 mg three times daily in 3 oz water
    - Efavirenz: 600 mg at night
  - Nucleotide reverse transcriptase inhibitor: Tenofovir: 300 mg daily
  - Fusion inhibitor: Enfuvirtide: twice-daily subcutaneous injection
  - Protease inhibitors
    - Saquinavir: 1200 mg three times daily
    - Ritonavir: 600 mg twice daily
    - Indinavir: 800 mg every 8 hours
    - Nelfinavir: 750 mg three times daily
    - Amprenavir: 1200 mg twice daily
    - Lopinavir + ritonavir: 400 mg lopinavir + 100 mg ritonavir
    - Fosamprenavir calcium: 700 mg twice daily
    - Atazanavir sulfate: 400 mg daily

REFERENCES

Balfour HH Jr, Kelly JM, Suarez CS: Acyclovir treatment of varicella in otherwise healthy children. *J Pediatr* 1990;116(4):633–639.

Bernstein DI, Aoki FY, Tyring SK, et al. Safety and immunogenicity of glycoprotein-D adjuvant genital herpes vaccine. *Clin Infect Dis* 2005;40:1271–1281.

Beutner KR, Tyring SK, Trofatter KF, et al: Imiquimod, a patient applied immune response modifier for the treatment of external genital warts. *Antimicrob Agents Chemother* 1998;42:789–794.

Carrasco DA, Trizna Z, Colome-Grimmer M, et al: Verrucous herpes of the scrotum in a human immunodeficiency virus-positive man: Case report and review of the literature. *JEADV* 2002;16:511–515.

Carrasco D, Vander Straten M, Tyring SK: Treatment of anogenital warts with imiquimod 5% cream followed by surgical excision of residual lesions. *J Am Acad Dermatol* 2002;47(4 Suppl):S212–216.

Chen J, Wang L, Chen JJ, et al: Detection of antibodies to human immunodeficiency virus (HIV) that recognize conformational epitopes of glycoproteins 160 and 41 often allows for early diagnosis of HIV infection. *J Infect Dis* 2002;186(3):321–331.

Corey L, Langenberg AGM, Ashley R, et al: Recombinant glycoprotein vaccine for the prevention of genital HSV-2 acquisition: Two double-blind, placebo-controlled trials. *JAMA* 1999;282:331–340.

Corey L, Wald A, Patel R, et al: Once-daily valacyclovir to reduce the risk of transmission of genital herpes. *N Engl J Med* 2004;350:11–20.

Dianzani F, Antonnelli G, Tyring SK, et al: The HIV RNA load in chronically infected patients circulates mainly as neutralized immune complexes. *J Infect Dis* 2002;185:1051–1054.

Freedberg IM et al. *Fitzpatrick's Dermatology in General Medicine*, 6th Ed. New York: McGraw-Hill; 2003.

Fuessel Haws AL, He Q, Rady PL, et al: Nested PCR with the PGMY09/11 and GP5(+)/6(+) primer sets improves detection of HPV DNA in cervical samples. *J Virol Methods* 2004;122:87–93.

Gonzalez L, Gaviria AM, Sanclemente G, et al: Clinical, histopathological and virological findings in patients with focal epithelial hyperplasia from Columbia. *Int J Dermatol* 2005;44:274–279.

McKee PH. *Pathology of the Skin: With Clinical Correlations*. London: Mosby-Wolfe; 1996.

Meadows KP, Tyring SK, Pavia AT, et al: Resolution of racalcitrant molluscum contagiosum lesions in HIV-infected patients treated with cidofovir. *Arch Dermatol* 1997;133:987–990.

Mertz GJ, Loveless MO, Levin MJ, et al: Oral famciclovir for suppression of recurrent genital herpes simplex virus infection in women. A multicenter, double blind, placebo-controlled trial. *Arch Int Med* 1997;157:343–349.

Patel R, Tyring SK, Strand A, et al: Impact of suppressive antiviral therapy on the health-related quality of life of patients with recurrent genital herpes infection. *Sex Trans Inf* 1999;75:398–402.

Patera A, Ali MA, Tyring SK, et al: Polymorphisms in the genes for herpesvirus entry. *J Infect Dis* 2002;186(3):444–445.

Rady PL, Hodak E, Yen A, et al: Detection of human herpesvirus 8 DNA in Kaposi's sarcomas from iatrogenically immunosuppressed patients. *J Am Acad Dermatol* 1998;38:429–437.

Reichman RC, Oakes D, Bonnez W, et al: Treatment of condyloma acuminatum with three different alpha interferon preparations administered parenterally: A double blind, placebo-controlled trial. *J Infect Dis* 1990;162: 1270–1276.

Reichman RC, Oakes D, Bonnez W, et al: Treatment of condyloma acuminatum with three different interferons administered intralesionally: A multicentered, placebo-controlled trial. *Ann Intern Med* 1988;108:675–679.

Reitano M, Tyring SK, Lang W, et al: Valaciclovir for the suppression of recurrent genital HSV infection: A large scale dose range-finding study. *J Infect Dis* 1998;178:603–610.

Roncalli W, Neto CF, Rady PL, et al: Clinical aspects of epidermodysplasia verruciformis. *J Eur Acad Venereol* 2003; 17:394–398.

Roncalli W, He Q, Rady PL, et al: HPV typing in Brazilian patients with epidermodysplasia verruciformis: High prevalence of EV-HPV 25. *J Cutan Med Surg* 2004;8:110–115.

Roncalli W, Rady PL, Grady J, et al: Association of p53 polymorphism with skin cancer. *Int J Dermatol* 2004; 43:489–493.

Roncalli W, Rady PL, Grady J, et al: Polymorphisms of the interleukin-10 gene promotor in epidermodysplasia verruciformis patients from Brazil. *J Am Acad Dermatol* 2003; 49:639–643.

Schell B, Rosen T, Rady P, et al: Verrucous carcinoma of the foot associated with human papillomavirus type 16. *J Am Acad Dermatol* 2001;45:49–55.

Shafran SD, Tyring SK, Ashton R, et al: Once, twice, or three times daily famciclovir compared with acyclovir for the oral treatment of herpes zoster in immunocompetent adults: A randomized, multicenter, double-blind clinical trial. *J Clin Virol* 2004;29:248–253.

Spruance SL, Tyring SK, DeGregorio B, et al: A large-scale placebo-controlled, dose-ranging trial of peroral valaciclovir for episodic treatment of recurrent herpes genitalis. *Arch Int Med* 1996;156:1729–1735.

Stanberry LR, Spruance SL, Cunningham L, et al: Glycoprotein D adjuvant vaccine to prevent genital herpes. *N Engl J Med* 2002;347:1652–1661.

Sterling J, Tyring S, eds. *Human Papillomaviruses*. New York: Oxford; 2001.

Trizna Z, Evans T, Bruce S, et al: A randomized phase II study comparing four different interferon therapies in patients with recalcitrant condylomata acuminata. *Sex Trans Dis* 1998;25:361–365.

Tyring S, ed. *Antiviral Agents, Vaccines and Immunotherapies*. New York: Marcel Dekker; 2005.

Tyring S, ed. *Mucocutaneous Manifestations of Viral Diseases*. New York: Marcel Dekker; 2002.

Tyring SK, Arany I, Stanley MA, et al: A molecular study of condylomata acuminata clearance during treatment with imiquimod: A randomized, double blind, vehicle-controlled study. *J Infect Dis* 1998;178:551–555.

Tyring SK, Diaz-Mitoma F, Shafran SD, et al: Oral famciclovir for the suppression of recurrent genital herpes: The combined data from two randomized controlled trials. *J Cutan Med Surg* 2003;7:449–454.

Tyring SK, Belanger R, Bezwoda W, et al: A randomized, double blind trial of famciclovir versus acyclovir for the treatment of localized dermatomal herpes zoster in immunocompromised patients. *Cancer Invest* 2001;19: 13–22.

Tyring SK, Beutner KR, Tucker BA, et al: Antiviral therapy for herpes zoster. *Arch Fam Med* 2000;9:863–869.

Tyring SK, Douglas J, Corey L, et al: A randomized, placebo-controlled comparison of oral acyclovir and valacyclovir HCl in patients with recurrent genital herpes infections. *Arch Dermatol* 1998;134:185–191.

Tyring SK, Edwards L, Friedman DJ, et al: Safety and efficacy of 0.5% podofilox gel in the treatment of external genital and/or perianal warts: A double blind, vehicle-controlled study. *Arch Dermatol* 1998;134:33–38.

Tyring S, Nahlik J, Cunningham A, et al: A double blind, randomized, placebo-controlled, parallel group study of oral famciclovir for the treatment of uncomplicated herpes zoster. *Ann Intern Med* 1995;123:89–96.

Tyring SK, Engst R, Corriveau C, et al: Famciclovir for ophthalmic zoster: A randomized acyclovir-controlled study. *Br J Ophthalmol* 2001;85:576–581.

Whitley RJ, Weiss H, Gnann Jr JW, et al: Acyclovir with and without prednisone for the treatment of herpes zoster: A randomized, placebo-controlled trial. *Ann Intern Med* 1996;125:376–383.

Yen-Moore A, Hudnall SD, Rady PL, et al: Differential expression of the HHV-8 vGCR cellular homolog gene in AIDS-associated and classic Kaposi's sarcoma: Potential role of HIV-1 Tat. *Virology* 2000;267:247–251.

Zong JC, Ciufo DM, Alcendor DJ, et al: High level variability in the ORF-K1 membrane protein gene at the left end of the Kaposi's sarcoma associated herpesvirus (HHV8) genome defines four major virus subtypes and multiple variants or clades in different human populations. *J Virol* 1999; 73:4156–4170.

Zong J, Ciufo DM, Viscidi R, et al: Genotypic analysis at multiple loci across Kaposi's sarcoma herpesvirus (KSHV) DNA molecules: clustering patterns, novel variants and chimerism. *J Clin Virol* 2002;23(3):119–148.

CHAPTER 18

BASIC SCIENCES

DANETTE M. PERSYN
MADELEINE DUVIC

EPIDERMIS AND DERMIS

Epidermis

- Stratified squamous epithelium
- Approximately 0.4 to 1.5 mm thick and consisting mostly of keratinocytes (Fig. 18-1)
- Renewal of the epidermis takes approximately 26 to 28 days (13 to 14 days for maturation from basal layer to corneum and another 13 to 14 days for shedding)
- Divided into four layers with characteristic cell shape, specialized intracellular structures, types of keratin, accessory cells, and proteins (Table 18-1)
- Stratum corneum, stratum granulosum, stratum spinosum, stratum germinativum
- Stratum lucidum is an additional layer present between the strata granulosum and corneum in palmoplantar skin. It appears as an electronlucent zone and contains nucleated cells
- Differentiation from basal cell to corneocyte involves the loss of the nucleus and extrusion of cellular contents except for keratin filaments and filaggrin matrix

SPECIALIZED CELLS

- Merkel cell
  - Type I mechanoreceptor (slow-adapting, low threshold)
  - Derived from ectoderm/neural crest
  - Mainly confined to basal layer
  - Present in areas with high tactile sensitivity (hairy and glabrous skin)
  - Typically found in epithelium of digits, lips, oral cavity, and outer root sheath of the hair follicle
  - Contain granules with neurotransmitter-like substances; nonspecific enolase present
  - Members of the amine precursor uptake and decarboxylation (APUD) system
  - K20 is specific for Merkel cell; also contain K18, K8, K19

- Melanocytes
  - Neural crest–derived dendritic cell
  - Mainly confined to basal layer
  - Extend above and below basal layer but do not form junctions with keratinocytes
  - Contains two types of the pigment melanin
    - Eumelanin (brown and black coloration)
    - Pheomelanin (red or yellow coloration)
- Langerhans cell
  - Dendritic, bone marrow–derived (mesoderm) antigen-presenting cell
  - Involved in T-cell responses (i.e., contact hypersensitivity and graft-versus-host disease)
  - Process antigen and present it to T cells in the presence of major histocompatability complex (MHC) class II
  - Produces interleukin 1 (IL-1)
  - Contains distinctive racket-shaped Birbeck granules that are formed when an antigen is internalized by endocytosis
  - Ultraviolet B (UV-B) decreases number and antigen-presenting ability of Langerhans cell
  - Can be infected with HIV
  - Reduced numbers in patients with psoriasis, sarcoidosis, and contact dermatitis

SPECIALIZED STRUCTURES

- Desmosomes
  - Prominent in the stratum spinosum
  - Anchoring junctions that connect adjacent keratinocytes (Fig. 18-2)
  - Keratin filaments extend from desmosome to desmosome to form keratin cytoskeleton
  - Structure consists of a desmosomal plaque on the interior of the cell membrane, transmembrane glycoproteins, and a central plate that crosses the intercellular space between two keratinocytes
  - Plaque contains six polypeptides
    - Desmoplakins 1 and 2—mediate attachment of keratins to plaque

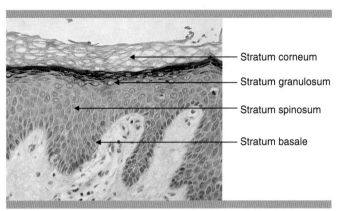

FIGURE 18-1 Epidermis. *(From Freedberg IM et al: Fitzpatrick's Dermatology in General Medicine, 6th ed. New York: McGraw-Hill, 2003, p. 92.)*

– Desmocalmin—important for calcium regulation
– Band 6 protein
– Plakoglobin—mediates attachment of keratins to plaque
– Desmoyokin—associated with cell membrane
• Transmembrane proteins are cadherins and provide adhesion.
    – Desmogleins 1 and 3
    – Desmocollins I and II
• Gap junctions
    • Allow for communication between cells
    • Made of connexin
• Adherens junctions
    • Made of "classic cadherins" (E-, P-, and N-cadherins)

TABLE 18-1 Layers of the Skin and Characteristics

	Cell Shape	Types of Cells	Types of Keratin	Additional Structures	Associated Proteins
Stratum corneum Stratum dysjuctum Stratum compactum	Flatttened polyhedral-shaped horny cells with loss of nucleus	Keratinocytes		Cornified cell envelope	Loricrin Profilaggrin Filaggrin Involucrin Cornifin Trichohyalin TGM 1/2/3 Envolplakin SPR 1/2
Stratum granulosum	Diamond-shaped with characteristic dense basophilic granules		K2 K11	Basophilic keratohyaline granules	Profilaggrin Loricrin
Stratum spinosum	Polyhedral with round nucleus; "spiny appearance"	Keratinocytes Langerhans cell Transient amplifying cells	K1 K10 K9	Lamellar granules Desmosomes Gap junctions	Desmoglein II/III Desmocollin I
Stratum germinativum	Columnar with round nucleus	Keratinocytes Stem cells (10%) Transient amplifying cells (50%) Postmitotic differentiated cells (40%) Melanocytes Merkel cell Langerhans cell	K5 K14 K19		BPAG 1

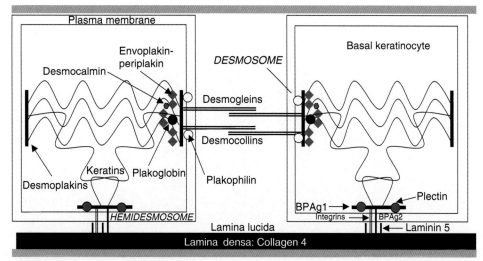

FIGURE 18-2 Desmosomes. *(From Freedberg IM et al: Fitzpatrick's Dermatology in General Medicine, 6th ed. New York: McGraw-Hill, 2003, p. 93.)*

- Sites of contact between neighboring keratinocytes or Langerhans cells
- Actin attaches to cadherins via alpha, beta, and gamma catenins
- Lamellar granules (Odland bodies)
  - First apparent in upper spinous layer, but primary site of action is the granular layer.
  - 0.2 to 0.3 μm in diameter, membrane-bound secretory granules
  - Contain glycoproteins, glycolipids, phospholipids, free sterols, acid hydrolases, and glucosylceramides (precursors to ceramides that contribute to corneum lipid layer)
  - Extrude their contents of lipids and enzymes into the intercellular space, where the lipid is rearranged to lipid sheets
  - Create a hydrophobic barrier between the granular and cornified layers
- Keratohyaline granules
  - Dense basophilic granules containing electrondense proteins of profilaggrin, keratin, and loricrin
  - Filaggrin (cleaved from profilaggrin) becomes the major protein of keratohyaline granules.
  - Involved in formation of cornified cell envelope
  - Rich in sulfur
- Cornified cell envelope (CCE)
  - An extremely durable protein-lipid polymer
  - Assembled on the interior of the keratinocyte
  - Eventually resides on the exterior of the corneocyte
  - Provides a mechanical and chemical barrier
  - CCE is 7 to 15 nm thick

- Impermeability of this layer is achieved by the action of calcium-dependent transglutaminases that bind (cross-link) loricrin, keratin, desmosomal proteins, involucrin, elafin, and other proteins to the cell membrane, creating a proteinaceous and insoluble shield
- Epsilon-gamma-glutamyl-lysine-isopeptide cross-links make the CCE insoluble

SPECIALIZED PROTEINS

- Profilaggrin/filaggrin
  - *Fi*lament *agg*regate prote*in*
  - Profilaggrin is a protein made up of 10 to 12 tandem repeat units of filaggrin
  - Profilaggrin is converted to monomers of filaggrin in a stepwise conversion by three proteases and dephosphorylation
  - Filaggrin is thought to provide a protein matrix for keratin filament aggregation in corneocytes
- Loricrin
  - A protein composing 70 percent of the CCE
  - Hydrophobic, cysteine-rich protein
  - Gene is located on chromosome 1q21 as part of the epidermal differentiation complex
  - Encoded along with other proteins required for the terminal differentiation of epidermis
  - Loricrin is localized to the desmosome in association with desmoglein
- Involucrin
  - Glutamine-rich, acidic protein
  - Resistant to denaturing and unchanged by retinoic acids
  - Early marker of keratin differentiation

- Serves as a scaffold for other proteins to bind during keratinization
- Diseases associated with abnormalities in epidermal proteins

Dermis

- Mesodermal origin
- Collagen is major protein composed of fibroblasts and products of dermis (type I in adult)
- Two regions
  - Papillary dermis
    - Superficial
    - Small collagen bundles
    - Fine meshwork of microfibrils (fibrillin) organized into elaunin and oxytalan fibers
  - Reticular dermis
    - Deeper
    - Large collagen bundles
    - Mature, branching elastic fibers
- Ground substance (mucopolysaccharides)
- Subpapillary vascular plexus
- Deeper vascular plexus that envelops hair follicles and eccrine sweat glands
- Fibroblasts, macrophages, and mast cells are located in the dermis
- Afferent nerves (stain for S-100)
  - Unmyelinated nerve fibers (C-type fibers)
    - Detect temperature, pain, and itch
    - Located in papillary dermis and possibly basal layer
    - Encapsulated nerve endings detect touch and pressure
  - Meissner corpuscles
    - Located in dermal papillae
    - Detect light pressure
    - More prevalent in palms and soles
    - "Pine cone" appearance
  - Vater-Pacini corpuscles
    - Located in deep dermis of palms, dorsum of hands, and soles; also skin of nipples and anogenital region
    - Detect deep pressure and vibration
    - "Pearl onion" appearance in cross section
  - Mucocutaneous end organs (Krause end bulbs)
    - Located in papillary dermis
    - Found in skin at mucocutaneous junction (vermilion border of lips, glans penis, clitoris)

DERMAL-EPIDERMAL JUNCTION

- Also referred to as the *basement membrane zone* (BMZ)
- Thickness of 0.5 to 1.0 mm

- Visualized with periodic acid–Schiff (PAS) staining, not hematoxylin and eosin (H&E) stain
- Most components arise from basal keratinocytes or fibroblasts
- Function
  - Supportive structure to anchor the epidermis to the dermis: Anchoring occurs through the cytoskeleton in keratinocytes binding to laminin 5 in lamina lucida, which, in turn, binds to type VII collagen in lamina densa
  - Regulates interactions between the dermis and epidermis
  - Provides a selective barrier between the dermis and epidermis
- Hemidesmosome (anchoring complex) (Fig. 18-3)
  - Attaches basal cells of epidermis to the basement membrane (link keratin cytoskeleton to laminin 5 in the lamina lucida)
  - Structurally different from desmosomes
  - Consists of a cytoplasmic portion (attachment plaque), transmembrane portion [bullous pemphigoid (BP) antigen 180 and integrin], and an extracellular portion (anchoring filaments and subbasal dense plate)
  - Cytoplasmic attachment plaque
    - Consists of BP antigen 230 and plectin (HD-1)
    - Keratin filaments (K5,14) attach to plaque
    - Desmocalmin and desmoplakin bind keratin to plaque
    - Intracellular portion of BP antigen 180 (BPAG2) and collagen XVII are also present
  - Transmembrane portion
    - Consists of BP antigen 180 (BPAG2)—type II transmembrane configuration
    - Contains $\alpha 6\beta 4$ integrin, which likely interacts with laminin 5 to form anchoring filaments
  - Subbasal dense plate and anchoring filaments
    - Located below the hemidesmosome in the lamina lucida
    - Integrins and BPAG2 cross the membrane and attach to plate
    - Anchoring filaments then extend from the subbasal plate into the lamina densa, providing a point of deeper attachment
- Three zones
  - Lamina lucida
    - Named for appearance on electron microscopy (EM) as electron-lucent
    - 8 nm wide
    - Weakest of layers—able to split with heat or salt
    - Composed of laminin 1, nidogen (entactin), and fibronectin
    - Anchoring filaments cross lamina lucida
      - ▲ Filaments contain laminin 5

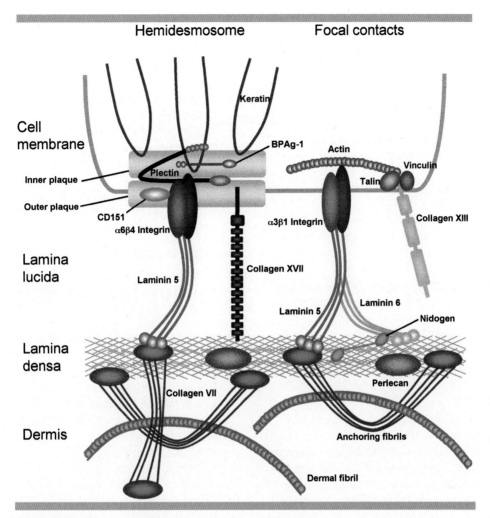

FIGURE 18-3 Hemidesmosome. *(From Freedberg IM et al: Fitzpatrick's Dermatology in General Medicine, 6th ed. New York: McGraw-Hill, 2003, p. 195.)*

▲ One side connects to attachement plaque of plasma membrane; the other side connects to the subbasal dense plate
• Lamina densa
  – Composed of type IV collagen (unique to dermal-epidermal junction)
  – Also contains entactin (nidogen): binds laminin, collagen IV, perlecan, and fibulins (calcium-binding extracellular matrix proteins)
  – Contains heparan sulfate proteoglycan, which is negatively charged owing to disulfide bridges and renders the dermal-epidermal junction impermeable to negatively charged substances
• Sublamina densa
  – Contains network of anchoring fibrils composed of type VII collagen
  – Anchoring fibrils originate in lamina densa, dip down into the dermis, and attach to an

anchoring plaque or loop back to reinsert into the lamina densa
  – Fibrils appear as "wheatstacks" on EM
  – Contains interstitial collagen fibers of types I, III, V, and VI
  – Contains microfibils composed of fibrillin: two types of microfibrils
    ▲ Elaunins—horizontal
    ▲ Oxytalins—perpendicular to elaunins
  – Contains microthread-like fibers of the glycoprotein linkin

KERATINS

Classification of Keratins

• Members of the structural protein group of intermediate filaments (named for their assembled diameter of 10 nm)

TABLE 18-2 Classification of Keratins

Type I	Type II
Acidic (pK 4.5–5.5)	Basic or neutral (pK 5.5–7.5)
Smaller in size (40–56.5 kDa)	Larger in size (52–67 kDa)
Keratins K9–K20 Hal to Ha4, Hax	Keratins K1–K8 Hb1 to Hb4, Hbx
Chromosome 17q12-21	Chromosome 12q11-13

- Six types of intermediate filaments (types I to VI)
- Keratins make up type I and type II intermediate filaments
- Approximately 40 varieties of keratin
- Spontaneously form pairs consisting of a type I and a type II (i.e., an acidic and a basic) (Table 18-2)

Structure of Keratins

- Polypeptides consisting of a central rod domain of approximately 310 amino acids (Fig. 18-4)
- Central domain is composed of four highly conserved alpha-helical regions (designated 1A, 2A, 1B, and 2B)
- Regions are connected by three nonhelical linking sequences thought to provide flexibility (designated L1, L12, and L2)
- Central domain is flanked by an amino head and carboxy tail

- Two keratin polypeptides (one type I and one type II) combine to form a parallel coiled coil
- Coil is stabilized by hydrophobic interactions between the two strands; structure is now a keratin heterodimer
- Keratin heterodimers form long chains in a head-to-tail sequence
- Two chains of keratin heterodimers then combine in antiparellel fashion to form a protofilament (2 to 3 nm)
- Two protofilaments combine to form a protofibril (4.5 nm)
- Protofibrils then assemble in groups of three or four strands to form a 10-nm intermediate filament of keratin

Keratins in Disease

- Mutations affecting the ends of the central domain prove the most deleterious (Table 18-3)

ADHESION MOLECULES

- Adhesion molecules contribute to
  - Cell-to-cell adhesion
  - Interaction between cells
  - Cell signaling
  - Inflammation
  - Migration of cells
  - Wound healing
  - Embryogenesis
- Families of adhesion molecules
  - Cadherins
    - Calcium-dependent cell-cell adhesion molecules
    - Main adhesion molecule in early embryogenesis

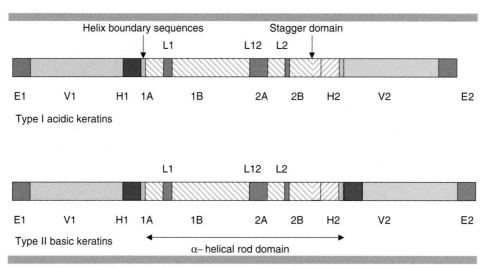

FIGURE 18-4 Polypeptides. *(From Freedberg IM et al: Fitzpatrick's Dermatology in General Medicine, 6th ed. New York: McGraw-Hill, 2003, p. 96.)*

TABLE 18-3 Keratin Expression Patterns and Keratin-Associated Diseases

Type II	Type I	Physiologic Location of Expression	Hereditary Diseases
1	10	Suprabasal keratinocytes	Bullous congenital ichthyosiform erythroderma
1	9	Palmoplantar suprabasilar keratinocytes	Epidermolytic PPK Diffuse nonepidermolytic PPK Epidermolytic PPK with polycyclic psoriasiform plaques
2e	10	Upper spinous and granular layer	Ichthyosis bullosa of Siemens
3	12	Cornea	Meesmann's corneal dystrophy
4	13	Mucosal epithelium	White sponge nevus
5	14	Basal keratinocytes	Epidermolysis bullosa simplex
6a	16	Outer root sheath, hyperproliferative keratinocytes, palmoplantar keratinocytes	Pachyonychia congenita type I Focal nonepidermolytic PPK
6b	17	Nail bed, epidermal appendages	Pachyonychia congenita type II Steatocystoma multiplex
8	18	Simple epithelium	Cryptogenic cirrhosis
	19	Embryonic	
Hb, 1, 3, 5, 6	Ha 1, 2, 3a, 3b, 4–8	Hair follicle	Monilethrix (Hb1 and 6)

Source: From Freedberg IM et al: *Fitzpatrick's Dermatology in General Medicine* 6th ed. New York McGraw-Hill, 2003, p. 91.

- Structure: single-pass transmembrane glycoprotein
- Bind to catenins (link cytoskeleton to adherens junction)
- Two types
  - ▲ Classic cadherins—found at adherens junctions and interact with cytoplasmic anchoring structures
    - △ E cadherin
      - ◆ Found on all epithelium
      - ◆ Chromosome 16q
    - △ N cadherin: found on nerve, muscle, epithelium
    - △ P cadherin: found on placenta and basal epithelium
  - ▲ Desmosomal cadherins—found in desmosomes; associate with keratin filaments via plakoglobin and desmoplakin
    - △ Desmoglein—membrane-bound
      - ◆ Pemphigus vulgaris—autoimmunity against desmoglein 3

- ◆ Pemphigus foliaceous—autoimmunity against desmoglein 1
- △ Desmocollins—membrane bound
- △ Plakoglobin—cytoplasmic
- △ Desmoplakin—cytoplasmic: only molecule known to be present in both desmosomes and adherens junctions
- Integrins—integrate intracellular cytoskeleton with extracellular matrix
  - Large family of transmembrane molecules composed of two noncovalently bound polypeptide subunits (α, β)
  - Most integrins recognize and bind peptide sequence of arginine-glycine-aspartic acid (commonly found on matrix proteins like collagen)
  - Subfamily depends on β
  - $\beta 1$—binds cells to extracellular matrix: This subfamily is also known as VLA (very late activation) 1–6
  - $\beta 2$—binds leukocytes to endothelium or other inflammatory cells

▲ Three members leukocyte function antigen-1 (LFA-1), macrophage activation antigen 1 (Mac 1), and p150,95
▲ Abnormality leads to leukocyte adhesion problems and chronic infection/abscess
- $\beta3$—interaction between platelets and neutrophils at sites of inflammation or vascular damage: contains two members: platelet glycoprotein IIb/IIIa and vitronectin receptor
- $\beta4$—$\alpha^6\beta_4$ is the most notable of this subfamily

▲ Localized to hemidesmosomes of basement membrane
▲ Binds to laminin 5 in anchoring filaments
▲ Plays an important role in junctional epidermolysis bullosa
• Summary of integrins (Table 18-4)
  • Selectins
    - Family of proteins that function in cell-cell adhesion; mediate recruitment of inflammatory cells

TABLE 18-4 Summary of Integrins

Integrin	Alternate Name	Expressed on	Matrix Ligand	Endothelial Ligand
$\beta1$ Subfamily				
$\alpha^1\beta_1$	VLA-1	T cells	Collagen I, IV Laminin	
$\alpha^2\beta_1$	VLA-2	T cells	Collagen I, IV Laminin	
$\alpha^3\beta_1$	VLA-3	T cells	Collagen Laminin 1, 5 Fibronectin Epiligrin	
$\alpha^4\beta_1$	VLA-4	T cells	Fibronectin	VCAM-1
$\alpha^5\beta_1$	VLA-5	T cells	Fibronectin	
$\alpha^6\beta_1$	VLA-6	T cells	Laminin	
$\beta2$ Subfamily				
$\alpha^1\beta_2$	LFA-1	Neutrophils Monocytes		ICAM-1 ICAM-2
$\alpha^m\beta_2$	Mac-1	Neutrophils Monocytes	C3bi Fibronectin	ICAM-1
$\alpha^x\beta_2$	P150, 95	Neutrophils Monocytes	C3b Fibronectin	
$\beta3$ Subfamily				
Platelet Glycoprotein Iib/IIIa		Platelets	Fibrinogen Fibronectin Von Willebrand factor Vitronectin	
Vitronectin Receptor			Vitronectin Fibrinogen vWF	
$\beta4$ Subfamily				
$\alpha6\beta4$		Keratinocytes (basal)	Laminin 1, 5	

- Three classes
  - ▲ L-selectin (leukocyte): expressed on leukocytes
  - ▲ P-selectin (platelet)
    - △ Stored preformed in Weibel-Palade bodies of endothelium; released rapidly to membrane in response to stimulation and then can be reinternalized
    - △ Also found on alpha-granules of platelets and megakaryocytes
  - ▲ E-selectin (endothelial): produced on endothelial cells in response to IL-1 and tumor necrosis factor (TNF)
- Immunoglobulin supergene family
  - Extensive group of cell surface-binding proteins that contain one or more Ig/Ig-like domain (disulfide-bridged loops)
  - Primary function is antigen recognition and cell-cell adhesion
  - Can be inducible or constitutively expressed on endothelium
  - Also referred to as *cellular adhesion molecule* (CAM)
  - Members
    - ▲ Intercellular adhesion molecule 1 (ICAM 1) CD 54
      - △ Expressed constitutively on endothelial cells, certain epithelial cells, and antigen presenting cells
      - △ Can be induced for surface expression on other cells by cytokines (αIFN)
      - △ ICAM 1 allows inflammatory cells to attach and infiltrate lesions in skin (e.g., psoriasis)
      - △ Ligand is LFA-1
      - △ Interaction of LFA-1 and ICAM allows T cells to come into close contact with an antigen-presenting cell (APC), which is a key step in activating a T-lymphocyte
      - △ ICAM 1 is the receptor for rhinovirus on respiratory epithelium
    - ▲ Intercellular adhesion molecule 2 (ICAM 2)
      - △ Constitutively expressed
      - △ A second ligand for LFA-1
    - ▲ Leukocyte function antigen 3 (LFA-3) CD 58
      - △ Expressed on APCs and forms a ligand with CD2 receptor on T-cell surface
      - △ This is a secondary signal in the activation of T cells
      - △ Important target for current psoriasis therapies
    - ▲ Vascular cell adhesion molecule 1 (VCAM 1)
      - △ Expressed on endothelial cells on activation
      - △ Expression induced by IL-1 and TNF-α
      - △ Directly involved in endothelium-lymphocyte interactions
      - △ Mediates recruitment of lymphocytes into areas of inflammation

COLLAGEN

- Produced by ribosomes within fibroblasts
- Provides structural stability
- Represents 70 to 80 percent of dry weight of the dermis
- Basic collagen structure is three alpha chains combined in a triple-helix formation with cross-linking hydrogen bonds
- Nineteen types of collagen
- Typical sequence of collagen: GLY—X—Y (Fig. 18-5)

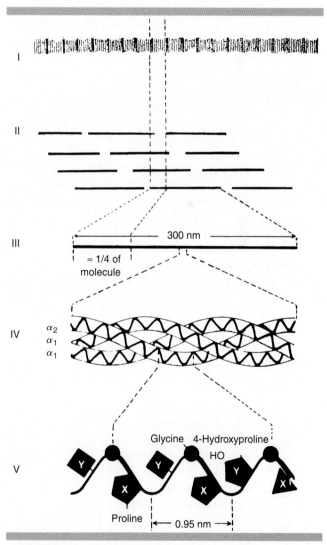

FIGURE 18-5 Typical sequence of collagen. *(From Freedberg IM et al: Fitzpatrick's Dermatology in General Medicine, 6th ed. New York: McGraw-Hill, 2003, p. 166.)*

- GLY = glycine, always the third residue, 33 percent of amino acids in collagen
- X = frequently proline
- Y = frequently hydroxyproline or hydroxylysine
- Four classes of collagen
  - Fibrillar collagen—types I, II, III, and XI
  - Network-forming collagens (nonfibrillar)—type IV
  - Microfibrillar—VI, VII
  - FACIT (fibril-associated collagens with interrupted triple helices)—IV, XII, XIV
- Collagen biosynthesis (Fig. 18-6)
  - Pretranslational
    - Occurs in the nucleus
    - Transcription of genes for procollagen
    - mRNA is formed
  - Cotranslational
    - mRNA is transferred to ribosomes of rich endoplasmic reticulum (RER)
    - Pre-procollagen is formed and contains a signal peptide that indicates that the peptide is to be excreted from the cell
    - During passage through the RER the following occurs
      - ▲ Hydrolytic cleavage of signal peptide
      - ▲ Hydroxylation of proline and lysine residues by prolyl hydroxylase or lysyl hydroxylase (deficient in type VI Ehlers-Danlos syndrome); hydroxylation requires oxygen, vitamin C, ferrous iron, α-ketoglutarate
      - ▲ Glycosylation of hydroxylysine residues and asparagine with N-linked oligosaccharides
  - Postranslational
    - While in the RER, three procollagens are aligned and form disulfide bonds between chains to stabilize the structure; this occurs first on the amino end and then on the carboxy end
    - Three procollagens form a triple helix (carboxy-to-amino end)
    - Procollagen is transferred from the RER to the Golgi complex and is secreted continuously from the cell into the extracellular space
    - Once excreted, neutral calcium-dependent proteinases cleave the extra peptide extensions on the end of the procollagen to form tropocollagen
    - Tropocollagen then combines to form collagen fibrils, which are stabilized by cross-links
    - Cross-linking is catalyzed by lysyl oxidase, which uses copper as a required cofactor (enzyme is defective in type IX Ehlers-Danlos syndrome)
    - Fibrils combine to create a collagen fiber
- Factors that affect collagen production
  - Ascorbic acid—stimulates
  - Transforming growth factor β (TGF-β)—stimulates
- IL-1—inhibits by stimulating PGE2
- Glucocorticoids—inhibit collagen gene transcription
- Retinoic acid—decreases in photoaging
- Interferon-γ (INF-γ)—potent inhibitor of collagen gene transcription
- TNF-α—inhibits gene transcription
- D-Penicillamine—interferes with collagen cross-linking
- Minoxidil—inhibits expression of lysyl hydroxylase
- Distribution of types of collagens (Table 18-5)
- Heritable connective tissue diseases (Table 18-6)

ELASTIC TISSUE

- Allows skin to return to normal shape after being deformed or stretched
- Composed of elastic fibers
- Elastic fibers are visualized with special stains: Verhoeff-van Gieson, Orcein, or Resorcin-Fuchsin
- Elastic fibers are made of protein filaments embedded in an amorphous matrix of mostly elastin; this elastin core is surrounded by microfibrils that contain fibrillin
- Papillary dermis—Elastic fibers are thin and run perpendicular to the skin surface; named *oxytalan fibers*
- Reticular dermis—Elastic fibers are thick and run parallel to the skin surface; named *elaunin fibers*
- Elastin
  - Secreted mainly by skin fibroblasts
  - Elastin is mapped to chromosome 7
  - Composed primarily of glycine, alanine, valine, proline, and lysine
  - Elastin contains the unique amino acids of desmosine and isodesmosine
    - These amino acids provide sites for cross-linking (catalyzed by lysyl oxidase); cross-linking creates stability and insolubility
    - Desmosine is formed in the extracellular space by oxidative deamination of lysyl residues to allysine and then the fusion of three allysines with a lysyl residue
    - This is catalyzed by the enzyme lysyl oxidase, with copper and oxygen as cofactors
    - Anetoderma = loss and fragmentation of skin owing to decreased desmosine
- Expression of elastin is activated early in embryogenesis and continues at a steady rate until age 40, when it drops off precipitously
- Degradation of elastic fibers occurs by elastases (proteolytic enzymes)
  - Classic elastases—degrade insoluble elastic fibers at neutral or mildly alkaline pH; found in

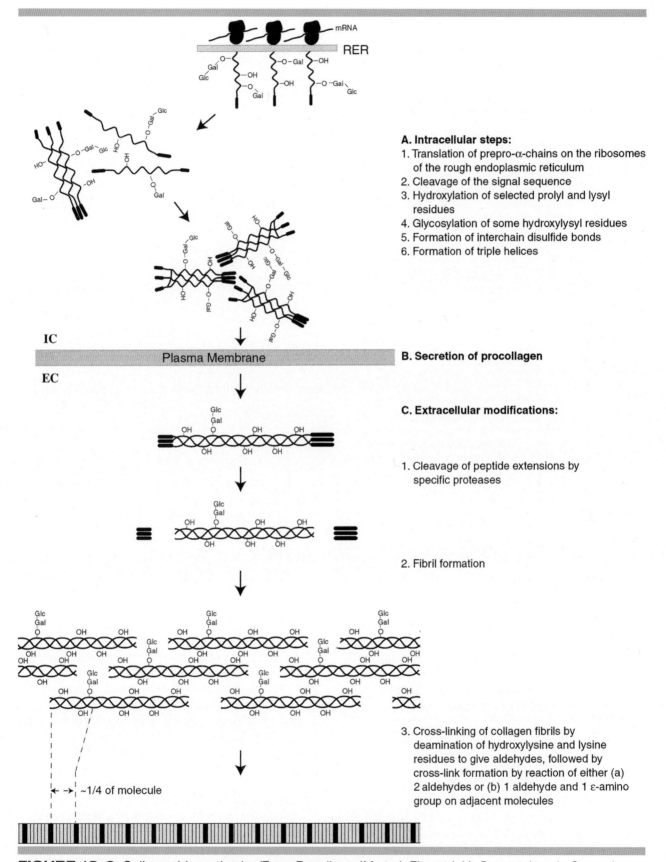

FIGURE 18-6 Collagen biosynthesis. *(From Freedberg IM et al: Fitzpatrick's Dermatology in General Medicine, 6th ed. New York: McGraw-Hill, 2003, p. 171.)*

TABLE 18-5 Distribution of Types of Collagens

Collagen	Distribution
I	Skin, bone, tendon, dentin (80% of total adult collagen)
II	Cartilage, vitreous
III	Blood vessels, gut, fetal skin (predominant cartilage), chorioamnion
IV	Basement membrane (lamina densa), epidermal appendages, blood vessels
V	Wide spread except in hyaline cartilage
VI	Aortic intima, placenta, widespread
VII	Anchoring fibrils, amnion
VIII	Endothelial cells, cornea
IX	Cartilage
X	Cartilage (hypertrophic)
XI	Cartilage
XII	Cartilage, fibroblasts, FACIT collagen, perichondrium, periosteum, cornea
XIV	Cartilage, skin, tendons, muscle, placenta, FACIT collagen
XV	Placenta, basement membrane
XVI	Placenta
XVII	Hemidesmosomes (Bullous pemphigoid antigen 2)
XVIII	Placenta, liver, kidney, basement membrane
XIX	Rhabdomyosarcoma, basement membrane

polymorphonuclear cells (PMNs); inhibited by α_1-antitrypsin, α_2-macroglobulin
- Elastase-like metalloproteases—degrade soluble elastin, oxytalan, and elaunin fibers; cannot degrade insoluble elastases; requires calcium
- Diseases with elastic fiber abnormalities (Table 18-7)

GROUND SUBSTANCE

- Component of connective tissue of dermis
- Consistency of a viscous solution or thin gel
- Stains with PAS reaction for carbohydrates or with toluidine blue
- Consists of several types of proteoglycans
- Proteoglycans (PGs)

- Macromolecule with a core of protein and covalently attached glycosaminoglycans (GAGs)
- Abundance of hydroxyl, carboxyl, and sulfate groups make proteoglycans hydrophilic and polyanionic; this creates an intensely hydrated molecule that can bind up to 1000 times of its own volume
- This hydration affects volume and compressibility of the dermis
- PGs also play a role in binding growth factors and acting as adhesion sites for other molecules
- Glycosaminoglycans—repeating units of disaccharides (Table 18-8)
- Mucopolysaccharidoses (Hunter's, Hurler's, San Filipo) result from defective lysosomal enzymes; the defect causes accumulation of GAGs in many tissues
- Aging results in increases of dermatan sulfate and decreases in chondroitin-6-sulfate

TABLE 18-6 Heritable Connective Tissue Diseases with Cutaneous Involvement

Disease	Inheritance*	Mutated Genes‡	Affected Protein
Ehlers-Danlos syndrome	AD, AR ~	COL1A1, COL1A2, COL3A1, COL5A1, COL5A2 PLOD ADAMTS-2 TNX B4GALT-7	α Chains of types I, III, and V collagens Procollagen-lysine 2-oxoglutarate 5-dioxygenase (lysylhydroxylase), Procollagen N-peptidase Tenascin-X Xylosylprotein 4-beta-galactosyl-transferase
Osteogenesis imperfecta	AD, AR,	COL1A1, COL1A2	α_1 and α_2 Chains of type I collagen
Cutis laxa	AD, AR, XR†	ELN MNK-1 (ATP7A)	Elastin ATP-dependent copper transporter
Homocystinuria	AR	CBS	Cystathionine β-synthase
Menkes' syndrome	XR	MNK-1 (ATP7A)	ATP-dependent copper transporter
Focal dermal hypoplasia	XD	ND	
Tuberous sclerosis (shagreen patches)	AD	TSK-1 TSC 1 plus 2	Hamartin 1 Tuberen
Familial cutaneous collagenoma	AD	ND	
Epidermolysis bullosa VII and XVII collagens	AD, AR	COL7A1 COL17A1	α_1 Chains of types

*AD, autosomal dominant; AR, autosomal recessive; XD, X-linked dominant; XR, X-linked recessive; ND, not determined.
†Most cases involve abnormalities in the elastic fibers, and in some cases, mutations in the elastin gene (ELN) have been disclosed. Occipital horn syndrome, a copper deficiency syndrome, allelic to the Menkes' syndrome gene (MNK-1), was previously known as x-linked cutis laxa and also Ehlers-Danlos syndrome IX (see Chap. 154).
‡For detailed discussion on these genes, see Refs. 4 and 87.
Source: From Freedberg IM et al: *Fitzpatrick's Dermatology in General Medicine* 6th ed. New York McGraw-Hill, 2003, p. 178.

- In wound healing, hyaluronic acid increases shortly after injury and then decreases as chondroitin sulfate increases

MELANOCYTES

- Melanocytes are derived from neural crest cells.
- Migrate dorsoventrally in the eighth week of fetal development
- Melanin synthesis begins in the head region in the third month of fetal development
- Melanin is also found in the retina, uvea, cochlea/vestibular apparatus, and leptomeninges; therefore, diseases of skin pigmentation also may have abnormalities in these areas
- In all races, density of melanocytes is a consistent ratio of about one melanocyte for every ten keratinocytes
- Melanocytes reside in the basal layer and send dendrites containing melanosomes (containing the pigment melanin) into contact with keratinocytes
- Melanocytes do not form desmosomes with adjacent keratinocytes; they may form contact via E-cadherin adhesion molecules
- Melanocytes do not form hemidesmosomes with the basement membrane
- Melanosomes

TABLE 18-7 Clinical Features, Histopathology, Inheritance, Associated Biochemical Findings, and Predisposing Clinical Conditions in Cutaneous Diseases with Elastic Fiber Abnormalities*

Disease	Inheritance[†]	Clinical Manifestations	Histopathology of Skin	Biochemical Findings[‡] Related to Elastic Fibers and Predisposing Clinical Conditions
Pseudoxanthoma elasticum	AR, sporadic[§]	Yellowish papules coalescing into plaques Inelastic skin Cardiovascular and ocular abnormalities	Accumulation of pleiomorphic and calcified elastic fibers in the mid-dermis	Deposition of calcium apatite crystals, excessive accumulation of glycosaminoglycans on elastic fibers; D-penicillamine treatment; mutations in the *ABCC6* gene
Buschke-Ollendorf syndrome	AD	Dermatofibrosis lenticularis disseminata and osteopoikilosis	Accumulation of interlacing elastic fibers in the dermis	Increased desmosine content in the skin
Cutis laxa	AR, AD, or NH	Loose, sagging, inelastic skin Pulmonary emphysema Tortuosity of aorta Urinary and gastrointestinal tract diverticuli	Fragmentation and loss of elastic fibers	Decreased desmosine content and reduced elastin mRNA levels; increased elastase activity in some cases; D-penicillamine treatment, inflammatory and urticarial skin lesions (e.g., drug reaction); mutations in the *ELN* or *FBLN5* gene in limited cases
DeBarsy syndrome	AR	Cutis laxa-like skin changes Mental retardation Dwarfism	Rudimentary, fragmented elastic fibers	Reduced elastin mRNA levels
Wrinkly skin syndrome	AR	Decreased elastic recoil of the skin Increased number of palmar and plantar creases	Decreased number and length of elastic fibers	
Mid-dermal elastolysis	NH	Fine wrinkling of the skin, primarily in exposed areas	Fragmentation and loss of elastin in the mid-dermis	Inflammatory; sun exposure
Anetoderma	NH	Localized areas of atrophic, saclike lesions	Loss and fragmentation of elastic fibers in the dermis	Reduced desmosine content in the lesions; often secondary to inflammatory lesions

(Continued)

TABLE 18-7 *(Continued)*

Disease	Inheritance[†]	Clinical Manifestations	Histopathology of Skin	Biochemical Findings[‡] Related to Elastic Fibers and Predisposing Clinical Conditions
Elastosis perforans serpiginosa	NH	Hyperkeratotic papules, commonly on the face and neck	Accumulation and transepidermal elimination of elastic fibers	D-Penicillamine–induced abnormalities in elastin cross-linking
Elastoderma	Unknown	Loose and sagging skin with loss of recoil	Accumulation of pleiomorphic elastotic material without calcification in the mid- and lower dermis and the subcutaneous tissue	
Isolated elastomas	NH	Dermal papules or nodules	Accumulation of thick elastic fibers in the dermis	
Elastofibroma dorsi	NH	Deep subcutaneous tumor, usually on subscapular area	Accumulation of globular elastic structures encased in collagenous meshwork	Trauma on the lesional area
Actinic elastosis	NH	Thickening and furrowing of the skin	Accumulation of irregularly thickened elastic fibers in upper dermis	Chronic sun exposure
Marfan's syndrome	AD	Skeletal, ocular, and cardiovascular abnormalities, hyperextensible skin; striae distensae	Fragmentation of the elastic structure in the aorta	Mutations in the FBN1 gene Fibrillin 1 protein
Congenital contractural arachnodactyly	AD	Camptodactyly and joint contractures		Mutations in the FBN2 gene Fibrillin 2 protein

(Continued)

TABLE 18-7 (Continued)

Disease	Inheritance[†]	Clinical Manifestations	Histopathology of Skin	Biochemical Findings[‡] Related to Elastic Fibers and Predisposing Clinical Conditions
Williams syndrome	AD	Supravalvular aortic stenosis; velvety skin; dysmorphic facies	Disruption of smooth muscle and matrix relationship affecting blood vessels	Allelic deletion of the *ELN* gene; contiguous gene deletion syndrome

*Most of these conditions represent a group of diseases with clinical, genetic, and biochemical heterogeneity.
[†]AD, autosomal dominant; AR, autosomal recessive; NH, not a heritable disease.
[‡]The biochemical abnormalities have been demonstrated in only a limited number of patients in each group, and it is not known whether the biochemical changes are the same in each patient with given disease.
[§]Rare cases with a distinct acquired form of pseudoxanthoma elasticum have been described.
Source: From Freedberg IM et al: *Fitzpatrick's Dermatology in General Medicine* 6th ed. New York McGraw-Hill, 2003, p. 187.

- Melanosomes are secretory organelles developed from specialized exocrine cells of neural crest origin
- Each melanocyte secretes melanosomes into a set number of keratinocytes (approximately 36); this relationship is known as the *epidermal melanin unit*
- Differences in skin pigmentation are due to differences in size and distribution of melanosomes

- Dark = small and single melanosomes
- Light = small and grouped melanosomes
- Four stages of melanosome development
  - Stage I—premelanosome
    - ▲ Round in shape
    - ▲ No organized structure
    - ▲ Few filaments present
  - Stage II—melanosome
    - ▲ Eumelanosomes with oval, lamellar structure

TABLE 18-8 Glycosaminoglycans

Glycosominoglycan	Distribution and Collagen Interaction
Hyaluronic acid	Found in dermins, umbilical cord, synovial fluid, cartilage, vitreous No interaction with collagen High levels associated with nonscarring wound healing (i.e., fetal)
Dermatan sulfate	Found in structures formed by collagen fibers; dermins, tendon, ligaments, heart valves, arteries, fibrous cartilage Interaction with type I collagen **Decorin**—small dermatan sulfate, found along surface of collagen fibrils and assist with lateral fibrils into fibers; low levels in hypertrophic scars
Chondroitin 4- to 6-sulfate	Hyaline and elastic cartilage, arterial medial layer, nucleus pulposus Interact with type II collagen
Heparan sulfate	**Basement** membrane, structures with reticular fibers: smooth muscle, liver, spleen nerves Interact with type III collagen

- ▲ Pheomelanosomes with round, irregular structure
- ▲ Start of melanin deposition
- ▲ Tyrosinase activity
  - Stage III—melanosome
    - ▲ Partially melanized
    - ▲ Decrease in tyrosinase activity
    - ▲ Acid phosphatase present
  - Stage IV—melanosome
    - ▲ Complete melanization
    - ▲ Very little tyrosinase activity
    - ▲ Acid phosphatase present
- Pathway of melanin formation
  - Melanosome structure is formed within melanocyte
  - Tyrosinase enzyme necessary for melanin formation is formed from Golgi apparatus of melanocyte
  - Tyrosinase is transported to melanosome and begins melanin formation
  - Melanosome is transferred to keratinocyte
  - Melanosome is degraded during ascent to cornified layer
  - Melanin is ultimately removed with loss of stratum corneum
- Melanin
  - Pigment that absorbs UV and visible light over a wide range of wavelengths without a distinct peak of absorption
  - Able to absorb free radicals
  - Tyrosinase is the main enzyme for melanin formation and catalyzes the first step: hydroxylation of tyrosine to dopa
  - Tyrosinase is copper-dependent
  - Tyrosine → dopa → dopaquinone: Both these steps are catalyzed by tyrosinase
  - The type of melanin produced depends on presence of other factors
    - Eumelanin—brown-black pigment
      - ▲ Formed if divalent cations are present with dopaquinone
      - ▲ Found in dark, oval melanosomes
    - Pheomelanin—yellow-red pigment
      - ▲ Formed if cysteine (or glutathione) is present with dopaquinone
      - ▲ Found in round, lamellar melanosomes
- Control of melanin production
  - Pigmentation is either constitutive (level of pigment determined genetically) or facultative (inducible by UV, "tan")
  - Stimulated by melanocyte-stimulating hormone (MSH), which is derived from the larger precursor proopiomelanaocortin (POMC); POMC is also the precursor for adreno-corticotropic hormone (ACTH); this explains

the hyperpigmentation of Addison's disease
- Stimulated by estrogens and progesterones
- Melanocytic protein associated conditions:

ENDOTHELIAL CELLS

- Flattened epithelial-like cells
- Thickness <10 μm
- Usually form a continuous monolayer with gap junctions between cells
- Endothelial cells rest on a basal lamina of laminin 1, collagens, fibronectin, nidogen (entactin), and heparan sulfate
- Endothelial cells have a polarized structure with differences between apical (lumen) aspect and basal surface
  - Integrin receptors for ground substance/matrix molecules on basal surface
  - Leukocyte receptors on apical (lumen) side
- Endothelial cells have a number of specialized structures
  - Weibel-Palade bodies (WPBs)
    - Contain vWF, P selectin, and CD 63
    - P selectin (CD62P) mediates leukocyte adhesion
    - CD 63 is a lysosomal membrane glycoprotein that interferes with neutrophil adhesion
  - Fenestrae
    - Sieve-plate structure of membrane
    - 175 nm in diameter
    - Unique to endothelial cells
    - Capillaries composed of endothelial cells with fenestrae are more permeable to water and small-molecular-weight solutes
    - Located in capillaries in lymph nodes, renal glomerulus, intestine, hepatic sinusoids, and bone marrow sinusoids
    - Negative charge of fenestrae prevents transfer of negatively charged plasma proteins
  - Caveolae
    - "Little caves" or vesicles associated with the plasma membrane via the protein caveolin
    - Serve as storage compartments for growth factor receptors structural components
  - Tight (occludens) junctions
    - Provide dual function of sealing off paracellular space and dividing the cell into distinct apical and basolateral segments
    - Appear as continuous interlocking beltlike strands that associate laterally with tight junctions of adjacent cell
    - Consist of transmembrane proteins occludin and claudins
    - Also associated with cytoplasmic proteins ZO-1, ZO-2, and ZO-3

- Adherens junctions
  - Composed of cadherin adhesion molecules
  - Presence of junctions regulates paracellular transport and adhesion of molecules to one another
  - Cadherins link adjacent cells via a cytoplasmic plaque structure connected to the cytoskeleton
  - The plaque is composed of transmembrane proteins cadherin 5 (CD 144) and PECAM 1 (CD31)
  - Cadherin 5 is now renamed *vascular endothelial cadherin* (VE cadherin)
  - The cadherins are attached to the actin cytoskeleton by catenins
- Gap junctions
  - Clusters of transmembrane channels formed by six connexin monomers
  - Connexin 37, 40, and 43
  - Allow direct exchange of ions and small molecules between endothelial cells
- Complexus adherentes
  - Endothelial cells have no desmosomes
  - However, the desmosomal protein desmoplakin is located to complexus adherents and participates in a distinct type of cell contact separate from desmosomes
- Endothelial cells play a critical role in cutaneous inflammation
  - Endothelial cells produce a number of cytokines
    - IL-1
      - ▲ Responsible for upregulation of ICAM-1, VCAM-1, and E-selectin
      - ▲ Induces platelet-activating factor, prostaglandins, and nitric oxide
      - ▲ Activates T cells, serves as chemoattractant for lymphocytes, and stimulates proliferation of B cells
    - IL-6: has few effects on normal endothelium but plays a critical role as a growth factor for Kaposi sarcoma neoplasms
    - IL-8: likely plays a role as a chemoattractant for inflammatory cells
    - G-CSF
    - M-CSF
    - GM-CSF
  - Endothelial cells express a variety of adhesion molecules that play a vital role in inflammation
    - ICAM-1 (binds LFA-1 on leukocytes)
    - ICAM-2 (binds LFA-1 on leukocytes)
    - E-selectin (binds memory T cells, especially in chronic inflammation)
    - P-selectin (binds Lewis X, which is important in initial binding of PMNs to endothelium)
    - VCAM-1 (binds $\alpha4\beta1$ integrin of leukocytes)
    - MHC I, II (bind CD8 and CD4 on T cells)
    - LFA-3 (binds CD2 on T cells)
    - CD 44 (binds hyaluronic acid)

SWEAT GLANDS: ECCRINE AND APOCRINE

- Eccrine glands
  - Primary function of the eccrine unit is thermoregulation: cooling effects of evaporation of sweat on the skin surface
  - Highest density of eccrine glands is seen on the palms, soles, and axillae
  - Consists of two segments: secretory coil and a duct
  - Coil: composed of three distinct cell types: clear (secretory), dark (mucoid), and myoepithelial cells
  - Duct: outer ring of peripheral cells (basal) and an inner ring of luminal cells (cuticular); the coiled duct (proximal) is more active than the distal (straight) portion
  - Duct is referred to as the *acrosyringium* because it spirals through the epidermis and opens directly onto the skin surface
  - Eccrine sweat is produced via merocrine secretion in the coiled gland and is composed of water, sodium, potassium lactate, urea, ammonia, serine, ornithine, citrulline, aspartic acid, heavy metals, organic compounds, and proteolytic enzymes
  - Stimulation of eccrine sweat production is mediated predominantly through postganglionic C fiber production of acetylcholine
- Apocrine sweat gland
  - Outgrowths of the superior portions of pilosebaceous units
  - Respond mainly to cholinergic stimuli
  - It consists of a coiled gland in the deep dermis or at the junction of the dermis and subcutaneous fat and a straight duct that traverses the dermis and empties into the isthmus (uppermost portion) of a hair follicle
  - Secretion is decapitation, a process where the apical portion of the secretory cell cytoplasm pinches off and enters the lumen of the gland
  - Sweat consists mainly of sialomucin; although odorless initially, as apocrine sweat comes in contact with normal bacterial flora on the surface of the skin, an odor develops
  - Specialized variants: the Moll's glands seen on the eyelids, the cerumen (ear wax–producing) glands of the external auditory canal, and the milk-producing glands of the breasts
- Fox Fordyce disease
  - Chronic pruritic disease
  - Usually in women
  - Characterized by small follicular papular eruptions in apocrine areas
  - Caused by obstruction and rupture of intraepidermal apocrine ducts

TABLE 18-9 Matrix Metalloproteinases

Enzyme	MMP Number	Alternate Name	Proenzyme Mol. Wt.	Known Matrix Substrates
Interstitial collagenase	MMP-1	Type 1 collagenase	52,000	Collagens I, II, III, VII, VIII, X, entactin, tenascin, aggrecan, denatured collagens, IL-1β, myelin basic protein, L-selectin
Neutrophil collagenase	MMP-8		75,000	Collagens, I, II, III, V, VII, VIII, X, gelatin, aggrecan, fibronectin
Collagenase-3	MMP-13		52,000	Collagens, I, II, IV, IX, X, XIV, aggrecan
Gelatinase A	MMP-2	72-kDa type IV collagenase	72,000	Denatured collagens, collagens IV, V, VII, X, XI, XIV, collagen 1, species-dependent, elastin, fibronectin, laminin, aggrecan, myelin basic protein
Gelatinase B	MMP-9	92-Kda type IV collagenase	92,000	Denatured collagens, collagens IV, V, VII, X, XIV, elastin, entacin, aggrecan, fibronectin, osteonectin, IL-1β, plasminogen, myelin basic protein
Stromeylsin-1	MMP-3	Proteoglycanase	57,000	Proteoglycan core protein, laminin, fibronectin collagens I, IV, V, IX, X, XI, gelatin, elastin, tenascin, aggrecan, myelin basic protein, entactin, decorin, osteonectin
Stromelysin-2	MMP-10	Transin-2	55,000	Proteoglycan core protein, collagens III, IV, V, laminin, fibronection, elastin, aggrecan
Stromelysin-3	MMP-11		61,000	α_1 proteinase inhibitor
Martrilysin	MMP-7	PUMP Matrilysin-1	28,000	Collagen IV, denatured collagens, laminin, fibronectin, elastin, aggrecan, tenascin, myelin basic protein
Matrilsyin-2	MMP-26	Endometase	28,000	Gelatin, α_1 proteinase inhibitor
Membrane type matrix metallo-proteinase-1	MMP-14	MT1-MMP	63,000	Progelatinase A, denatured collagen, fibronectin, laminin, vitronectin, entactin, proteoglycans
Membrane type matrix metallo-proteinase-2	MMP-15	MT2-MMP	72,000	Progelatinase A
				(Continued)

Table 18-9 *(Continued)*

Enzyme	MMP Number	Alternate Name	Proenzyme Mol. Wt.	Known Matrix Substrates
Membrane type matrix metallo-proteinase-3	MMP-16	MT3-MMP	64,000	Progelatinase A
Membrane type matrix metallo-proteinase-4	MMP-17	MT4-MMP	70,000	Unknown
Membrane type matrix metallo-proteinase-5	MMP-24	MT5-MMP	73,000	Progelatinase A
Membrane type matrix metallo-proteinase-6	MMP-25	MT6-MMP	63,000	Unkown
Metalloelastase	MMP-12		54,000	Elastin, collagen IV, vitronectin, plasminogen, laminin, entactin, fibrinogen, fibrin, fibronectin
Enamelysin	MMP-20		54,000	Amelogenin, aggrecan
MMP-19	MMP-19	RASI-1	57,000	Gelatin, aggrecan, fibronectin
MMP-21	MMP-21		Unknown	Unknown
MMP-22	MMP-22		Unknown	Unknown
MMP-23	MMP-23		44,000	Unknown
Epilysin	MMP-28		56,000	Unknown

Source: From Freedberg IM et al: *Fitzpatrick's Dermatology in General Medicine* 6th ed. New York McGraw-Hill, 2003, p. 201.

- Apoeccrine sweat gland
  - Readily distinguished from classic eccrine and apocrine glands
  - Develop during puberty from eccrine-like precursor glands and are found in as many as 50 percent of the axillary glands in patients with hyperhidrosis
  - Long duct, opens onto skin surface (similar to eccrine glands)
  - Cholinergic and adrenergic, secretory rate is 10 times that of the eccrine glands because of its large glandular size
  - Thick segment of the duct is similar in morphology to apocrine glands
- Disorders of the eccrine glands and apocrine glands
  - Hyperhidrosis, or excessive eccrine sweat secretion
  - Localized hyperhidrosis of the palms and soles is often due to emotional stressors
  - Hypohidrosis: decreased eccrine sweating; anhidrosis: absent sweating seen in hereditary disorders such as the ectodermal dysplasias or in acquired conditions such as heat stroke or heat exhaustion
  - Miliaria crystalline: Excessive heat and humidity causes duct obstruction within the stratum

corneum, asymptomatic superficial vesicles, and no surrounding inflammation
- Miliaria rubra (prickly heat): Obstruction is found deeper in the epidermis; pruritic or tender red macules or papules that are often located on the thorax and neck
- Miliaria profunda: duct obstruction at or below the dermal-epidermal junction; asymptomatic skin-colored papules
- Apocrine miliaria: Inflammation follows intraepidermal rupture of apocrine ducts
- Hidradenitis suppurativa: intense inflammation owing to follicular obstruction
- Syringomas: most common benign sweat gland tumor; skin-colored papules on lower eyelids of adult

MATRIX METALLOPROTEINASES

- Group of zinc-dependent enzymes (endopeptidases) that degrade varying components of the extracellular matrix in both normal and diseased tissue
- Includes collaganases, gelatinases the stomelysins, the matrilysins, metalloelasstases, enamelysins, and the membrane-type matrix metalloproteinases (MMPs) (Table 18-9)
- Synthesized as inactive proenzymes; limited proteolysis or treatment with an organomercurial compound sets up a chain of events causing conversion to the fully active form by complete removal of a propeptide (gelatinalse A,MMP-2, can only be activated by the second mechanism)
- Cells secrete extracellular matrix (ECM) metalloproteinases in a complex pattern of response to multiple growth factors and oncogenes
- Inhibitors can modulate proteolysis once proenzymes have been activated
- α_2-Macroglobulin, a nonspecific antiproteinase, accounts for more than 95 percent of the inhibitory activity
- Tissue inhibitors of metalloproteinases (TIMPs) are considered to be the major tissue inhibitors; these are secreted proteins that are tightly regulated during tissue remodeling and physiologic processes

HAIR DEVELOPMENT

(See Chap. 1, "Hair Findings.")

NAIL DEVELOPMENT

(See Chap. 3, "Nail Findings.")

REFERENCES

Alberts B, et al: *Molecular Biology of the Cell,* 4th ed. New York: Garland Science, 2002.

Amagai M: Adhesion molecules: I. Keratinocyte-keratinocyte interactions; cadherins and pemphigus. *J Invest Dermatol* 1995; 104:146–152.

Burgeson RE, Christiano AM: The dermal-epidermal junction. *Curr Opin Cell Biol* 1997; 9:651–658.

Freedberg IM, et al (eds): *Fitzpatrick's Dermatology in General Medicine,* 5th ed. New York: McGraw-Hill, 1999.

Frienkel RK, Woodley D: *The Biology of the Skin.* New York: Parthenon, 2001.

Fuchs E, Weber K: Intermediate filaments: Structure, dynamics, function, and disease. *Annu Rev Biochem* 1994; 63: 345–382.

Katz AM, Rosenthal D, Sauder DN: Cell adhesion molecules: Structure, function, and implication in a variety of cutaneous and other pathologic conditions. *Int J Dermatol* 1991; 30:130–161.

Kimayai-Asadi A, Kotcher LB, Jih MH: The molecular basis of hereditary palmoplantar keratodermas. *J Am Acad Dermatol* 2002; 47(3):327–343.

Paus R, Cotsarelis G: Mechanisms of disease: The biology of hair follicles. *N Engl J Med* 1999; 341(7):491–497.

Roitt I, Brostoff J, Male D: *Immunology,* 6th ed. St. Louis: Mosby, 2001.

Smack DP, Korge BP, James WD: Keratin and keratinization. *J Am Acad Dermatol* 1994; 30(1):85–102.

Swerlick RA, Lawley TJ: Role of microvascular endothelial cells in inflammation. *J Invest Dermatol* 1993; 100(1): 111S–114S.

Vestweber D: Molecular mechanisms that control endothelial cell contacts. *J Pathol* 2000; 190:281–291.

Yaar M, Gilchrest BA: Human melanocyte growth and differentiation: A decade of new data. *J Invest Dermatol* 1991; 97(4):611–617.

CHAPTER 19

NUTRITION-RELATED DISEASES

HOLLY BARTELL
ASRA ALI

VITAMIN DEFICIENCIES

Vitamin B₃ (Niacin/Nicotinic Acid) Deficiency

- Results in pellagra
- Niacin is required for adequate cellular function and metabolism
- Secondary to niacin or tryptophan deficiency → precursor amino acid needed for oxidation/reduction reactions
- Constituent of nicotinamide–adenine dinucleotide
- Risk factors for pellagra genesis
  - Drugs: 6-mercaptopurine, sulfapyradine, 5-flurouracil, phenobarbitol, ethionamide, pyrazinamide, hydantoins, isoniazid therapy (pyridoxine deficiency secondary to isoniazid treatment could cause pellagra because pyridoxine is required for the conversion of tryptophan to niacin)
  - Carcinoid → tryptophan diverted to serotonin
  - Intestinal parasites (hookworms)
  - Gastrointestinal (GI) disorders: Crohn's, GI surgery
  - Prolonged intravenous (IV) supplementation
  - Poverty
  - Poor nutrition
  - Chronic alcoholism
  - Food faddism
  - Malabsorptive states
  - Hartnup disease: This is an inborn error (autosomal recessive) of tryptophan metabolism and a cause of infantile pellagra
  - Cirrhosis of the liver
  - Diabetes mellitus
  - Prolonged febrile illness
- Clinical
  - Pathologic changes in the skin include vascular dilatation, proliferation of endothelial lining, perivascular lymphocytic infiltration, hyperkeratinization and subsequent atrophy of the epidermis, erythema, and edema
  - Glossitis: atrophy of the papillae of the tongue
  - Acute inflammation of the small intestine and colon
  - In the sun, exposed sites form dry, brown scaling skin (goose skin)
  - Patchy demyelinization and degeneration of the various affected parts of the nervous system
  - Three D's: (1) dermatitis, (2) dementia, (3) diarrhea
  - Four types of dermatitis
    - Photosensitive eruptions
    - Perineal lesions
    - Thickening and pigmentation over bony prominences
    - Seborrheic-like dermatitis on the face
  - Skin lesions may be earliest sign: Parts of the body usually involved include the dorsal hands, feet, forearms, and legs; the face presents with a butterfly distribution over the cheeks, forehead, tip of the nose, and V of the neck (Casal's necklace)
  - Neuropsychiatric symptoms of pellagra include depression, anxiety, irritability, and poor concentration
- Diagnosis
  - Low serum niacin, tryptophan, NAD levels, and NADP levels
- Treatment: nicotinomide 100 mg PO q6h for several days or until resolution of major acute symptoms, followed by 50 mg PO q8-12h until all skin lesions heal
  - Dietary animal proteins, eggs, milk, vegetables

Vitamin B₂ (Riboflavin) Deficiency

- Riboflavin deficiency is usually associated with other vitamin B complex deficiencies, and isolated deficiency is rare

- Alcoholic patients, acute boric acid ingestion, hyperthyroidism, chlorpromaquine
- Oral: perleche, glossitis, cheilosis, vermilion border
- Genital: vuvla/scrotum with scaling (intertrigo)
- Eye
  - Conjunctivitis
  - Cataracts may occur more frequently
  - Photophobia
- Other associations of deficiency include
  - Fatigue and/or dizziness
  - Dermatitis with a dry yet greasy or oily scaling
  - Nervous tissue damage
  - Retarded growth in infants and children
- Treatment
  - Riboflavin 5 mg/day
  - Brewer's yeast is the richest natural source of riboflavin
  - Liver, tongue, and other organ meats are excellent sources
  - Oily fish, eggs, shellfish, millet, wild rice, dried peas, beans, and some seeds

Vitamin B_{12} (Cyanocobalamin) Deficiency

- Total-body stores are 2 to 5 mg, of which half is stored in the liver
- Cobalamin binds with gastric intrinsic factor (IF), a 50-kDa glycoprotein produced by the gastric parietal cells, the secretion of which parallels that of hydrochloric acid
- In states of achlorhydria, IF secretion is reduced, leading to cobalamin deficiency
- Absorbed in distal ileum after binding to intrinsic factor in acidic pH
- Caused by
  - Deficiency of intrinsic factor
  - Achlorhydria
  - Ileal disease
  - Malabsorption syndrome
- Triad of weakness, sore tongue, and paresthesias
- Sensation of cold, numbness, or tightness in the tips of the toes and then in the fingertips
- Paresthesias are ascending and occasionally involve the trunk
- Gait abnormalities occur in 12 percent
- Psychiatric or cognitive symptoms were noted in 3 percent
- Pigmented nails
- Symmetric hyperpigmentation of the extremities
- Megaloblastic anemia
- Diagnosis
  - Serum cobalamin levels are the initial test
  - Abnormally low vitamin B_{12} levels
  - Test for pernicious anemia by measuring antibodies against IF

- Schilling test is used to determine the etiology of vitamin B_{12} deficiency in patients with normal IF antibodies
- Treatment
  - Vitamin B_{12}: 1000 μg/d IM/SC for 5 days or 1000 μg IM two times per week for 2 weeks, then 1000 μg/wk IM/SC for 5 weeks, then 100 to 1000 μg IM/SC every month
  - Dietary replacement: animal proteins, eggs, milk, vegetables

Vitamin C (Ascorbic Acid) Deficiency (Fig. 19-1)

- Causes scurvy
- Symptoms develop after at least 3 months of severe or total vitamin C deficiency
- Elderly male alcoholics, psychiatric patients on restrictive diets
- Clinical = four Hs
  - Hemorrhagic signs
  - Hyperkeratosis of hair follicles: leads to corkscrew hairs
  - Hypochondriasis
  - Hematologic abnormalities
- Can cause a secondary defect in collagen formation
- Vitamin C is a reducing agent: maintains hydroxylating enzymes in an active form; therefore, deficiency results in decreased hydroxylation of protocollagen (lysyl hydroxylase)
- Perifollicular petechiae
- Tender nodules with subcutaneous (SQ) and intramuscular (IM) hemorrhage
- Bleeding into the joints causes exquisitely painful hemarthroses
- Subperiosteal hemorrhage
- Woody edema
- Sicca syndrome
- Cortical thinning, which is sometimes described as a "pencil-point cortex"
- Depression
- Delayed wound healing
- Anemia develops in 75 percent of patients
- Epistaxis
- Hemorrhagic gingivitis after 6 months, redness, swelling, necrosis
- Treatment with vitamin C
  - Infants: 30 to 40 mg
  - Children and adults: 45 to 60 mg
  - Pregnant women: 70 mg
  - Lactating mothers: 90 to 95 mg

Vitamin B_1 (Thiamine) Deficiency

- Results in the condition Beriberi
- Persons may become deficient in thiamine either by
  - Decreased amount: not ingesting enough vitamin B_1 through the diet; prolonged diarrhea may

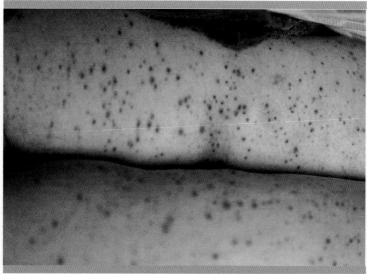

FIGURE 19-1 Vitamin C (ascorbic acid) deficiency. *(From Freedberg IM et al: Fitzpatrick's Dermatology in General Medicine, 6th ed. New York: McGraw-Hill, 2003, p. 1409.)*

impair the body's ability to absorb vitamin B_1, and severe liver disease impairs its use

- Increased depletion
  - Hyperthyroidism
  - Pregnancy
  - Lactation
  - Fever
  - Diarrhea
  - Diuretic therapies
  - Peritoneal dialysis
  - Hemodialysis
- Decreased absorption
  - Chronic intestinal disease
  - Alcoholism
  - Malnutrition
  - Folate deficiency
- Clinical
  - Early: anorexia, irritability, weight loss
  - Dry beriberi = nervous system defects, red burning tongue
  - Peripheral neuropathy: symmetric impairment of sensory, motor, and reflex functions of the extremities, especially in the distal aspects of the lower limbs
  - Wernicke encephalopathy: vomiting, horizontal nystagmus, palsies of the eye muscles, fever, ataxia, and progressive mental impairment leading to Korsakoff syndrome
  - Korsakoff amnestic state is observed in a small number of patients; individuals present alert and responsive; it is characterized by both anterograde

(i.e., learning) and retrograde (i.e., memory of past events) amnesia
- Wet beriberi = high-output cardiac failure secondary to peripheral vasodilatation
- Chronic form of wet beriberi consists of three stages
  - First stage: Peripheral vasodilation occurs, leading to a high-output cardiac state
  - Second stage: Salt and water retention are mediated through the renin-angiotensin-aldosterone system in the kidneys
  - Third stage: As the vasodilation progresses, the kidneys detect a relative loss of volume and respond by conserving salt; with the salt retention, fluid is also forced into the circulatory system; the resulting fluid overload leads to edema of the dependent extremities
- Shoshin beriberi (acute fulminant cardiovascular beriberi): The predominant injury is to the heart, and rapid deterioration follows the inability of the heart muscle to satisfy the body's demands because of its own injury
- Treatment: thiamine
  - Mild neuropathy: 10 to 20 mg/day IM divided bid for 2 weeks
  - Mild to advanced neuropathy: 20 to 30 mg/day IM divided bid for several weeks after symptoms resolve
- Shoshin: 100 mg IV qd for several days, followed by 50 to 100 mg IV/IM bid for several days, and then 10 to 20 mg IM qd until full response

Pyridoxine (Vitamin B$_6$) Deficiency

- Pyridoxine 5'-phosphate is an essential cofactor in various transamination, decarboxylation, and synthesis pathways involving carbohydrates, sphingolipids, sulfur-containing amino acids, heme, and neurotransmitters
- Tryptophan is a precursor to several neurotransmitters and is required for niacin production; thus pyridoxine deficiency can cause a syndrome indistinguishable from pellagra
- Conditions that increase risk for pyridoxine deficiency
  - Advanced age
  - Medical conditions
    - Severe malnutrition
    - Hospitalization
    - Celiac disease
    - Hepatitis and extrahepatic biliary obstruction
    - Hepatocellular carcinoma
    - Chronic renal failure
    - Kidney transplant
    - Hyperoxaluria types I and II
    - High serum alkaline phosphatase level, such as in cirrhosis and tissue injury
    - Catabolic state
  - Medical procedures
    - Hemodialysis
    - Peritoneal dialysis
    - Phototherapy for hyperbilirubinemia
  - Medications
    - Cycloserine
    - Hydralazine
    - Isoniazid
    - D-Penicillamine
    - Pyrazinamide
  - Social-behavioral conditions
    - Excessive alcohol ingestion (except for pyridoxine-supplemented beer)
    - Tobacco smoking
    - Severe malnutrition
- Occurs in cases of uremia, cirrhosis, drug related
- Clinical
  - Oral
    - Glossitis
    - Cheilosis
  - Dermatologic, such as seborrheic dermatitis
  - Adult neurologic
    - Distal limb numbness and weakness
    - Impaired vibration and proprioception
    - Preserved pain and temperature
    - Sensory ataxia
    - Generalized seizures
  - Neonatal and young infant, neurologic
    - Hypotonia
    - Irritability
    - Restlessness
    - Focal, bilateral motor, or myoclonic seizures
    - Infantile spasms
    - Secondary niacin deficiency
  - Skin
    - Dermatitis over sun-exposed areas
    - Blisters and vesicles
    - Beefy red, raw tongue
  - Central nervous system
    - Confusion
    - Dementia
    - Disorientation
    - Rigid tone
    - Primitive reflexes
- Treatment: supplementation of pyridoxine hydrochloride
  - Cirrhosis—50 mg/day
  - Hemodialysis—5 to 50 mg/day
  - Peritoneal dialysis—2.5 to 5 mg/day
  - Chronic renal failure—2.5 to 5 mg/day
  - Sideroblastic anemia—50 to 600 mg/day
  - Pyridoxine-dependent seizures—100 mg/day
  - Homocystinuria—100 to 500 mg/day

Vitamin D$_3$ (Cholecalciferol) Deficiency

- Causes rickets
- Vitamin D [cholecalciferol (vitamin D$_3$), a steroid compound] is formed in the skin under the stimulus of ultraviolet light
- Ultraviolet light was the only significant source of vitamin D until early in the twentieth century, when ergosterol (vitamin D$_2$), which is contained in fish liver oil or as an irradiated plant steroid, was discovered
- Synthesis
  - Cholecalciferol (vitamin D$_3$) is formed in the skin from 5-dihydrotachysterol
  - Undergoes hydroxylation in two steps
    - First step: occurs at position 25 in the liver, producing calcidiol (25-hydroxycholecalciferol), which is the circulating reserve compound
    - Second step: occurs in the kidney at the 1 position, where it undergoes hydroxylation to the active metabolite calcitriol (1,25-dihydroxycholecalciferol), a hormone
  - Calcitriol [1,25(OH)$_2$ D$_3$] acts at three known sites
    - Promotes absorption of calcium and phosphorus from the intestine
    - Increases reabsorption of phosphate in the kidney
    - Acts on bone to release calcium and phosphate
- Clinical
  - Weight bearing produces deformities
  - Generalized muscular hypotonia
  - Thickening of the skull develops

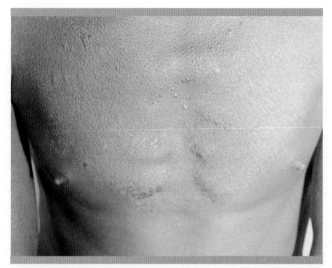

FIGURE 19-2 Vitamin A deficiency. *(From Freedberg IM et al: Fitzpatrick's Dermatology in General Medicine, 6th ed. New York: McGraw-Hill, 2003, p. 1404.)*

- In the chest, knobby deformity results in the rachitic rosary
- Only dermatologic manifestation is alopecia
- Treatment: adequate ultraviolet light or 10 μg (400 units) PO daily of a vitamin D preparation

Vitamin A Deficiency (Fig. 19-2)

- Causes phyrnoderma
- Fat-soluble vitamin
- Caused by disease of fat malabsorption: Crohn's disease, celiac disease, cystic fibrosis, cholestatic liver disease
- Skin eruption = phrynoderma = toad skin
  - Resembles keratosis pilaris
  - Keratotic papules of various sizes
  - Comedomes on face
  - Diffuse xerosis
- Eye findings
  - Night blindness
  - Photosensitivity
  - Xerophthalmia
  - Xerosis corneae
  - Keratomalacia
  - Myctalgsia: delayed adaptation to dark
  - Bitot's spots: circumscribed areas of xerosis of the conjunctiva, lateral to cornea; these are triangular with apex toward canthus
- Diagnosis: serum vitamin A level
- Treatment: vitamin A 100,000 IU/day for two days plus 200,000 IU for one day and then recommended dietary supplement

Hypervitaminosis A

- Loss of hair, coarseness of hair
- Exfoliative cheilitis
- Generalized exfoliation and pigmentation
- Clubbing of fingers
- Hepatomegaly, splenomegaly
- Hyperchromic anemia, depressed serum proteins, elevated liver function tests
- Bone growth may be retarded by premature closure of the epiphyses in children
- Pseudotumor cerebri with papilledema may occur early: bulging fontanelle in children.
- Treatment: vitamin A 100,000 IU/day for two days plus 200,000 IU for one day and then recommended dietary supplement

Vitamin K Deficiency

- Vitamin K is an essential lipid-soluble vitamin that plays a vital role in the production of coagulation proteins
- Low dietary intake owing to chronic illness, malnutrition, alcoholism, multiple abdominal surgeries, long-term parenteral nutrition
- Malabsorption, cholestatic disease, inflammatory bowel disease
- Parenchymal liver disease
- Cystic fibrosis
- Drugs: antibiotics (cephalosporin), coumadin, salicylates, anticonvulsants, certain sulfa drugs
- Clinical: secondary to decrease in vitamin K–dependent clotting factors. II, VII, IX, and X
  - Hemorrhage
  - Echymosis
  - Purpura
- Diagnosis
  - Elevated serum prothrombin time (PT) and activated partial thromboplastin time (aPTT)
  - High level of des-gamma-carboxy prothrombin (DCP)
- Treatment: phytonadione: promotes liver synthesis of clotting factors
- 5 to 25 mg/day PO, usual dose is 5 to 10 mg/day for blood clotting or dietary supplement; may repeat in 12 to 48 hours, 10 mg/day IM; may repeat in 8 to 12 hours
- Acute crisis: fresh frozen plasma

MINERAL DEFICIENCIES

Zinc Deficiency

- Two types
  - Hereditary: acrodermatitis enteropathica (AE) (Fig. 19-3)
    - A defect in zinc metabolism (especially in intestinal absorption or bioavailability of zinc in the intestinal lumen) is a possible pathway
    - Autosomal recessive most common type (zinc found in all tissues)

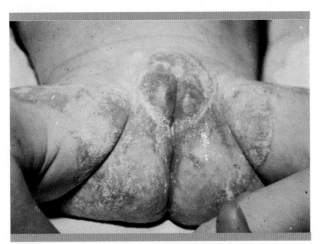

FIGURE 19-3 Acrodermatitis enteropathica. *(From Freedberg IM et al: Fitzpatrick's Dermatology in General Medicine, 6th ed. New York: McGraw-Hill, 2003, p. 1413.)*

- In infants with AE, an absence of a binding ligand may contribute to zinc malabsorption during weaning
- Premature infants at risk because of inadequate body zinc stores, suboptimal absorption, high zinc requirements
- Human breast milk usually has adequate zinc content
- Weaning will precipitate zinc deficiency in premature babies
- Acral and perioral vesiculobulous, pustular, eczematous skin lesions; alopecia; nail dystrophy; diarrhea; glossitis; stomatitis; behavior changes; secondary infections
- Triad: Diarrhea, dermatitis, alopecia occurs at the time of weaning from breast milk to cow's milk secondary to decreased zinc (human milk has picolinic acid, which increases absorption of milk)
- Small, moist, erythematous lesions around the orifices also located symmetrically on the buttocks, extensor surfaces of major joints, scalp, fingers, and toes
- Drooling, change of hair color to red (zebra striped), perleche, pustular paryonichia
- Decreased alkaline phosphatase secondary to zinc-dependent enzyme
- Acquired
  - Alcoholics
  - Complication of malabsorption
  - Inflammatory bowel disease, jejunoileal bypass
  - Metabolic stress (e.g., following surgery)

- Normal infants who are breast-feeding still may show signs of zinc deficiency secondary to
  ▲ Decreased zinc in breast milk
  ▲ Higher zinc requirements for infant
- Diagnosis: Plasma zinc concentrations are low (<50 μg/dl) but not diagnostic
- Treatment
  - Zinc gluconate or sulfate oral at 1 to 3 mg/kg per day, IV 300 to 1000 μg/kg per day
  - Warm compresses and petrolatum applied tid to areas of weeping or crusted dermatitis may enhance reepithelialization when used concurrently with zinc replacement

Iron Deficiency

- Decreased total-iron body content
- Iron balance is achieved largely by regulation of iron absorption in the proximal small intestine
- Diminished absorbable dietary iron or excessive loss of body iron can cause iron deficiency
- Hemorrhage is the most common cause of excessive loss of body iron, but it can occur with hemoglobinuria from intravascular hemolysis; malabsorption of iron is relatively uncommon in the absence of small bowel disease
- Women lose about 500 mg iron during pregnancy; 4 to 100 mg during menses
- Clinical
  - Pallor of the mucous membranes
  - Koilonychia: spoon-shaped deformity of the fingernails/toenails
  - Glossitis
  - Angular chelitis, pruritus, telogen effluvium
  - Plummer-Vinson syndrome: microcytic anemia, dysphagia, and anemia in middle-aged women
  - Splenomegaly may occur with severe, persistent, untreated iron-deficiency anemia
- Diagnosis: Check serum iron levels
- Treatment: iron sulfate 325 mg tid

Copper Metabolism Defect

- X-linked recessive (Xq13); results in Menke's kinky hair disease (MKHD)
- Typically occurs in males ages 2 to 3 months
- Biochemical phenotype in MKHD involves (1) low levels of copper in plasma, liver, and brain because of impaired intestinal absorption, (2) reduced activities of numerous copper-dependent enzymes, and (3) paradoxical accumulation of copper in certain tissues (i.e., duodenum, kidney, spleen, pancreas, skeletal muscle, placenta)
- Loss of previously obtained developmental milestones and the onset of hypotonia, seizures, and failure to thrive

- Scalp hair of infants short, sparse, coarse, and twisted; often less abundant and even shorter on the sides and the back of the head than on the top; may be lightly pigmented and may demonstrate unusual colors
- Light microscopy of patient's hair illustrates pathognomonic pili torti (i.e., 180-degree twisting of the hair shaft) and often other abnormalities, including trichoclasis (i.e., transverse fracture of hair shaft) and trichoptilosis (i.e., longitudinal splitting of shaft)
- Skin often appears loose and redundant, particularly at the nape of the neck and on the trunk
- Decreased lysyl oxidase, tyrosine rate
- Diagnosis: low copper and ceruloplasmin; decreased copper in cultured fibroblasts
- Treatment
  - Parenteral administration of copper in any form restores circulating copper and ceruloplasmin to reference range levels and oral copper does not
  - Copper chloride: <12 months: 0.5 ml SC bid; >12 months: 0.5 ml SC qd

Folic Acid Deficiency

- *Humans do not generate folate endogenously*
- Associated with
  - Increased destruction: Superoxide, an active metabolite of ethanol metabolism, is known to inactivate folate
  - Pregnancy (20 percent of pregnant women are folate-deficient owing increased requirement)
  - Impaired absorption (celiac disease and tropical sprue)
  - Impaired metabolism
  - Antimetabolites (methotrexate and trimethoprim both are folate antagonists that inhibit dihydrofolate reductase)
  - Hypothyroidism
  - Increased excretion/loss: Increased excretion of folate can occur subsequent to vitamin B_{12} deficiency
- Biologically active form of folic acid is tetrahydrofolic acid (THFA), which is derived from the two-step reduction of folate involving dihydrofolate reductase
- Signs and symptoms
  - Hyperpigmentation: patchy distribution should resolve gradually after weeks or months of folate treatment
  - Glossitis
  - Cheilitis
  - Megaloblastic anemia
- Diagnosis: serum folate (reference range: 2.5 to 20 ng/ml) and serum cobalamin (reference range: 200 to 900 pg/ml)
- Treatment: folic acid
  - Megaloblastic anemia: 0.4 mg PO/IM/SC qd for 4 to 5 days; not to exceed 1 mg/day

- Pregnancy: 1 mg PO/IM/SC qd
- Nutritional supplementation: 0.15 to 0.2 mg PO/IM/SC qd for men; 0.15 to 0.18 mg PO/IM/SC qd for women
- Foods: green leafy vegetables, citrus fruits, and animal products

OTHER DEFICIENCIES

Biotin Deficiency

- Universally available; produced by intestinal bacteria
- Deficiency is rare but can occur in patients with short gut or malabsorption of avidin—found in raw egg white: may bind biotin, leading to deficiency
- Prolonged use of certain drugs, especially phenytoin, primidone, and carbamazepine; anticonvulsants inhibit biotin transport across the intestinal mucosa
- Prolonged oral antibiotic therapy
- Two inherited syndromes
  - Multiple carboxylase deficiency: holocarboxylase synthetase deficiency (neonatal type)
  - Biotinidase deficiency (juvenile type)
  - Dermatitis similar to zinc deficiency and essential fatty acid deficiency
  - Periorificial: patchy, red, eroded lesions
  - Alopecia
  - Conjunctivitis
  - Neurologic findings: depression, lethargy, hallucinations, limb paresthesia
  - Infants: hypotonia, lethargy, withdrawn behavior, seizures, developmental delay
  - Neurologic defects may be permanent
  - Urine organic acid analysis may be performed
  - Treatment: 10 to 40 mg/day PO/IV/IM; adjust dose depending on severity of deficiency and response to therapy

Essential Fatty Acid Deficiency

- Infants with low birth weight, gastrointestinal anomalies, inflammatory bowel disease, intestinal surgery, prolonged parenteral nutrition without essential fatty acid (EFA) supplementation
- Increased risk of infection
- Hair becomes lighter in color
- Poor wound healing, growth failure
- Dermatitis: generalized xerosis
- Widespread erythema
- Intertrigenous weeping eruption
- EFAs: constitute one-quarter of the fatty acids of the stratum corneum and are required for normal epidermal barrier function
- Treatment: IV lipid therapy with Intralipid 10%

Marasmus

- Protein-energy malnutrition
- Marasmus results from a negative energy balance
- Fat stores can decrease to as low as 5 percent of the total body weight
- Potassium deficit: contributes to hypotonia, apathy, and impaired cardiac function
- Skin: dry, wrinkled, loose
- "Monkey facies": loss of buccal fat pad
- Treatment: adequate diet
- Overall goal of nutrition rehabilitation is to overcome the anorexia

Kwashiorkor

- Kwashiorkor represents a maladaptive response to starvation
- Adequate carbohydrate consumption and decreased protein intake lead to decreased synthesis of visceral protein
- Hypoalbuminemia contributes to extravascular fluid accumulation
- Serum levels of zinc have been implicated as the cause of skin ulceration in many patients
- Dermatologic findings appear more significant and occur more frequently among darker-skinned people
- Hair: hypopigmented, dry, lusterless, scaling
- Flag sign: alternating light and dark bands, dark hair during normal nutrition, hair grown during malnutrition is pale
- Impaired growth
- Poor weight gain or weight loss
- Potbelly
- Skin: red color
- Hypopigmented lesions appear in areas of friction of pressure
  - Flexures
  - Groin
  - Buttocks
  - Elbows
- Desquamation: "crazy pavement," "crackled skin," "mosaic skin," "enamel paint"
- Nails: soft, thin
- Edema
- Atrophy of the papillae on the tongue, angular stomatitis, xerophthalmia, and cheilosis can occur
- Treatment: fluid and electrolyte abnormalities and treatment for any infections

IRON EXCESS: HEMOCHROMATOSIS

- Toxicity owing to excess iron can occur either acutely after a single large dose of iron or chronically owing to excessive accumulation of iron in the body from either diet or blood transfusions or both

- Tetrad: cirrhosis, diabetes, hyperpigmentation, cardiac failure
- Main manifestations
  - Liver disease
  - Skin pigmentation
  - Diabetes mellitus
  - Arthropathy
  - Impotence in males
  - Cardiac enlargement, with or without heart failure or conduction defects
  - Early symptoms include
    - Severe fatigue (74 percent)
    - Impotence (45 percent)
    - Arthralgia (44 percent)
  - Later patients may experience
    - Skin bronzing or hyperpigmentation (70 percent):
    - Diabetes mellitus (48 percent)
    - Cirrhosis
    - Hemosiderosis: stainable iron in tissues
- Diagnosis
  - A persistently elevated transferrin saturation in the absence of other causes of iron overload
  - Serum ferritin levels elevated higher than 200 μg/liter in premenopausal women and 300 μg/liter in men and postmenopausal women indicate primary iron overload owing to hemochromatosis
  - Liver biopsy with determination of hepatic iron concentration and histologic evaluation with iron staining were considered the standard for diagnosis
- Treatment
  - Weekly therapeutic phlebotomy of 500 ml whole blood (equivalent to approximately 200 to 250 mg iron)
  - Deferoxamine mesylate (Desferal): drug of choice used in primary and secondary iron overload syndromes; 20 to 50 mg/kg per day by continuous SC infusion over 10 to 12 hours

REFERENCES

Freedberg IM et al. *Fitzpatrick's Dermatology in General Medicine*, 6th Ed. New York: McGraw-Hill; 2003.

Hegyi J, Schwartz RA, Hegyi V. Pellagra: dermatitis, dementia, and diarrhea. *Int J Dermatol* 2004; 43(1):1–5.

Hirschmann JV, Raugi GJ. Adult scurvy. *J Am Acad Dermatol* 1999; 41(6):895–906; quiz 907-910. Review.

MacDonald A, Forsyth A. Nutritional deficiencies and the skin. *Clin Exp Dermatol* 2005; 30(4):388–390.

McKee PH. *Pathology of the Skin: With Clinical Correlations.* London: Mosby-Wolfe; 1996.

Perafan-Riveros C, Franca LF, Alves AC, Sanches JA Jr. Acrodermatitis enteropathica: case report and review of the literature. *Pediatr Dermatol* 2002; 19(5):426–431. Review.

Sheehy TW. Vitamin deficiency and toxicity. Garden Grove, California: Medcom, Inc.; 1985.

CHAPTER 20

CUTANEOUS FINDINGS RELATED TO PREGNANCY

HOLLY BARTELL
ASRA ALI
VASEEM ALI

INTRAHEPATIC CHOLESTASIS OF PREGNANCY (PRURIGO GRAVIDARUM)

- Hepatic condition of unknown cause that usually occurs in the third trimester of pregnancy
- Severe puritus (localized at first and then generalized) followed by clinical jaundice (about 4 weeks later) in 10–20 percent of patients
- Hormonally induced in susceptible individuals
- No primary cutaneous lesion, although secondary excoriations may occur
- Laboratory tests: reveal elevations in total serum bile salts and hepatic transaminases
- Treatment: ursodeoxycholic acid, cholestyramine
- Symptoms remit a few days after delivery: maternal outcomes are goal
- Fetal complications include prematurity and intrauterine demise
- Recurs with other pregnancies 60–70 percent

PRURITIC URTRICARIAL PAPULES AND PLAQUES OF PREGNANCY (PUPPP) (FIG. 20-1)

- Most common dermatosis of pregnancy affects $1/160$ to $1/300$
- Erythematous papules and plaques; small vesicles often are noted
- Begin as 1- to 2-mm lesions within abdominal striae
- Spread over the course of a few days to involve abdomen, buttocks, and thighs
- Lesions coalesce to form urticarial plaques
- Spongiotic vessels are present occasionally
- Intensely pruritic
- Primigravids: 75 percent

- Does not recur with subsequent pregnancies
- Begins late in third trimester and resolves with delivery
- Postpartum onset or exacerbation is rare
- Histology: focal spongiosis and parakeratosis; lymphohistiocytic infiltrate and dermal eosinophils and dermal edema
- Treatment: topical or oral steroids, diphenhydramine

PUSTULAR PSORIASIS OF PREGNANCY (IMPETIGO HERPETIFORMIS) (FIG. 20-2)

- No previous history of psoriasis, can occur anytime during pregnancy
- Extremely rare condition
- Recurrences in subsequent pregnancies, menses, and oral contraceptives
- Erythematous patches with pustules on the inner thighs and groin; pustules join and spread to the trunk and extremities, usually sparing the face, hands, and feet
- Constitutional signs: fever, chills, nausea, vomiting, diarrhea, and fatigue
- Tetany, secondary hypocalemia
- Histology: same as pustular psoriasis; polymorphonuclear neutrophils in spongiotic foci in the epidermis (spongiform pustules of Kogoj); parakeratosis; elongation of rete ridges
- Laboratory tests: increased white blood cell (WBC) count, increased erythrocyte sedimentation rate (ESR), hypocalcemia, hypoalbuminemia
- Course: remits after delivery; increased morbidity of fetus secondary to placental insufficiency
- Treatment: systemic steroids; antibiotics are only used if the rash becomes secondarily infected

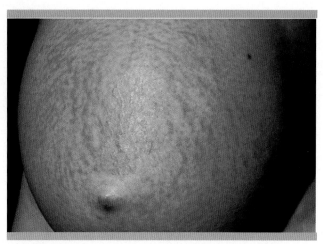

FIGURE 20-1 Pruritic urtricarial papules and plaques of pregnancy (PUPPP). *(From Freedberg IM et al: Fitzpatrick's Dermatology in General Medicine, 6th ed. New York: McGraw-Hill, 2003, p. 1363.)*

HERPES GESTATIONIS (PEMPHIGOID GESTATIONIS)

- Autoimmune dermatosis of pregnancy
- Second trimester of pregnancy
- Urticarial plaques and papules develop around the umbilicus and extremities; spread peripherally to abdomen, back, chest, and palms/soles
- Face, scalp, oral mucosa are spared
- Disease flares a few days after delivery and then remits spontaneously within 3 months
- Recurrences triggered by oral contraceptives, subsequent menstrual periods, subsequent pregnancies

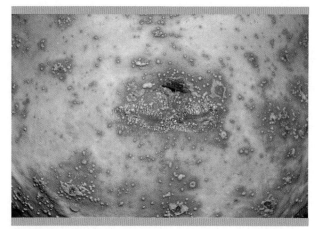

FIGURE 20-2 Impetigo herpetiformis. *(From Freedberg IM et al: Fitzpatrick's Dermatology in General Medicine, 6th ed. New York: McGraw-Hill, 2003, p. 1364.)*

- No residual scarring
- Maternal health not affected
- Infant morbidity: premature, small for gestational age; fewer than 5 percent of infants have urticarial lesions or bullae that clear spontaneously
- HG factor: Heat-stable IgG that binds normal human complement to the basement membrane zone is believed to trigger an immune response that leads to the formation of subepidermal vesicles and blisters
- Antigen: bullous pemphigoid antigen 2 (BPAG2)/MCW-1 domain, 180 kDa/collagen XVII
- Increased HLA-DR3, -DR4
- Histology: subepidermal blister with an eosinophil-predominant infiltrate
- Direct immunofluorescence (DIF): IgG and C3 at the dermal-epidermal junction
- Treatment: topical steroids, prednisone, diphenhydramine, cyclosporine

PAPULAR DERMATITIS OF PREGNANCY

- Rare
- Pruritic, generalized eruption of 3- to 5-mm erythematous papules surrounded by a small, firm central crust
- May erupt at any time during pregnancy
- Resolves after delivery
- Diagnosis: elevation of 24-hour urinary gonadotropin
- Treatment: systemic corticosteroids

PRURIGO GESTATIONIS

- Recently called prurigo of pregnancy
- Pruritic, excoriated papules of proximal limbs and upper trunk
- Usually begins in second–third trimester
- Clears postpartum and does not recur
- No adverse effects on maternal or fetal health
- May be an expression of atopic dermatitis in pregnancy
- Treatment: topical steroids and antihistamines

POLYMORPHIC ERUPTIONS OF PREGNANCY

- Term that encompasses all pruritic inflammatory dermatoses of pregnancy
- Toxemic rash of pregnancy
- Prurigo annularis
- Erythema multiforme gestationes
- Late-onset prurigo of pregnancy
- Pruritic urticarial papules and plaques of pregnancy

- Prurigo gestationis
- Early-onset prurigo of pregnancy
- Papular dermatitis of pregnancy
- Pruritic folliculitis of pregnancy

OTHER CONDITIONS

- Melasma: brown, clearly defined patches on the face, typically on the cheekbones and forehead
- Darkening of the nipples and external genitals (pubic area)
- Darkening of existing moles
- Linea nigra: a dark line that appears on the abdomen running midline from the umbilicus
- Striae gravidarum (stretch marks of pregnancy): red lines or bands that can appear on the abdomen during pregnancy or the breasts after breast-feeding that later become white, smooth, shiny, and flattened
- Varicose veins can appear on the legs
- Pyogenic granuloma
- Melanoma

REFERENCES

Aronson IK, Bond S, Fiedler VC, et al.: Pruritic urticarial papules and plaques of pregnancy: clinical and immunopathologic observations in 57 patients. *J Am Acad Dermatol* 1998; 39(6):933–939.

Bacq Y, Sapey T, Brechot MC, et al.: Intrahepatic cholestasis of pregnancy: a French prospective study. *Hepatology* 1997; 26(2):358–364.

Charles-Holmes R: Skin diseases specifically associated with pregnancy, in Harahap M, Wallach RC (eds.): *Skin Changes and Diseases in Pregnancy*. New York: Marcel Dekker, 1996:55.

Freedberg IM et al. *Fitzpatrick's Dermatology in General Medicine*, 6th Ed. New York: McGraw-Hill; 2003.

Kenyon AP, Piercy CN, Girling J, et al.: Obstetric cholestasis, outcome with active management: a series of 70 cases. *BJOG* 2002; 109(3):282–288.

McKee PH. *Pathology of the Skin: With Clinical Correlations*. London: Mosby-Wolfe; 1996.

Roger D, Vaillant L, Fignon A, et al.: Specific pruritic diseases of pregnancy. A prospective study of 3192 pregnant women. *Arch Dermatol* 1994; 130(6):734–739.

Vaughan Jones SA, Black MM: Pregnancy dermatoses. *J Am Acad Dermatol* 1999; 40(2 Pt 1):233–241.

CHAPTER 21

HISTOLOGIC STAINS AND SPECIAL STUDIES

A. HAFEEZ DIWAN
VICTOR G. PRIETO

- Hematoxylin and eosin (H&E)
  - Used for elucidation of basic histologic features, prior to the use of special stains or immunohistochemical studies as needed; among other features, calcification and microorganisms such as fungi and bacteria may be detected by H&E and confirmed by additional studies

STAINS FOR CARBOHYDRATES

- Periodic-acid Schiff (PAS)
  - Stains glycogen red—diastase labile; therefore diastase pretreatment will remove glycogen
  - Stains mucopolysaccharides red—diastase stable
  - Stains fungi red—diastase stable
  - Stains basement membrane red—diastase stable
- Colloidal iron
  - Stains mucin blue
- Alcian blue
  - Stains mucopolysaccharides blue
    - At pH 2.5: acid (carboxylated or sulfated mucopolysaccharides)
    - At pH 1.0: acid (sulfated mucopolysaccharides)
    - With hyaluronidase: only epithelial mucins will stain (connective tissue mucins will be digested and will not stain)
    - With PAS: acid mucopolysaccharides will stain blue and neutral polysaccharides will stain magenta; also, the yeast of *Cryptococcus* will stain red and the capsule will stain blue with this method
- Mucicamine
  - Stains epithelial mucins red (also stains capsule of *Cryptococcus* red)

STAINS FOR PIGMENTS

- Fontana-Masson
  - Stains melanin and argentaffin granules black (nuclei will be red); useful for quantifying melanocytes (e.g. in vitiligo)
  - Also stains *Cryptococcus*
- Grimelius argyrophil stain
  - Argentaffin and argyrophil substances will stain black
- Tyrosinase (DOPA-oxidase)
  - Requires fresh tissue
  - Stains melanin-containing cells brownish-black (due to tyrosinase acting on DOPA, the substrate for this reaction)

STAINS FOR MINERALS

- Von-Kossa
  - Stains calcium salts black; useful for detecting calcification of vessel walls and elastic tissue (elastosis and elastofibroma)
- Alzarin red S
  - Stains calcium red
- Prussian blue stain
  - Stains iron blue (the Prussian blue reaction: tissue treated with dilute hydrochloric acid and potassium ferrocyanide)
- Gomorri methenamine silver (GMS)
  - Stains urates black; *note:* urates are lost if tissue is processed in formalin
  - Tissue must be processed with alcohol to prevent loss of urates
  - Stains fungi

STAINS FOR CONNECTIVE TISSUE COMPONENTS

- Trichrome
  - Stains collagen blue or green and muscle red, depending on the type of reagents used
- Verhoeff-van Gieson
  - Stains elastic fibers black, collagen red, and muscle yellow (also red cells will stain yellow)

STAINS FOR AMYLOID

- Congo red
  - Stains amyloid pinkish-red; gives apple-green birefringence to amyloid (the most specific method for amyloid)
- Thioflavin T
  - Amyloid shows yellow fluorescence
- Crystal violet
  - Stains amyloid purple-violet

STAINS FOR FAT

- Oil red O
  - Stains fat red; needs frozen/fresh tissue (once tissue is fixed and processed into paraffin blocks, this method does not work)
- Osmium tetroxide
  - Paraffin-embedded tissue; stains fat black
- Sudan black B
  - Paraffin-embedded tissue; stains fat black

STAINS FOR MICRO-ORGANISMS

- H&E
  - May demonstrate fungi, bacteria
- Gram
  - Stains gram-positive bacteria (also *Nocardia*) blue and gram-negative organisms red
- Giemsa
  - For *Leishmania* and granuloma inguinale
- Gomori methenamine silver (GMS)
  - Stains fungi, *Pneumocystis jiroveci* (formerly *carinii*), and protothecosis black
- PAS
  - Stains fungi and protothecosis pink
- Fontana-Masson
  - Stains *Cryptococcus* black
- Warthin-Starry
  - Stains spirochetes black
- Ziehl-Neelson stain
  - Uses carbol fuchsin; stains mycobacteria red

- Fite stain
  - Modification of Ziehl-Neelson; stains *Mycobacterium leprae* and *Nocardia*

STAINS FOR MAST CELLS

- Giemsa and toluidine blue are metachromatic stains for mast cells; also chloroacetate esterase (Leder stain)
- Mast cell tryptase
  - Immunohistochemical study for mast cells

IMMUNOHISTOCHEMICAL STUDIES

- Uses primary antibodies (polyclonal or monoclonal) to a particular antigen, followed by secondary antibody complexed to an enzyme; subsequently, a chromagen is added, which is acted on by the enzyme, releasing a colored product that is evaluated histologically

STUDIES FOR EPITHELIA

- Cytokeratins (CK) are intermediate filaments found in epithelial cells; the following antibodies and cocktail antibodies are useful
  - AE1/AE3—a cocktail antibody recognizing a broad spectrum of keratin; it labels most squamous cell carcinomas (SCC), basal cell carcinoma (BCC), adnexal tumors, and Merkel cell carcinoma but it may not label spindle cell SCC
  - CAM5.2—useful for eccrine tumors, Paget's disease (PD), extramammary Paget's disease (EMPD), and will also label sebaceous carcinoma and a minority of BCC; SCC is mostly negative, however
  - CK5/6—useful for SCC, including spindle cell SCC; it has been shown to label the majority of primary cutaneous adnexal neoplasms and may be useful in distinguishing these from metastatic adenocarcinoma to the skin (fewer of these are reactive with anti-CK5/6)
  - CK7—Very useful for demonstrating PD and EMPD; present in less than a quarter cases of Merkel cell carcinoma
  - CK20—Merkel cell carcinoma will typically exhibit dot-like positivity
- CEA (carcinoembryonic antigen)
  - Antibody to CEA, which is an oncofetal antigen, will demonstrate glandular differentiation (helpful in eccrine and apocrine adnexal neoplasms)
  - It will also be positive in the ducts of sebaceous carcinoma

- It is extremely useful to demonstrate EMPD but may not be as good for PD
- EMA (epithelial membrane antigen)
  - Positive in numerous tumors: EMPD, PD, adnexal neoplasms especially sebaceous neoplasms, perineuriomas, and focally positive in most SCC and in epithelioid sarcoma; also positive in plasma cells
- GCDFP (gross cystic disease fluid protein)
  - Positive in PD, EMPD, and adnexal neoplasms; breast carcinomas are also labeled

STUDIES FOR MESENCHYMAL TISSUE

- Actin antibodies (smooth muscle actin)
  - Useful in demonstrating leiomyoma/leiomyosarcoma, glomus tumors, and dematomyofibroma
  - Cellular neurothekeoma will also exhibit positivity in 50% of cases
- Desmin
  - For leiomyoma/leiomyosarcoma
- CD34
  - Very useful for dermatofibrosarcoma protuberans (DFSP); it is positive in vascular tumors such as hemangioma, angiosarcoma, Kaposi's sarcoma, and lymphangioma and is also positive in nearly half the cases of epithelioid sarcoma
- CD31
  - It is positive in vascular neoplasms: angiosarcoma, hemangioma, lymphangioma, Kaposi's sarcoma; also positive in macrophages

STUDIES FOR NEUROECTODERMAL LESIONS

- S-100
  - Not very specific but extremely sensitive for primary melanoma (including desmoplastic melanoma), metastatic melanoma, and nevi; also positive in a variety of other tumors such as breast carcinoma, Rosai-Dorfman disease, granular cell tumor, neurofibroma, schwannoma, myxoid neurothekeoma, chondroid syringoma, syringoma, and Langherhans cell histiocytosis
  - S-100A6 is positive in cellular neurothekeomas and some melanocytic lesions
- MART-1 (melanoma antigen recognized by T-cells)
  - Less sensitive and more specific than S-100 for melanocytic lesions; only a minority of cells in a proportion of desmoplastic melanoma label with this marker
  - It is also positive in adrenocortical carcinoma and angiomyolipoma (among others)

- Melan-A is a similar antibody, except it does not label adrenocortical carcinoma
- HMB45 and Ki-67
  - HMB45 is less sensitive and more specific than S-100 for melanocytic lesions; it reacts with gp100, a glycoprotein present in premelanosomes
  - Only a minority of cells in a proportion of desmoplastic melanoma label with this marker
  - This is a useful marker to demonstrate maturation in melanocytic lesions: i.e., melanocytic cells in the dermis label at the top of benign melanocytic lesions but not at the bottom; in suspicious lesions, demonstration of maturation may be helpful in arguing against a diagnosis of melanoma
  - Regarding blue nevi versus spindle cell melanoma, the former are strongly, diffusely positive with HMB45; HMB45 is especially useful in this context when used together with Ki-67, a marker of proliferation
  - Melanocytic cells in the dermis that show maturation with HMB45 and show low proliferation (less than approximately 5% of cells reacting with Ki-67) are less likely to be melanoma; of course, it is not possible to be absolutely certain about this, but in the appropriate clinical context, it may provide helpful information
- CK20 (see above)
- Synaptophysin and chromogranin
  - Both of these markers may be positive in Merkel cell carcinoma
- CD57
  - Labels a small proportion of cellular neurothekeoma and neurofibroma
- PGP9.5
  - It is positive in cellular neurothekeoma; it is not very specific, though, and is positive in many other tumors, including Merkel cell carcinoma and dermatofibroma
- NKI/C3
  - It is positive in cellular neurothekeoma, but is not very specific

STUDIES FOR HEMATOPOEITIC LESIONS

- CD1a
  - Marker for Langerhans cells (and therefore useful in Langerhans cell histiocytosis)
- CD3
  - Marks T-cells
- CD4
  - Marks T-cells (T-helper cells), Langerhans cells, and macrophages; in mycosis fungoides, typically CD4 predominates over CD8

- CD5
  - Marks T-cells; it is also positive in B-cells in chronic lymphocytic leukemia (CLL) and mantle zone lymphoma
- CD7
  - Marks T-cells
  - It may be useful in MF in the following manner: it may not be present on cells that mark with CD4 and CD3, for example, suggesting loss of expression; however, inflammatory lesions may also exhibit this feature
- CD8
  - Marks T-cells (T-cytotoxic/suppressor cells) (see CD4 above)
- CD20
  - Marks B-cells; may be useful, along with CD3, Kappa and Lambda in showing that a lymphoid infiltrate in the skin is composed of heterogenous cells, and therefore likely to be reactive rather than neoplastic (not always true, however)
- CD21
  - Marks B-cells and follicular dendritic cells; positive in follicular dendritic cell sarcoma
- CD30
  - Marks activated T-cells (among others)
  - It labels the majority of cells in anaplastic T-cell lymphoma (ALCL) (primary cutaneous ALCL shows less positivity for ALK-1 as compared to systemic ALCL; nevertheless, ALK-1 may be positive in a minority of primary cutaneous ALCL)
  - CD30 also labels large cells in lymphomatoid papulosis (Types A and C; also, to a lesser extent, Type B)
  - It is very rarely found in cutaneous B-cell lymphoma
- CD34
  - Helpful marker for leukemia cutis
- CD35
  - Marks follicular dendritic cells; positive in follicular dendritic cell sarcoma

- CD45
  - Marks most hematopoeitic cells; ALCL may be negative, however
- CD56 (neuronal cell adhesion marker-NCAM)
  - Marker for NK cell lymphoma
  - Leukemic cells may be positive as well; also positive in neural neoplasms such as neurofibroma myxoid neurothekeoma and in desmoplastic melanoma
- CD57 (see above)
- Mast cell tryptase
  - Positive in mast cells
- MPO (myeloperoxidase)
  - Antibody to MPO may label leukemic cells; also labels neutrophils and monocytes (note that there is a histochemical stain for MPO as well, with similar usefulness)

STUDIES FOR INFECTIOUS DISEASES

- The following is a list of useful antibodies:
  - HHV-8:   Kaposi's sarcoma
  - Spirochetal antibody: Syphilis
  - Herpes-simplex antibody: For demonstrating *Herpes simplex* virus
  - Herpes-zoster antibody: For demonstrating zoster

REFERENCES

Carson FL. *Histotechnology. A Self-Instructional Text*, 2nd ed. Chicago: ASCP Press; 1997.

Elder DE, Elenitsas R, Johnson BL Jr, Murphy BG. *Lever's Histopathology of the Skin*, 9th ed. Philadelphia: Lippincott Williams & Wilkins; 2005.

Rosai J. *Rosai and Ackerman's Surgical Pathology*, 9th ed. Edinburgh: Mosby; 2004.

Smoller B. *Practical Immunopathology of the Skin*. Totowa, NJ: Humana Press; 2002.

CHAPTER 22

GENITAL DERMATOLOGY

VICTORIA G. ORTIZ
NISHATH ALI

Lichen Sclerosus et Atrophicus (LS) (Fig. 22-1)

- Atrophic white papules or plaques, usually anogenital skin
- Figure-of-eight lesion when perineum involved
- Females affected more often than males
- Secondary problems: candidiasis or atrophic vaginitis
- Severe cases can lead to scarring of vaginal vault and introitus and urethral meatus (balanitis xerotica obliterans); squamous cell carcinoma
- Penile LS
  - Common in middle age
  - Glans and inner aspect of the prepuce or circumferentially around the urethral meatus (can cause phimosis in uncircumcised males)
- Squamous cell carcinoma can arise in lesions
- Histology: orthokeratosis, hyperkeratosis, atrophy, basal cell layer vacuolation, edema and homogenization of collagen in the upper dermis; a focal perivascular or bandlike mononuclear cell infiltrate containing plasma cells is seen beneath the edema
- Treatment: high-potency topical glucocorticoids, topical antibiotics, circumcision for phimosis

Pyronie's Disease (Penile Fibromatosis)

- Idiopathic disorder
- Angulation of erect penis in middle age
- Caused by fibrosis of tunica albuginea, covers the corpora cavernosa

Vulvodynia

- Diagnosis of exclusion
- Vulvar discomfort, usually burning pain
- Q-tip test to localize pain
- Treatment: topical estrogen, tricyclic antidepressant

Pearly Penile Papules (Fig. 22-2)

- Normal variant
- Small pearly papules along the coronal rim; may extend to the frenulum and urethral meatus

- Histology: angiofibromas with dense connective tissue and a rich vascular complex
- No treatment is indicated

Scrotal Cysts

- Common
- Epidermal inclusion cyst
- Medical raphe cyst lined with epithelium of combined epidermal and urothelial origin

Scrotal Calcinosis

- May arise from epidermoid cysts
- Cysts with white chalky material seen after incision

Fournier's Gangrene

- Necrotizing soft tissue infection of the genital and anorectal regions
- Tissue necrosis: cellulitis, fasciitis, and myositis
- Involves scrotum and penis with edema, erythema, skin necrosis, crepitus, and bulla formation
- Progression is rapid
- Etiologic factors: diabetes mellitus, periurethritis with urinary extravasation, indwelling catheter placement, traumatic injury

Diaper Dermatitis

- Primarily perianal
- Related to the irritant substances found in stool
- Presents with a bright red perianal acute dermatitis
- Superinfection with *Candida albicans*
- Treatment: topical antibacterial creams, topical antifungals, emollients

Angiokeratoma of Fordyce

- Found on the scrotum and penis
- Asymptomatic, occasionally bleed spontaneously or during intercourse

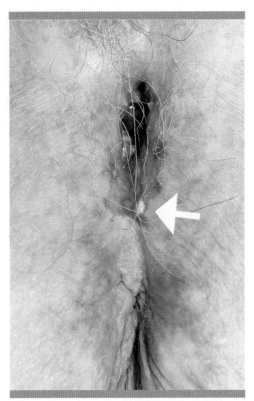

FIGURE 22-1 Lichen sclerosus et atrophicus. *(From Freedberg IM et al: Fitzpatrick's Dermatology in General Medicine, 6th ed. New York: McGraw-Hill, 2003, p. 1111.)*

- Purple 1- to 5-mm papules
- Histology: dilated dermal blood vessels surrounded by a thinned epidermis
- Treatment: None needed; bleeding lesions can be ablated easily by electrocoagulation

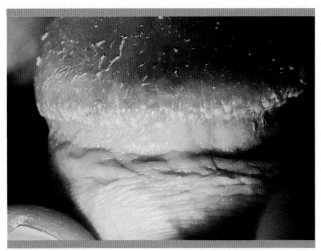

FIGURE 22-2 Pearly penile papules. *(From Freedberg IM et al: Fitzpatrick's Dermatology in General Medicine, 6th ed. New York: McGraw-Hill, 2003, p. 1092.)*

MALIGNANT CONDITIONS

Bowen's Disease/Erythroplasia of Queyrat

- Most common etiologic factor: human papilloma virus infection
- Erythroplasia of Queyrat
  - Squamous cell carcinoma (SCC) in situ confined to the mucosa of the glans penis
  - Sharply demarcated, velvety, bright reddish plaque
- Bowen's disease
  - SCC in situ of the nonmucosal areas
  - Five percent develop invasive carcinoma
  - Extends through most of the thickness of the epidermis; basement membrane remains intact
- Clinical
  - Erythematous, sharply demarcated, scaly, hyperkeratotic, macule, papule, or plaque
  - Vulvar lesions are associated with a high incidence of uterine, cervical, and upper vaginal cancer
- Histology: parakeratotic hyperkeratosis; keratinocytes with atypia and mitoses, producing a "wind blown" appearance; upper dermis with infiltrate of lymphocytes, histiocytes, and plasma cells
- Usually seen in uncircumcised men
- Good penile hygiene or early circumcision would reduce the incidence of this disorder
- Progresses slowly
- Treatment: electrosurgery, cryosurgery, laser surgery, topical application of 5-fluorouracil, as well as Imiquimod cream; Mohs' micrographic surgery

Extramammary Paget's Disease

- Intraepidermal adenocarcinoma in situ with potential to become invasive
- May present as pagetoid spread of an underlying adnexal tumor or of a local internal malignancy, common ones found in males is adenocarcinoma of the sweat glands and rectal carcinoma
- Eroded macular, slightly raised plaque with well-demarcated borders, pink, red, tan or brown
- Histology: intraepithial neoplastic proliferative cells with large, atypical cells with pale-staining cytoplasm and atypical nuclei; mitoses; pagetoid cells distributed singly or in clusters in the epithelium with variable extension into hair follicles and sweat gland ducts
- Immunohistiochemistry: cytokeratin 7, carcinoembryonic antigen
- Treatment: excision

INFLAMMATORY CONDITIONS

- Inverse psoriasis
  - Occurs in intertriginous areas
  - Genital psoriasis is frequently accompanied by perianal and intergluteal cleft psoriasis
  - Vulvar psoriasis affects fully keratinized skin, sparing the modified mucous membrane
  - Dusky red, well-demarcated plaques; with moist, fine scale or a glazed, shiny surface texture
  - Frequently complicated by *Candida* infection
  - Treatment: hydrocortisone or other mild topical glucocorticoid

Lichen Planus

- Violaceous, flat-topped, polygonal papules with Wickham's striae (fine, whitish puncta or reticulated networks)
- Commonly affects oral mucosa, glans penis, wrists
- Associated with hepatitis C
- Histology: lichenoid infiltrate with basal cell vacuolarization, sawtooth rete ridges, Max-Joseph spaces
- Treatment: topical or intralesional steroids, calcinuerin inhibitors

Lichen Nitidus

- Small skin-colored papules with a glistening appearance
- Often on the penis, abdomen, and arms
- Histology: clawlike extension of rete ridges around a focal mixed dermal infiltrate
- Resolves spontaneously after months to years

Plasma Cell Balanitis (Balanitis Circumscripta Plasmacellularis, Zoon's Balanitis) (Fig. 22-3)

- Solitary, glistening, red or cayenne pepper–colored plaque on the glans penis and/or prepuce of uncircumcised men
- Female equivalent is plasma cell vulvitis; oral mucosal equivalent is plasma cell orificial mucositis
- Histology: dense bandlike or lichenoid infiltrate with a predominance of plasma cells
- Treatment: low-potency topical steroids, circumcision

Lichen Simplex Chronicus

- Scrotum and/or penis, vulva
- Results from chronic rubbing and scratching
- Areas of hypo- and hyperpigmentation may result
- Treatment: Castellani's paint, intralesional or topical mild- to moderate-strength glucocorticoid, and oral antipruritic agents

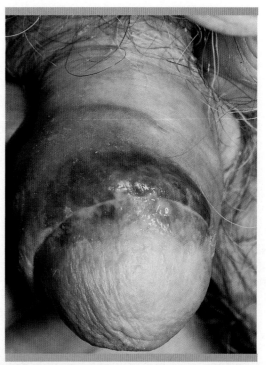

FIGURE 22-3 Plasma cell balanitis. *(From Freedberg IM et al: Fitzpatrick's Dermatology in General Medicine, 6th ed. New York: McGraw-Hill, 2003, p. 1093.)*

Hidradenitis Suppurativa

- Chronic, inflammatory, scarring disease of apocrine gland–bearing skin (axillae, buttocks, inguinal region, breasts)
- Follicular-occlusion triad: acne conglobata, hidradenitis suppurativa, dissecting cellulitis of the scalp
- Early lesion is a tender dermal abscess; recurrent episodes cause scarring and sinus tract formation
- Rectal, urethral, and vaginal fistulas may develop rarely
- Staging:
  - Stage I: solitary or multiple isolated abscess formation without scarring or sinus tracts
  - Stage II: recurrent abscesses, single or multiple widely separated lesions with sinus tract formation and cicatrization
  - Stage III: diffuse or broad involvement across a regional area with multiple interconnected sinus tracts and abscesses
- *Staphylococcus, Streptococcus,* and *E. coli* are most commonly cultured
- Histology: follicular plugging with various degrees of inflammation and fibrosis, dermal abscess
- Treatment: intralesional steroids, antibiotics, incision and drainage, isotretinoin; wide local excision may be performed in recalcitrant cases

Fixed Drug Eruption

- Follows ingestion of a sensitizing hapten: barbiturates, carbamazepine, dapsone, griseofulvin, nonsteroidal anti-inflammatory drugs, phenazones, sulfonamides, tetracycline
- Sharply demarcated, dusky, erythematous macules or erosions
- Heals with postinflammatory hyperpigmentation
- Recurs in the same location with rechallenge
- Common on glans and distal shaft of the penis, vulva, labia
- Fixed eruption heals in 2 to 3 weeks

INHERITED DISEASES

Cystic Fibrosis

- Autosomal recessive
- Exocrine glands affected: involves the tracheobronchial tree, pancreas, and gastrointestinal tract
- Viscid mucous plugs may cause fecal impaction, intussusception, and rectal prolapse in infancy
- Pancreatic insufficiency
- Progressive lung disease with chronic bronchitis, emphysema, and cor pulmonales
- Cutaneous features: increased amounts of electrolyte in the sweat lead to excessive skin wrinkling when the palms and soles are immersed in water
- It can present with a groin rash similar to acrodermatitis enteropathica

Acrodermatitis Enteropathica

- Autosomal recessive
- Inability to absorb sufficient zinc from the diet
- Triad: acral dermatitis, alopecia, and diarrhea
- Distribution: face, hands, feet, anogenital area
- Dry, scaly, eczematous plaques, perlèche
- Progresses to vesicobullous, pustular, and erosive lesions
- Alopecia: worsens with time
- Diarrhea is the most variable, intermittent or totally absent
- Treatment: supplementation with zinc salts

Hailey-Hailey (Familial Benign Pemphigus)

- Autosomal dominant, chromosome 3q
- Axillae, groin, intertriginous areas; mucosal surfaces are rarely involved
- Flaccid vesicles and blisters on an erythematous background
- Friction breaks blisters, resulting in erosions

- Frequent exacerbations, precipitated by friction and infection
- Histology: suprabasal cleavage, acantholysis, and intercellular edema ("dilapidated brick wall")
- Treatment: tetracyclines, fusidic acid, imidazoles, topical or systemic glucocorticoids

INFECTIONS AND INFESTATIONS

Candidiasis

- Usually caused by *C. albicans*
- Vaginal and vuvovanginal candidiasis
  - Thick vaginal discharge associated with burning, itching, and dysuria
  - Whitish plaques on the vaginal wall with underlying erythema and surrounding edema; can extend to labia and perineum
- Balanitis or balanoposthitis
  - Small papules on glans or coronal sulcus
  - Erythematous erosions with a colleratte of whitish scale
  - Infection may spread to the scrotum and inguinal areas
  - Confluent and discrete erythematous areas with pustular and erosive satellite lesions
- Treatment: oral or topical azoles

Crab Louse (Pediculosis Pubis)

- Parasite *Phthirus pubis,* the pubic louse
- Transmitted sexually; mites cling to pubic and facial hair/eyelashes
- Nits (egg casings) of head and crab lice are firmly cemented to the hairs of the host
- Main symptom is pruritus; bites are painless, rarely detected
- Maculae ceruleae: blue macules
- Treatment
  - Permethrin 1% cream rinse
  - Lindane 1% shampoo (potential for central nervous system toxicity; not recommended for use on infants, young children, or pregnant or nursing women)
  - Sexual contacts should be treated simultaneously

Tinea Cruris

- Dermatophytosis involving the groin area
- Causative dermatophytes: *Epidermophyton floccosum, Trichophyton rubrum*
- Dermatophytoses elsewhere on the body provide a reservoir for autoinfection in tinea cruris
- Clinical: multiple, erythematous papulovesicles with a well-marginated, raised border

- Scrotum usually appears completely normal (*Candida* may spread to the scrotum)
- Treatment: decrease occlusion and moisture in the involved area; tolnaftate, and topical imidazoles, powder or minimally occlusive cream base

SEXUALLY TRANSMITTED DISEASES (DESCRIBED IN OTHER CHAPTERS)

- Bacterial vaginosis
- Chancroid
- Gonorrhea
- Granuloma inguinale
- Human immunodeficiency virus infection
- Syphilis
- Donovanosis
- Lymphogranuloma venereum
- Genital herpes
- Molluscum contagiosum
- Nongonococcal urethritis
- Pubic lice
- Trichomoniasis
- Human papilloma virus infection

REFERENCES

Freedberg IM et al. *Fitzpatrick's Dermatology in General Medicine,* 6th Ed. New York: McGraw-Hill; 2003.

Jansen I, Altmeyer P, Piewig G: Acne inversa (alias hidradenitis suppurativa). *J Eur Acad Dermatol Venereol* 2001; 15(6): 532–540.

Lewis FM: Vulval lichen planus. *Br J Dermatol* 1998; 138(4): 569–575.

McKee PH. *Pathology of the Skin: With Clinical Correlations.* London: Mosby-Wolfe; 1996.

Moyal-Barracco M, Lynch PJ: 2003 ISSVD terminology and classification of vulvodynia. *J Reprod Med* 2004; 49:772.

Shepherd V, Davidson E J, Davies-Humphreys J: Extramammary Paget's disease. *BJOG* 2005; 112(3):273–279.

Sobel JD: Candida vaginitis. *Infect Dis Clin Pract* 1994; 3:334.

Thomas RH, Ridley CM, McGibbon DH, et al: Anogenital lichen sclerosus in women. *J R Soc Med* 1996; 89(12):694–698.

CHAPTER 23

CUTANEOUS MALIGNANCIES

MADELEINE DUVIC
TRI H. NGUYEN
ASRA ALI

NONMELANOMA SKIN CANCER

- Tumor suppressor genes
  - Negative cancer regulators
  - Cause apoptosis of DNA-damaged cells and blocks cell division
  - Encode cell-cycle regulators, adhesion molecules, DNA repair enzymes, or signal transduction pathway molecules
  - Are recessive
  - Even if heterozygosity exists, tumor suppression continues
  - p53 (Fig. 23-1)
    - Found on chromosome 17p
    - Mutation of a single copy of the two copies is enough for the deleterious effect
    - Most common cancer mutation
    - Ninety percent of squamous cell carcinomas (SCCs) and in most basal cell carcinomas (BCCs) and actinic keratosis
    - Extrinsic and intrinsic apoptotic pathways
      - ▲ Lead to the activation of the aspartate-specific cysteine proteases (caspases) that mediate apoptosis
      - ▲ Extrinsic pathway
        - △ Involves engagement of particular "death" receptors that belong to the tumor necrosis factor receptor (TNF-R) family (e.g., Fas, DR5, and PERP)
        - △ Also causes the formation of the death-inducing signaling-complex (DISC)
      - ▲ Intrinsic pathway
        - △ Triggered in response to DNA damage
        - △ Associated with mitochondrial depolarization and release of cytochrome c from the mitochondrial intermembrane space into the cytoplasm
        - △ Cytochrome c, apoptotic protease-activating factor 1 (APAF-1), and procaspase-9 form a complex termed the *apoptosome* (caspase-9 is activated and promotes activation of caspase-3, caspase-6, and caspase-7)
    - Mutation is not the only way to inactivate tumor suppressor genes; function also can be blocked by methylation of their promoter
- Oncogenes
  - Genes with growth-promoting activity
  - Mutated gene causes cellular products to become constitutively active
  - Are dominant
  - If a normal gene (protooncogene) is present at a locus along with one mutated gene (oncogene), the abnormal product takes control
  - May derive from viruses (e.g., *Src, ras, cmyc*)
- Carcinogenesis
  - Two-hit theory of Knudsen
  - First: inheriting a defect in the familial form (5 to 10 percent of cancers result from germ-line mutations) or exposure to a carcinogen
  - Second: ongoing exposure to the carcinogen that acts as a tumor promoter or cocarcinogen
  - Repeated assault on the DNA leads to mutations that cause the cell cycle to lose control
  - Mutations from ultraviolet B (UV-B) light cause cytosine (C) to change to thymine (T)
- AP-1 (activating protein-1)
  - Negative regulator for procollagen transcription; blocked by retinoids
  - Collective term referring to dimeric transcription factors composed of *Jun, Fos,* or *ATF* subunits (protooncogenes)
  - UV-B induces AP-1 binding to DNA at the AP-1-binding site

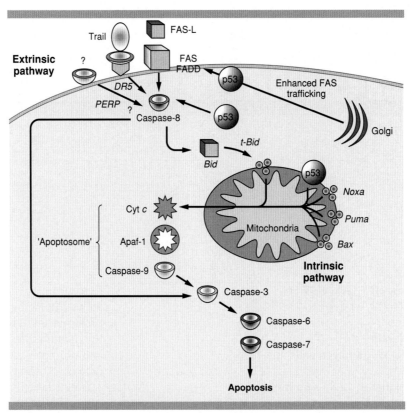

FIGURE 23-1 A model for p53-mediated apoptosis. *(From Haupt S, Berger M, Goldberg Z, Haupt Y: Apoptosis: The p53 network. J Cell Sci 2003; 116(20):4080.)*

- AP-1 upregulates mRNA expression for gelatinase and collagenase
- AP-1 blocks collagen gene expression in dermal fibroblasts
- AP-1 proteins regulate the expression and function of cell-cycle regulators such as p53
- Absence of c-Jun results in elevated expression of the tumor suppressor gene *p53*
- Overexpression of c-Jun supresses p53

Basal Cell Carcinoma

- Clinical
  - Most common malignancy in humans
  - Mutations in the *p53* tumor suppressor gene, which resides on chromosome 17p
    - Clinical and histologic subtypes
      - ▲ Nodular (Fig. 23-2)
      - ▲ Pigmented
      - ▲ Cystic
      - ▲ Superficial
      - ▲ Micronodular*
      - ▲ Morpheaform/sclerosing and infiltrating*

*Aggressive subtypes: higher risk of recurrence and subclinical extension

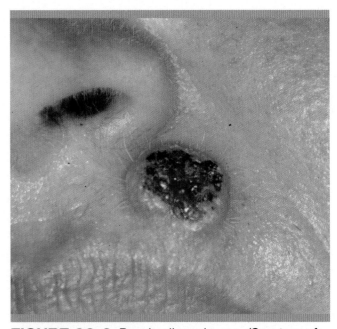

FIGURE 23-2 Basal cell carcinoma. *(Courtesy of Dr. Adelaide Hebert.)*

- Causes
  - Ultraviolet radiation
  - Other radiation: x-rays and Grenz rays
  - Arsenic exposure
  - Xeroderma pigmentosum
- Nevoid BCC syndrome
  - Also known as basal cell nevus syndrome, Gorlin syndrome
  - Autosomal dominant; abnormalities in the *patched* (*PTCH*) gene, chromosome 9
  - Starts at an early age; third decade or earlier
  - Characteristic facies: broad nasal root, frontal bossing, hypertelorism
  - Multiple BCCs
  - Opacity and cataract or glaucoma
  - Odontogenic keratocysts
  - Palmoplantar pitting
  - Intracranial calcification; calcification of the falx
  - Bifid ribs
  - Various tumors: medulloblastomas, meningioma, fetal rhabdomyoma, ameloblastoma
- Acrokeratosis paraneoplastica of Bazex
  - Bazex-Dupre-Christol syndrome
  - X-linked dominant
  - Follicular atrophoderma ("ice pick" marks, especially on dorsal hands)
  - Multiple BCCs: face, the neck, and the upper part of the trunk
  - Local anhidrosis
  - Respiratory tract or digestive tract carcinomas
- Course
  - Incidence of new NMSC after initial skin cancer diagnosis
  - 35 percent at 3 years
  - 50 percent at 5 years
- Staging
  - TNM classification
  - Stage 0: Tis, N0, M0
  - Stage I: T1, N0, M0
  - Stage II: T2, N0, M0; T3, N0, M0
  - Stage III : T4, N0, M0; any T, N1, M0
  - Stage IV: any T, any N, M1
- Low-risk tumors
  - Borders are well defined; primary tumor; nonimmunosuppressed; nodular or superficial subtype
  - Location
    - Trunk and extremities: <2 cm
    - Cheek/forehead/scalp/neck: <1 cm
- High-risk tumors
  - Features
    - Aggressive histology: recurrent, micronodular, metatypical, sclerosing/morpheaform, infiltrative, perineural
    - Recurrent, immunosuppressed, BCCNS, ill-defined borders, setting of irradiated skin
  - Location
    - ▲ Trunk and Extremities: >2m
    - ▲ Cheek/forehead/scalp/neck: ≥1 cm
    - ▲ Mask areas of face [central face (nose, periorbital, cutaneous and mucosal lips, chin), periauricular, temple]
- Treatment
  - Electrodesiccation and curettage
  - Cryotherapy
  - Imiquimod cream
  - Photodynamic therapy (PDT)
  - Radiation therapy: nonsurgical candidates, debilitated patients
  - Excision
  - Mohs micrographic surgery
  - Intralesional interferon

Squamous Cell Carcinoma

- Second most common form of skin cancer
- Malignant tumor of keratinocytes
- Predisposing conditions
  - Immunosuppression [especially solid-organ transplant recipients, chronic lymphocytic lymphoma, human immunodeficiency virus infection]
  - Psoralen and ultraviolet A light (>300 treatments)
  - Chemical carcinogens (tar, soot, arsenic)
  - Smoking
  - Genetic syndromes (ie, xeroderma pigmentosum)
  - Chronic inflammatory conditions (ie, discoid lupus erythematosus, erosive oral lichen planus)
  - Chronic infections (ie, osteomyelitis)
  - Chronic scarring conditions (ie, burn scars, thermal injury, irradiated skin [ionizing radiation])
  - Human papillomavirus-associated SCC
- Types
  - SCC in situ: referred to as Bowen's disease (Fig. 23-3)
  - Invasive SCC
  - Nodular SCC
  - Periungual SCC
  - Keratoacanthoma
    - Well-differentiated SCC
    - Solitary, rapidly growing, dome-shaped papulonodule with a central, horn-filled, crater-like depression
  - Verrucous carcinoma
    - Indolent form of SCC that presents as an exophytic verrucous tumor
    - Oral cavity (oral florid papillomatosis)
    - Foot (epithelioma cuniculatum)
    - Genitals (giant condyloma of Buschke and Löwenstein)

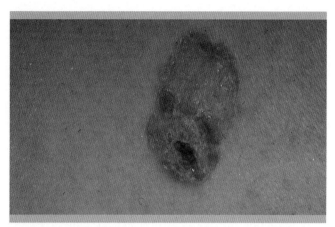

FIGURE 23-3 Bowen's disease. *(Courtesy of Dr. Robert Johnson.)*

- Marjolin ulcer: SCC arising in a chronic site of inflammation: old burn scar or a draining sinus tract
- High-risk SCCs and metastatic rate
  - Metastasis to primary or first echelon draining lymph nodes
  - Location
    - External ear: 11 percent
    - Lip: 10 to 14 percent
  - Depth >4 mm or less than Clark level IV: 45 percent
  - Marjolin ulcer: 18 to 38 percent
  - Organ transplant patient metastatic rate is 18 to 36 times that of the general population
  - Perineural invasion: 35 percent.; local recurrence rate as high as 47 percent
  - Poorly differentiated: 33 percent
- Treatment
  - Excision
  - Radiation
  - Mohs' micrographic surgery
  - Patients with regional disease
    - Focused neck dissection
    - Superficial parotidectomy
    - Adjuvant radiation therapy
    - Primary radiation if inoperable tumor
  - Cryosurgery
  - Electrodesiccation and curettage
  - Photodynamic therapy (PDT)
  - Topical therapy (imiquimod, florouracil)

Melanoma

- Accounts for 4 percent of all skin cancer; accounts for >70 percent of deaths related to skin cancer
- More than 50 percent of cases are believed to arise de novo
- 10 to 20 percent of all patients with melanoma have a family history of melanoma

- Risk factors for cutaneous melanoma
  - Dysplastic nevi in familial melanoma
  - Greater than 50 nevi 2 mm or greater in diameter
  - One family member with melanoma
  - Previous history of melanoma
  - History of acute, severe, blistering sunburns
  - Freckling
- Clinical types
  - Superficial spreading (Fig. 23-4): most common type (70 percent)
  - Lentigo maligna: 10 percent of all melanomas
  - Acrolentiginous
    - 2 to 8 percent of melanoma in white persons
    - 29 to 72 percent of melanoma in dark-skinned individuals
  - Amelanotic melanoma: <2 percent of melanomas
  - Mucosal: approximately 3 percent
  - Nodular: 10 to 15 percent

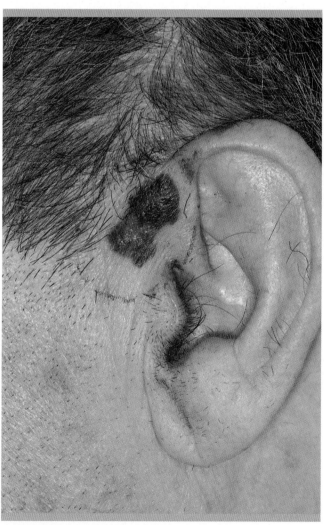

FIGURE 23-4 Superficial spreading melanoma. *(Courtesy of Dr. Tri Nguyen.)*

- Genes implicated in the development of melanoma
  - Cyclin-dependent kinase inhibitor 2A (CDKN2A) resides on chromosome 9p
    - Cell-cycle regulatory gene
    - Protein target: inhibitor of cyclin-dependent kinase 4 (CDK4)
    - Encodes two distinct gene products that are regulators of cell division cycle
      - ▲ p16(INK4a): INK4 proteins inhibit complexes formed by the cell cycle kinases CDK4 and CDK6 and the D-type cyclins
      - ▲ p19 (ARF): acts on the p53 pathway
    - Associated with 25 to 60 percent of familial melanoma
- Prognosis
  - Ulceration, Breslow depth, and tumor thickness, important histologic determinants
  - Breslow depth: measured vertically in millimeters from the top of the granular layer (or base of superficial ulceration) to the deepest point of tumor involvement
- Immunohistochemical staining
  - Homatropine methylbromide 45 (HMB-45)
    - Spindle cell and desmoplastic variants fail to react with HMB-45
    - Shown to react with other neural crest-derived tumors and occasionally with adenocarcinomas and other neoplasms
    - Specificity for detecting melanoma is 96.9 percent
  - S-100: specificity of 70 percent
  - Microphthalmia transcription factor (Mitf): nuclear transcription factor critical for melanocyte development and survival
  - Tyrosinase: enzyme involved in the early stages of melanin production
  - Melan-A (or MART-1)
    - Product of the *MART-1* gene
    - Cytoplasmic protein that is expressed in mature melanocytes
  - Ki67: Proliferating cell nuclear antigen
- Revised AJCC TNM classification and staging
  - T classification
    - T1: ≤ 1.0 mm
      - ▲ a: without ulceration
      - ▲ b: with ulceration or level IV or V
  - T2: 1.01–2.0 mm
    - a: without ulceration
    - b: with ulceration
  - T3: 2.01–4.0 mm
    - a: without ulceration
    - b: with ulceration
  - T4: >4.0 mm
    - a: without ulceration
    - b: with ulceration

- N classification
  - N1: one lymph node
    - a: micrometastasis
    - b: macrometastasis
  - N2: 2–3 lymph nodes
    - a: micrometastasis
    - b: macrometastasis
    - c: in-transit metastasis(-es)/satellite(s) without metastatic lymph nodes
  - N3: 4 or greater metastatic lymph nodes, malted lymph nodes, or combinations of in-transit metastasis(-es)/satellite(s) and metastatic lymph nodes
- M classification
  - M1: distant skin, subcutaneous, or lymph node metastasis
  - M2: lung metastasis
  - M3: all other visceral or any distant metastasis with elevated LD14
- Treatment: wide local excision
  - Tumors ≤ 1 mm depth: 1 cm margin
  - Tumors 1 to 4-mm in depth: 2–3 cm margins
  - Overall survival rates: Delayed lymph node dissection was not statistically significant compared with immediate node dissection
- Sentinel lymph node biopsy/lymphatic mapping
  - Absence of clinically palpable nodes
  - Thicker melanomas (≥1 mm in depth)
  - Determines presence of micrometastasis; if positive sentinel lymph node, then therapeutic lymph node dissection proceeds
  - Lymphoscintigraphy: preoperative radiographic mapping and vital blue dye injection around the primary melanoma or biopsy scar; isosulfan blue dye plus sulfur-colloid-labeled technetium isotope increase accuracy of finding sentinel node
  - Performed at the time of wide local excision/reexcision
  - Identifies and removes the initial draining regional node(s)
  - Yields prognostic information but no evidence SLN; removal improves survival (current studies ongoing)
- Risk of primary tumor recurrence
  - Desmoplastic subtype
  - Positive microscopic margins
  - Recurrent disease
  - Thick primary lesions with ulceration or satellitosis
- High risk of nodal relapse
  - Extracapsular extension
  - Involvement of four or more lymph nodes
  - Lymph nodes measuring at least 3 cm
  - Cervical lymph node location
  - Recurrent disease

- Interferon alfa (IFN-α)
  - Approved by the Food and Drug Administration (FDA) for treatment of melanoma
  - Adjuvant treatment after excision in patients who are free of disease but are at high risk for recurrence: stages IIB and III
  - For primary tumors > 4 mm depth and regional nodal disease
  - Binds to cell surface receptors, interacting with specific gene sites in both normal and neoplastic cells
  - Modulates the expression of host natural killer cells, T cells, monocytes, dendritic cells, and class I and II major histocompatibility (MHC) antigens in both neoplastic and nonneoplastic host tissues
  - Shown to have a growth-inhibitory effect when added to tumor cells in vitro
  - 11 percent increase (26 to 37 percent) in survival rates at 5 years in the IFN-α treatment group compared with the observation arm
- Interleukin 2 (IL-2): indirectly causes tumor cell lysis by proliferating and activating cytotoxic T-lymphocytes
- Dacarbazine (DTIC)
  - Approved by FDA for treatment of melanoma
  - Response rate of 10 to 20 percent
  - Combination therapy
    - Cisplatin, vinblastine, and DTIC (CVD) regimen
    - Cisplatin, DTIC, carmustine, and tamoxifen
- Radiation
  - Adjuvant treatment of regional node metastasis with extracapsular extension
  - Palliative treatment of distant metastatic disease: bone or brain
- Factors predicting response to treatment:
  - Good performance status
  - Soft-tissue disease or only a few visceral metastases
  - Age younger than 65 years
  - No prior chemotherapy
  - Normal hepatic and renal function
  - Normal complete blood count (CBC)
  - Absence of central nervous system metastases
- Melanoma vaccines
  - *Active* immunization: elicits specific or nonspecific reactivity against a tumor antigen by stimulating the patient's own immune system
  - *Passive* immunization: administration of antitumor antibodies or cells against a tumor antigen
  - Autologous (killed cell and recombinant types): Heat shock protein extracts purified from autologous tumor cells also have been shown to have antitumor reactivity
  - Allogeneic
    - Generated using established stable cultured cell lines derived from tumors previously obtained from patients

- Shed from tumor
- Antigen-directed or genetically engineered
- Polyvalent or univalent
- Whole-cell preparations: immunizing with diverse antigens that are present on the tumor surface without knowing the exact antigen(s)
- Gangliosides: tumor antigens that are created synthetically: GM2
- Peptides/proteins
  - Direct loading of peptide fragments onto APCs
  - Antigenic epitopes responsible for eliciting an antitumor response consist of small peptide fragments
- Dendritic cell vaccines
  - Recombinant viral and bacterial vaccines
  - Direct transduction
- Cytokine and growth factor modulation
  - IL-2, interferons (IFN-α, IFN-β, IFN-γ), GM-CSF, and TNF
  - Allow sustained local release of cytokines to enhance a potent local inflammatory response
- DNA and RNA vaccines
  - Induce activation of APCs, which then present antigens to T cells

Merkel Cell Carcinoma (MCC)

- Neuroendocrine carcinoma of the skin
- Mortality rate is approximately 25 percent
- Most frequent sites: head, neck region, and extremities
- Located in or near the basal layer of the epidermis
- Clinical
  - Painless, indurated, solitary dermal nodule, slightly erythematous to deeply violaceous color
  - Regional lymph nodes at presentation: 10 to 45 percent
  - Regional lymph node metastases during course of disease: 50 and 75 percent
  - Distant metastases: 50 percent
    - Common sites: lymph nodes, liver, bone, brain, lung, and skin
  - Local recurrence develops in 25 to 44 percent after primary tumor excision
- Histology: three distinct subtypes
  - Trabecular
  - Intermediate
  - Small cell type
- Staging: classification based on clinical presentation
  - Stage IA: primary tumor ≤ 2 cm, with no evidence of spread to lymph nodes or distant sites
  - Stage IB: primary tumor > 2 cm, with no evidence of spread to lymph nodes or distant sites
  - Stage II: regional node involvement but no evidence of distant metastases
  - Stage III: presence of systemic metastases beyond the regional lymph nodes

- Treatment
  - Stage I
    - Wide local excision: 2-cm margins
    - Elective lymph node dissection (ELND)
      ▲ Larger tumors, tumors with greater than 10 mitoses per high-power field, lymphatic or vascular invasion, and the small cell histologic subtypes
    - Sentinel lymph node (SLN) biopsy
      ▲ MCC sites with indeterminate lymphatic drainage
      ▲ Effective in preventing short-term regional nodal recurrence
    - Adjuvant radiation therapy
      ▲ Primary site and to the regional lymph node basin
      ▲ Larger tumors, tumors with lymphatic invasion, tumors approaching the surgical margins of resection, and locally unresectable tumors
      ▲ 50 Gy to the surgical bed and the draining regional lymphatics: delivered in 2-Gy fractions
  - Stage II
    - Wide local excision of the primary tumor
    - Regional lymph node dissection
    - Adjuvant radiation therapy: primary site and to the regional lymph node basin
      ▲ Larger tumors, tumors with lymphatic invasion, tumors approaching the surgical margins of resection, and locally unresectable tumors
      ▲ 50 Gy to the surgical bed and the draining regional lymphatics: delivered in 2-Gy fractions
    - Adjuvant chemotherapy: regimens similar to patients with small cell lung cancer
      ▲ Cyclophosphamide, doxorubicin, and vincristine and etoposide plus cisplatin are the most commonly used regimens
      ▲ Impact on survival uncertain
  - Stage III
    - Chemotherapy: unresectable recurrent tumors
    - Regional lymph node dissection and adjuvant radiation therapy if the regional draining nodes have not been treatedpreviously
    - Adjuvant radiation therapy: site of recurrence as well as regional lymph node beds

Cutaneous T-Cell Lymphoma (CTCL)

- Mycosis fungoides (MF): most common type of CTCL
- Sézary syndrome (SS)
  - Leukemic form of MF
  - 5 to 10 percent of all cases of MF
- Expansion of a clone of CD4+/helper memory skin-homing T cells

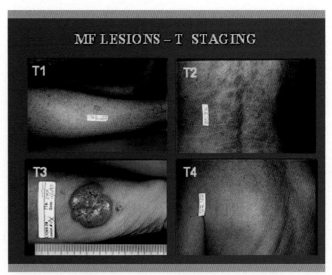

FIGURE 23-5 TNM. *(Courtesy of Dr. Madeline Duvic.)*

- Frequently lack other normal T-cell antigens: CD4+ CD7−, CD4+ CD26−
- Cutaneous lymphocyte antigen (CLA)—positive cells
  - Home to the skin
  - Travel to lymph nodes and then through efferent lymphatics back to the blood
- MF initially presents as eczematous or psoriasiform skin involvement; is systemic but not measurable early on
- Natural history of MF is indolent
- Clinical
  - Patches, plaques, tumors, or erythroderma; hypopigmented, folliculocentric, granulomatous
  - TNM definitions (Fig. 23-5)
    - Primary tumor (T)
      ▲ T1: eczematous patches, papules, or limited plaques covering less than 10 percent of the skin surface
      ▲ T2: erythematous patches, papules, or generalized plaques covering 10 percent or more of the skin surface
      ▲ T3: tumors, one or more
      ▲ T4: generalized erythroderma
    - Nodal involvement (N)
      ▲ N0: no clinically abnormal peripheral lymph nodes; pathology negative for CTCL
      ▲ N1: clinically abnormal peripheral lymph nodes; pathology negative for CTCL
      ▲ N2: no clinically abnormal peripheral lymph nodes; pathology positive for CTCL
      ▲ N3: clinically abnormal peripheral lymph node with effacement of architecture; pathology positive for CTCL

- Distant metastasis (M)
  - ▲ M0: no involvement of visceral organs
  - ▲ M1: visceral involvement (must have confirmation of pathology; organ involved should be specified)
- The TNM classification includes a subcategory for patients with CTCL
  - ▲ Blood involvement (B)
    - △ B0: <5 percent atypical lymphocytes
    - △ B1: ≥5 percent atypical lymphocytes
    - △ B2: >10 percent atypical cells, T cell abnormal > 1000 m^2; FACS clone present > 30 percent, CD4/CD8 is > 10
- Stage I
  - Stage IA is defined as the following TNM grouping: T1, N0, M0
  - Stage IB is defined as the following TNM grouping: T2, N0, M0
- Stage II
  - Stage IIA is defined as either of the following TNM groupings: T1 or T2, N1, M0
  - Stage IIB is defined as either of the following TNM groupings: T3, N0 or N1, M0
- Stage III: Stage III is defined as either of the following TNM groupings: T4, N0 or N1, M0
- Stage IV
  - Stage IVA is defined as any of the following TNM groupings: T1-T4, N2 or N3, M0
  - Stage IVB is defined as any of the following TNM groupings: T1-T4, N0-N3, M1
- Diagnosis
  - Laboratory studies
    - HIV
    - Human T-cell lymphotrophic virus type I (HTLV-I)
    - Liver-associated enzymes
    - Buffy coat smear for Sézary cells
      - ▲ Flow cytometry is preferred
      - ▲ >30 percent CD4+ CD26− or CD4+ CD7−, or CD4/CD8 ratio is greater than 10
      - ▲ MF/SS cells (convoluted lymphocytes)
    - Flow cytometric
      - ▲ Study of the blood (include available T-cell-related antibodies)
      - ▲ Identifies circulating malignant clone
      - ▲ Circulating Sézary cells can be confirmed by T-cell receptor gene analysis or by flow cytometry
  - Imaging
    - Chest radiograph
    - Computed tomographic (CT) scan of the abdomen and pelvis
  - Skin biopsy
    - Formalin-fixed for light microscopy
    - T-cell receptor gamma gene rearrangement by polymerase chain reaction (PCR)
    - Bandlike upper dermal infiltrate and epidermal infiltrations with Pautrier's abscesses (collections of neoplastic lymphocytes)
    - Early on: epidermotrophic lymphocytes along basal cell layer with single cells in the epidermis; atypical cells and nuclear halos are present
- Lymph node biopsy and bone marrow examination
  - If palpable nodes are present
  - Bone marrow if blood is abnormal
- Treatment
  - Stage I
    - Class I steroids
    - Topical bexarotene
    - Psoralen and ultraviolet A radiation with or without interferon-α
    - Topical mechlorethamine, nitrogen mustard
    - Total-skin electron-beam irradiation
      - ▲ Electron irradiation of appropriate energies will penetrate only to the dermis, and thus the skin alone can be treated without systemic effects
  - Stage II
    - Psoralen and ultraviolet A radiation along with interferon-α or retinoids
    - Total-skin electron-beam irradiation or local electron-beam irradiation
    - Topical mechlorethamine, nitrogen mustard
    - Interferon-α alone or in combination with topical therapy
    - Bexarotene, an oral or topical retinoid
    - Adjuvant therapy with topical steroids
  - Stage III
    - Extracorporeal photochemotherapy plus interferon and bexarotene
    - Bexarotene with an oral or topical retinoid
    - Interferon-α alone or in combination
    - Denileukin diftitox (interleukin-2 fusion toxin) for CD25
    - Systemic chemotherapy
    - Chlorambucil and prednisone or methotrexate
    - 2-Chlorodeoxyadenosine and pentostatin
    - Psoralen and ultraviolet A radiation as adjuvant therapy
    - Total-skin electron-beam irradiation or local electron-beam irradiation
  - Stage IV
    - Systemic chemotherapy
    - Mechlorethamine, cyclophosphamide, methotrexate, combination chemotherapy, total-skin electron-beam irradiation
    - Adjuvant psoralen and ultraviolet A radiation
    - Fludarabine, 2-chlorodeoxyadenosine, and pentostatin if erythrodermic

- Denileukin diftitox (interleukin-2 fusion toxin) for CD25
- Extracorporeal photochemotherapy alone or in combination with total-skin electron-beam irradiation for Sézary syndrome
- Bexarotene, an oral or topical retinoid
- Gencitabine, doxorubicin

REFERENCES

Ballo MT, Ang KK: Radiotherapy for cutaneous malignant melanoma: Rationale and indications. *Oncology* 2004; 18(1):99–107; discussion 107-10, 113–114.

Becker M, Hoppe RT, Knox SJ: Multiple courses of high-dose total skin electron beam therapy in the management of mycosis fungoides. *Int J Radiat Oncol Biol Phys* 1995; 32(5):1445–1449.

Duvic M, Hymes K, Heald P, et al: Bexarotene is effective and safe for treatment of refractory advanced-stage cutaneous T-cell lymphoma: Multinational phase II-III trial results. *J Clin Oncol* 2001; 19(9):2456–2471.

Freedberg IM et al. *Fitzpatrick's Dermatology in General Medicine*, 6th Ed. New York: McGraw-Hill; 2003.

Goessling W, McKee PH, Mayer RJ: Merkel cell carcinoma. *J Clin Oncol* 2002; 20(2):588–598.

Gollard R, Weber R, Kosty MP, et al: Merkel cell carcinoma: Review of 22 cases with surgical, pathologic, and therapeutic considerations. *Cancer* 2000; 88(8):1842–1851.

Haag ML, Glass LF, Fenske NA: Merkel cell carcinoma: Diagnosis and treatment. *Dermatol Surg* 1995; 21(8):669–683.

Haigh PI, DiFronzo LA, McCready DR. Optimal excision margins for primary cutaneous melanoma: a systematic review and meta-analysis. *Can J Surg* 2003; 46(6):419–426.

Herrmann JJ, Roenigk HH Jr, Hurria A, et al: Treatment of mycosis fungoides with photochemotherapy (PUVA): Long-term follow-up. *J Am Acad Dermatol* 1995; 33(2 pt 1): 234–242.

Kim YH, Jensen RA, Watanabe GL, et al: Clinical stage IA (limited patch and plaque) mycosis fungoides: A long-term outcome analysis. *Arch Dermatol* 1996; 132(11):1309–1313.

Lui et al: Affected members of melanoma-prone families with linkage to 9p21 but lacking mutations in *CDKN2A* do not harbor mutations in the coding regions of either *CDKN2B* or *p19*[ARF] *Genes Chromosomes Cancer* 1997; 19:52–54.

Marks ME, Kim RY, Salter MM: Radiotherapy as an adjunct in the management of Merkel cell carcinoma. *Cancer* 1990; 65(1):60–64.

McKee PH. *Pathology of the Skin: With Clinical Correlations*. London: Mosby-Wolfe; 1996.

Nghiem P, McKee PH, Haynes HA: Merkel cell (cutaneous neuroendocrine) carcinoma. In Sober AJ, Haluska FG (eds): *Skin Cancer*. Hamilton, Ontario: BC Decker, Inc., 2001., pp. 127–141.

Platz et al: Screening of germline mutations in the *CDK4*, *CDKN2C*, and *TP53* genes in familial melanoma: A clinic-based population study. *Int J Cancer* 1998; 78:13–15.

Thomas JM, Newton-Bishop J, A'Hern R, et al: Excision margins in high-risk malignant melanoma. *New Engl J Med* 2004; 350(8):757–766.

Walker GL et al: Mutations of the *CDKN2/p16* gene in Australian melanoma kindreds. *Hum Mol Genet* 1995; 4:1845–1852.

Zuo L et al:Germline mutations in the p16 binding domain in familial melanoma. *Nature Genet* 1996; 12:97–99.

CHAPTER 24

DERMOSCOPY

ASRA ALI
MARK NAYLOR

DERMOSCOPY

- Also known as
  - Epiluminescence microscopy
  - Dermatoscopy
  - Amplified surface microscopy
  - Noninvasive method of evaluating skin lesions using either
    - Optical magnification and liquid oil immersion
      - ▲ Oil removes normal scattering of light at the stratum corneum.
      - ▲ Epidermis then becomes more translucent
    - Optical magnification and polarized light

DIAGNOSTIC DERMATOSCOPIC FEATURES OF PIGMENT IN THE SKIN

- Melanin location and lesion color
  - Stratum corneum, stratum spinosum: black
  - Dermal-epidermal junction: light to dark brown
  - Papillary dermis: slate blue
  - Reticular dermis: steel blue
- Pigment network
  - Gridlike/honeycomb-like network of pigmented "lines" (tips of the dermal papillae) and hypopigmented "holes" (suprapapillary plates)
  - Formed by melanin in basal keratinocytes and melanocytes along the dermal-epidermal junction
  - Network represents the rete ridge pattern of the epidermis
  - Regular/discrete/typical network (Fig. 24-1)
    - Uniform, regularly meshed, homogeneous in color, thinning out at the periphery
    - Benign melanocytic lesions
  - Irregular network (Fig. 24-2)
    - Irregular prominent network
    - Nonuniform, darker, and/or broadened lines and holes heterogeneous in area and shape
    - Found in dysplastic nevi and in in situ and invasive melanoma

- Broadened network
  - Broad-width grids are present
  - Occurs in 49 percent of lentigo maligna (rhomboidal structures), absent in the majority of benign pigmented macules of the face
- Pseudo-broadened network
  - Due to dilated follicular openings on the face
  - Benign pigmented macule: ephilis, lentigo, junctional nevus
- Negative pigment network: elongated hypomelanotic rete pegs: Spitz and melanoma (specificity of 95 percent and sensitivity of 22 percent)
- Volar site patterns
  - Parallel furrow: Pigment follows the surface skin markings
  - Lattice-like: Pigment crosses the surface skin markings.
  - Fibrillar: meshlike crossing of the surface skin markings
- Pigmentation pattern symmetry
  - Symmetric pigmentation pattern (Fig. 24-3): mirror symmetry across any axes through the center of lesion
  - Asymmetric pigmentation pattern (Fig. 24-4)
    - Found in lesions that lack symmetry of one or more axes through its center
    - Specificity: 46 percent; sensitivity: 100 percent for invasive melanoma
  - Blue-white veil (Fig. 24-5)
    - Irregular, indistinct, confluent blue pigmentation with an overlying white "ground-glass" haze
    - Does not occupy the entire lesion
    - Aggregation of heavily pigmented cells or melanin in the dermis (blue color) in combination with a compact orthokeratosis (whitish color)
    - Can represent invasive melanoma: sensitivity 51 percent, specificity 97 percent

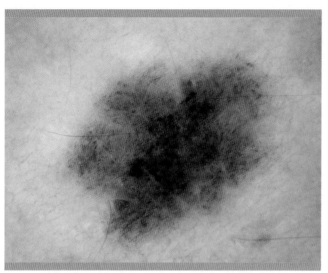

FIGURE 24-1 Regular pigment network in an atypical nevus.

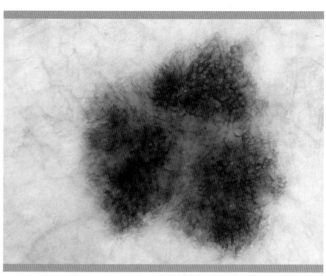

FIGURE 24-3 Pigment symmetry in an atypical nevus.

- Dots
  - Small, round structures of less than 0.1 mm in diameter
  - Represent pigment accumulation in the stratum corneum and the upper part of the epidermis
  - Color varies depending on the level of pigment in the skin.
  - Increased specificity for melanoma when found at the periphery of a lesion

- Black dots (Fig. 24-6)
  - Pigment in the stratum corneum
  - Found in benign pigmented lesions (tend to be central); also found in invasive melanoma (tend to be peripheral): sensitivity 60 percent and specificity 81 percent (any position of dots)
- Multiple brown dots (Fig. 24-7)
  - Well-defined dark brown dots of intraepidermal pigment

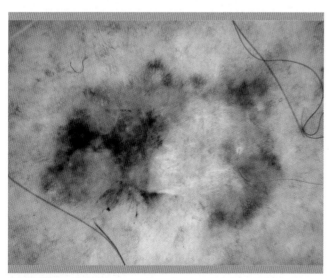

FIGURE 24-2 Irregular pigment network in a very atypical nevus.

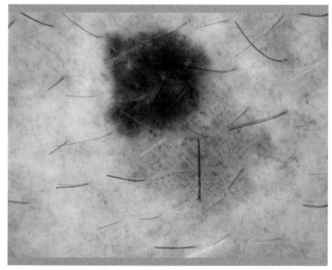

FIGURE 24-4 Asymmetric pigment pattern in an atypical nevus.

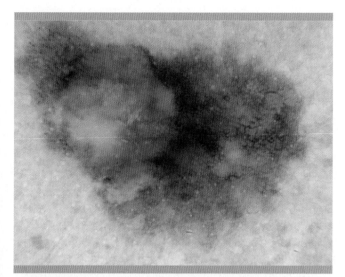

FIGURE 24-5 Prominent blue-white veil over the invasive portion of this superficial spreading melanoma.

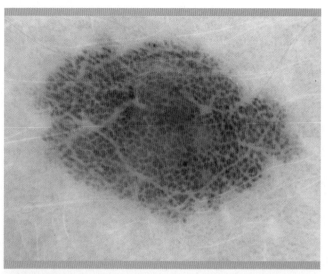

FIGURE 24-7 Regular brown dots in a benign lesion (atypical nevus).

- Invasive melanoma: specificity 97 percent and sensitivity 30 percent
- Brown dots (Fig. 24-8)
  - Focal melanin accumulations or pigmented cell nests at the dermal-epidermal junction
  - Regular appearance in size in benign lesions
  - Irregular appearance in size and distribution in dysplastic nevi and melanomas
- Multiple gray-blue dots/granules
  - White scarlike depigmentation
  - "Peppering": diffuse presence of melanophages in the papillary dermis

- May represent regression; can be seen in any pigmented lesion
- Globules
  - Symmetric, round to oval, well-demarcated structures that are brown, black, or red
  - More than 1 mm in diameter
  - Correspond to nests of pigmented benign or malignant
    - Melanocytes
    - Clumps of melanin
    - Melanophages
  - Multiple blue-gray globules

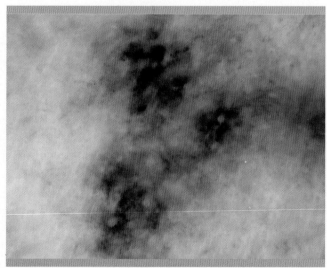

FIGURE 24-6 Lentigo maligna. Note regular dots in the upper left-hand corner of image.

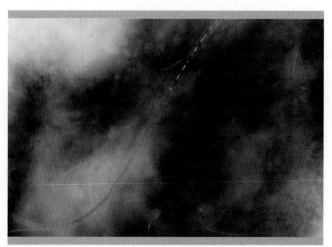

FIGURE 24-8 Irregular, peripheral dots in a melanoma.

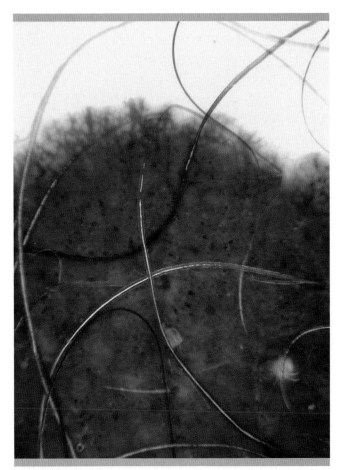

FIGURE 24-9 Pseudopods marking the radial growth phase at the border of this melanoma.

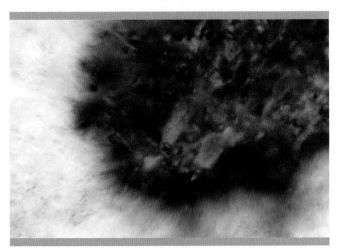

FIGURE 24-10 Radial streaming marking the advancing edge of the radial growth phase of this melanoma.

- – Larger and better circumscribed compared with blue-gray dots
- – Specific for pigmented basal cell carcinomas (if absent pigment network) or melanoma
- Multiple peripheral brown globules: may represent Spitz or dysplastic nevi
- Pseudopods (Fig. 24-9)
  - Curved, bulbous, fingerlike projections
  - Predominantly dark brown or black
  - Located at the periphery of a lesion
  - Intraepidermal or junctional pigment
  - Can represent radial growth phase of melanoma
- Radial streaming (Fig. 24-10)
  - Radial linear extensions asymmetrically arranged and parallel
  - Found at the periphery of a lesion
  - Confluent pigmented junctional nests of pigmented melanocytes
  - Depth determines the colors, which are brown, dark brown, blue-gray, and black

- Can represent radial growth phase of melanoma: specificity 96 percent and sensitivity 18 percent
- Large blue-gray ovoid nests (Fig. 24-11)
  - Larger than globules and not intimately connected to a pigmented tumor body
  - Large, confluent or near-confluent pigmented ovoid areas
  - Highly suggestive of pigmented basal cell carcinoma
- Lesion edge and shape
  - Irregular edge
  - Abrupt edge

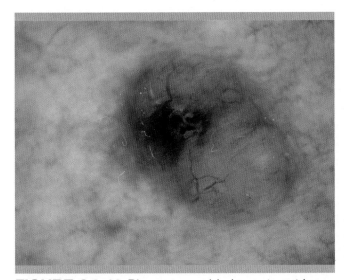

FIGURE 24-11 Blue-gray ovoid pigment nest in a basal cell carcinoma.

- Moth-eaten edge
  - Well-defined, punched-out concave areas at the edge of a lesion
  - Flat seborrheic keratosis
- Regular shape
- Fingerprint-like structures
  - Tiny ridges (thinner than a pigment network)
  - Run in parallel and produce a "fingerprint" pattern
  - Flat seborrheic keratosis, benign lentigo
- Leaflike areas
  - Gray-blue, discrete, bulbous, leaflike pattern
  - Represent nests of pigmented basal cell carcinoma cells: specificity 100 percent; only found in 10 percent of basal cell carcinomas
- Spoke wheel–like structures
  - Brown to gray/blue/brown radial projections meeting at a darker central hub
  - Absence of a pigment network highly suggestive of basal cell carcinoma
- Vascular pattern
  - Erythema: diffuse pink-red area
  - Telangiectasia
    - Comma vessels: some dermal nevi
    - Point vessels: amelanotic melanoma
    - Treelike vessels (arborizing): found in basal cell carcinomas (52 percent), invasive melanoma (23 percent), benign pigmented lesions (8 percent)
    - Wreathlike vessels
    - Hairpin-like vessels: pigmented seborrheic keratosis, invasive melanoma
  - Lacunae (Fig. 24-12)
    - Red-blue dilated vascular spaces in dermis

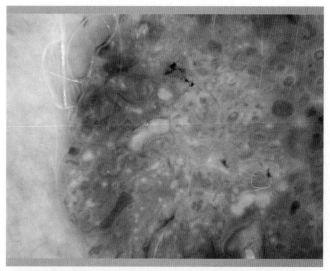

FIGURE 24-13 Small white milia-like cysts in a seborrheic keratosis. This lesion demonstrates yellow and brown-colored comedo-like openings that are also characteristic of seborrheic keratoses.

- Oval, sharply demarcated
- Represent hemangiomas
- Milia-like cysts (Fig. 24-13)
  - Discrete, round, whitish or yellowish structures
  - Intraepidermal keratin-filled cysts
  - Found in seborrheic keratosis, compound or dermal nevi, pigmented BCC
- Fissures and crypts
  - Crypts: irregularly filled craters
  - Fissures: confluent irregular linear keratin-filled depressions (clefts)
  - Found in seborrheic keratosis and dermal nevi with congenital patterns
- Depigmentation
  - May indicate histopathologic regression
  - Irregular depigmentation may indicated invasive melanoma: specificity 92 percent and sensitivity of 46 percent
  - Scarlike depigmentation: significant feature of invasive melanoma: specificity of 93 percent and sensitivity of 36 percent

TWO-STEP PROCEDURE FOR THE DIAGNOSIS OF PIGMENTED SKIN LESIONS

- First step: identify the lesion as either melanocytic or nonmelanocytic (if lesion is identified as melanocytic, then proceed to the second step)
- Second step: differentiate between benign melanocytic lesions and melanoma

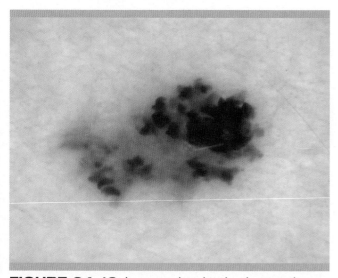

FIGURE 24-12 Lacunae in a benign hemangioma.

- First step: diagnostic algorithm
  - Criteria for a melanocytic lesion: pigment network or pseudonetwork (also can be seen in dermatofibroma or seborrheic keratosis)
    - Aggregated brown or black globules
    - Pseudopods or radial streaming
    - Homogeneous blue pigmentation (also can be seen in hemangiomas and basal cell carcinomas, intradermal melanoma metastases)
    - Parallel pattern on palms and soles
  - Criteria for seborrheic keratosis
    - Multiple milia-like cyst (also can be seen in dermal nevi)
    - Fissures and ridges
    - Light-brown fingerprint-like structures
  - Criteria for basal cell carcinoma
    - Absent pigment network and one or more of the following
    - Arborizing vessels
    - Maple leaf–like areas
    - Large blue-gray ovoid nests
    - Multiple bule-gray globules (also can be seen in seborrheic keratosis)
    - Spoke wheel areas
    - Ulceration
  - Criteria for vascular lesions
    - Widespread red-blue lacunes
    - Red-bluish to red-black homogeneous areas
- Second step: diagnosis of invasive melanoma
  - Negative features (one or the other)
    - Symmetric pigmentation pattern
    - Presence of only a single color
  - Positive features (at least one feature found)
    - Blue-white veil
    - Multiple brown dots
    - Pseudopods
    - Radial streaming
    - Scarlike depigmentation
    - Peripheral black dots/globules
    - Multiple colors (five to six)
    - Multiple blue-gray dots
    - Broadened network
  - Additional positive features for diagnosis of Lentigo maligna
    - Rhomboidal structures
    - Asymmetric pigmented follicular openings
    - Slate gray dots/globules

REFERENCES

Braun RP, Rabinovitz HS, Oliviero M et al. Dermoscopy of pigmented skin lesions. *J Am Acad Dermatol* 2005;52(1):109–121.

Grin CM, Friedman KP, Grant-Kels JM. Dermoscopy: a review. *Dermatol Clin* 2002;20(4):641–646, viii.

Menzies SW et al. *An Atlas of Surface Microscopy of Pigmented Skin Lesions: Dermoscopy*, 2nd Ed. Sydney: McGraw-Hill; 2002.

Rubegni P, Burroni M, Andreassi A, Fimiani M. The role of dermoscopy and digital dermoscopy analysis in the diagnosis of pigmented skin lesions. *Arch Dermatol* 2005;141(11):1444–1446.

Zalaudek I, Argenziano G, Di Stefani A et al. Dermoscopy in general dermatology. *Dermatology* 2006;212(1):7–18. Review.

CHAPTER 25

CUTANEOUS MANIFESTATIONS OF RHEUMATOLOGIC DISEASES

A. SOHAIL AHMED
SYLVIA HSU
ASRA ALI

CONNECTIVE TISSUE DISEASES

- Represent classic models of systemic autoimmune diseases
- Screening
  - When the clinical assessment of a patient suggests the presence of an autoimmune disease, an antinuclear antibody (ANA) test is usually performed
  - Patient serum is incubated with a tissue substrate to which any autoantibodies to nuclear antigens will bind
  - A fluoresceinated antibody is added, and the tissue is observed under fluorescence microscopy to check for a specific staining pattern
  - A positive ANA test is defined as a level (titer) exceeding that found in 95 percent of normal individuals (5 percent of normal individuals can be ANA-positive with titers usually ≤ 1:320 and a speckled or homogeneous pattern)
- Rim pattern (anti–double stranded DNA and anti-laminin antibodies): systemic lupus erythematosus (most specific) but also may be seen in chronic active hepatitis
- Homogeneous pattern (Fig. 25-1) (antihistone, anti-DNA antibodies)
  - Systemic lupus erythematosus (very specific) but also may be seen in drug-induced lupus
  - Further evaluation for SLE includes testing for antibodies to
    - dsDNA (double-stranded DNA or native DNA) 60 percent

  - SS-A (Ro) 30 percent, SS-B (La) 15 percent
  - Sm (Smith) 30 percent
  - RNP (ribonucleoprotein) 30 percent
- Speckled pattern (Fig. 25-2)
  - Indicates antibodies to
    - Smith
    - RNP (ribonucleoprotein antibody)
    - Scl-70 (topoisomerase I)
    - SS-A and SS-B
  - Disorders
    - Systemic lupus erythematosus (SLE)
    - Mixed connective tissue disease (MCTD)
    - Scleroderma [progressive systemic sclerosis (PSS)]
    - Sjögren's syndrome
- Nucleolar pattern (homogeneous, speckled, or clumpy staining of nucleolus)
  - Suggest antibodies to RNA polymerase I (RNA pol 1), clumpy (U3 RNP, fibrillarin), homogeneous (Pm–Scl), NOR 90 (nucleolar organizing region)
  - Disorders
    - PSS/polymyositis (50 percent)—homogeneous staining of PM-Scl
    - PSS (3 to 6 percent)—clumpy staining of fibrillarin
  - Further evaluation
    - Scl-70 (topoisomerase I)—seen in 20 to 28 percent of patients with PSS
    - Creatinine phosphokinase (CPK), erythrocyte sedimentation rate (ESR), C-reactive protein, anti-Jo-1 (seen in 25 to 44 percent patients with myositis)

331

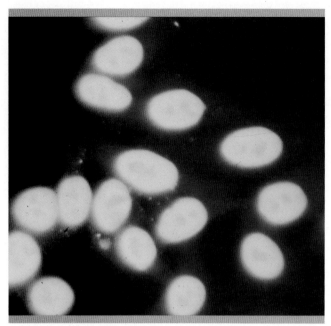

FIGURE 25-1 Homogeneous pattern. *(Courtesy of Dr. Robert Jordon.)*

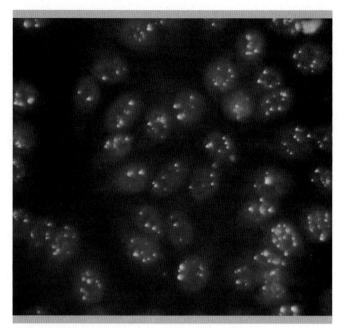

FIGURE 25-2 Speckled pattern. *(Courtesy of Dr. Robert Jordon.)*

- Centromere pattern (antibodies to kinetichore proteins)
  - Seen in limited scleroderma primarily (60 to 90 percent) as opposed to diffuse scleroderma
  - Can be associated with CREST (calcinosis, Raynaud's, esophageal dysmotility, sclerodactyly, telangiectasias) variant

Lupus Erythematosus

- Autoimmune disorder with a spectrum of presentations
  - Chronic cutaneous lupus erythematosus (CCLE)
  - Subacute cutaneous lupus erythematosus (SCLE)
  - Systemic lupus erythematosus (SLE)

SYSTEMIC LUPUS ERYTHEMATOSUS (SLE)

- Autoimmune disorder that affects many organ systems
- Associated with human leukocyte antigens DR2 and DR3
- Skin findings
  - Malar rash
    - Lasts from days to weeks
    - Flat or raised over the malar eminence, tending to spare nasolabial folds
    - Often is painful or pruritic
    - Temporal association with sun exposure is common
  - Generalized erythema and bullae can be present

- Alopecia (while seen does not count for diagnostic criteria)
  - Patchy or generalized
  - Can arise independent of cutaneous manifestations and may be associated with flares of disease
- Leukocytoclastic vasculitis
- Urticaria
- Lupus panniculitis
- Livedo reticularis: especially in patients with antiphospholipid antibodies
- Mucous membrane lesions (hard palate and nasopharyngeal erythema and ulceration) that are usually painless and have to be observed by a physician to be counted for diagnostic criteria
- Raynaud's phenomenon (20 to 30 percent of patients)
- Diagnostic criteria (4 of 11)
  - Mucocutaneous
    - Malar rash
    - Naso-oral ulcers (have to be observed by physician)
    - Photosensitivity rash (owing to unusual reaction to sunlight)
    - Discoid rash (erythematous raised patches with adherent keratotic scaling and follicular plugging with atrophic scarring in older lesions)
  - Systemic
    - Nonerosive arthritis of two or more joints characterized by tenderness, swelling, or effusion

- Serositis
  - ▲ Pleuritis: convincing history of pleuritic pain or rub heard by physician or evidence of pleural effusion
  - ▲ Pericarditis: documented by electrocardiogram (ECG), rub, or evidence of pericardial effusion)
- Renal involvement: proteinuria >0.5 g/day or >3 + protein in urinalysis (UA) or cellular casts in UA (red cell, hemoglobin, granular, tubular, or mixed)
- Hematologic disease (hemolytic anemia with reticulocytosis or leukopenia < 4000 white blood cells (WBCs; two occasions) or lymphopenia < 1500 (2 occasions) or thrombocytopenia < 100,000 in the absence of offending drug
- Neurologic disorders (seizures or psychosis in the absence of offending drugs or known metabolic disorderor psychosis)
- Laboratory
  - ANA (more than 99 percent of patients) in the absence of drugs known to induce "drug-induced lupus"
  - Other laboratory tests
    - ▲ Anti-dsDNA
      - △ Highly specific; lower sensitivity than ANA; 70 percent test positive
      - △ Levels may correlate with disease activity, particularly with SLE nephritis
    - ▲ Anti-Smith: highly specific for SLE; 30 to 40 percent test positive
    - ▲ Positive LE preparation (old method of measuring ANA that was considered positive if a PMN was seen containing phagocytosed nuclear material)
    - ▲ Positive findings of antiphospholipid antibodies based on (1) abnormal serum levels of IgG or IgM anticardiolipin antibodies, (2) positive test for lupus anticoagulant, or (3) false-positive serologic test for syphilis (positive for at least 6 months) confirmed by TPI or FTA-ABS
      - △ Associated with livedo reticularis, arterial and venous thrombosis without vasculitis or active SLE, and increased incidence of fetal wastage
- Other immunologic changes (not part of the criteria)
  - Deficiencies of complement components, including C3, C4, and C1q
  - Anti-Ro, anti-La antibodies (15 to 20 percent)
  - Antiribonucleoprotein (anti-RNP) antibodies
- Histologic findings: focal liquefactive degeneration of the basal cell layer; perivascular and periadnexal lymphocytes

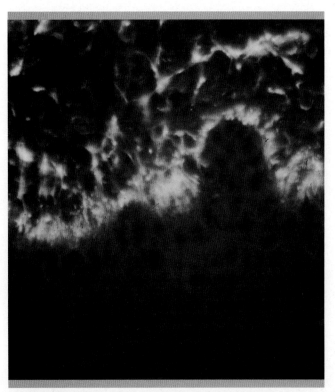

FIGURE 25-3 Immunohistology of systemic lupus erythematosus. *(Courtesy of Dr. Robert Jordon.)*

- Immunohistology (Fig. 25-3): IgG, C3 along dermal-epidermal junction in a continous granular or linear bandlike array (lupus band: lesional or nonlesional)
- Treatment
  - Prednisone
  - Azathioprine
  - Cyclophosphamide
  - Thalidomide
  - Hydroxychloroquine
  - Intravenous IgG (IVIG)

DRUG-INDUCED LUPUS ERYTHEMATOSUS (DILE)

- Differs from classic SLE: autoantibody profile; spares the kidneys and central nervous system (CNS); malar and discoid lesions unusual in DILE
- Antihistone antibody–positive
- Increased frequency in association with HLA-DR4
- Patients who are slow acetylators have a higher incidence of DILE
- Can appear in up to one-fifth of patients with SLE
- Patients have one or more clinical symptoms of SLE
- Noninflammatory joint pain (90 percent of patients)
- Etiologic agents
  - Antiarrhythmics (procainamide and quinidine)
  - Antibiotics (minocycline, isoniazid, and griseofulvin)
  - Anticonvulsants (valproate, ethosuximide, carbamazepine, and hydantoins)

- Hormonal therapy (leuprolide acetate)
- Antihypertensives (hydralazine, methyldopa, and captopril)
- Anti-inflammatories (D-penicillamine and sulfasalazine)
- Antipsychotics (chlorpromazine)
- Cholesterol-lowering agents (lovastatin, simvastatin, and gemfibrozil)
- Anitibody profile
  - Positive ANA (95 percent)
    - Homogeneous pattern: procainamide, isoniazid, timolol, hydralazine, and phenytoin
    - Speckled pattern (anti-SSA/Ro): thiazide diuretics, terbinafine
  - Antihistone antibodies
    - Detected by a homogeneous pattern of ANAs
    - More than 75 percent of patients
    - Also seen in 50 to 70 percent of patients with SLE (however, dsDNA are highly specific for SLE)
  - Complement levels normal
- Treatment: not needed; symptoms usually clear up within weeks of stopping the implicated drug

SUBACUTE CUTANEOUS LUPUS ERYTHEMATOSUS (SCLE)

- Associated with HLA-B8, HLA-DR3, HLA-DRw52, and HLA-DQ1
- Drugs also may induce SCLE: most commonly hydrochlorothiazide, calcium channel blockers, angiotensin-converting enzyme inhibitors, griseofulvin, terbinafine

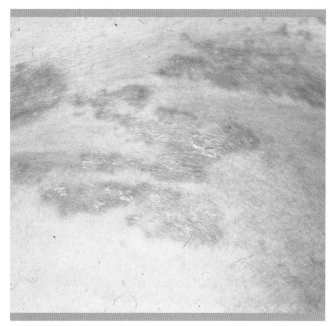

FIGURE 25-4 Subacute cutaneous lupus erythematosus. *(Courtesy of Dr. Robert Jordon.)*

- Clinical (Fig. 25-4)
  - Begin as erythematous papules or plaques
  - Evolve either into annular lesions or into diffuse scaling
  - Tend to occur on sun-exposed areas of the body but can be generalized
  - Nonfixed and nonscarring; follow a waxing and waning course
  - May occur with few other SLE features except for musculoskeletal symptoms and laboratory abnormalities
  - Tumid lupus erythematosus (TLE): involves a deeper, more nodular lesion in which little or no scaling is seen
- Laboratory studies
  - Antinuclear antibody (ANA)
  - Anti-Ro (SS-A)
  - Antinative DNA
  - Cytopenias may be present.
  - Elevated erythrocyte sedimentation rate (ESR)
  - Rheumatoid factor may be positive
  - Complement levels may be depressed
- Histology: similar to SLE; TLE lacks epidermal involvement; little or no vacuolar degeneration
- Treatment
  - Sun-protection methods
  - Hydroxychloroquine, thalidomide, azathioprine, interferon-α2a and -α2b, acitretin

CHRONIC CUTANEOUS LUPUS ERYTHEMATOSUS (CCLE)/DISCOID LUPUS

- Localized skin changes: occur in the absence of other systemic symptoms or organ involvement
- Clinical
  - Begin as erythematous papules or plaques, progress to atrophic patches with follicular plugging (Fig. 25-5)
  - Photosensitive dermatosis
  - Fewer than 5 percent with DLE progress to SLE
  - Can result in permanent alopecia
  - Subsets
    - Localized DLE: head and neck affected
    - Widespread DLE: skin affected below the neck in addition to head and neck
  - Laboratory studies
    - ANA: 20 percent
    - Anti-Ro (SS-A): 1 to 3 percent of patients
- Histology: similar to SLE with follicular plugging
- Treatment
  - Corticosteroids (topical or intralesional)
  - Antimalarials
  - Thalidomide
  - Oral retinoids
  - Interferon
  - Immunosuppressive agents

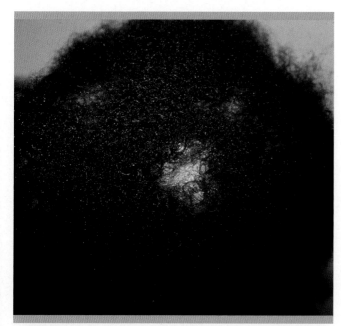

FIGURE 25-5 Clinical observational findings of chronic cutaneous lupus erythematosus (CCLE). *(Courtesy of Dr. Robert Jordon.)*

LUPUS PANNICULITIS (FIG. 25-6)

- Primarily affects subcutaneous fat (2 to 5 percent)
- Lupus profundus: affects epidermis and dermis in addition to fat
- Preceding, subsequent, or concomitant lesions of discoid lupus erythematosus (in 70 percent of patients)
- 50 percent eventually develop SLE

- Deep, erythematous plaques, nodules, and ulcers
- Tender and painful and frequently heal with atrophy and scars
- Usually involves the proximal extremities, trunk, breasts, buttocks, and face
- Histologic features: epidermal atrophy, hydropic degeneration of the basal cell layer, and perivascular and periappendageal lymphocytic inflammation that extends into the subcutaneous fat (lobular panniculitis) and that may be accompanied by hyalinized fat necrosis

NEONATAL LUPUS ERYTHEMATOSUS (NLE)

- Nonscarring form of LE in neonates
- 1 percent of infants with positive maternal autoantibodies develop NLE
- Mother with anti-Ro autoantibodies; incidence in subsequent pregnancies is approximately 25 percent
- Usually resolves by age 4 to 6 months
- Clinical (Fig. 25-7)
  - Well-demarcated erythematous, mild, scaling plaque that is often annular
  - Appears predominately on the scalp, neck, or face
  - Two-thirds have congenital skin lesions
  - Lesions worsened by UV light
  - Congenital heart block (15 to 30 percent)
  - Complete heart block requires a pacemaker; patients may develop heart failure
  - Hepatosplenomegaly may occur
- Laboratory studies
  - Cytopenias: leukopenia, thrombocytopenia

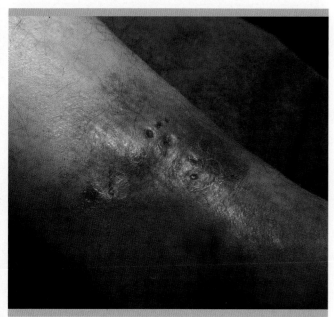

FIGURE 25-6 Lupus panniculitis. *(Courtesy of Dr. Robert Jordon.)*

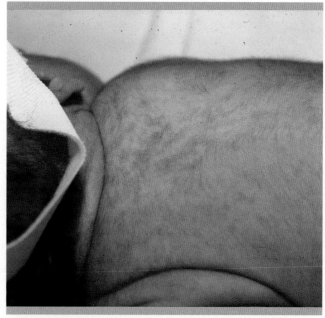

FIGURE 25-7 Clinical observational findings of neonatal lupus erythematosus (NLE). *(Courtesy of Dr. Robert Jordon.)*

- Anti-SSA/Ro52 autoantibodies recognize the Ro52 protein cardiac 5-HT4 serotoninergic receptor and inhibit serotonin activated L-type calcium currents (I_{Ca})
- Antigen B8 (HLA-B8) and human leukocyte antigen DR3 (HLA-DR3) in the mother
- Maternal autoantibodies: Ro (SSA), La (SSB), and/or U1-RNP; they are transported passively across the placenta
- Treatment
  - Photoprotection
  - Mild topical steroids
  - Congestive heart failure: early placement of a pacemaker
  - Neonatal mortality rate is 20 to 30 percent

Antiphospholipid Syndrome (APS)

- Production of antibodies against coagulation factors, including prothrombin, protein C, and protein S
- Vascular thrombosis
- Frequent miscarriages or premature births
- Cutaneous findings
  - Livedo reticularis
  - Superficial thrombophlebitis
  - Leg ulcers
  - Painful purpura
  - Splinter hemorrhages
  - Venous thrombosis
  - Leg swelling (DVT)
  - Ascites (Budd-Chiari syndrome)
  - Arterial thrombosis
  - Abnormal neurologic examination (e.g., cerebrovascular accident)
  - Digital ulcers
  - Gangrene of distal extremities
- Laboratory studies
  - Antiphospholipid (aPL) antibodies
  - Anticardiolipin (aCL) antibodies
  - Anti-β_2-glycoprotein I antibodies
  - Activated partial thromboplastin time (aPTT)
  - Lupus anticoagulant (LA) test such as dilute Russell viper venom time (DRVVT)
  - False-positive serologic test result for syphilis
  - Complete blood cell count (thrombocytopenia, Coombs-positive hemolytic anemia)
- Diagnostic criteria: one clinical and one laboratory criterion should be met from the following
  - One or more episodes of arterial, venous, or small-vessel thrombosis in any tissue and organ and thrombosis confirmed by histopathology or Doppler studies
  - Pregnancy morbidity (involving unexplained deaths, premature births, or unexplained consecutive spontaneous abortions based on length of pregnancy)

- Anticardiolipin antibody or lupus anticoagulant on two occasions at least 6 weeks apart
- Treatment
  - After thrombosis
    - Full anticoagulation with intravenous heparin is followed by warfarin.
    - Heparin or low-molecular-weight (LMW) heparin also may be used
  - Pregnancy with a history of recurrent fetal loss: followed closely as high-risk obstetric patients and treated with subcutaneous heparin 7500 to 12,000 units twice daily along with aspirin 81 mg daily; no controlled evidence that corticosteroids improve fetal survival

Sjögren's Syndrome (SS)

- HLA-DR3 and HLA-DR52 in patients with primary SS
- Secondary SS has xerophthalmia and xerostomia and occurs with rheumatoid arthritis or SLE
- Primary SS has xerophthalmia and xerostomia only
- Clinical findings
  - Xerophthalmia and xerostomia (Fig. 25-8)
  - Bilateral parotid swelling is the most common sign of onset in children.
  - Unstimulated salivary flow less than 1.5 ml/min
  - Annular erythematous rash with scales, localized especially on the face and neck, is recognized as a cutaneous manifestation of SS
- Extraglandular symptoms
  - Hepatitis (13 percent)
  - Arthritis (42 percent)

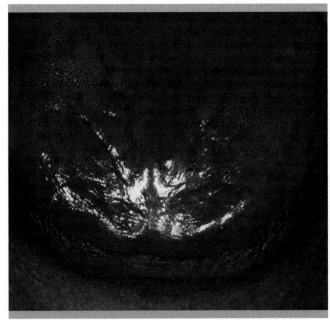

FIGURE 25-8 Sjögren syndrome (SS). *(Courtesy of Dr. Toth.)*

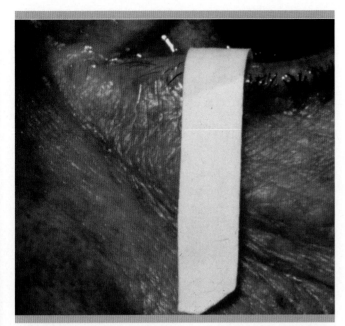

FIGURE 25-9 Positive Schirmer test. *(Courtesy of Dr. Robert Jordon.)*

- Laboratory studies
  - Anti-Ro/SS-A ± anti-La/SS-B (95 percent)
  - Rheumatoid factor
  - Antithyroglobulin antibodies (25 percent)
  - Anti-120-kDa α-fodrin (actin binding protein)
  - Bax and caspase 3 are overexpressed in the salivary gland epithelial cells: proapoptotic molecules
  - B-lymphocyte infiltration (20 to 25 percent) and CD4+ T-cell infiltration (70 to 80 percent) localized in the salivary glands
- Positive Schirmer test (Fig. 25-9)
  - Induces a lacrimation response in the eye
  - Filter paper strip placed in lower conjunctival sac and the wetting length achieved in 5 minutes is measured
  - Greater than 8 mm in 5 minutes is abnormal
- Histopathologic findings: minor salivary gland: mononuclear inflammatory infiltrates, interstitial fibrosis, and acinar atrophy
- Diagnostic criteria: presence of three of six of the following criteria establish probable diagnosis of Sjögren's syndrome [high sensitivity (99.1 percent); insufficient specificity (57.8 percent)]
  - Ocular symptoms of dryness
  - Oral symptoms of dryness
  - Ocular signs (e.g., positive Schirmer)
  - Focus score ≥ 1 on minor salivary gland biopsy
  - Salivary gland involvement (scintigraphy, sialography, salivary flow)
  - Autoantibodies (Ro, La, ANA, RF)

- Treatment
  - No curative agents exist.
  - Topical cyclosporine A 0.05% to 0.1%
  - Pilocarpine HCl (Salagen)
    - 5-mg tablets
    - Cholinergic agonist
  - Plaquenil (hydroxychloroquine)
  - Cevimeline HCI (Evozac)
    - Cholinergic agonist that bonds to muscarinic receptors
    - 30-mg capsules

MIXED CONNECTIVE-TISSUE DISEASE (MCTD)

- (HLA) HLA-DR4 or HLA-DQB1
- Defined by a combination of clinical and serologic findings
  - Raynaud phenomenon
  - Swollen hands
  - Synovitis
  - Acrosclerosis with or without proximal scleroderma
  - Histologically proven myositis
  - Anti-U1-RNP antibodies > 1:1600 titer
- Other findings
  - Abnormal capillaries in the nail fold (50 percent)
  - Palpable purpura (25 percent)
  - Vascular disturbances may lead to peripheral gangrene and leg ulcers
  - Arthralgias (60 percent)
  - Dysphagia and dysfunction of esophageal motility
  - Pleuropulmonary complications (20 to 85 percent)
- Laboratory studies
  - Dependent on the spectrum of CTD symptoms
  - ANA: speckled staining pattern; usually these are very high titer ANAs
  - Lupus band test (LBT) might be positive
  - Antibodies to extractable nuclear antigens (ENAs)
  - Antibodies against U1—70-kDa small nuclear ribonucleoprotein (snRNP) at titer >1:1600
- Diagnostic criteria: one serologic criteria and three of five clinical criteria (or five of five clinical criteria if RNP titer is less than 1:1600)
- Treatment
  - Corticosteroids
  - Plasmapheresis
  - Chronic and usually mild disease that responds to corticosteroids

Dermatomyositis (DM)

- Autoimmune condition affecting muscles and skin
- Diagnostic criteria (two of five)
  - Symmetric proximal weakness

- Elevated muscle enzymes
- Abnormal ECG
- Abnormal muscle biopsy
- Cutaneous findings
- Clinical
  - Cutaneous findings
    - Typically develops 2 to 3 months before muscle weakness
    - Heliotrope rash first cutaneous sign: periorbital, symmetric, violaceous patches with or without edema
    - Gottron papules
      - ▲ Elevated violaceous papules and plaques
      - ▲ Bony prominences (metacarpophalangeal joints, proximal interphalangeal joints, and/or the distal interphalangeal joints)
    - Periungual telangiectases
    - Poikiloderma
      - ▲ May occur on exposed skin, upper part of the back (shawl sign)
      - ▲ V of the neck
    - Scalp: psoriasiform dermatitis
  - Extracutaneous findings
    - Proximal symmetric muscle weakness
    - Joint swelling
    - Raynaud's phenomenon
- Other types of DM
  - DM sine myositis
    - Amyopathic dermatomyositis (ADM)
    - Cutaneous disease without muscle involvement
    - Serum muscle enzyme levels are normal
  - Juvenile DM
    - Onset more insidious
    - May manifest all the features of classic DM
    - Vasculopathic lesions are more common: poorer prognosis
    - Calcinosis may be a complication at the site of inflammation; found in 40 percent of children
    - Lipodystrophy also is seen more commonly in juvenile DM
    - Thrombospondin-1, a mediator of angiogenesis, is increased in patients with juvenile DM
  - DM associated with malignancy
    - May precede, coincide with, or follow the diagnosis
    - Ovarian cancer in female patients
  - Anitbody-related syndromes
    - Antisynthetase syndrome
      - ▲ Aminoacyl-tRNA synthetases (most commonly anti-Jo-1)
      - ▲ Mechanic's hands: scaly, dry patches on extensor surfaces of finger joints
      - ▲ Myositis
      - ▲ Interstitial lung disease
      - ▲ Chronic joint involvement

- ▲ Raynaud's phenomenon
- ▲ Patients can be refractory to treatment
  - Autoantibodies to Mi-2
    - ▲ Myositis-specific antibodies directed against a nuclear helicase
    - ▲ V-sign, shawl sign, and cuticular overgrowth
    - ▲ Good prognosis with a good response to therapy
- Laboratory studies
  - Elevated creatine kinase level
  - Liver enzyme elevations: aldolase, aspartate aminotransferase (AST), and lactate dehydrogenase (LDH)
  - Antinuclear antibody
  - Anti-Mi-2
  - Anti-Jo-1
  - Anti-Ku
  - Anti-polymyositis/Scl (PM/Scl)
  - Annexin XI (56-kDa): most sensitive for juvenile DM
  - Electromyographis detect: inflammation of the muscles
  - Muscle biopsy
- Histologic findings (skin biopsy): similar to lupus erythematosus; interface dermatitis, mucin, perivascular and periadnexal lymphocytic infiltrate
- Treatment
  - Systemic corticosteroids
  - Methotrexate
  - Hydroxychloroquine and chloroquine

Systemic Sclerosis (SSc)

- Systemic connective tissue disease with excessive collagen deposition HLA-B8, HLA-DR5, HLA-DR3, HLA-DR52, and HLA-DQB2
- Also associated with the following exposures
  - Organic solvents
  - L-5-Hydroxytryptophan
  - Drugs (e.g., bleomycin, carbidopa, pentazocine, cocaine, penicillamine, vitamin K)
  - Vibration injury
  - Silica
  - Aliphatic hydrocarbons (e.g., hexane, vinyl chloride, trichloroethylene)
- Clinical findings
  - Raynaud's phenomenon (digits): blanching, cyanosis, and hyperemia on exposure to cold
  - Begins as joint pain in 15 percent of patients
  - Skin sclerosis that affects the arms, face, and/or neck
  - Sclerodactyly, erosions (Fig. 25-10)
  - Bilateral lung fibrosis
  - Cutaneous involvement has three phases: (1) edematous, (2) indurative, and (3) atrophic

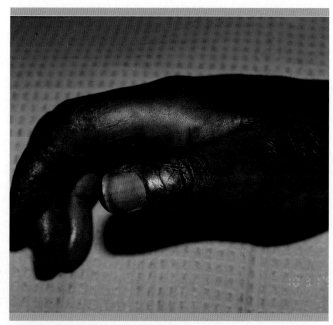

FIGURE 25-10 Sclerodactyly. *(Courtesy of Dr. Robert Jordon.)*

- Diffuse scleroderma
  - Topoisomerase I DNA (Scl 70) in approximately 30 percent
  - Generalized skin fibrosis of the chest and limbs
  - Involvement of the lungs, kidneys, digestive system, and heart: 30 to 60 percent of patients, fibrosis of the basal parts of the lungs
  - Limited scleroderma
    - ▲ Anticentromere antibodies in approximately 70 to 80 percent of patients
    - ▲ Mainly affects hands, face, feet, and forearms
    - ▲ More commonly associated with pulmonary hypertension
- Laboratory studies
  - Antibodies against fibrillarin, a 34-kDa protein of ribonucleoprotein U3 RNP
  - Antibodies against the ribonucleoprotein nucleolar 7-2 RNA protein particle Th RNP
  - Antibodies to 20- to 110-kDa proteins related to preribosomes (PM-Scl)
- Histologic findings
  - Loss of rete ridges, atrophy of epidermal skin appendages, marked increase in the number of compact collagen fibers in the reticular dermis
  - Subintimal proliferation of small arteries and arterioles causing lumen narrowing
  - Dermis is thickened because of the excessive deposition of collagen fibrils
- Diagnostic criteria
  - One major or two or more minor criteria are present

- Major: proximal scleroderma, thickening of skin, of fingers and skin proximal to metacarpophalangeal and metatarsophalangeal joints, and also may include the entire extremity, face, neck, and trunk
- Minor
  - Sclerodactyly
  - Digital pitting scar or loss of substance of finger pad
  - Bibasilar pulmonary fibrosis on x-ray
- Treatment
  - Lung involvement: calcium-channel blockers (e.g., nifedipine), prostaglandins (e.g., prostacyclin), and cyclophosphamide
  - Calcinosis: colchicine
  - Intralesional steroids
  - Calcium-channel blockers
  - Antifibrotic agents *may* be helpful
    - D-Penicillamine
    - Interferon-α and interferon-γ
  - Photopheresis
  - Corticosteroids (inflammatory myositis, pericarditis, refractory arthritis, or alveolitis)
  - Methotrexate (15 mg/week)
  - Chlorambucil
  - Cyclosporine
  - FK506 (tacrolimus)
  - Thalidomide
- Gastrointestinal tract involvement: proton pump inhibitors (e.g., omeprazole), H_2 blockers, cisapride, and metoclopramide

CREST Syndrome

- Variant of scleroderma
- Clinical findings
  - Calcinosis cutis (Fig. 25-11): calcium apatite crystals found in tissue
  - Raynaud's phenomenon: endothelial injury is believed to result in intimal hyperplasia and fibrosis
  - Esophageal dysmotility: dysmotility secondary to nerve injury, smooth muscle atrophy
  - Sclerodactyly: mucopolysaccharide, glycoprotein, and collagen (types I and III) deposition in the dermis
  - Telangiectasia
- Laboratory studies: Anticentromere antibodies are found in approximately 50 to 90 percent
- Treatment
  - D-Penicillamine
  - Raynaud's: calcium channel blockers, topical nitropaste
  - Telangiectasia: laser ablation, sclerotherapy
  - Esophageal dysmotility: H_2 blockers

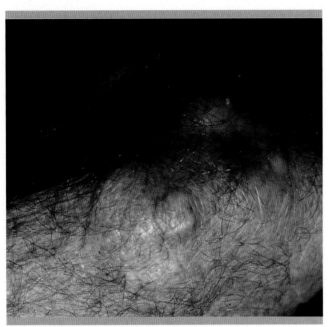

FIGURE 25-11 Calcinosis cutis. *(Courtesy of Dr. Robert Jordon.)*

Morphea

- Also known as localized scleroderma
- Clinical findings
  - Thickening and induration of the skin and subcutaneous tissue owing to excessive collagen deposition
  - Indurated plaques 1 to 30 cm in diameter
  - Begins as an area of erythema
  - Surface becomes smooth and shiny
  - Skin eventually softens and becomes atrophic
- Types
  - Plaque-type
    - Most common
    - Single and unilateral in 95 percent of cases
    - Atrophoderma of Pasini and Pierini: represents an end-stage form of plaque-type morphea
  - Generalized: widespread morphea plaques
  - Linear
    - En coup de sabre: affects frontoparietal scalp
    - Parry-Romberg syndrome: progressive hemifacial atrophy; primary lesion occurs in the subcutaneous tissue, muscle, and bone
  - Deep
    - Subcutaneous morphea or morphea profunda
    - Deep dermis, subcutaneous tissue, fascia, muscle, and bone
- Laboratory studies
  - ANA
    - 50 percent plaque-type or generalized morphea
    - 67 percent linear morphea

- Anti-single-stranded DNA
  - 27 percent plaque-type morphea
  - 75 percent generalized morphea
  - 53 percent with linear morphea
- Antihistone antibodies (AHAs)
  - 42 percent plaque-type morphea
  - 87 percent generalized morphea
- Soluble interleukin 2 (IL-2) receptors: levels may correlate with disease activity
- Treatment
  - Plaque-type morphea
    - Topical or intralesional corticosteroids have limited benefit.
    - Topical calcipotriene may be attempted
  - Generalized, linear, and deep morphea: systemic corticosteroids, antimalarial agents, D-penicillamine, cyclophosphamide, azathioprine
  - Low-dose UV-A phototherapy
  - Tranilast (Rizaben), an antifibrotic agent
  - Physical therapy

Eosinophilic Fasciitis (EF)

- Peripheral eosinophilia and fasciitis
- Thickening of subcutaneous tissue that mimicks PSS, but unlike PSS, EF usually spares the fingers, hands, and face
- Increased expression of genes for transforming growth factor β (TGF-β) and extracellular matrix proteins in fibroblasts
- Associated with L-tryptophan ingestion
- Eosinophilic fasciitis, eosinophilia-myalgia syndrome, and toxic oil syndrome (TOS) share common clinical and histopathologic features
- Clinical findings
  - Swelling and progressive induration of the skin (peau d'orange skin)
  - Onset may be acute following some sort of strenuous exercise, or it may be subacute
  - Contractures (75 percent of patients)
  - Groove sign: vertically linear depressions following the course of vessels that occurs between muscle groups
  - Neuromuscular features: myalgia/myopathy, severe cramps, distal sensorimotor neuropathy, mononeuritis multiplex, cognitive symptoms
  - Cardiopulmonary features: pneumonitis, respiratory muscle dysfunction, pulmonary hypertension
- Laboratory signs
  - Peripheral blood eosinophilia (64 percent of patients)
  - Hypergammaglobulinemia (75 percent of patients)
  - Erythrocyte sedimentation rate (50 to 70 percent)
- Histologic findings: inflammation, edema, thickening, and sclerosis of the fascia; infiltrate

consists of lymphocytes, plasma cells, histiocytes, and eosinophils
- Treatment: prednisone (20 to 40 mg/day; taper according to symptoms, ESR, and eosinophil count)

Cryoglobulinemia

- Cryoglobulins: immunoglobulins that precipitate at cold temperatures; reversible reaction
- Type I
  - Monoclonal immunoglobulin, usually IgM or IgG
  - Associated with
    - Waldenstrom's macroglobulinemia
    - Multiple myeloma
    - Monoclonal gammopathy of undetermined significance
  - Clinical findings
    - Inflammatory macules and papules
    - Raynaud's phenomenon
    - Cold urticaria
    - Hemorrhagic crusts
    - Cutaneous ulcerations
    - Infarctions
    - Livedo reticularis
    - Cutaneous ischemic necrosis (40 percent)
- Type II and type III (mixed cryoglobulinemia)
  - Contain rheumatoid factors (RF) (usually IgM)
  - Form complexes with the fragment, crystallizable (Fc) portion of polyclonal IgG
  - Monoclonal (in type II) immunoglobulin
  - Polyclonal (in type III) immunoglobulin
  - Associated with
    - Chronic lymphocytic leukemia (CLL)
    - Chronic liver disease
    - Coexisting connective tissue diseases (i.e., SLE)
    - Infections
      ▲ Streptococcal infections, syphilis, Lyme disease, leprosy, Q fever, coccidioidomycosis, malaria, toxoplasmosis
      ▲ Hepatitis A, B, and C (associated with type II in 30 to 98 percent of cases)
  - Clinical findings
    - Arthralgias and arthritis in the proximal interphalangeal (PIP) joints, metacarpophalangeal (MCP) joints, knees, and ankles
    - Renal immune-complex disease (diffuse glomerulonephritis)
    - Palpable purpura (60 to 70 percent)
- Laboratory studies
  - Serum evaluation: Specimen must be obtained in warm tubes
  - Type I precipitates within the first 24 hours
  - Type III cryoglobulins may require 7 days
  - RF is positive in types II and III
- Histology: leukocytoclastic vasculitis in patients with skin vasculitic purpura; intraluminal cryoglobulin

deposits may be observed, especially in renal glomeruli
- Treatment
  - Nonsteroidal anti-inflammatory drugs (NSAIDs)
  - Immunosuppressives: corticosteroid therapy and/or cyclophosphamide or azathioprine, interferon-α (IFN-α)

Cryofibrinogenemia

- Cryofibrinogen
  - Plasma complex of fibrin, fibrinogen, and fibronectin
  - Reversibly precipitates on cooling at 4°C
  - Associated with
    - Carcinomas, infections, collagen-vascular diseases, thromboembolic diseases
    - Can be primary or essential
- Clinical findings
  - Purpura
  - Livedo reticularis
  - Ulcerations: usually on the legs
- Histology: fibrin thrombi within superficial dermal vessels
- Treatment
  - Symptomatic
  - Usually unresponsive to treatment
  - Heparin, sodium warfarin, dicumarol, streptokinase, plasmapheresis, dapsone, azathioprine, prednisone, and stanozolol

Seronegative Spondyloarthropathies

- Chronic inflammatory diseases
- Involve the sacroiliac joints, axial skeleton, and peripheral joints
- HLA class I gene, HLA-B27
- Results in a cytotoxic CD8+ T-cell response
- Ankylosing spondylitis, spondyloarthropathy associated with inflammatory bowel disease (IBD), psoriatic arthritis, reactive arthritis (ReA)/Reiter syndrome (RS)
- Reactive arthritis (ReA): previously called Reiter's syndrome with or without extraarticular symptoms 1 month following a gastrointestinal or genitourinary infection
- Human leukocyte antigen HLA-B27 (65 to 96 percent of patients)
- Usually follows gastrointestinal infections with
  - Shigella
  - Salmonella
  - Campylobacter
  - Genitourinary infections: Chlamydia trachomatis
- Clinical findings
  - Triad: nongonococcal urethritis, conjunctivitis, and arthritis (lasting longer than 1 month)
  - Arthritis or enthesitis or spondylitis

- Asymmetric, mainly lower extremity oligoarthritis
- Low back pain occurs in 50 percent of patients
- Enthesopathy
- Renal: immunoglobulin A (IgA) nephropathy
- Mucocutaneous lesions
  - Keratoderma blennorrhagica: palms and soles: clinically appears similar to pustular psoriasis
  - Circinate balanitis
    - Gyrate white plaques eventually cover the entire surface of the glans penis
    - In women: circinate vulvitis
  - Painless shiny patches in the palate, tongue, and mucosa of the cheeks and lips
  - Ocular: bilateral conjunctivitis
  - Severe psoriasiform dermatitis: RS in association with HIV infection
- Histology: similar to psoriasis vulgaris: elongation of rete ridges, psoriasiform hyperplasia, subcorneal abscesses, and spongiform pustules; dermis shows a mixed inflammatory infiltrate with neutrophils
- Laboratory studies
  - Elevated erythrocyte sedimentation rate (ESR) and C-reactive protein (CRP)
  - Synovial fluid: leukocytosis; Gram stain and culture results are negative
  - Throat, stool, or urogenital tract cultures
- Treatment
  - Self-limited course, with resolution of symptoms by 3 to 12 months
  - NSAIDs
  - Intraarticular injection of or systemic corticosteroids
  - Antibiotic treatment does not change the course of the disease.
  - Sulfasalazine
  - Methotrexate

Psoriatic Arthritis

- Undulating course
- Found in 5 percent of patients with psoriasis; precedes the onset of psoriatic arthritis in 60 to 80 percent of patients
- Clinical findings
  - Dactylitis
  - Entheopathy
  - Tendonitis
  - Asymmetric oligoarthritis (70 percent of patients)
  - Arthritis mutilans: 5 percent of patients
  - Spondylitis: 5 percent of patients, often asymptomatic
  - Psoriatic-onychopachydermoperiostitis (POPP)
    - Psoriatic nail lesions
    - Soft tissue thickening above the terminal phalanx and radiologic involvement of the phalanx with periosteal reaction

- Laboratory studies
  - Elevated ESR and CRP
  - Leukocytosis of synovial fluid
- Radiologic findings: x-ray—pencil-in-cup deformity, fluffy periosteal bone formation
- Treatment
  - NSAIDs
  - Mycophenolate mofetil, methotrexate, sulfasalazine, and cyclosporine
  - Infliximab, etanercept

Scleredema

- Benign self-limited skin disease
- Unknown etiology
- Associated with antecedent febrile illness, diabetes mellitus, or blood dyscrasia
- Clinical findings
  - Nonpitting induration of face, neck, or upper part of back
  - Group 1
    - History of a preceding febrile illness
    - Onset of the skin lesions is rapid
    - Clears in 6 months to 2 years
  - Groups 2 and 3
    - Insidious
    - Risk of developing paraproteinemias
    - Prior history of diabetes mellitus
    - Unremitting course
- Histology: thickened dermis with deposition of mucin between thickened collagen bundles
- Treatment
  - Treat underlying infection or diabetes
  - Physical therapy

REFERENCES

Clements PJ, Furst DE, eds. *Systemic Sclerosis.* Baltimore: Williams & Wilkins; 1996.

Fernandez-Madrid F, Mattioli M. Antinuclear antibodies (ANA): immunologic and clinical significance. *Semin Arthritis Rheum* 1976;6:83.

Freedberg IM et al. *Fitzpatrick's Dermatology in General Medicine,* 6th Ed. New York: McGraw-Hill; 2003.

Fritzler MJ. Antinuclear antibodies in the investigation of rheumatic disease. *Bull Rheum Dis* 1987;35:127–136.

Klippel JH, ed. *Primer on the Rheumatic Diseases,* 12th Ed. Atlanta: Arthritis Foundation; 2001.

Klippel JH, Dieppe PA, eds. Rheumatology, 2nd Ed. London: Mosby; 1998.

McKee PH. *Pathology of the Skin: With Clinical Correlations.* London: Mosby-Wolfe; 1996.

Tan EM. Antinuclear antibodies: diagnostic markers for autoimmune diseases and probes for cell biology. *Adv Immunol* 1989;44:93.

Wallace DJ, Hahn BH, eds. *Dubois' Lupus Erythematosus,* 5th Ed. Baltimore: Williams & Wilkins; 1997.

CHAPTER 26

BIOSTATISTICS

TAHNIAT S. SYED
RAJESH BALKRISHNAN
ASRA ALI

STATISTICAL ANALYSIS

Test Sensitivity

- General: assesses the validity of a test
- Definition: ability of screening test to identify correctly those who *have* the disease:
  = $TP/(TP + FN)$ (Table 26-1)
- Properties
  - Test with high sensitivity has few false-negative results
  - Independent of disease prevalence in the community

Test Specificity

- General: assesses the validity of a test
- Definition: ability of screening test to identify correctly those who do *not* have the disease:
  = $TN/(TN + FP)$ (Table 26-1)
- Properties
  - Test with high specificity has few false-positive results.
  - Independent of disease prevalence in the community

Positive Predictive Value (PPV)

- General: assesses reliability of positive test
- Definition: probability that patient has disease when test is positive: $PPV = TP/(TP + FP)$
- Properties
  - Affected by two factors
    - Disease prevalence
    - Specificity (only when disease in infrequent)
  - Higher disease prevalence results in higher PPV
  - Higher specificity results in higher PPV (with infrequent diseases)

Negative Predictive Value (NPV)

- General: assesses reliability of negative test

- Definition: probability that patient does *not* have disease when the results are negative:
  $NPV = TN/(TN + FN)$
- Properties
  - Affected by two factors
    - Disease prevalence
    - Specificity (only when disease is infrequent)
  - Lower disease prevalence results in higher NPV
  - Test sensitivity effect minimized at low prevalence
  - Results in more reliable negative test

Relative Risk or Risk Ratio (RR)

- Definition: ratio of incidence of disease in exposed individuals to incidence of disease in *non*exposed individuals
- Can only be derived directly from cohort studies (because incidence of disease in exposed and nonexposed individuals can be determined)
- Meaning of results
  - RR = 1: No evidence for increased risk in exposed individuals compared with nonexposed individuals
  - RR > 1: Risk in exposed individuals is greater than the risk in nonexposed (i.e., there is a positive association)
  - RR < 1: Risk in exposed individuals is less than the risk in nonexposed (i.e., there is a negative association; suggests a "protective" effect)

Odds Ratio (OR) (Table 26–2)

- Derived from cohort study or case-control study
- Definition depends on type of study
  - Cohort: odds of disease developing in exposed individuals
  - Case-control: odds that cases were exposed versus odds that controls were exposed
- Results are interpreted the same as RR (see "Meaning of results" under RR)
- Measure of whether a certain *exposure* is associated with a specific disease

343

TABLE 26-1 Calculating Sensitivity and Specificity

Test Results	Disease +	Disease −
+	A (TP)	B (FP)
−	C (FN)	D (TN)

Note: TN = true negative; FN = false negative; TP = true positive; FP = false positive.
Sensitivity = TP/TP + FN
Specificity = TN/TN + FP

- The OR approximates the RR when
  - Cases studied are representative of people with disease in the population.
  - Controls studied are representative of people without disease in the population
  - The disease being studied does not occur frequently

Statistics Equations Review

- Sensitivity = A/(A + C)
- Specificity = D/(B + D)
- PPV = A/(A + B)
- NPV = D/(C + D)
- Relative risk = [A/(A + B)]/[C/(C + D)]
- Odds ratio = (A × D)/(B × C)
- Attributable risk = [A/(A + B)] − [C/C + D)]

P-Value

- The level of statistical significance
- Alpha or type I error
- Definition: probability that a difference between two groups could have arisen by chance alone
- Commonly set at 0.05: this means that the probability that the difference between the two groups occurred by chance alone was 0.05, or 1 in 20

TABLE 26-2 Calculating Odds Ratio

	Disease Develops	Disease Does Not Develop
Exposed	A	B
Not exposed	C	D

Note: OR = AD/BC.

- The lower the *p*-value, the lower the chance that the difference occurred by chance alone as opposed to the intervention being tested

Power (P)

- Definition: how good the study is at correctly identifying a difference between therapies if, in reality, they are different
- 1 − Beta (probability of making a type II error) = P
- Probability of correctly concluding that the treatments differ
- Power is commonly set at 80 or 90 percent
- Increases when the sample size and true unknown effect increases and when the intersubject variability decreases

Null Hypothesis (H_0)

- The assumption that there is no difference in parameters (mean, variance) for two or more entities
- Any observed difference in samples is due to chance or sampling error
- Assumes that a hypothesis may not be correct (i.e., no effect of a treatment) and attempts to gather evidence against that assumption (i.e., tries to reject H_0)
- H_0 usually specifies a single point, such as a 0 mmHg reduction in blood pressure, but it can specify an interval: blood pressure reduction between −1 and +1 mmHg
- Statisticians often use H_0 to indicate the statistical hypothesis being tested

Type I Error (Alpha)

- In hypothesis testing, rejecting the null hypothesis (no difference) when it is in fact true
- There was an assumed relationship where none existed (Table 26-3)

Type II Error (Beta)

- In hypothesis testing, failing to reject a false null hypothesis
- It is assumed that no relationship exists when in fact it does (Table 26-3)

Variance

- A measure of the spread or variability of a distribution
- Equaling the average value of the squared difference between measurements and the population mean measurement
- Variances are typically useful only when the measurements follow a normal or at least a symmetric distribution

TABLE 26-3 Understanding Hypothesis Testing

Study Results	Reality	
	Treatments Are Really Not Different	Treatments Are Really Different
Treatments are *not* different	Correct decision (1 − alpha)	Type II error (probability = beta)
Treatments *are* different	Type I error (probability = alpha)	Correct decision (probability = 1 − beta) (power)
Note: Only pertains to outcomes of a randomized controlled trial.		

Confidence Interval

- If the 95 percent confidence limits for an unknown quantity are [a; b], then 95 percent of similarly constructed confidence limits in repeated samples from the same population would contain the unknown quantity
- One could say that there is 95 percent confidence that the unknown value is in the interval [a; b]
- A confidence interval should be symmetric about a point estimate only when the distribution of the point estimate is symmetric

Mean

- Arithmetic average
- Sum of all the values divided by the number of observations

Median

- Middle point of a data set; 50 percent of the values are below this point, and 50 percent are above this point
- Not heavily influenced by outliers, so it can be more representative of typical subjects
- When the data happen to be normally (gaussian) distributed, the median is not as precise as the mean in describing the central tendency

Standard Deviation (SD)

- A measure of the variability (spread) of measurements across subjects
- Standard deviation has a simple interpretation only if the data distribution is gaussian (normal), and in that restrictive case, the mean 2 standard deviations is expected to cover 95 percent of the distribution of the measurement; 1 SD holds 68 percent of values, and 3 SDs holds 99.7 percent of values
- Standard deviation is the square root of the variance (the sum of the squared deviations from the mean divided by the sample size minus one)

Normal (gaussian) Distribution

- Spread of information (such as product performance or demographics)
- The most frequently occurring value is in the middle of the range, and other probabilities tail off symmetrically in both directions
- Graphically categorized by a bell-shaped curve, also known as a *gaussian distribution*
- For normally distributed data, the mean and median are very close and may be identical
- For a normal distribution, the probability that a measurement will fall within 1.96 standard deviations of the mean is 0.95

Multivariable Model/Multivariate Analysis

- A model relating multiple predictor variables (risk factors, treatments, etc.) to a single response or dependent variable
- Multivariate analyses are used to examine the relationship between a single response and a dependent variable and multiple predictor variables
- One can ascertain the relationship between a predictor variable and the dependent variable independently and account for the effects of other predictor variables

Intention to Treat

- Subjects are analyzed according to the treatment group to which they were assigned, even if they did not receive the intended treatment or received only a portion of it
- This analysis reflects real-world nonadherence to treatment

Disease Incidence

- Number of *new* disease cases per population at risk
- The number of new disease cases in the population during a specific time divided by the number of individuals at risk of developing the disease during that specific time

- High incidence implies high disease occurrence
- Low incidence implies low disease occurrence
- Measured over a given time interval
- Determines probability of developing a specific disease
- Used to detect etiologic factors

Disease Prevalence

- Number of *current* cases per population at risk: the number of current disease cases at a specific time divided by the number of individuals in the population at that specific time
- Old: persistent active disease contracted previously
- New: onset of active disease
- Point prevalence: disease prevalence at a point in time
- Period prevalence: disease prevalence over a given period of time
- Measures amount of illness in the community
- Determines health care needs of the community

Reliability

- Precision of a test
- Measures the reproducibility and consistency of a test
- Reduced by random error

Test Validity

- Accuracy of a test
- Measures the trueness of measurement
- Reduced by systematic error
- Four types
  - Internal validity: Is there in fact a causal relationship between the experimental treatment and the observed effect?
  - Construct validity of cause: infers that the observed effect is attributable to the specific experimental intervention and not other variables of effect; infers that the conceptual dependent variable is accurately reflected by the dependent variable as operationalized and measured
  - External validity: Could the observed effect be produced in other settings, with other populations at other times?
  - Statistical conclusion validity: Are the conclusions reached justifiable on statistical grounds?

Correlation Coefficient

- Measures how related are two values
- The range of the coefficient is −1 to +1
- The important point in determining the strength of the relationship between two variables is how far the number is from zero (absolute value)
- Zero equals no association, +1 equals a perfect positive correlation, and −1 equals a perfect negative correlation

Research Error

- Two types of research error
  - Random error: handled with the use of statisitcal tests and methods
  - Systematic error: uncontrolled error that may change the results and/or interpretation of research

Selection Bias

- Introduction of error due to systematic differences in the characteristics of those selected to participate in a study or receive an intervention and/or allowing potential participants to self-select for the intervention
- Two types
  - Sampling bias: Error results from failure to ensure that all members of the reference population have a known chance of being selected for inclusion in the sample
  - Allocation bias: Error results from systematic differences in the characteristics of those assigned to treatment versus control groups in a controlled study

Randomization

- Best means of avoiding allocation bias
- Balances the groups for prognostic factors (i.e., disease severity)
- Eliminates overrepresentation of any one characteristic within the study group
- Should be concealed from the clinicians and researchers of the study to help eliminate conscious or unconscious bias

Blinding

- People involved in the study do not know which treatments are given to which patients
- With double blinding, neither the patient nor the clinician knows which treatment is being administered
- Eliminates bias and preconceived notions as to how the treatments should be working

Sample Size

- Specifications needed to estimate sample size in a randomized trial
  - Differences in response rates to be detected
  - Estimate of the response rate in one of the groups
  - Level of statistical significance (alpha)
  - Level of power (1 − beta)
  - Whether test should be one- or two-tailed
- Large enough number needed to reject a null result (i.e., to be sure that there is some treatment effect)

"Gold Standard"

- Provides objective criteria (e.g., laboratory test not requiring interpretation) or a current clinical standard (e.g., a venogram for deep venous thrombosis) for diagnosis

CLINICAL TRIALS: TYPES OF STUDIES

Case-Control Study (Retrospective Study)

- A group of individuals with the *disease* (cases) and a group of people *without disease* (controls) are identified
- The proportion of cases and controls that were exposed and the proportion that were not exposed are determined by looking in the past
- Patients in the present who have the specific condition in question are then compared with people who do not with respect to the exposure in question.
- Less reliable than randomized controlled trials and cohort studies because a statistical relationship does not mean that one factor necessarily caused the other
- Can only determine odds ratio (OR)

Case Report

- A report on a single patient
- Reports of cases with no control groups with which to compare outcomes; they have no statistical validity

Case Series

- Consists of collections of reports on the treatment of individual patients

Cohort Study (Prospective Study)

- Groups of *exposed* and *nonexposed* individuals are followed to compare the incidence of disease (or rate of death from disease) in the two groups
- Can determine incidence (new cases) of disease and determine if a temporal relationship exists
- Types of cohort studies
  - Concurrent (concurrent prospective or longitudinal): Original population is defined at the start of the study, and subjects are followed through time until the disease does or does not develop
  - Retrospective cohort (historical cohort, nonconcurrent prospective): Exposed population is defined by historical records, and outcome is determined at the time the study begins
- Not as reliable as randomized controlled studies because the two groups may differ in ways other than the variable under study
- Can determine relative risk (RR) or odds ratio (OR)

Crossover Trial

- Each subject receives both treatments being compared or the treatment and control

- Used for patients who have a stable, usually chronic condition during both treatment periods

Meta-Analysis

- Uses statistical techniques to combine the results of several studies as if they were one large study

Phases of Clinical Trials

- Phase 1
  - Studies to obtain preliminary information on dosage, absorption, metabolism, and the relationship between toxicity and the dose-schedule of treatment
- Phase II
  - Studies to determine feasibility and estimate treatment activity and safety in diseases (or, for example, tumor types) for which the treatment appears promising
  - Generates hypotheses for later testing
- Phase III
  - Comparative trial to determine the effectiveness and safety of a new treatment relative to standard therapy
  - These trials usually represent the most rigorous proof of treatment efficacy (pivotal trials) and are the last stage before product licensing
- Phase IV: postmarketing studies of licensed products

Practice Guidelines

- Evidence-based developed statements to assist practitioners about appropriate health care for specific clinical circumstances
- Guidelines review and evaluate the evidence and then make explicit recommendations for practice

Randomized Controlled Trials

- Study the effect of a therapy or test on real patients
- Include methodologies that reduce the potential for bias and that allow for comparison between intervention groups and control groups (no intervention)
- Evidence for questions of diagnosis is found in prospective trials that compare tests with a reference or "gold standard" test

Retrospective Study

- Uses data that existed prior to the date that the study was designed

Systematic Reviews

- Focus on a clinical topic and answer a specific question

- Extensive literature searches are conducted to identify studies with sound methodology
- The studies are reviewed, assessed, and summarized according to the predetermined criteria of the review question

COMPARISON OF DATA

Analysis of Variance

- Used to determine if samples are actually from a single population
- Does not allow you to compare which groups are more like to differ from the other (that's the *t* test)

t Test

- Used to test for differences between the mean values of two treatment groups
- Employs the statistic (t): t = difference of sample means/standard error of the difference in sample means

Chi-Square Test

- Used to determine if differences exist between observed and expected frequencies of results that are tabulated in a 2×2 contingency table
- Statistical test that consists of three different types of analysis
  - Goodness of fit: determines if the sample under analysis was drawn from a population that follows some specified distribution
  - Test for homogeneity: answers the proposition that several populations are homogeneous with respect to some characteristic
  - Test of independence: tests the null hypothesis, which states that two criteria of classification, when applied to a population of subjects, are independent; if they are not independent, then there is an association between them

REFERENCES

Glantz S: *Primer of Biostatistics,* 5th Ed. New York: McGraw-Hill; 2002.
Gordis L: *Epidemiology,* 3rd Ed. Philadelphia: Saunders, 2004.

CHAPTER 27

CUTANEOUS MANIFESTATIONS OF METABOLIC DISEASES

VICTOR R. LAVIS
ASRA ALI

PORPHYRIAS

- Porphyrias are metabolic disorders of heme synthesis
- Partial enzymic deficiencies result in excessive accumulation and excretion of 5-aminolevulinic acid (ALA), porphobilinogen (PBG), and/or porphyrins
- Photosensitivity is caused by absorption of ultraviolet (UV) radiation in the Soret band (400 to 410 nm)
- Two groups: the "hepatic" and "erythropoietic" types
- Cutaneous porphyrias: porphyrias with skin manifestations
- Acute porphyrias: characterized by sudden attacks of pain and other neurologic manifestations
- Heme synthesis: partly in the mitochondria and partly in the cytoplasm
  - Initial reaction in heme biosynthesis takes place in the mitochondrion
  - Condensation of 1-glycine and 1-succinylCoA by Δ-aminolevulinic acid synthase (ALA synthase): rate-limiting reaction of heme biosynthesis
  - Mitochondrial Δ-aminolevulinic acid (ALA) is transported to the cytosol
  - ALA dehydratase (also called *porphobilinogen synthase*) dimerizes two molecules of ALA to produce porphobilinogen
  - Uroporphyrinogen I synthase, also called *porphobilinogen deaminase* or *PBG deaminase,* causes condensation of four molecules of porphobilinogen to produce intermediate hydroxymethylbilane
  - Hydroxymethylbilane undergoes enzymatic conversion to uroporphyrinogen III by uroporphyrinogen synthase plus a protein known as *uroporphyrinogen III cosynthase*

- In the cytosol, the acetate substituents of uroporphyrinogen (normal uroporphyrinogen III or abnormal uroporphyrinogen I) are decarboxylated by uroporphyrinogen decarboxylase
- The resulting coproporphyrinogen III intermediate is transported to the interior of the mitochondrion, where, after decarboxylation, protoporphyrinogen IX results
- In the mitochondrion, protoporphyrinogen IX is converted to protoporphyrin IX by protoporphyrinogen IX oxidase
- Final reaction in heme synthesis takes place in the mitochondrion by ferrochelatase

Erythropoietic Porphyria (EP)

- Gunther's disease: congenital erythropoietic porphyria
- Inheritance/defect: autosomal recessive defect of uroporphyrinogen III cosynthetase
- Clinical
  - Appears soon after birth
  - Severe photosensitivity with burning, edema, bullae, mutilating scars
  - Red urine
  - Erythrodontia (seen with Wood's lamp)
  - Hypertrichosis
  - Splenomegaly
  - Hemolytic anemia
- Laboratory findings
  - Urine: uroporphyrin I, coproporphyrin I
  - Stool: coproporphyrin I
  - Blood: uroporphyrin I, protoporphyrin
- Course/management
  - Strict photoprotection

349

- Splenectomy
- Blood transfusions

Erythropoietic Protoporphyria (EPP)

- Inheritance/defect
  - Autosomal dominant
  - *FECH* gene
  - Ferrochelatase deficiency
- Clinical
  - Mainly affects the skin
  - Painful erythematous, edematous plaques after exposure to UV light
  - Aged appearance, scarring
  - Porphyrin gallstones
  - Liver disease in 10 percent
- Laboratory findings
  - Urine: normal
  - Stool: protoporphyrin
  - Blood: protoporphyrin
- Course/management
  - Photoprotection
  - Beta-carotene
  - Normal life span if liver spared

Porphyria Cutanea Tarda (PCT) (Fig. 27-1)

- Inheritance/defect
  - Autosomal dominant
  - Uroporphyrinogen decarboxylase deficiency
  - Most common of the porphyrias
- Features
  - Bullae, erosions on sun-exposed skin
  - Hypertrichosis, milia

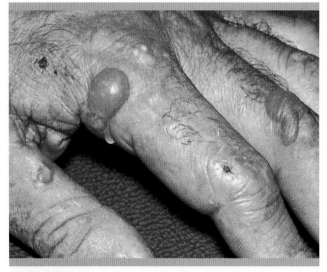

FIGURE 27-1 Porphyria cutanea tarda. *(From Freedberg IM et al: Fitzpatrick's Dermatology in General Medicine, 6th ed. New York: McGraw-Hill, 2003, p. 1453.)*

- Coral-pink fluorescence of urine under Wood's lamp
- Associated with hepatitis C, hepatocellular carcinoma, increased liver iron stores, HIV (human immunodeficiency virus) infection, dermatomyositis
- Laboratory findings
  - Urine: uroporphyrin I–III > coproporphyrin
  - Stool: isocoproporphyrins, tetracarboxyl porphyrins
  - Blood: normal
  - Serum iron: increased
  - Liver biopsy: hepatocellular damage with fatty infiltration and hemosiderosis
- Course/management
  - Phlebotomy
  - Antimalarials (hydroxychloroquine or chloroquine)
  - Avoidance of alcohol, estrogen, iron supplements
  - Photoprotection
  - Interferon for hepatitis C

Acute Intermittent Porphyria (AIP)

- Inheritance/defect
  - Autosomal dominant
  - Porphobilinogen (PBG) deaminase deficiency
- Features
  - No skin findings
  - Periodic attacks of abdominal colic
  - Neurologic disorders (neuropathy, palsy, seizures, coma)
  - Psychiatric disorders (confusion)
  - Attacks may be precipitated by drugs, hormones, fever, or starvation
  - Risk of hepatic carcinoma
  - Hyponatremia: inappropriate release of antidiuretic hormone
- Laboratory findings
  - Urine: aminolevulinic acid (ALA) and porphobilinogen (PBG)
  - Erythrocyte PBG deaminase activity: to help distinguish acute intermittent porphyria from variegate porphyria and hereditary coproporphyria
  - Stool: normal
  - Blood: normal
- Course/management
  - Avoid precipitators
  - Glucose loading and hematin infusions during attacks; supportive care
  - Acute attacks may be life-threatening and leave residual neurologic deficits

Variegate Porphyria (VP)

- Mixed porphyria
- Inheritance/defect
  - Autosomal dominant

- Protoporphyrinogen oxidase deficiency
- Most common in South Africans
- Features
  - Skin lesions of PCT
  - Gastrointestinal and neurologic symptoms similar to AIP
  - Attacks may be precipitated by alcohol, hormones, and drugs (dapsone, anticonvulsants, barbiturates)
- Laboratory findings
  - Urine: ALA, PBG during attacks; coproporphyrin > protoporphyrin (acute and asymptomatic periods: helps distinguish from PCT)
  - Stool: protoporphyrin
  - Blood: porphyrin (fluoresces at 626 nm)
- Course/management
  - Avoid precipitators
  - Photoprotection
  - Treat acute attacks as AIP

Hereditary Coproporphyria (HCP)

- Inheritance/defect
  - Autosomal dominant
  - Coproporphyrinogen oxidase deficiency
- Features
  - Similar to AIP and VP, with gastrointestinal and neurologic attacks
  - Thirty percent develop photosensitive bullae
  - Homozygous deficiency of coproporphyrinogen oxidase
  - Photosensitivity, hypertrichosis, and hemolytic anemia beginning in childhood
- Course/management
  - Urine: coproporphyrin III, ALA, PBG during attacks
  - Stool: coproporphyrin III
  - Blood: normal
- Course/management
  - Avoid precipitators
  - Photoprotection
  - Treat acute attacks as with AIP

Hepatoerythropoietic Porphyria (HEP)

- Inheritance/defect
  - Autosomal dominant
  - Uroporphyrinogen decarboxylase deficiency (homozygous form of PCT)
- Features
  - Severe photophotosensitivity with burning, erythema, vesicles, bullae
  - Mutilating scar formation
  - Hypertrichosis
  - Hemolytic anemia, splenomegaly
  - Dark urine at birth
  - Erythrodontia

- Laboratory findings
  - Urine: uroporphyrin I–III
  - Stool: uroporphyrin, coproporphyrin, isocoproporphyrin
  - Blood: protoporphyrin
  - Erythrodontia
- Course/management
  - Photoprotection
  - Oral charcoal
  - Normal lifespan

ALA Dehydrogenase—Deficiency Porphyria

- Inheritance/defect
  - Autosomal recessive
  - ALA dehydrogenase deficiency
- Features
  - No skin lesions
  - Symptoms similar to AIP
- Laboratory findings
  - Urine: ALA, coproporphyrin, uroporphyrin
  - Stool: coproporphyrin, protoporphyrin
  - Blood: protoporphyrin
- Course/management: Alcohol and stress may precipitate

SPHINGOLIPIDOSES (LIPID STORAGE DISORDERS)

- Inherited disorders with a deficiency of a lysosomal hydrolase
- Leads to lysosomal accumulation of the enzyme's specific sphingolipid substrate

Fabry's Disease (Angiokeratoma Corporis Diffusum)

- X-linked recessive, Xq22
- Defective α-galactosidase A
- Results in accumulation and deposition of glycosphingolipids (globotriaosylceramide) in plasma and lysosomes of vascular endothelial and smooth muscle cells
- Presents in adolescence
- Clinical
  - Ischemia
  - Angiokeratomas at lower trunk, thighs, oral/ocular mucosa (Fig. 27-2)
  - Painful crises, acroparesthesias
  - Coronary artery disease
  - Renal failure
  - "Maltese crosses" in urine: lipid inclusions with characteristic birefringence
  - Cerebrovascular accident (CVA), peripheral neuropathy
  - Corneal opacities
- Course/management
  - Death by fifth decade from myocardial infarction, CVA, and renal failure

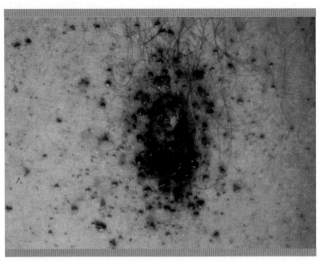

FIGURE 27-2 Angiokeratomas. *(From Freedberg IM et al: Fitzpatrick's Dermatology in General Medicine, 6th ed. New York: McGraw-Hill, 2003, p. 1476.)*

- Dialysis
- Pain management of crises
- Phenytoin and carbamazepine for paresthesias

Gaucher Disease

- Autosomal recessive
- Decreased β-glucocerebrosidase activity with resulting accumulation of glucocerebroside in histiocytes (Gaucher cells)
- Clinical
  - Type I (adult)
    - Diffuse hyperpigmetation
    - Bone pain, fractures, aseptic necrosis of femoral head hepatosplenomegaly, lymphadenopathy, pingueculae
    - Pancytopenia
  - Type II (infantile)
    - CNS involved with hypertonicity, neck rigidity, laryngeal spasm, dysphagia
    - Hepatosplenomegaly
    - Aspiration pneumonia
  - Type III: rapid deterioration
- Laboratory studies
  - Gaucher cell in the reticuloendothelial system
    - Wrinkled-paper appearance resulting from presence of intracytoplasmic inclusions
    - Erlenmeyer flask deformity of the distal femur
- Course/management
  - Type I: imiglucerase (Cerezyme), a recombinant-derived analogue of β-glucocerebrosidase
  - Bone marrow transplant, splenectomy
  - Type II: supportive care, antibiotics (enzyme replacement is unable to cross blood-brain barrier); death at 1 to 2 years owing to aspiration

Niemann-Pick Disease (NPD)

- Autosomal recessive
- High incidence in Ashkenazi Jews
- Sphingomyelinase deficiency with sphingomyelin accumulation (foam cells)
- Clinical
  - Type A (most common): xanthomas, psychomotor deterioration, hepatosplenomegaly, failure to thrive, lymphadenopathy, blindness, cherry red spots in fovea, deafness, pneumonia
  - Type B: central nervous system spared
  - Type C
    - Developmental delay, psychomotor deterioration, hepatosplenomegaly
    - Cholesterol esterification defect (normal sphingomyelinase)
- Laboratory studies: Niemann-Pick cells: lipid-laden foam cells
- Course/management
  - Type A: death by 2 to 3 years with failure to thrive, pneumonia
  - Type B: death in adolescence or adulthood
  - Type C: death in adolescence

Fucosidosis

- Autosomal recessive
- Alpha-L-fucosidase deficiency: abnormal accumulations of glycosphingolipids, glycolipids, and glycoproteins (fucose-containing compounds)
- Clinical
  - Type I: neurologic changes, cardiomegaly, severe mental retardation, respiratory tract infections, hyperhidrosis
  - Type II
    - Late infantile onset
    - Short stature
    - Coarse facies, mental retardation, hypertonia
    - Angiokeratomas (similar distribution to Fabry's disease)
    - Longer survival than type I

Farber (Acid Ceramidase Deficiency, Lipogranulomatosis)

- Autosomal recessive
- Clinical
  - Subcutaneous, periarticular swelling
  - Visceral nodules (lipogranulomatosis)
  - Mental retardation
  - Mild macular degeneration
  - Arthropathy
  - Hoarse cry
  - Pulmonary failure

Mucopolysaccharidoses (MPS) (Lysosomal Storage Diseases)

- Inherited deficiency of enzymes
- Involved in the degradation of glycosaminoglycans (GAGs); also refered to as *acid mucopolysaccharides*
  - Dermatan sulfate, heparan sulfate, keratan sulfate (KS), and chondroitin sulfate are the main GAGs in tissues
  - Composed of sulfated sugar and uronic acid residues (except for KS)
  - Degraded by a series of lysosomal enzymes
- Diseases are autosomal recessive, except for MPS type II, which is X-linked

Hurler's Syndrome (MPS-IH, Gargoylism)

- Autosomal recessive
- Defect in alpha-L-iduronidase
- Dermatan, heparan sulfate accumulation
- Classic form of MPS
- Clinical
  - Coarse facies with macrocephaly, hypertelorism
  - Hirsutism
  - Valvular disease
  - Umbilical hernias
  - Upper respiratory infections
  - Corneal opacities
  - Short stature, fingers, dysostosis multiplex
  - Scheie MPS-IS
    - Onset at 5 or 6 years
    - Mild form of the MPS-IH
    - Aortic valve disease
    - Joint stiffness, claw hands, deformed feet, genu valgum
    - Deafness
    - Corneal clouding
    - Normal intelligence and life span
  - Scheie and Hurler compound syndromes (MPS-IH/S)
    - Clinically intermediate between types IH and IS
    - Healthy at birth; onset of symptoms at 3 to 8 years
    - Corneal clouding, joint stiffness, dysostosis multiplex, and heart disease
- Course
- Deaths caused by upper airway obstruction and pulmonary complications
- Treatment
  - Bone marrow transplantation for Hurler's syndrome (not helpful for Hunter)
  - Laronidase: increases catabolism of glycosaminoglycans (GAGs)
  - Corrective surgery for joint contractures

Hunter Syndrome (MPS II)

- Inheritance
- X-linked recessive
- Defect of iduronate 2-sulfatase
- Accumulation of heparan and dermatan sulfate
- Clinical
  - Type A
    - Severe form
    - Clinical features similar to MPS-IH
    - Ivory papules distributed symmetrically between the angles of the scapulae and posterior axillary lines
    - Marker for the disease
    - Hypertrichosis may result in synophrys
    - Atypical retinitis pigmentosa
  - Type B
    - Mild form
    - Clinical features similar to MPS-IS
    - Airway obstruction secondary to accumulation of mucopolysaccharide in the trachea and bronchi
    - Deafness
- Treatment: symptomatic care

Sanfilippo Syndrome (MPS Type III)

- Heparan sulfate sulfamidase deficiency
- Accumulation of heparan sulfate
- Clinical
  - Regression of psychomotor development
  - Neurologic signs (e.g., hyperactivity, autistic features, behavioral disorder)

Morquio Syndrome (MPS Type IVA)

- Classic form
- Galactosamine-6-sulfatase deficiency
- Accumulation of keratan sulfate and chondroitin-6-sulfate
- Clinical
  - Abnormalities of the skeletal system (e.g., kyphoscoliosis, pectus carinatum, subluxation of the hips)
  - Aortic valvular disease
  - Dental abnormalities

Morquio Syndrome (MPS Type IVB)

- β-Galactosidase deficiency
- Accumulation of chondroitin-6-sulfate

Maroteaux-Lamy Syndrome (MPS Type VI)

- First clinical signs usually appear in the first 2 years of life
- Psychomotor retardation
- Resembles Hurler syndrome

Sly Syndrome (MPS Type VII)

- Arylsulfatase B
- Hepatosplenomegaly

- Clinical: facial deformities: hypertelorism, prominent maxilla, depressed bridge of the nose
- Diagnosis: mucopolysaccharide staining
  - Acid: hematoxylin and eosin, Giemsa, colloidal iron mucicarmine, Alcian blue, pH 2.5, methyl and toludine blue
  - Neutral: periodic acid Schiff, gamori methinamine silver
  - Sulfated: aldehyde fuschin, Alcian blue, pH 0.5

DISORDERS OF AMINO ACID METABOLISM

Alkaptonuria/Ochronosis

- Autosomal recessive
- Deficient homogentisic acid oxidase
- Presents childhood to adulthood
- Clinical
  - Ochronosis
    - Macular blue-gray pigmentation on face, sclera, cartilage, and tendons
    - Papules, milia, and nodules also can occur
  - Black cerumen and sweat
  - Dark urine at pH > 7
  - Large joint arthropathy
  - Calcification of intervertebral discs
  - Localized exogenous
    - No joint involvement
    - Secondary to chemicals that inhibit homogentisic acid oxidase
    - Quinacrine, carbolic acid, hydroquinone, phenol, resorcinol, picric acid
- Diagnosis
  - Urinary homogentisic acid level
  - Darkening of urine with NaOH
- Histology: ochronotic (yellow-brown) pigment in dermis, "yellow bananas," and within macrophages, homogenization and swelling of collagen bundles
- Treatment
  - Arthritis: analgesics, physical therapy
  - Pigment changes persist

Phenylketonuria (PKU)

- Autosomal recessive
- Chromosome arm 12q
- Presents at birth
- Deficiency of phenylalanine hydroxylase
- Malignant PKU
  - Patients also have a deficiency in the enzyme's cofactor, tetrahydrobiopterin
  - Cofactor required for
    - Hydroxylation of tyrosine (a precursor of dopamine)
    - Hydroxylation of tryptophan (a precursor of serotonin)
- Clinical
  - Toxic CNS effects
  - Mental retardation, seizures, hyperreflexia
  - Generalized hypopigmentation, blond hair, blue eyes; due to tyrosine deficiency
  - Eczema, sclerodermoid skin
  - Urine has "mousy" odor
- Diagnosis: routine neonatal screening
- Treatment: begin low-phenylalanine diet early to prevent CNS and skin changes
- Course: Normal life span if treated early

Homocystinuria

- Autosomal recessive
- Cystathionine β-synthetase deficiency
- Defect in methionine metabolism
- Accumulation of homocystine
- Competitive inhibitor of tyrosinase
- Presents in early childhood
- Clinical
  - Marfanoid habitus
  - Malar rash, livedo reticularis
  - Pale and pink skin: due to tyrosine deficiency
  - Buccal skin shows red macules
  - Hyperhidrosis, dry skin, and acrocyanosis
  - Ectopia lentis with downward displacement, glaucoma
  - Mental retardation, seizures, cerebrovascular occlusions
  - Leg ulcers, deep venous thrombosis
- Treatment
  - Low methionine
  - High-cystine diet
  - Pyridoxine (300 to 600 mg/day)
  - Folic acid, betaine, cyanocobalamin
- Course: death in third to fourth decade from vascular events

Richner-Hanhart Syndrome (Tyrosinemia II)

- Hepatic tyrosine aminotransferase
- Clinical
  - Herpetiform corneal ulcers, blindness
  - Focal or diffuse palmoplantar keratoderma
  - Hyperkeratotic lesions of the digits, palms, and soles
  - Mental retardation
  - Erosions, bullae
  - Hyperkeratotic plaques on elbows, knees
- Treatment
  - Topical therapy, oral retinoids
  - Low-phenylalanine/tyrosine diet can prevent skin and eye manifestations

Lipoid Proteinosis (Urbach-Wiethe Disease, Hyalinosis Cutis et Mucosae)

- Autosomal recessive
- Defect in extracellular matrix protein 1
- *ECM1* gene
- Accumulation of eosinophilic material composed of mucopolysaccharides, hyaluronic acid, neutral fat, lipids, and cholesterol
- Clinical
  - Patchy areas of alopecia may develop where hyaline deposits are present
  - Oral cavity: cobblestone appearance to mucosa
  - Earliest sign: hoarse cry owing to vocal cord infiltration
  - Early bullae formation: the face and distal extremities
  - Heal with ice-pick scarring
  - Beaded papules along the eyelid margins (moniliform blepharitis) (Fig. 27-3)
  - Infiltrative papules on mucous membranes, large "wooden" tongue, parotiditis
  - Verrucous nodules on elbows, knees, and hands
  - Patchy alopecia, dental anomalies
  - Skin becomes waxy, thickened, and yellow
- Diagnosis: computed tomography or x-ray: hippocampal "bean-shaped" calcifications
- Treatment: oral dimethylsulfoxide may be helpful
- Course: chronic course

Wilson Disease (Hepatolenticular Degeneration)

- Autosomal recessive
- Defect of *ATP7B* gene: copper-transporting adenosine triphosphatase (ATPase) in the liver

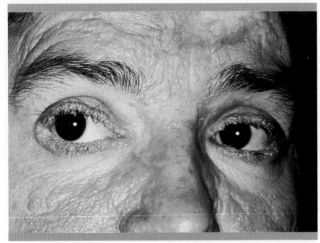

FIGURE 27-3 Lipoid proteinosis. *(From Freedberg IM et al: Fitzpatrick's Dermatology in General Medicine, 6th ed. New York: McGraw-Hill, 2003, p. 1487.)*

- Excessive absorption of copper from the small intestine
- Decreased excretion of copper by the liver
- Clinical
  - Copper accumulates in liver, brain, and cornea
  - Seen in childhood to adulthood
  - Hepatomegaly, cirrhosis
  - Dysarthria, ataxia, dementia
  - Kayser-Fleischer ring: deposition of copper in Descemet membrane of cornea
  - Pretibial hyperpigmentation
  - Blue lunulae
  - Jaundice, varices, spider angiomas, and palmar erythema
- Treatment
  - D-Penicillamine, copper chelators, liver transplant, decreased copper intake
  - Symptoms reverse (except CNS) with early treatment

Hemochromatosis

- Autosomal recessive
- Mutations in the *HFE* gene
- Chromosome 6
- Increased iron absorption with solid-organ iron deposition
- Presents in fifth decade
- Clinical
  - Diffuse gray hyperpigmentation
  - Sparse hair
  - Koilonychia
  - Hepatomegaly
  - Cardiac failure, arrhythmias, diabetes, hypogonadism, polyarthritis
- Treatment: serial phlebotomy, deferoxamine, supportive care of diabetes, arrhythmias
- Course: premature death owing to hepatic failure, hepatocellular carcinoma, heart disease

Amyloidosis

- Insoluble protein fibrils accumulate extracellularly
- Diagnosis
  - Amorphous eosinophilic appearance on light microscopy after hematoxylin and eosin (H&E) staining
  - Bright green fluorescence observed under polarized light after Congo red staining
  - Regular fibrillar structure as observed by electron microscopy
  - Beta-pleated sheet structure as observed by x-ray diffraction
  - Solubility in water and buffers of low ionic strength

Systemic Amyloidosis

Fibril Protein and Related Diseases

- A amyloidosis protein (AA)
- Apo-SAA (serum amyloid A protein)
- Acute-phase protein secondary to inflammation
- Precursor protein is a normal sequence
- Non-immunoglobin-related protein
- Clinical
  - Secondary systemic
  - Chronic inflammation is associated with amyloid deposition
    - Leprosy
    - Osteomyelitis
    - Tuberculosis
    - Rheumatoid arthritis
    - Familial Mediterranean fever
    - Hodgkin's disease
    - Renal cell carcinoma
  - No skin findings
  - Also associated with
    - Familial Mediterranean fever
      - ▲ Autosomal recessive
      - ▲ Chromosome 16, mutation in the gene *pyrin* (*Marenostrin*)
      - ▲ Self-limited attacks of fever accompanied by peritonitis, pleurisy, and arthritis
      - ▲ Erysipelas, eruption on lower legs
      - ▲ Urticaria
      - ▲ Henoch-Schonlein purpura
      - ▲ Treatment: colchicine (preventative)
      - ▲ NSAIDs
    - AA Muckle-Wells
      - ▲ Autosomal dominant
      - ▲ Urticaria, fever, paresthesias, limb pain, deafness, renal
- Histology: AA amyloid first in interstitium and blood vessel wall, then replacement of parenchyma, deposition within glomeruli and peritubular, renal failure
- Treatment: control underlying disorder, etretinate, psoralen and UVA light, dimethyl sulfoxide

Amyloid Light Chain (AL)

- Primary systemic
- Monoclonal plasma cell disorders closely related to multiple myeloma
- Most commonly lambda light chain (88 percent)
- Clinical
  - Renal: nephrotic syndrome with peripheral edema
  - Cardiac: restrictive cardiomyopathy
  - Soft tissues enlarged ("shoulder pad sign")
  - Mucocutaneous
    - Petechiae, ecchymoses, pinch purpura (posttrauma around orbits, umbilicus, axillae, perianal) (Fig. 27-4)
    - Papules, plaques (waxy, shiny)/neuropathies, arrhythmias
    - Macroglossia
  - Carpal tunnel, 17 percent
  - Hepatosplenomegaly
  - Gastrointestinal bleeding
  - Neuropathy: Deposition occurs in the peripheral nerves
  - Localized
    - Cutaneus nodular form (see below)
    - Tumefactive: organ-limited (lungs)
  - Associated with AL Waldenstrom's macroglobulinemia, benign monoclonal gammopathy, heavy-chain disease, angioimmunoblastic lymphadenopathy, nodular malignant lymphoma, agammaglobulinemia
- Diagnosis
  - Biopsy of abdominal fat (capillaries involved) or biopsy of an affected organ
  - Histology
    - Eosinophilic, amorphous, fissured masses of amyloid in dermis and subcutaneous tissue, extravasated red blood cells, no lymph, intradermal bullae around blood vessels; amyloid rings (amyloid around individual fat cells)
    - Stains:
      - ▲ *Congo red* (brick red, apple-green birefringence)
      - ▲ *Cystal violet* (metalchromasia [red])

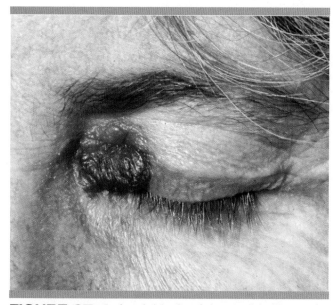

FIGURE 27-4 Amyloidosis of the eyelid. *(From Freedberg IM et al: Fitzpatrick's Dermatology in General Medicine, 6th ed. New York: McGraw-Hill, 2003, p. 1430.)*

▲ *Methyl violet* (metachromasia)
▲ *PAS+ and diastase-resistant*
- Indirect immunofluouresence: differentiates AA/AL
- Bone marrow: 10 percent plasma cells in 40 percent of patients
- Monoclonal Ig light chain 90 percent in serum or urine (Bence-Jones protein)
- Immunoelectrophoresis: monoclonal protein
- Treatment
  - Chemotherapy
    - Melphalan, vincristine, cyclophosphamide
  - Prednisone
  - Colchicine
  - Penicillamine
  - Azathioprine

TRANSTHYRETIN (TTR)

- Transport protein synthesized in the liver and choroid plexus
- Transports thyroxine and retinol
- Familial amyloidosis: deposits primarily in the peripheral nerves, heart, gastrointestinal tract, and vitreous of eyes
- Senile cardiac amyloidosis
  - Forms amyloid deposits in the cardiac ventricles of elderly people
  - Increases progressively with age, affecting 25 percent or more of the population

BETA-2 MICROGLOBULIN (AB2M)

- Hemodialysis-associated
- Protein accumulates in the serum
- Organs involved
  - Carpal ligament, possibly, the synovial membranes: arthropathies and bone cysts
  - Heart, gastrointestinal tract, liver, lungs, prostate, adrenals, and tongue

Localized Amyloid

ALTERED KERATIN

- Amyloid deposits bind to antikeratin antibodies
- Lichen amyloidosis
  - Closely set, discrete brown-red papules, pruritic
  - Commonly on the legs
- Macular amyloidosis
  - Due to constant scratching
  - Brown-gray, reticulated, rippled, macules/patches mainly on upper back
  - Notalgia paresthetica
  - Some postinflammatory hyperpigmentation
- Diagnosis: direct immunoflouresence: IgM, C3, Ig, light chains

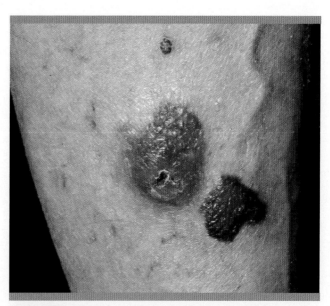

FIGURE 27-5 Nodular amyloidosis. *(From Freedberg IM et al: Fitzpatrick's Dermatology in General Medicine, 6th ed. New York: McGraw-Hill, 2003, p. 1431.)*

- Histology
  - Amyloid deposits in papillary dermis, globular, colloid deposition in dermis
  - Lichen type with epidermal hyperplasia
- Treatment
  - Class I/II topical steroids, intralesional steroids, Dimethyl sulfoxide (DMSO)
  - Macular—UV-B, antihistamines

NODULAR AMYLOIDOSIS

- Localized to skin
- Deposition of AL protein
- One or several nodules on legs/face (Fig. 27-5)
- Histology: atrophic epidermis, masses of amyloid dermis, subcutaneous fat, appears as "cracks in mud," lymphocytoplasmic infiltrate scattered through, Russell bodies: round hyaline, eosinophilic bodies inside/outside of plasma cells (with Ig), foreign-body giant cells
- Treatment
  - Surgical excision, CO₂ laser + recurrence
  - Can develop systemic amyloidosis

SENILE AMYLOIDOSIS

- Associated with Alzheimer's disease
- Senile/neuritic plaques: neurofibrillary tangles, vascular lesions
- Due to β amyloid = major fibril protein
- Amyloid precursor protein (APP)
- No skin lesions

XANTHOMAS

- Accumulations of lipid-laden macrophages
- Lipids transported in plasma as complexes with specific apoproteins, forming lipoproteins
- Lipoproteins: may be classified according to their buoyant density
  - Chylomicrons
  - Very low density lipoproteins (VLDLs)
  - Intermediate-density lipoproteins (IDLs)
  - Low-density lipoproteins (LDLs)
  - High-density lipoproteins (HDLs)

Phenotypic Classification of Hyperlipidemias

- Hyperchylomicronemia
  - Example: familial lipoprotein lipase deficiency
  - Frederickson type I
  - Eruptive xanthomas
- Isolated increased LDL
  - Frederickson type IIA
  - Tendinous or tuberous xanthomas, as well as xanthelasmas
- Increased LDL and VLDL
  - Frederickson type IIB
  - Tuberous xanthomas, as well as xanthelasmas
- Dysbeta-lipoproteinemia
  - Various mutations of apoprotein E
  - Elevated β-VLDL
  - Frederickson type III
  - Xanthomas, particularly planar (palmar) xanthomas
- Isolated increased VLDL
  - Familial hypertriglyceridemia; Frederickson type IV
  - Hypertriglyceridemia; elevated VLDL and LDL, usually secondary causes
  - Tuberous xanthomas
- Elevated chylomicrons and VLDL
  - Example: defects of the apolipoprotein C-II gene. Apo C-II deficiency also can cause simple hyperchylomicronemia
  - Frederickson type V
  - Eruptive xanthomas

Types of Cutaneous Xanthomas

- Xanthelasma palpebrarum
  - Most common of the xanthomas
  - Fifty-five percent of the patients may have hyperlipidemia
  - Symmetric soft, velvety, yellow, flat, polygonal papules around the eyelids
  - Upper eyelid near the inner canthus
- Tuberous xanthomas (Fig. 27-6)
  - Firm, painless, red-yellow nodules
  - Can coalesce to form multilobated tumors
  - Develop in pressure areas, such as the extensor surfaces of the knees, the elbows, and the buttocks

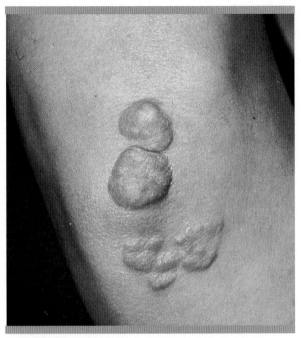

FIGURE 27-6 Tuberous xanthoma. *(From Freedberg IM et al: Fitzpatrick's Dermatology in General Medicine, 6th ed. New York: McGraw-Hill, 2003, p. 1471.)*

- Tendinous xanthomas
  - Subcutaneous nodules related to the tendons or the ligaments
  - Most common locations are the extensor tendons of the hands, the feet, and the Achilles tendons
  - Often related to trauma
- Eruptive xanthomas
  - Crops of small, red-yellow papules on an erythematous base
  - Most commonly arise over the buttocks, the shoulders, and the extensor surfaces of the extremities
  - May resolve spontaneously over weeks
  - Pruritus is common
- Planar xanthomas
  - Macular
  - Can occur in any site: Palmar crease is characteristic of type III dysbetalipoproteinemia
  - Generalized plane xanthomas: cover large areas of the face, neck, thorax, and flexures
  - May be associated with monoclonal gammopathy
- Xanthoma disseminatum
  - Occur in normolipemic patients
  - Red-yellow papules and nodules with a predilection for the flexures
  - Mucosa of the upper part of the aerodigestive tract is involved
  - Usually resolves spontaneously
- Verruciform xanthoma

- Occurs in normolipemic patients
- Oral cavity of adults as a single papillomatous yellow lesion
- Reactive condition with benign behavior
- Histology
  - Vacuolated macrophages filled with lipid (foamy macrophages)
  - Lipids dissolved and removed from the tissue during histologic processing
  - Multinucleated histiocytes (Touton giant cells) are present
- Treatment
  - Local excision
  - Topical trichloroacetic acid
  - Electrodesiccation
  - Laser therapy
  - Recurrences can occur

DIABETES-ASSOCIATED DISEASES

Acanthosis Nigricans

- Marker of insulin resistance
- Excessive amounts of circulating insulin bind with insulin-like growth factor receptors on keratinocytes and dermal fibroblasts
- Activation of tyrosine kinase receptors
  - Epidermal growth factor receptor (EGFR)
  - Insulin-like growth factor receptor
  - Fibroblast growth factor receptor
  - Exert antiapoptotic and mitogenic effects on keratinocytes
- Associated conditions
  - Obesity: most common type
  - Syndromic
    - Insulin resistance
    - Type A syndrome: (HAIR-AN syndrome)
      ▲ Hyperandrogenemia, insulin resistance, and acanthosis nigricans syndrome
      ▲ Polycystic ovaries or signs of virilization
    - Type B syndrome: due to antibodies directed against the insulin receptor: uncontrolled diabetes mellitus, ovarian hyperandrogenism, or an autoimmune disease
  - Familial
    - Autosomal dominant
    - Progresses until puberty, then stabilizes or regresses
  - Drug-induced: nicotinic acid, systemic corticosteroids, oral contraceptives
  - Malignant: most commonly adenocarcinoma of gastrointestinal tract
- Clinical
  - Symmetric, hyperpigmented, velvety plaques (Fig. 27-7)

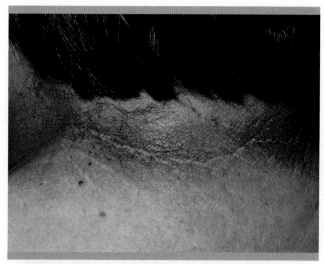

FIGURE 27-7 Acanthosis nigricans. *(From Freedberg IM et al: Fitzpatrick's Dermatology in General Medicine, 6th ed. New York: McGraw-Hill, 2003, p. 1797.)*

- Intertriginous areas of the axilla, groin, and posterior neck
  - Acrochordons (skin tags) often are found
  - Tripe palms
    - Thickening of the palms with accentuation of the ridges and furrows
    - Paraneoplastic sign
    - Seventy-seven percent occurred in association with acanthosis nigricans
    - Ninety-four percent were associated with cancer
- Histology: hyperkeratosis, papillomatosis, and slight irregular acanthosis with minimal or no hyperpigmentation; the dermal papillae project upward as finger-like projections
- Treatment
  - Correct the underlying disease
  - Topical tretinoin

Necrobiosis Lipoidica Diabeticorum (NLD) (Fig. 27-8)

- Degenerative disease of collagen in the dermis and subcutaneous fat
- Diabetics account for perhaps two-thirds of all cases
- One percent of diabetics have some degree of NLD
- Clinical
  - Patches on pretibial areas, symmetric, well circumscribed
  - Initially red-brown and progress to yellow, depressed atrophic plaques
  - Telangiectatic vessels on the surface
  - Koebner phenomenon present
  - Typically multiple and bilateral

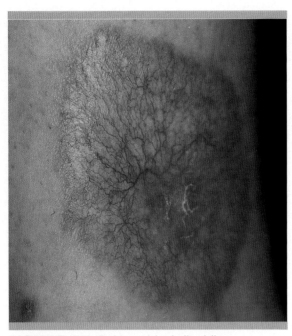

FIGURE 27-8 Necrobiosis lipoidica diabeticorum. *(From Freedberg IM et al: Fitzpatrick's Dermatology in General Medicine, 6th ed. New York: McGraw-Hill, 2003, p. 1657.)*

- Histology
  - Neutrophilic vasculitis; granulomas are arranged in a tierlike fashion and are admixed with areas of collagen degeneration
  - Thickening of the blood vessel walls
  - Direct immunofluorescence: immunoglobulin M, immunoglobulin A, C3, and fibrinogen in the blood vessels
- Treatment
  - Topical and intralesional steroids
  - Antiplatelet aggregation therapy with aspirin and dipyridamole
  - Excision and grafting

Diabetic Dermopathy

- Most common cutaneous finding in diabetes
- Clinical
  - Round to oval atrophic hyperpigmented lesions on the pretibial ares of the lower extremities
  - Brownish hyperpigmentation hemosiderin deposits
- Histology: edema of the papillary dermis, thickened superficial blood vessels, extravasation of erythrocytes, mild lymphocytic infiltrate
- Course: resolves spontaneously

Diabetic Bullae

- Confined to the hands and feet
- Occur spontaneously

- Types
  - Sterile with fluid
    - Heals without scarring
    - Histology: intraepidermal cleavage without acantholysis
  - Hemorrhagic
    - Heals with scarring
    - Histology: cleavage below the dermal-epidermal junction, destruction of anchoring fibrils
  - Multiple nonscarring bullae
  - Sun-exposed areas
  - Histology: cleavage at lamina lucida

Diabetic Ulcers

- Ischemic ulcers
- Neuropathic ulcers in patients with diminished sensation

Acquired Perforating Dermatosis

- Seen in patients with kidney failure associated with diabetes
- Kyrle's disease (reactive perforating collagenosis)
  - Extensor surfaces of the lower extremities
  - Papules with a keratotic plug owing to elimination of collagen and elastin
- Histology: hyperkeratosis surrounding a plug of degenerated material

Glucagonoma Syndrome

- Caused by glucagon-secreting tumors of the alpha cells of the pancreas
- Associated with
  - Hyperglucagonemia
  - Diabetes mellitus
  - Hypoaminoacidemia
  - Cheilosis
  - Normochromic, normocytic anemia
  - Venous thrombosis
  - Neuropsychiatric features
- Clinical: mucocutaneous findings
  - Necrolytic migratory erythema (NME)
    - Predilection for the perineum, buttocks, groin, lower abdomen, and lower extremities
    - Annular erythematous patches with blisters that erode
  - Atrophic glossitis, cheilosis, dystrophic nails, and buccal mucosal inflammation

Carotenemia

- Associated with ingestion of yellow and green vegetables
- Slow conversion of beta-carotene (provitamin A) to vitamin A
  - Accelerated by thyroxine and hyperthyroidism

- Conversion occurs in the mucosal cells of the small intestine
- Diagnosis: carotene excreted in the stool, skin, and urine
- Clinical
  - Xanthoderma
    - Yellow color of skin
    - Greatest concentration is in areas with increased sweating
    - Lipophilic: may take months before color of skin returns to normal
  - Sclera and mucous membranes are spared (unlike in jaundice)

THYROID DERMOPATHY

- Associated with Graves' disease
- Stimulatory autoantibodies directed at the TSH receptor are the cause of hyperthyroidism
- Clinical
  - Characterized by hyperthyroidism, goiter, and exophthalmos
  - Pretibial myxedema (PTM) (Fig. 27-9)
    - Deposition of hyaluronic acid in the dermis and subcutis
    - IgG antibodies directed at the thyroid stimulating harmone receptor (thyroid stimulating immunoglobulins; thyroid receptor blocking antibodies) are present in the serum of at least 80 percent of patients

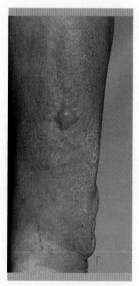

FIGURE 27-9 Thyroid dermopathy. *(From Freedberg IM et al: Fitzpatrick's Dermatology in General Medicine, 6th ed. New York: McGraw-Hill, 2003, p. 1663.)*

- Lateral or anterior aspect of the legs: pink to purple-brown bilateral, firm, nonpitting, asymmetric plaques or nodules, peau d'orange texture
  - Elephantiasic form: verruciform plaques
- Majority of patients with dermopathy have ophthalmopathy
- Histology: hyperkeratosis, mucin (glycosaminoglycans) in the reticular dermis, and a Grenz zone of relatively normal papillary dermis; blue with Alcian blue, at a pH of 2.5, and colloidal iron stains; metachromasia with toluidine blue stain
- Laboratory tests: serum thyroid function tests, thyroid-stimulating immunoglobulins
- Treatment: topical or intralesional corticosteroids

OSTEOMA CUTIS

- Presence of bone within the skin in the absence of a preexisting or associated lesion
- Associated with
  - Albright hereditary osteodystrophy
    - Patients with pseudohypoparathyroidism and pseudopseudohypoparathyroidism
    - Complex inheritance, with imprinting
    - Short stature, round face, defective teeth, mental retardation, brachydactyly (short fourth metacarpals and metatarsals)
    - Tetany in patients with hypocalcemia
    - Osteomas of the soft tissue and skin
    - Miliary osteomas of the face, following acne, neurotic excoriation
    - Congenital plaquelike osteomatosis
  - Secondary types of cutaneous ossification: occur by metaplastic reaction to inflammatory, traumatic, and neoplastic processes
- Laboratory findings
  - Serum calcium and parathyroid hormone (PTH) for hypoparathyroidism and pseudohypoparathyroidism
  - Excisional biopsy for diagnosis
- Treatment: excision or laser resurfacing

Nephrogenic Fibrosing Dermopathy

CLINICAL

- Indurated plaques with brawny hyperpigmentation
- Distinct papules and subcutaneous nodules
- Extremities more common than trunk; face usually spared
- Patients with renal insufficiency, pathogenesis unknown
- Histology: thickened collagen bundles with surrounding clefts, mucin deposition, proliferation of fibroblasts and elastic fibers
- Occasional CD34-positive dendritic fibroblasts

REFERENCES

Badiu C, Cristofor D, Voicu D, et al: Diagnostic traps in porphyria: case report and literature review. *Rev Med Chir Soc Med Nat Iasi* 2004; 108(3):584–591.

Chemmanur AT, Bonkovsky HL: Hepatic porphyrias: diagnosis and management. *Clin Liver Dis* 2004; 8(4):807–838, viii.

Cowper SE, Su LD, Bhawan J, et al: Nephrogenic fibrosing dermopathy. *Am J Dermatopathol* 2001; 23:383–393.

Freedberg IM et al. *Fitzpatrick's Dermatology in General Medicine,* 6th Ed. New York: McGraw-Hill; 2003.

Jabbour SA: Cutaneous manifestations of endocrine disorders: a guide for dermatologists. *Am J Clin Dermatol* 2003;4(5): 315–331.

Jensen TG: Strategies for long-term gene expression in the skin to treat metabolic disorders. *Expert Opin Biol Ther* 2004; 4(5):677–682.

McKee PH. *Pathology of the Skin: With Clinical Correlations.* London: Mosby-Wolfe; 1996.

Perez MI, Kohn SR: Cutaneous manifestations so diabetes mellitus. *J Am Acad Dermatol* 1994; 30(4):519–531.

Schneider JB, Norman RA: Cutaneous manifestations of endocrine-metabolic disease and nutritional deficiency in the elderly. *Dermatol Clin* 2004; 22(1):23–31, vi.

Somorin AO, Al Harbi A, Subaity Y, et al: Calciphylaxis: case report and literature review. 2002; 31(2):175–178. *[sic Pub Med]*

CHAPTER 28

ORAL PATHOLOGY

ASRA ALI

Black Hairy Tongue (Fig. 28-1)

- Inadequate hygiene or microbial overgrowth stimulates elongation of filiform papillae (cover entire anterior dorsal tongue)
- Clinical: black or brown hairlike projections on dorsal tongue
- Histology: elongation of filiform papillae; many microbial colonies between them
- Treatment: proper hygiene and search for cause

Actinic Cheilosis/Chelitis

- Due to ultraviolet (UV) light (actinic radiation)
- Clinical findings
  - Thickening and crusting of the lower lip
  - May progress to overt invasive squamous cell carcinoma
- Histology: hyperkeratosis usually is accompanied by dysplasia and superficial invasion
- Treatment: liquid nitrogen, imiquimod cream 5%, 5-fluorouracil

Aphthous Stomatitis

- Clinical findings
  - Several painful ulcers on the lining mucosa
  - Ulcers heal in 7 to 10 days without scarring
  - Recurrent aphthous ulcers (RAU)
  - Three clinical forms
    - RAU minor
      - ▲ Accounts for 80 percent of all RAUs
      - ▲ Discrete, painful, shallow, recurrent ulcers
    - RAU major
      - ▲ Oval-shaped ulcers that are 1 to 3 cm in diameter
      - ▲ Severe form, 1 to 10 major aphthae may be present
    - Herpetiform RAU: tends to occur in clusters that may consist of tens or hundreds of minute ulcers
- Causes
  - Genetic
  - Vitamin deficiency: iron, folic acid, or vitamin B_{12}

- Immune dysregulation
- Stress
- Environmental factors
- Local, chemical, or physical trauma (pathergy)
- Contact allergy
- HIV infection (associated with lesions)
- Behçet syndrome (associated with lesions)
- Histology: ulceration of lining mucosa
- Treatment
  - Topical corticosteriods
  - Systemic agents
    - Colchicine (0.6 mg tid)
    - Cimetidine (200 mg bid/qid)
    - Azathioprine (50 mg qd)
    - Thalidomide

Cicatricial Pemphigoid

- Clinical findings
  - Gingival bullaus
  - Rupture leaving a slough covering a shallow ulcer
  - Also may affect the eyes and occasionally the skin
  - Caused by autoantibodies to bullous pemphigoid antigens I and II; directed against the basement membrane of oral mucosa
- Histology: subepidermal separation with eosinophilic infiltrate
- Treatment: corticosteroid therapy: oral and/or topical; immunosuppressive therapy

Squamous Carcinoma In Situ

- Associated with tobacco use
- Can lead to invasive squamous cell carcinoma
- Clinical finding: white and/or red patch or soft ulcer
- Histology: anaplasia with or without hyperkeratosis; no invasion
- Treatment: surgical excision and/or radiation

Fissured Tongue (Scrotal Tongue, Lingua Plicata)

- Developmental etiology
- Seen in
  - Melkersson-Rosenthal syndrome
  - Down syndrome

363

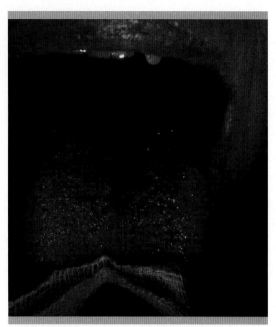

FIGURE 28-1 Black hairy tongue.
(Courtesy of Dr. Robert Jordon.)

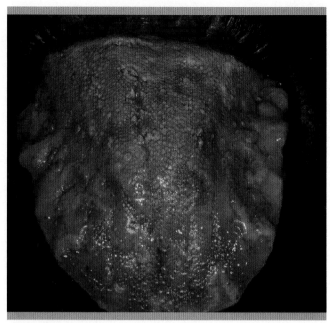

FIGURE 28-2 Geographic tongue. *(Courtesy of Dr. Bela Toth.)*

- Frequently associated with benign migratory glossitis (geographic tongue)
- Clinical findings
  - Irregular clefts are observed in the tongue dorsum
  - Food debris and *Candida albicans* colonies may form in the fissures
- Treatment: none

Fordyce's Spots

- Clinical findings
  - Yellow papules
  - Buccal mucosa (often bilateral), the vermilion upper lip
- Histology: ectopic sebaceous glands
- Treatment: none

Focal Melanosis (Melanoacanthoma, Melanoacanthosis)

- Clinical findings: scattered brown pigmentation of gingiva, tongue, palate
- Histology: local concentration of melanin pigment in the epidermis
- Treatment: none

Geographic Tongue (Benign Migratory Glossitis) (Fig. 28-2)

- Clinical findings
  - Atrophy of the filiform papillae of the tongue
  - Atrophic area surrounded by a serpiginous, white, hyperkeratotic border

- Heals and develops again elsewhere ("migration")
- Burning sensation or an irritation of the tongue noted with hot or spicy foods
- Unknown cause: In patients with psoriasis, geographic tongue occurred in 10 percent
- Histology: psoriasiform mucositis; elongation of the rete ridges is noted with associated hyperparakeratosis and acanthosis; absence of filiform papillae in center; clustering of neutrophils within the epithelium (Munro microabscesses)
- Treatment: none
- Prognosis: excellent; often self-limited

Granular Cell Tumor (GCT)

- Cells are of neural derivation (Schwann cells)
- Tongue is affected in approximately 25 percent of cases
- Gastrointestinal tract harbors approximately 5 percent of all GCTs
- Malignant GCTs are present if cells show cytologic features of malignancy
- Clinical findings: submucosal nodule covered with normal mucosa
- Histology
  - Tumor cells with abundant granular eosinophilic cytoplasm with centrally located vesicular or pyknotic nuclei and markedly enlarged lysosomes
  - Periodic acid–Schiff (PAS) staining; Sudan black B. trichrome preparations
  - Immunohistochemical stains: S-100 protein, neuron-specific enolase, and NK1-C3, myelin-

associated P0 and P2 proteins, myelin basic protein, and Leu-7
- Treatment: surgical excision
- Prognosis
  - Benign lesions; recurrence rates are 2 to 8 percent
  - Ki-67 immunoreactivity of 10 percent or more tumor cells is an adverse prognostic factor

Oral Lichen Planus (OLP) (Fig. 28-3)

- Chronic inflammatory disease
- Lymphocytic infiltrate is composed of activated CD8+ lymphocytes
- May trigger keratinocyte apoptosis
- 15 percent of patients with OLP have coincident skin lesions
- Clinical findings
  - Affects buccal, vestibular, lingual mucosa
  - Intersecting white lines in a netlike pattern; irregular white plaques
  - Erythema (mucosal atrophy), erosions (shallow ulcers), or blisters
  - Erosive form: ulceration and sloughing; potential for cancer formation (fewer than 5 percent of patients)
  - OLP related to
    - Medications
      - ▲ Nonsteroidal anti-inflammatory drugs (NSAIDs), sulfonylureas, antimalarials, beta-blockers, and some angiotensin-converting enzyme (ACE) inhibitors
    - Dentures, amalgams; allergy to metals or components of dental appliances

- Hepatic causes: hepatitis C virus (HCV) infection, autoimmune chronic active hepatitis, and primary biliary cirrhosis
- Histology
  - Hyperkeratosis, parakeratosis, acanthosis, and sawtooth rete pegs
  - Chronic inflammation; bandlike subepithelial mononuclear infiltrate consisting of T cells and histiocytes
  - Basal cell liquefaction, degenerating basal keratinocytes that form colloid (Civatte, hyaline, cytoid) bodies
- Treatment
  - Eliminate local exacerbating factors
  - Topical steroids, topical tacrolimus or cyclosporine

Lymphangioma

- Congenital malformation of the lymphatic system
- Clinical findings
  - Oral lesions: tongue, cheek most common sites
  - Small clusters of vesicles measuring about 2 to 4 mm
- Histology
  - Dilated lymph channels; papillary dermis expands
  - Channels lined by flat endothelial cells (stain positive for *Ulex europaeus* agglutinin-I)
- Treatment: surgical excision or produce scarring with chemicals or lasers

Median Rhomboid Glossitis (Fig. 28-4)

- Inflammatory lesion of the tongue secondary to candidiasis

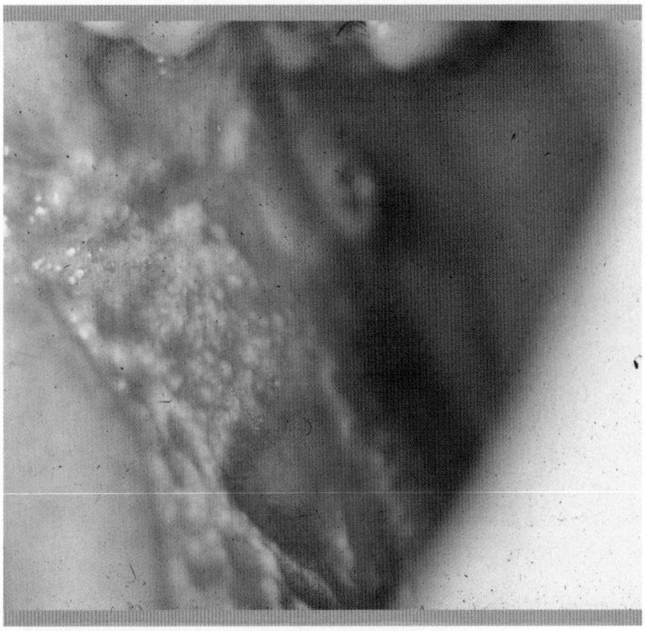

FIGURE 28-3 Oral lichen planus. *(Courtesy of Dr. Bela Toth.)*

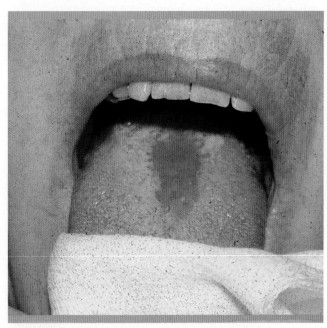

FIGURE 28-4 Median rhomboid glossitis. *(Courtesy of Dr. Bela Toth.)*

- Clinical findings
  - Dorsal surface of the tongue along the midline, anterior to the foramen cecum
  - 1- to 3-cm rhomboid or oval, red, smooth, depapillated, asymptomatic patch
- Treatment: topical or systemic antifungal drugs

Odontogenic Keratocyst (OKC)

- Associated with nevoid basal cell carcinoma syndrome
- Cyst derived from the remnants of the dental lamina
- Benign
- 70 to 80 percent involve the mandible
- Histology
  - Distinctive lining of 6 to 10 cells in thickness
  - Exhibits a basal cell layer of palisaded cells and a surface of corrugated parakeratin
- Radiologic findings: well-demarcated area of radiolucency with a scalloped, radiopaque margin

Drug-Induced Gingival Hyperplasia

- Clinical findings
  - Increase in the fibrous component of the gingiva
  - Long-term phenytoin (Dilantin), cyclosporine, and nifedipine
- Treatment
  - Good oral hygiene with regular dental cleanings
  - Discontinuation of precipitating drugs when possible
  - Surgical or laser resection of tissue for severe cases

Xerostomia (Dry Mouth)

- Clinical findings: dry, glossy atrophic mucosa
- Causes
  - Medications: anticholinergic effects: diuretics, sedatives, hypnotics, antihistamines, antihypertensives, antipsychotics, antidepressants, anticholinergics, and appetite suppressants
  - Radiation therapy to head and neck
  - Salivary gland surgery
  - Autoimmune disorders
  - Human immunodeficiency virus (HIV) infections, systemic lupus erythematosus, rheumatoid arthritis, and Sjögren's syndrome
  - Endocrine disorders: diabetes and hyperthyroidism
- Treatment
  - Discontinue offending medication
  - Commercial saliva substitute
  - Fluoride supplementation

Leukoplakia (Leukokeratosis, Erythroleukoplakia) (Fig. 28-5)

- Clinical term describes mucosal conditions that produce a whiter than normal coloration of the mucous membranes

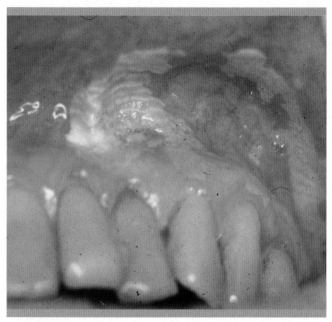

FIGURE 28-5 Leukoplakia. *(Courtesy of Dr. Bela Toth.)*

- Potentially precancerous disease
- Clinical findings: White patch varies from flat, smooth, and slightly translucent macular areas to thick, firm, rough-surfaced, and fissured raised plaques
- Etiology: tobacco, alcohol, ultraviolet radiation, microorganisms, trauma
- Histology: thickened surface; keratin layer; a thickened spinous layer of chronic inflammatory cells in the connective tissue
- Treatment: based on the exact nature of the lesion

Osteoma

- Associated with Gardner syndrome; autosomal dominant
- Gastrointestinal polyps, multiple osteomas, and soft tissue tumors
- Clinical findings
  - Osteoma
  - Exophytic nodular growth of dense cortical bone on or within the mandible or maxilla in locations other than those occupied by tori or exostoses
  - Develops first within the angle of the mandible
- Radiographic features: well-delineated or spherical calcifications
- Treatment: Osteomas may require excision if severely deforming or interfere with function

Kaposi's Sarcoma

- Related to human herpes virus type 8
- Clinical findings

- Hard palate hyperpigmented macular lesions are most common and may include the gingiva, tongue, uvula, tonsils, pharynx, and trachea
- Larger nodular lesions may become exophytic and ulcerated
- Histology
  - Spindle cells
  - Slit-like vascular spaces containing erythrocytes
  - Inflammatory cell infiltrate
- Treatment: antiretroviral therapy

Hutchinson's Incisors

- Screwdriver-shaped central incisors seen in congenital syphilis

Mulberry Molars

- Berry-like molars seen in congenital syphilis

Linea Alba

- Clinical findings
  - Linear white streak on the buccal mucosa at the occlusal line
  - Initiated by irritation from rough buccal cusps, bruxism, or habitual clenching of teeth
- Histology: parakeratosis of tissue

Oral-Facial-Digital Syndrome Type I

- X-linked dominant
- Malformations of the face, oral cavity, and digits
- Clinical findings: oral anomalies: lobed tongue, hamartomas or lipomas of the tongue, cleft of the hard or soft palate, accessory gingival ferrule, hypodontia

Papillon-Lefèvere Syndrome

- Autosomal recessive disorder
- Clinical findings
  - Destructive periodontal disease
  - Affects both primary and permanent dentitions
  - Premature shedding of both deciduous and permanent teeth
- Radiographic findings: Teeth appear to float in the soft tissue
- Treatment: periodontal therapy and antibiotics

Pyogenic Granuloma

- Clinical findings
  - Smooth or lobulated red to purple masses that may be either pedunculated or sessile; commonly on the gingiva
  - Fast-growing reactive proliferation of endothelial cells
  - In response to chronic irritation
- Histology: proliferating vascular channels and a mixed inflammatory infiltrate
- Treatment: excision, laser

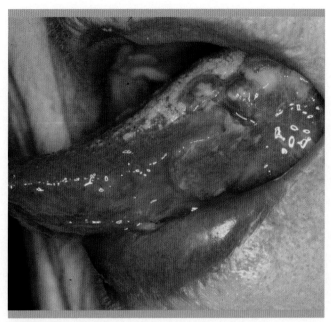

FIGURE 28-6 Squamous cell carcinoma. *(Courtesy of Dr. Bela Toth.)*

Squamous Cell Carcinoma (Fig. 28-6)

- Malignant neoplasm of stratified squamous epithelium
- Capable of locally destructive growth and distant metastasis
- Clinical findings
  - Early lesion: leukoplakias and erythroplakias
  - Late lesion: painless ulcer, tumorous mass, or verrucous (papillary growth)
- Histology
  - Keratin pearls (abnormal keratinization)
  - Increased mitotic activity
  - Chronic inflammation
- Treatment: surgical excision, radiation therapy

Verrucous Carcinoma

- Papillary, superficial, nonmetastasizing form of well-differentiated squamous cell carcinoma
- Clinical findings: broad-based, exophytic, indurated lesion
- Histology: well-differentiated; basement membrane intact; papillary surface
- Treatment: excision, radiation

Amalgam Tattoo (Fig. 28-7)

- Clinical findings: bluish gray permanent area of pigmentation
- Histology: pigmented fragments of metal within the connective tissue
- Treatment: generally not indicated

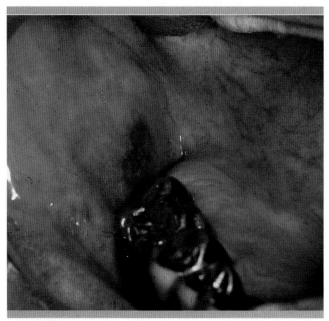

FIGURE 28-7 Amalgam tattoo. *(Courtesy of Dr. Bela Toth.)*

White Sponge Nevus (Fig. 28-8)

- Autosomal dominant
- Defect of keratins 4 and 13
- Clinical findings
    - Symmetric, thickened, white, corrugated or velvety, diffuse plaques
    - Buccal mucosa, ventral tongue, labial mucosa, soft palate, alveolar mucosa, or floor of the mouth
- Histology: acanthosis, spongiosis, hyperkaeratosis
- Treatment: No treatment is necessary

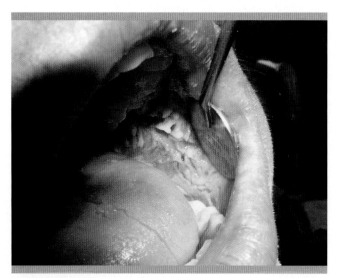

FIGURE 28-8 White sponge nevus. *(Courtesy of Dr. Kelly Peters.)*

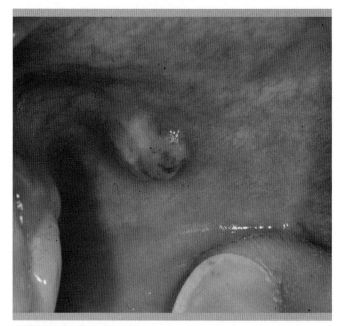

FIGURE 28-9 Mucocele. *(Courtesy of Dr. Bela Toth.)*

Mucocele (Fig. 28-9)

- Foreign-body reaction to saliva
- Caused by traumatic injury to a minor salivary gland
- Clinical findings: Duct appears as a raised, soft, translucent bluish lesion
- Histology: chronic inflammation with macrophages surrounding spilled saliva
- Treatment: surgical excision

Tori, Exostoses, and Enostoses (Fig. 28-10)

- Overgrowth of mature bone
- Clinical findings
    - Elevated hard lesions extending out from the jaws
    - Midline hard palate, buccal or lingual mandible
- Treatment: usually not treated; may be surgically removed

Oral Hairy Leukoplakia (Fig. 28-11)

- Secondary to Epstein-Barr virus (EBV)
- Located mainly on the sides of the tongue
- Clinical findings
    - White thickening or coating of the lining of the mouth; does not scrape off
    - 40 percent of patients with HIV may develop this
- Treatment: may respond to acyclovir or ganciclovir, topical retinoids

Thrush

- Caused by *Candida albicans*
- Clinical findings
    - Velvety white plaques in the mouth and on the tongue

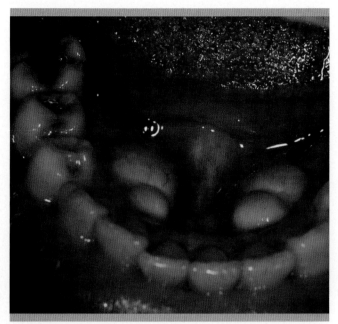

FIGURE 28-10 Tori. *(Courtesy of Dr. Bela Toth.)*

- Lesions are difficult to remove and leave behind an inflamed base that may be painful and may bleed
- Usually a mild and self-limited illness
- Predisposing factors
  - Underlying immunodeficiency
  - Antibiotics, steroids
  - Excessive use of antibacterial mouthwash
  - Dry mouth

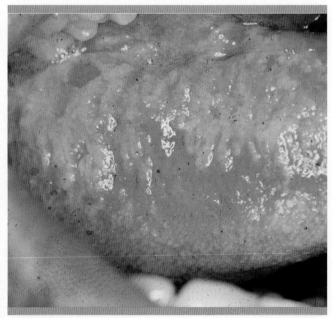

FIGURE 28-11 Oral hairy leukoplakia. *(Courtesy of Dr. Bela Toth.)*

- Medication-induced: antidepressants, antipsychotics, chemotherapy, radiotherapy, or Sjögren's syndrome
  - Trauma to oral cavity
  - Diabetes mellitus
  - Vitamin deficiency: iron, folate
- Treatment: nystatin suspension, diflucan

Actinomyces

- Facultatively or strictly anaerobic gram-positive bacilli
- Bacteria with fungi-like structures
- Normal flora of the upper respiratory, gastrointestinal and female genital tracts
- Causes opportunistic disease following disruption of mucosal barriers by trauma, surgery, or infection
- Clinical findings
  - Multiple abscesses and interconnecting sinus tracts: contain granules of microcolonies
    - Imbedded in tissue elements
    - Macroscopic masses of filamentous bacterial cells that are "cemented" together by calcium phosphate
    - Known as *sulfur granules* owing to their yellow or orange appearance
  - Chronic suppuration results in granuloma formation and a fibrotic "walling off" of the lesion
  - Cervicofacial actinomycosis
    - Most common form
    - Associated with poor oral hygiene, an invasive dental procedure, or oral trauma
    - Tissue swelling with fibrosis and draining sinus tracts along the jawline
- Laboratory studies
  - Difficult to culture and identify because the numbers of organisms are limited in affected tissues and are sequestered in sulfur granules
  - Fastidious and slow growth (up to 2 weeks or more)
- Treatment
  - Surgical debridement
  - Long-term antibiotic therapy (susceptible to penicillin)
  - Maintain good oral hygiene
  - Prophylactic antibiotics prior to invasive oral or abdominal surgical procedures

Chemotherapy-Induced Oral Mucositis

- Clinical findings
  - Localized areas of full-thickness erosions occur
  - Can become covered by a fibrinous pseudomembrane
  - May become colonized by mixed flora
  - Dose-limiting toxicity for antimetabolites
  - Fluorouracil, methotrexate, and purine antagonists
  - Chemotherapeutic insult

- Causes release of inflammatory cytokines, resulting in local tissue damage and increased vascularity
- Decrease rates of cell division in the oral basal epithelium
- Leads to reduced cell renewal, atrophy, and ulceration
- Treatment
  - Analgesics and nutritional support
  - Antimicrobial treatment for secondary infection
  - Tocopherol (vitamin E) accelerates mucosal healing
  - Ice chips
  - Induce local vasoconstriction; reduce amount of fluorouracil delivered to oral mucosal cells
  - Reduces the severity and duration of mucositis by 50 percent
  - Palifermin-synthetic kevatinocyte growth factor

REFERENCES

Deshpande RB, Bharucha MA: Median rhomboid glossitis: Secondary to colonization of the tongue by *Actinomyces* (a case report). *J Postgrad Med* 1991; 37:238–240.

Fanburg-Smith JC, Meis-Kindblom JM, Fante R, Kindblom LG: Malignant granular cell tumor of soft tissue: Diagnostic criteria and clinicopathologic correlation. *Am J Surg Pathol* 1998; 22(7):779–794.

Freedberg IM et al. *Fitzpatrick's Dermatology in General Medicine*, 6th Ed. New York: McGraw-Hill; 2003.

McKee PH. *Pathology of the Skin: With Clinical Correlations*. London: Mosby-Wolfe; 1996.

Seo IS, Azzarelli B, Warner TF, et al: Multiple visceral and cutaneous granular cell tumors: Ultrastructural and immunocytochemical evidence of Schwann cell origin. *Cancer* 1984; 53(10):2104–2110.

CHAPTER 29

PIGMENTARY DISORDERS

ASRA ALI
FRAN E. COOK-BOLDEN

MELANOCYTES

- Epidermal melanocytes are dendritic cells
  - Provide melanin for 36 neighboring basal and spinous layer keratinocytes
  - Number and distribution are the same in all skin types
  - Production and distribution/retention of melanin cause different skin colors
- Types of melanin
  - Phaeomelanin: red-yellow
  - Eumelanin: brown-black
- Constitutive synthesis
  - Refers to the basal, unstimulated rate of melanogenesis
- Facultative synthesis
  - Induced or stimulated rate
  - Following ultraviolet (UV) exposure, hormonal stimulation, postinflammatory
- Melanosomes
  - Move from melanocytes to keratinocytes = epidermal melanin unit
  - Membrane-bound spherical organelles, site of melanin synthesis and storage
  - Synthesized in the cytoplasm and travel to the ends of dendrites
  - Four stages
    - Stage I melanosomes
      ▲ Found in the cytoplasm, contain tyrosinase
      ▲ Enzymatic activity, no melanin
    - Stage II melanosomes
      ▲ Found in the cytoplasm
      ▲ Round or oval, with longitudinally oriented filaments
      ▲ Tyrosinase present
    - Stage III melanosomes
      ▲ Found in the cytoplasm or dendrite
      ▲ Round or oval, electron dense, melanin partially obscures the internal filament network

      ▲ Tyrosinase activity becomes positive
      ▲ Melanization begins at this stage
    - Stage IV melanosomes
      ▲ Found in the cytoplasm or dendrite
      ▲ Round or oval, electron opaque
      ▲ Formed by progressive melanization
      ▲ Possess melanin, no enzymatic activity
- Tyrosinase
  - Cofactor: copper (Cu^{2+})
  - Catalyzes two reactions
    - Hydroxylation of tyrosine to dopa (dihydroxyphenylalanine)
    - Oxidation of dopa to dopaquinone

PIGMENTED LESIONS

Melasma (Fig. 29-1)

- Increased number of melanocytes, increased melanized melanosomes
- Enhanced by hormones (oral contraceptive pills, pregnancy), sun exposure
- Clinical findings
  - Blue-gray hyperpigmented macules, which can be confluent or punctate
  - Most commonly seen centrofacial/malar/mandibular
  - Epidermal, dermal, or mixed
- Diagnosis
  - History/clinical: distribution
  - Wood's light (wavelength, 340 to 400 nm): locates pigment
  - Epidermal pigment enhanced, dermal pigment is not
- Treatment
  - Sunscreen
  - Hydroquinone
  - Tretinoin
  - Chemical peels/microdermabrasion
  - Azelaic acid
  - Compounded agents
  - Kojic acid
  - Lasers

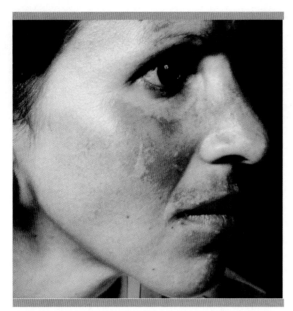

FIGURE 29-1 Melasma. *(From Freedberg IM et al: Fitzpatrick's Dermatology in General Medicine, 6th ed. New York: McGraw-Hill, 2003, p. 869.)*

Becker's Nevus (Fig. 29-2)

- Increase in the number of basal melanocytes occasionally can be detected; melanosomes are increased in keratinocytes
- Acquired lesion in adolescent males
- Increased number of testosterone receptors
- Clinical findings
  - Large, focal, brown, hair-bearing verrucous plaque
  - Back, shoulder, submammary
  - Associated with underlying smooth muscle hamartomas (arrecter pilli)

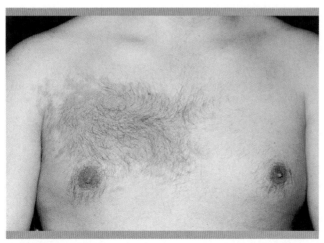

FIGURE 29-2 Becker's nevus. *(From Freedberg IM et al: Fitzpatrick's Dermatology in General Medicine, 6th ed. New York: McGraw-Hill, 2003, p. 867.)*

- Histology: increased pigment of basal layer, increased number of melanocytes, pigment incontinence, no nevus cells in dermis, mature hair follicles, thick bundles of smooth muscles

Congenital Nevomelanocytic Nevus (CNN)

- Presence of a pigmented lesion is noted at birth or soon thereafter
- Categorized by size
  - Small (<1.5 cm in diameter)
  - Medium (1.5 to 20 cm)
  - Large or giant (>20 cm in adolescents and adults or comprising 5 percent of the body surface area or greater in infants, children, and preadolescents): Lifetime risk of developing a melanoma for patients with a large CNN is 6.3 percent
- Leptomeningeal melanocytosis/neurocutaneous melanosis
  - Giant pigmented nevi with concurrent involvement of meninges and/or central nervous system
  - Can lead to a communicating hydrocephalus
  - Symptoms: irritability, photophobia, papilledema, nerve palsies
  - Contrast-enhanced MRI
    - Most sensitive imaging method to document CNS metastases
- Histology
  - Cells around and within adnexal components
  - Splaying of nevus cells as solitary units between reticular dermal collagen (in "Indian file")
  - Cells in a horizontal band in a thickened papillary dermis
- Treatment
  - Surgical excision
  - Chemotherapy for metastatic disease

Spitz Nevus (Spindle Cell Nevus)

- Clinical findings
  - Solitary dome-shaped red/brown papule with a smooth surface/face
  - Red color due to ectatic blood vessels
  - Fifty percent of cases occur in children younger than 10 years of age
- Histology: Predominantly compound, although junctional and intradermal lesions are also observed; large and/or spindle-shaped melanocytes, usually in nests, periodic acid Schiff-positive globules (Kamino bodies or colloid bodies), and nondisruptive (Indian-file-like) infiltration of collagen are important
- Treatment: excision

Cronkhite-Canada Syndrome

- Sporadically occurring
- Mutations of a tumor suppressor gene *PTEN* (phosphatase and tensin homologue deleted on chromosome 10)

- Most patients are older than age 50 at the time of presentation
- Clinical findings
  - Patchy alopecia
  - Circumscribed hypermelanosis with lentigo-like macules on extremities
  - Nail dystrophy
  - Sessile or semipedunculated polyps in the colon but also in the stomach and small intestine with malignant potential
- Histology: increase in melanin within the basal layer without the melanocyte proliferation

Blue Nevus (Fig. 29-3)

- Dermal arrest in embryonal migration of neural crest melanocytes that fail to reach the epidermis
- Blue color due to Tyndall effect: preferential absorption of long wavelengths of light by melanin and the scattering of shorter wavelengths
- Three main types
  - Common blue nevus: blue-black papule
  - Cellular blue nevus: gray-blue solitary, larger than common blue nevus and usually smooth-surfaced papules; buttocks, the sacral region
  - Combined: blue nevus with a nevomelanocytic nevus
  - Malignant blue nevus may develop in contiguity with a cellular blue nevus; expanding dermal nodule with or without ulceration
- Carney syndrome (complex)
  - Autosomal dominant
  - Cardiac, cutaneous, and mammary myxomatous masses; lentigines, blue nevi, endocrine disorders, and testicular tumors
- LAMB: lentigines, atrial myxomas, mucocutaneous myxomas, and blue nevi
- NAME: nevi, atrial myxomas, myxoid tumors (neurofibromas), and ephelides
- Familial multiple blue nevi
  - Autosomal dominant
  - Multiple lesions are present on the head and the neck, the trunk, the extremities, and the sclera
  - Not associated with other cutaneous or systemic findings
- Histology
  - *Common:* dermal melanocytes, melanin contain fibroblast-like in irregular bundles

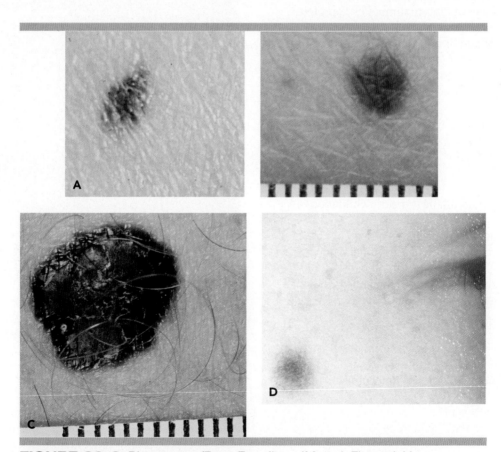

FIGURE 29-3 Blue nevus. *(From Freedberg IM et al: Fitzpatrick's Dermatology in General Medicine, 6th ed. New York: McGraw-Hill, 2003, p. 898.)*

- *Cellular:* common blue nevus exists with fascicles of spindle-shaped cells with ovoid nuclei and pale cytoplasm with little or no melanin
  - *Combined:* macrophages with melanin, ultimately forming fibrous tissue that may extend down to fat
- Treatment: simple excision

Café-Au-Lait Macules (Fig. 29-4)

- Discrete, pale brown macules
- Serrated or irregular margins
- Appear at or soon after birth and disappear with age
- Isolated lesions occur in up to 20 percent of the population
- Increased melanin in melanocytes and basal keratinocytes without melanocytic proliferation
- Associated diseases
  - Neurofibromatosis; Silver-Russel sydrome; Bloom's, Watson's, and Westerhof's syndromes; multiple lentigines syndrome; multiple endocrine neoplasia type IIb; Banyan-Riley-Ruvalcaba and Maffucci's syndromes
  - McCune-Albright syndrome (Albright's syndrome)
    - Sporadic
    - *GNAS1* gene mutation (stimulates G protein, which increases cAMP)
    - Large café-au-lait macule with "coast of Maine" border
    - Polyostotic fibrous dysplasia (pseudocysts of long bones), recurrent fractures, limb-length discrepancies
    - Precocious puberty
    - Hyperthyroidism
    - Normal life span

Nevus Spilus

- Presents during late infancy or early childhood
- Clinical findings
  - Circumscribed, lightly pigmented patch
  - Darkly pigmented, speckled nevomelanocytic elements
- Histology: increased number of melanocytes resembling a lentigo, collection of nevus cells

Lentigo

- Brown to dark variegated to uniformly colored macules
- Basilar hyperpigmentation with melanocyte proliferation
- Acquired brown macule
- Few in number, evenly pigmented
- Types
  - Lentigo simplex: not induced by sun exposure and not associated with systemic disease

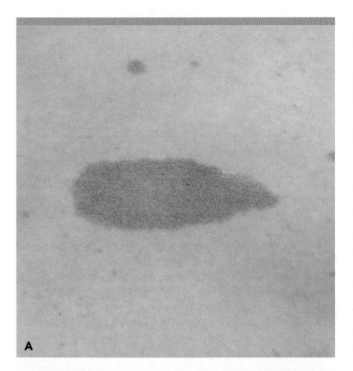

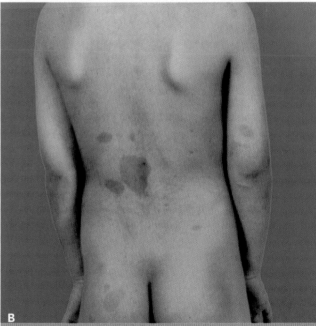

FIGURE 29-4 Café-au-lait macules. *(From Freedberg IM et al: Fitzpatrick's Dermatology in General Medicine, 6th ed. New York: McGraw-Hill, 2003, p. 867.)*

- Solar lentigo: slowly increase in number and in size
- Ink-spot lentigo: reticulated black solar lentigo
- Psoralen and ultraviolet A light lentigo: persist for 3 to 6 months after therapy is discontinued

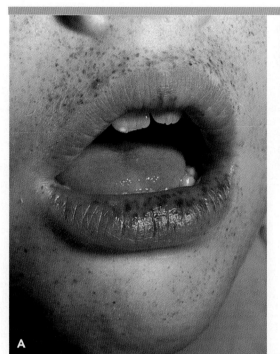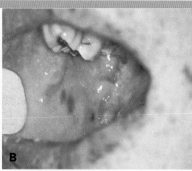

FIGURE 29-5 Peutz-Jehgher's syndrome. *(From Freedberg IM et al: Fitzpatrick's Dermatology in General Medicine, 6th ed. New York: McGraw-Hill, 2003, p. 866.)*

- Peutz-Jeghers syndrome (Fig. 29-5)
  - Autosomal dominant
  - Benign gastrointestinal polyps
  - Oral and labial melanotic macules: can be associated with
    - LEOPARD syndrome: lentigines, electrocardiographic conduction defects, ocular hypertelorism, pulmonary stenosis, abnormal genitalia, retardation of growth, and deafness
- Laugier-Hunziker syndrome: absence of intestinal polyps
- Histology: mild acanthosis with hyperpigmentation of basal layer
- Treatment
  - Cryosurgery: Melanocytes freeze at –4 to –7°C
  - Laser
  - Tretinoin cream and hydroquinone
  - Chemical peel

Ephelides (Freckles)

- Increased melanogenesis, no increase in number of melanocytes
- Light brown macules
- Occur on sun-exposed areas
- Appear in the summer months, and they may persist throughout life

- Color of the lesions tends to deepen after sun exposure
- Histology: Epidermis is unchanged

Nevocellular Nevus

- Benign neoplasms
- Nests of melanocytes
- Stimulated by exposure to sunlight
- Junctional nevi
  - Brown to brown/black macules
  - Melanocytes are positioned at epidermal-dermal junction
- Compound nevi
  - Papules, tan to light brown
  - Melanocytes in dermis and at epidermal-dermal junction
- Dermal nevi
  - Papules display no melanin
  - Melanocytes in dermis

Dysplastic or Atypical Nevi

- Also known as Clark nevi: clinically are asymmetric, with irregular borders, variegate in color
- Familial atypical multiple mole and melanoma (FAMMM) syndrome
  - Also known as the dysplastic nevus syndrome

- Presence of the following features
  - Occurrence of malignant melanoma in one or more first- or second-degree relatives
  - Presence of numerous (often > 50) melanocytic nevi, some of which are clinically atypical
  - Many of the associated nevi show certain histologic features and have an elevated lifetime risk for the development of melanoma
- Histology
  - Single melanocytes
  - Elongation of rete ridges
  - Cytologic atypia of melanocytes with enlarged, hyperchromatic nuclei
  - Bridging: melanocytes aggregate into variably sized nests, which fuse with adjacent rete ridges
  - Dermal fibroplasias: lamellar and concentric
  - Lymphocytic infiltrate
  - Shouldering: junctional component extends beyond the last dermal nest

Halo Nevus

- Nevomelanocytic nevus that develops a depigmented halo around it
- Occasionally the central nevus will regress
- Histology: melanocytic nevus with an acquired surrounding zone of hypopigmentation, dermal lymphocytic infiltrate

Nevus of Ota

- Melanocytes that have not migrated completely from the neural crest to the epidermis during the embryonic stage
- Asian population most commonly affected
- Clinical findings
  - Blue to gray speckled macules or patches
  - Unilateral (90 percent)
  - Forehead, temple, malar area, or periorbital skin
  - Oculodermal melanosis: blue-black macules, most commonly on skin innervated by cranial nerve five (V1,V2 branches)
  - Risk of glaucoma
- Histology
  - Dendritic melanocytes are present and surrounded by fibrous sheaths
- Five types based on the locations of the dermal melanocytes, which are (1) superficial, (2) superficial dominant, (3) diffuse, (4) deep dominant, and (5) deep
  - Dermal melanophages
- Treatment: Q-switched: alexandrite, Nd:YAG, ruby lasers

Nevus of Ito

- Blue to gray speckled macules or patches

- Presents over the shoulder girdle region
- Histology and treatment similar to nevus of Ota

Mongolian Spot

- Congenital dermal melanosis (CDMs)
- Entrapment of melanocytes in the dermis during their migration from the neural crest into the epidermis
- Clinical findings: blue-gray macules, lumbosacral skin, buttocks
- Histology: dermal melanocytes with fully melanized melanosomes; usually oriented parallel to the epidermis

Dowling-Degos Disease (DDD)

- Autosomal dominant
- Clinical findings
  - Reticular, macular hyperpigmentation
  - Initially affects axillae and groin, other flexural areas
  - Comedo-like lesions and pitted acneiform scars near angle of mouth, neck, and back
- Histology: acanthosis, irregular elongation of thin branching rete ridges with a concentration of melanin at the tips, no increase in melanocytes, but increase in melanosomes
- Treatment: erbium YAO laser
- Prognosis: slowly progressive but not life-threatening

HYPOPIGMENTED LESIONS (TABLE 29-1)

Nevus Depigmentosus

- Decreased number of melanosomes in keratinocytes, reduced dopa activity, underdeveloped dendrites, defect in melanosome transfer (melanin remains in melanocytes instead of transfering to keratinocytes)
- Clinical findings: unilateral hypopigmented macular lesion that can present as circumscribed irregular, oval, or round or as a unilateral band or streak with a blocklike configuration or arranged along one or more Blaschko lines

Nevus Anemicus (Fig. 29-6)

- Defect at motor end plate of smooth muscle effector cells of blood vessels
- Focal area of blood vessel with increased sensitivity to catecholamines
- Clinical findings
  - Vessels persistently vasoconstricted
  - Area of cutaneous blanching
- Diagnosis
  - Dermoscopy: obliterates border
  - Wood's lamp: no accentuation
- Histology: normal epidermis, dermis, no changes in vasculature

TABLE 29-1 Hypopigmented Diseases and Defects

Disease	Defect
Albinism	Decreased melanin synthesis
Nevus depigmentosus	Melanosome transfer
Menkes kinky hair	Decreased tyrosinase activity
Cross syndrome	Decreased number of melanocytes
Tuberous sclerosis	Decreased number of melanocytes, decreased melanin synthesis, decreased melanosome size
Vogt-Koyanagi-Harada	Decreased melanocytes

Pityriasis Alba

- Melanocytes decreased in number with fewer and small melanosomes
- Clinical findings
  - Pale pink/light brown macules with indistinct margins, powdery scale

- Eczematous dermatosis with hypomelanosis secondary to postinflammatory
- More apparent on darker skin
- Treatment: emollients

Ash-Leaf Macules (Fig. 29-7)

- Initial expression of tuberous sclerosis
- Normal or decreased number of melanocytes, underdeveloped dendrites

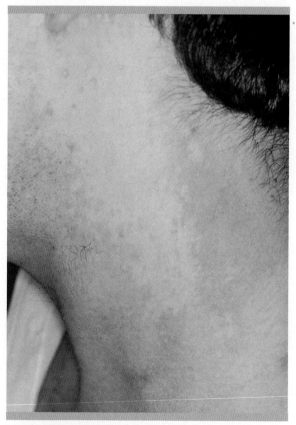

FIGURE 29-6 Nevus anemicus. *(From Freedberg IM et al: Fitzpatrick's Dermatology in General Medicine, 6th ed. New York: McGraw-Hill, 2003, p. 862.)*

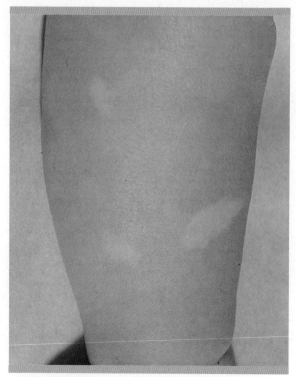

FIGURE 29-7 Ash-leaf macules. *(From Freedberg IM et al: Fitzpatrick's Dermatology in General Medicine, 6th ed. New York: McGraw-Hill, 2003, p. 1823.)*

- Small/poorly melanized melanosomes
- Clinical findings
  - Oval macules
  - Posterior trunk, upper and lower extremities
- Histology: mononuclear infiltrate concentrated in the area of hair follicles and sweat glands, absence of melanin

Idiopathic Guttate Hypomelanonis (Fig. 29-8)

- Common, acquired, discrete hypomelanosis
- Usually on extremities of darker-skinned patients
- Incidence increases with age
- Clinical: discrete, well-circumscribed, porcelain round macules
- Histology: flattening of the dermal-epidermal junction, moderate to marked reduction of the melanin granules in the basal layer, epidermal atrophy, hyperkeratosis
- Treatment: cryotherapy

Futcher's Lines (Voigt's Lines) (Fig. 29-9)

- Pigmentary demarcation lines
- Abrupt transitions from deeply pigmented skin to ligher-pigmented skin
- Often present at birth tend to darken with time

HYPOMELANOSIS SYNDROMES

Vogt-Koyanagi-Harada Syndrome

- Acquired absence of melanocytes
- Due to an aseptic meningitis or autoimmune etiology
- Adults, during third decade of life
- Clinical findings
  - Prodrome: fever, malaise, headache, nausea, vomiting
  - Ophthalmic and autditory stage: posterior uveitis, glaucoma, dysacusis, deafness, tinnitus (50 percent)
  - Poliosis stage (90 percent): symmetric vitiligo, white eyelashes and brows, alopecia
  - Cerebrospinal fluid: pleocytosis, meningeal symptoms

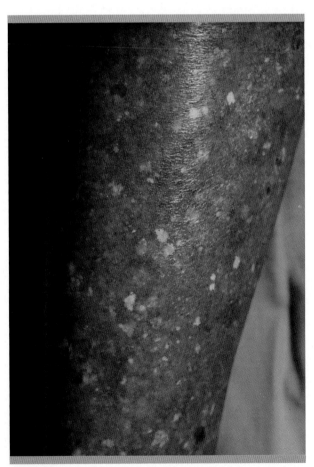

FIGURE 29-8 Idiopathic guttate hypomelanosis. *(From Freedberg IM et al: Fitzpatrick's Dermatology in General Medicine, 6th ed. New York: McGraw-Hill, 2003, p. 1823.)*

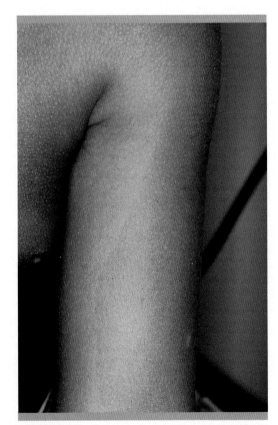

FIGURE29-9 Futcher's lines (Voigt's lines). *(From Freedberg IM et al: Fitzpatrick's Dermatology in General Medicine, 6th ed. New York: McGraw-Hill, 2003, p. 861.)*

Oculocutaneous Albinism (OCA)

- Hypopigmentary diseases
- Due in part to defects in the metabolism of tyrosine leading to failure to convert it into melanin
- OCA IA: (white), tyrosinase negative
- OCA IB: (yellow), pheomelanin, tyrosinase positive
- OCA II: (brown), *p* gene defect; most common form
- OCA III: (red), *TRP1* gene defect

OCULOCUTANEOUS ALBINISM IA

- Autosomal recessive
- Mutated tyrosinase (*TYR*) gene
  - complete loss of tyrosinase function; no pigmented lesions
- Melanosomes are normal
- Clinical findings
  - White hair and skin, blue-gray eyes at birth
  - Decreased visual acuity, photophobia
  - Complete absence of melanin in skin, hair, eyes
  - "Albino" phenotype, pink irides, no pigment

OCULOCUTANEOUS ALBINISM IB

- Some tyrosinase function
- Clinical findings
  - Develop varying pigment with age (pigmented lesions)
  - Minimum pigment, no eumelanin
  - Hair with pheomelanin (spherical yellow melanosomes) and decreased dopaquinone
  - Little or no pigment at birth

OCULOCUTANEOUS ALBINISM TS (TEMPERATURE-SENSITIVE)

- Enzyme temperature-sensitive (decreased activity of tyrosinase with increased temperature)
- Clinical: pigment at distal, cooler body parts

OCULOCUTANEOUS ALBINISM II

- Autosomal recessive, tyrosinase positive
- "Brown" OCA
- Mutation in *P* gene (membrane transport protein); transmembrane protein on melanocytes
- Chromosome 15
- Clinical findings
  - Hair pigment present at birth (different from OCA I)
    - Yellow to blond at birth owing to pheomelanin
  - Most common OCA worldwide
  - Production in eumelanin synthesis, ellipsoidal melanosomes with pheomelanin
  - Irises blue-gray
  - Pigmented nevi may develop
- Prader-Willi syndrome
  - Deletion of long arm of paternal chromosome 15 (70 percent of patients)

- Developmental syndrome
- Neonatal hypotonia
- Hyperphagia and obesity
- Hypogonadism
- Small hands and feet
- Mental retardation
- Skin hypopigmented, no ocular albinism
- Zangelman
  - Defect in the location of *P* gene of chromosome 15
  - Hypopigmentation, light skin and hair, iris translucency
  - Autosomal recessive ocular albinism
  - Nearly normal cutaneous pigmentation and ocular albinism
  - Might represent spectrum of OCA IB/OCA II

OCULOCUTANEOUS ALBINISM III

- Autosomal recessive
- Mutation in *TRP1* (tyrosinase-related protein)
  - *TRP* maps to the brown locus in the mouse: color change black-brown
  - Acts as a dihydroxyindole-2 carboxylic acid (CDHICA); oxidase needed in the eumelanin pathway
- Chromosome 9
- Common in South Africa
- "Rufus/red OCA"
- Clinical findings
  - Red to brownish skin, red hair
  - Hazel to brown eyes

OCULOCUTANEOUS ALBINISM IV

- Defect in *MATP* (membrane associated transport protein)
- Clinical: similar to OCA II

Hermansky-Pudlak Syndrome

- Autosomal recessive
- Chromosome 10q
- Lysosomal membrane defect: accumulation of ceroid lipofuscin in macrophages in lung and gastrointestinal tract
- Bleeding diathesis owing to impaired platelet aggregation
- Tyrosinase positive
- Clinical findings
  - Skin: pigment dilution, pigmented nevi, ecchymosis
  - Hair: cream, red/brown
  - Eyes: photophobia, nystagmus, decreased visual acuity, strabismus
  - Hematologic: epistaxis, gingival bleeding, prolonged bleeding
  - Lymphohistiocytic: ceroid (chromolipid) deposition in macrophages

- Lung: pulmonary fibrosis
- Gastrointestinal: granulomatous colitis
- Cardiac: cardiomyopathy
- Diagnosis
  - Prothrombin time/partial thromboplastin time (PT/PTT)
  - Platelet count
  - Pulmonary function test, chest x-ray, and colonoscopy if symptomatic
- Treatment: avoid aspirin and other blood thinners

Chediak-Higashi Syndrome

- Autosomal recessive
- *LYST* gene defect (lysosomal tansport protein)
- Incomplete oculocutaneous albinism, severe infections
- Decreased chemotaxis of neutrophils, decreased antibody-dependent cellular cytotoxicity
- Clinical findings
  - Eyes: ocular hypopigmentation causes photophobia, nystagmus, and strabismus
  - Hair: silvery sheen
  - Skin: pale, deep ulcerations, petechiae, bruising, gingival bleeding
  - Neurologic: seizures
  - Lymphoma: "accelerated phase" precipitated by viruses (e.g. Epstein-Barr virus); widespread infiltration of viscera
  - Other: hepatosplenomegaly, lymphadenopathy, pancytopenia, pseudomembrane, sloughing of the buccal mucosa
- Laboratory findings
  - Giant granules in circulating neutrophils, melanocytes, neurons, and renal tubular cells
  - Granules form secondary to delayed disorder of lysosomal enzymes from cells
- Treatment: bone marrow (or stem cell) transplant, acyclovir, interleukin, gammaglobulin, vincristine, prednisone
- Course: death at about 6 years old secondary to infection, lymphoma-like accelerated phase

Alezzandrini Syndrome

- Melanocytes originate in the neural crest and then migrate to the skin, leptomeninges, retinas, uvea, cochleae, and vestibular labyrinths
- Clinical findings: facial vitiligo, poliosis, deafness, unilateral tapetoretinal (retinal pigmented epithelia) degeneration

Piebaldism

- Autosomal dominant
- *C-kit* mutation, also seen in mastocytosis
- Protooncogene, tyrosine kinase; chromosome 4 codes for steel factor (*C-kit* ligand)

- Clinical findings
  - Present at birth, does not progress
  - Familial white spotting
  - Cutaneous: depigmented patches midforehead, extremities; pigmented islands present
  - Hair: white forelock (80 to 90 percent)
  - Gastrointestinal: Hirschsprung disease
  - Neurologic: mental retardation, cerebellar ataxia, deafness

Waardenburg Syndrome

- Autosomal dominant
- Defect in neural crest migration, absent melanocytes
- Types I and III: *PAX3* (paired box) gene
- Type II: *MITF* (microphthalmia-associated transcription factor) gene
- Type IV: *EDN3* (endothelin receptor) or *SOX10* (sex determining region) gene
- Clincal findings
  - Skin: depigmentation
  - Hair: white forelock at birth (80 percent), synophrys (70 percent)
  - Oral: tooth caries
  - Eyes: heterochromia, dystopia canthorum (99 percent), lateral displacement of medial canthi with normal interpupillary distance; inner/outer canthi > 0.6
  - Nose: broad nasal root
  - Ears: congenital sensorineural deafness (20 percent)
  - Gastrointestinal: Hirschsprung disease (<5 percent)
  - Type I: only dystopia canthorum, heterochromia
  - Type II: heterochromaia
  - Type III: musculoskeletal, limb abnormalities
  - Type IV: Hirschsprung disease

Vitiligo

- Various theories on etiology
  - Autoimmune hypothesis of melanocyte destruction
  - Neurochemical mediator destroys melanocytes
  - Intermediate or metabolic product of melanin synthesis causes melanocyte destruction
- Associated with: thyroid disease (especially women over age 40), diabetes mellitus, pernicious anemia, Addison's disease, and multiple endocrinopathy syndrome
- Clinical findings
  - Depingmented, sharply circumscribed macules or patches
  - Poliosis = leukotrichia = whiteness of hair; clinical finding in 9 to 45 percent of patients
  - Canities = premature graying of hair (37 percent)
- Types
  - Localized
  - Focal

- Segmental
- Mucosal
- Generalized
- Acrofacial
- Vulgaris
- Mixed: acrofacial and vulgaris or segmental and acrofacial and/or vulgaris
- Universal
- Diagnosis: Wood's lamp: bright white or blue white
- Histology: absence of melanocyte and melanin in the affected area
- Treatment
  - Narrow-band ultraviolet B
  - Oral or topical psoralen plus UV-A (PUVA)
  - Tacrolimus
  - Topical steroids
  - Donor grafts: punch grafts, minigrafts, suction blister

REFERENCES

Barnhill RL. Malignant melanoma, dysplastic melanocytic nevi, and Spitz tumors. Histologic classification and characteristics. *Clin Plast Surg* 2000;27(3):331–360, viii. Review.

Barnhill RL. The Spitzoid lesion: rethinking Spitz tumors, atypical variants, "Spitzoid melanoma" and risk assessment. *Mod Pathol* 2006;19(2 Suppl):S21–S33.

Cohen JB, Janniger CK, Schwartz RA. Cafe-au-lait spots. *Cutis* 2000;66(1):22–24.

Freedberg IM et al. *Fitzpatrick's Dermatology in General Medicine*, 6th Ed. New York: McGraw-Hill; 2003.

Grimes PE. Melasma. Etiologic and therapeutic considerations. *Arch Dermatol* 1995;131(12):1453–1457. Review.

McKee PH. *Pathology of the Skin: With Clinical Correlations*. London: Mosby-Wolfe; 1996.

Oetting WS, King RA. Molecular basis of oculocutaneous albinism. *J Invest Dermatol* 1994;103(5 Suppl):131S–136S.

Wick MR, Patterson JW. Cutaneous melanocytic lesions: selected problem areas. *Am J Clin Pathol* 2005;124 Suppl:S52–S83. Review.

9

CHAPTER 30

DISORDERS OF CORNIFICATION, INFILTRATION, AND INFLAMMATION

HOLLY BARTELL
ASRA ALI

CUTANEOUS DISORDERS OF CORNIFICATION

Ichthyoses

- Group of diseases characterized by excessive thickening of the stratum corneum, producing fishlike scales
- Pathogenesis: increased cohesiveness of cells of the stratum corneum, abnormal keratinization, and increased proliferation

ICHTHYOSIS VULGARIS (FIG. 30-1)

- Autosomal dominant
- Altered profilaggrin expression (component of keratohyalin granules)
- Retention hyperkeratosis
- Hereditary ichthyosis: associated with atopy (keratosis pilaris, hyperlinear palms)
  - Clinical signs: begins usually in early childhood, white scales cover trunk, extensor surfaces and face
- Acquired ichthyosis
  - Associated with internal disease
  - Associated with medications
  - Malignancies
- Clinical findings
  - Symmetric, hyperkeratotic brown scales, snake skin appearance, xerosis
  - Affects dorsal surfaces; mucuous membranes are not involved
  - Extent of the disease is variable
  - Hyperlinear palms

- Histology: compact hyperkeratosis; patchy parakeratosis, granular layer may be absent; decreased rete-papillae pattern
- Electron microscopy: absent keratohyalin granules
- Treatment: hydration, ointment to prevent evaporation
  - Keratolytics
  - Topical retinoids
  - Acquired ichthyosis vulgaris treatment of the underlying systemic condition

LAMELLAR ICHTHYOSIS (FIG. 30-2)

- Autosomal recessive
- Mutation in the gene for transglutaminase 1 (*TGM1*)
- Accelerated epidermal turnover with proliferative hyperkeratosis
- Clinical findings
  - Collodion membrane
  - Ectropion, eclabium, bilateral conjunctivitis, generalized erythroderma
  - Scales are dark and platelike, increased in flexural surfaces, scarring alopecia; nail dystrophy
- Histology: thickened granular layer, hyperkeratosis, increased mitoses, and a perivascular lymphocytic infiltrate
- Treatment: newborn—risk of hypernatremic dehydration, sepsis; hydration, oral retinoids, emollients

NONBULLOUS CONGENITAL ICHTHYOSIFORM ERYTHRODERMA (NONBULLOUS CIE)

- Transglutaminase defect
- Begins with collodion membrane

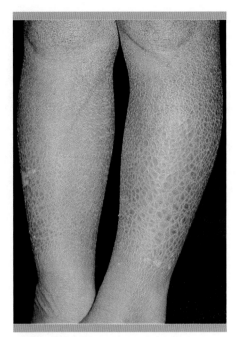

FIGURE 30-1 Ichthyosis vulgaris. *(From Freedberg IM et al: Fitzpatrick's Dermatology in General Medicine, 6th ed. New York: McGraw-Hill, 2003, p. 487.)*

- Accelerated epidermal turnover; on a spectrum with lamellar ichthyosis
- Generalized erythroderma with fine, white scale, palmoplantar keratoderma

- Alopecia, ectropion, or eclabian not as common as in lamellar ichthyosis
- Treatment: topical alpha-hydroxy acids, emollients, oral retinoids

X-LINKED ICHTHYOSIS

- X-linked recessive
- Steroid sulfatase deficiency (*STS*)
- Retention hyperkeratosis
- Clinical findings
  - Brown "dirty" scales
  - Comma-shaped corneal opacities
  - Cryptorchidism
  - Failure of labor progression in mother
- Laboratory findings: increase in cholesterol sulfate levels and reduction in serum cholesterol levels, decreased excretion of maternal urinary steroids
- Histology: orthokeratotic hyperkeratosis with a normal or slightly thickened granular layer
- Electron microscopy: keratohyaline granules are increased in size and number
- Treatment: topical keratolytics and emollients

ICHTHYOSIS BULLOSA OF SIEMENS

- Autosomal dominant
- Mutation in keratin 2e
- Clinical: erythema and superficial blistering with superficial "molting," flexural hyperkeratosis

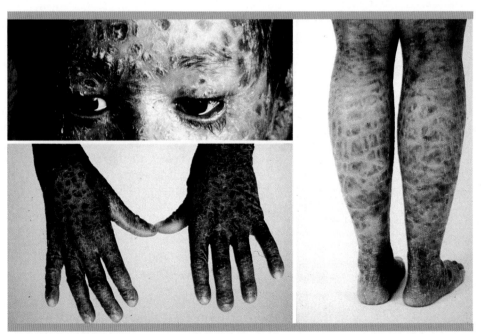

FIGURE 30-2 Lamella ichthyosis. *(From Freedberg IM et al: Fitzpatrick's Dermatology in General Medicine, 6th ed. New York: McGraw-Hill, 2003, p. 490.)*

EPIDERMOLYTIC HYPERKERATOSIS (BULLOUS CONGENITAL ICHTHYOSIFORM ERYTHRODERMA, BULLOUS ICHTHYOSIS)

- Autosomal dominant
- Keratins 1 and 10 gene mutations
- Newborn: widespread bullae, erythroderma
- Later: hyperkeratosis with "corrugated cardboard" appearance at flexures
- Palmoplantar keratoderma
- Treatment: avoid salicylic acid based keratolytics in newborns, emollients

HARLEQUIN FETUS

- Autosomal recessive
- Large hyperkeratotic plates with deep fissures present at birth
- Ectropion, eclabium, absent or deformed ears, nose, fingers, toes
- Electron microscopy: absent lamellar bodies
- Prognosis: death common within first days
- Treatment: Etretinate may improve survival

SJÖGREN-LARSON SYNDROME

- Autosomal recessive
- Fatty aldehyde dehydrogenase deficiency
- Infancy: generalized ichthyosis, erythrodema, pruritus
- Later: dark scale at flexures, abdomen
- Mental retardation, spastic diplegia with scissor gait, epilepsy
- "Glistening dots" of retina by 1 year of age
- Treatment: emollients, retinoids, dietary restriction of long-chain fatty acids

REFSUM SYNDROME

- Autsomal recessive
- *PHYH* gene; phytanic acid oxidase deficiency
- Mild ichthyosis begins in adolescence
- Neurologic symptoms: ataxia, peripheral polyneuropathy, anosmia
- "Salt and pepper" retinitis pigmentosa, night blindness, cataracts
- Cardiac arrhythmias
- Muscle wasting
- Treatment: dietary restriction or plasma exchange; removal of phytanic acid may halt disease progression
- Prognosis: early death

Conradi-Hunerman Syndrome (Chondrodysplasia Punctata)

- X-linked dominant
- Peroxisomal enzyme defect; *PEX7* gene
- Infancy: ichthyosiform erythroderma
- Follicular atrophoderma
- Patchy alopecia
- Focal cataracts
- Stippled epiphyses (chondrodysplasia punctata), asymmetric limb shortening
- Facial asymmetry
- Chondrodysplasia punctata improves with time

CHILD SYNDROME

- Congenital hemidysplasia with ichthyosiform erythroderma and limb defects
- X-linked dominant
- *NSDHL* gene
- Unilateral ichthyosiform erythroderma with midline cutoff
- Ipsilateral alopecia
- Hypoplasia/agenesis of ipsilateral limbs and organs
- Treatment: emollients for ichthyosis

NETHERTON SYNDROME (ICHTHYOSIS LINEARIS CIRCUMFLEXA)

- Autosomal recessive
- SPINK 5 defect
- Generalized erythroderma, scaling
- Migratory, serpiginous plaques with double-edged scale (ichthyosis linearis circumflexa)
- Trichorrhexis invaginata "bamboo hairs," most specific hair finding (trichorrhexis nodosa is most common)
- Associated with atopic dermatitis
- Risk of hypernatremia in newborns
- Treatment: topical emollients, retinoids

ERYTHROKERATODERMA VARIABILIS (MENDES DE COSTA SYNDROME)

- Autosomal dominant
- Connexin 31 defect, *GJB4* gene (gap junction protein)
- Migratory geographic patches of erythema, fixed focal hyperkeratotic plaques
- Treatment: topical corticosteroids, retinoids, emollients

KID SYNDROME (KERATITIS-ICHTHYOSIS-DEAFNESS SYNDROME)

- Autosomal dominant
- Connexin 26 defect, *GJB2* gene
- Mild, generalized hyperkeratosis
- Ichthyosis
- Sensorineural deafness
- Scarring alopecia
- Vascularized keratitis with secondary blindness
- Hypohidrosis
- Teeth and nail anomalies

Palmoplantar Keratodermas (PPKs)

UNNA-THOST SYNDROME

- Diffuse, nonepidermolytic palmoplantar keratoderma
- Autsomal dominant
- Keratin 1 defect
- Palmoplantar keratoderma (PPK) with painful fissuring, hyperhidrosis
- Histology: orthohyperkeratosis
- Treatment: topical emollients, oral retinoids

VORNER'S SYNDROME (EPIDERMOLYTIC PALMOPLANTAR KERATODERMA)

- Autsomal dominant
- Keratin 9 defect
- Like diffuse PPK
- Histology: epidermolytic hyperkeratosis
- Treatment: topical emollients, antifungals, oral retinoids

HOWEL-EVANS SYNDROME

- Autosomal dominant
- Palmoplantar keratoderma
- Increased risk of esophageal carcinoma
- Treatment: topical therapy, oral retinoids
- Prognosis depends on early detection of carcinoma

VOHWINKEL SYNDROME (PALMOPLANTAR KERATODERMA MUTILANS, KERATODERMA HEREDITARIA MUTILANS)

- Autsomal dominant
- Connexin 26, *GJB2* mutation, defective loricrin
- Diffuse honeycombed palmoplantar keratoderma
- Pseudoainhum
- Starfish-shaped keratotic plaques
- Scarring alopecia
- High-frequency hearing loss
- Olmsted syndrome: Vohwinkel's and perioral keratoderma (sporatic transmission)
- Treatment: topical emollients and retinoids, oral retinoids, auditory testing

MAL DE MELEDA (KERATODERMA PALMOPLANTARIS TRANSGREDIENS)

- Autosomal recessive
- *SLURP1* gene defect
- Infants: palmoplantar erythema and scaling
- Later: glove-and-stocking palmoplantar keratoderma
- Fissures, hyperhidrosis, malodorous palms and soles
- Hyperkeratotic plaques at elbows, knees
- Onychogryphosis
- Scrotal tongue
- Treatment: keratolytics, oral retinoids

PAPILLON-LEFEVRE SYNDROME (PALMOPLANTAR KERATODERMA WITH PERIODONTOSIS)

- Autosomal recessive
- Cathepsin C defect
- Sharply demarcated palmoplantar keratoderma
- Hyperkeratotic plaques at elbows, knees
- Hyperhidrosis, pyogenic infections
- Sparse hair
- Periodontitis with loss of teeth
- Calcification of dura mater
- Treatment: meticulous oral hygiene, antibiotics, topical keratolytics, oral retinoids

RICHNER-HANHART SYNDROME (TYROSINEMIA TYPE II)

- Autosomal recessive
- Hepatic tyrosine aminotransferase deficiency
- Severe keratitis, corneal ulcers, blindness
- Focal or diffuse palmoplantar keratoderma, erosions, bullae
- Hyperkeratotic plaques on elbows, knees
- Treatment: topical emollients and retinoids, low-phenylalanine/tyrosine diet

DARIER DISEASE (KERATOSIS FOLLICULARIS) (FIG. 30-3)

- Autosomal dominant
- Defective ATPase *2A2* gene
- *SERCA2* sarcoendoplasmic reticulum calcium ATPase
- Clinical: chronic
- Hyperkeratotic papules and warty plaques in seborrheic distribution; exacerbated by heat, humidity, stress, sunlight
- Acrokeratosis verruciformis of Hopf: verruciform-like lesions are present on the backs of the hands
- Palmoplantar punctate hyperkeratosis

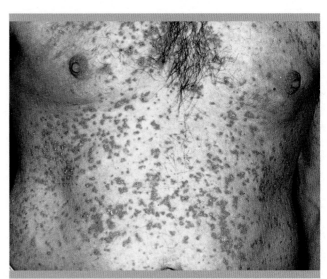

FIGURE 30-3 Darier disease. *(From Freedberg IM et al: Fitzpatrick's Dermatology in General Medicine, 6th ed. New York: McGraw-Hill, 2003, p. 524.)*

- Nails: red and white longitudinal bands, V-shaped nicking, subungual hyperkeratosis
- Cobblestone papules on mucous membranes
- Histology: hyperkeratosis, dyskeratotic cells (corps ronds), and corps grains; suprabasal acantholytic clefts
- Treatment: oral retinoids

POROKERATOSES

- Group of keratinization disorders
- Etiology: autosomal dominant in familial cases
- Clonal hyperproliferation of atypical keratinocytes: causes cornoid lamella, which expands peripherally and forms the raised boundary between abnormal and normal keratinocytes
- Five clinical variants
  - Classic porokeratosis (Mibelli)
    - Autosomal dominant
    - Childhood, asymptomatic
    - Irregularly shaped annular plaque with a raised, ridgelike border
  - Disseminated superficial (actinic) porokeratosis
    - Indistinct, light brown patches with a threadlike border
    - Predominantly on the extensor surfaces of the legs and the arms
    - Fair-skinned women in their third or fourth decade of life, with a history of excessive ultraviolet exposure
  - Linear porokeratosis
    - Infancy or early childhood
    - Unilateral, linear array of annular papules and plaques with the characteristic raised peripheral ridge
    - Follows a dermatomal distribution
  - Porokeratosis palmaris et plantaris disseminata (PPPD)
    - Autosomal dominant
    - Small, slightly hyperpigmented, atrophic center, and a minimally raised peripheral ridge
    - Mucosal lesions are small, annular or serpiginous, and pale
    - Palms and the soles, then generalized distribution
- Prognosis: formation of squamous or basal cell carcinomas has been reported in all forms of porokeratosis
- Histology
  - Cornoid lamella: thin column of tightly packed parakeratotic cells within a keratin-filled epidermal invagination; extends at an angle away from the center of the lesion
  - Epidermis, beneath the parakeratotic column, has keratinocytes that are irregularly arranged with atypical nuclei

- Papillary dermis with a moderately dense lymphocytic infiltrate and dilated capillaries
- Treatment: topical 5-fluorouracil, topical vitamin D_3 analogues, oral retinoids; excision if malignancy occurs
- Cryotherapy electrodesiccation and curettage

Pityriasis Rubra Pilaris (PRP) (Fig. 30-4)

- Clinical findings
  - Rare, onset at any age, chronic course
  - Orange-red or salmon-colored scaly plaques with sharp borders, islands of uninvolved skin
  - Juvenile, adult, limited forms
  - Tendency for erythroderma
  - Follicular hyperkeratosis
  - Palmoplantar keratoderma
  - Nails: distal yellow-brown discoloration, subungual hyperkeratosis, longitudinal ridging, nail plate thickening, and splinter hemorrhages
  - Mucous membrane: diffuse whitish appearance of the buccal mucosa, lacy whitish plaques, and erosions
- Griffith's classification
  - Type I: classic adult
  - Type II: atypical adult
  - Type III: classic juvenile
  - Type IV: circumscribed juvenile
  - Type V: atypical juvenile
  - Type VI: HIV-associated
- Histology: hyperkeratosis with alternating orthokeratosis and parakeratosis forming a

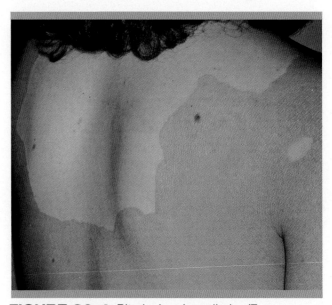

FIGURE 30-4 Pityriasis rubra pilaris. *(From Freedberg IM et al: Fitzpatrick's Dermatology in General Medicine, 6th ed. New York: McGraw-Hill, 2003, p. 444.)*

checkerboard pattern in the stratum corneum; focal or confluent hypergranulosis; follicular plugging with perifollicular parakeratosis forming a shoulder effect; thick suprapapillary plates; broad rete ridges; narrow dermal papillae; and sparse superficial dermal lymphocytic perivascular infiltration, acantholysis

- Treatment: topical corticosteroids, calcipotriol, emollients, acitretin, methotrexate, azathioprine

Lichen Simplex

- Caused by constant rubbing and scratching of skin
- Cause for pruritic skin usually cannot be determined
- Clinical findings
  - Prurigo nodularis of Hyde
  - Symmetric lichenified lesions on the extremities, upper back, neck, arms, legs (especially sites within reach of the patient)
  - Severe pruritus
  - Prolonged course
- Histology: hyperkeratosis, acanthosis, hypergranulosis, fibrosis and increased number of dilated capillaries; sometimes excoriations are found
- Treatment: topical or intralesional steroids, oral antihistamines, oral antianxiety medications and sedation, doxepine cream, and capsaicin cream, immunomodulators; for infected lesions, a topical or oral antibiotic

Tyloma, Callus

- Clinical findings: caused by chronic external pressure
- Histology: prominent hyperkeratosis, usually without parakeratosis

Clavus

- Clinical findings: hyperkeratotic lesion caused by chronic pressure at the sites of bony prominences
- Histology: hyperkeratosis with parakeratosis, epidermis is centrally atrophic, and on the periphery acanthotic, perivascular infiltration of upper dermis

Pityriasis Lichenoides (Mucha Habermann Disease) (Fig. 30-5)

- Occurs in two forms: chronic and acute
- Etiology unknown; most cases are idiopathic

PITYRIASIS LICHENOIDES ET VARIOLAFORMIS ACUTA (PLEVA)

- Clinical findings
  - Symmetric eruption on the trunk and extremities
  - Papules with central necrosis, hemorrhagic vesicles
  - No pruritus
  - Affects young individuals or children
  - Fine scale similar to (frosted glass); lesions at different stages of evolution (polymorphic)

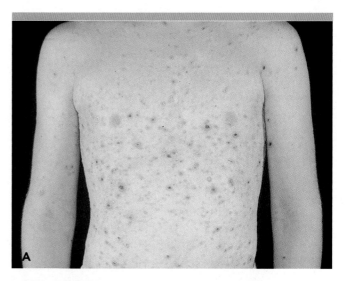

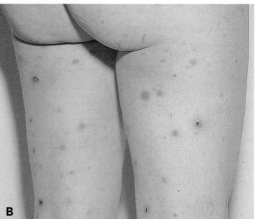

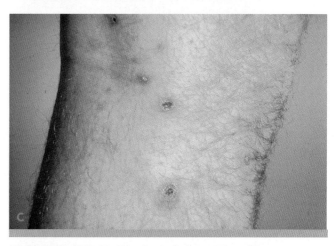

FIGURE 30-5 Pityriasis lichenoides. *(From Freedberg IM et al: Fitzpatrick's Dermatology in General Medicine, 6th ed. New York: McGraw-Hill, 2003, p. 459.)*

- Ulceronecrotic PLEVA presents with a sudden eruption of diffuse coalescent necrotic ulcerations associated with high fever

PITYRIASIS LICHENOIDES CHRONICA (PLC)

- Clinical findings
  - Symmetric eruption on the trunk and extremities
  - Lichenoid papules with scales, purpura, no pruritus
  - Duration: several weeks; heals with hyperpigmentation
- Histology: superficial and deep wedge-shaped perivascular infiltrate, vacuolar degeneration of basal layer, hemorrhage, epidermal necrosis
- Treatment: phototherapy, tetracycline, erythromycin, acitretin, methotrexate

Pityriasis Rosea (Fig. 30-6)

- Etiology: unknown, possibly herpesvirus
- Clinical findings
  - Symmetric involvement of the trunk and extremities
  - Pink macules and papules with central scaling making a collarette
  - Mild pruritus
  - Dissemination preceeded by a herald patch: single, red, slightly elevated patch, 2 to 5 cm
  - Lasts 1 or 2 months
- Histology: perivascular infiltrate in upper dermis (lymphocytes), slight epidermotropism, spongiosis, acanthosis, scattered necrotic keratinocytes, focal parakeratosis, dermal hemorrhage, diffuse infiltration of the upper dermis

Lichen Planus

- Etiology
  - Can be idiopathic
  - Linked to hepatitis virus C (HVC) infection
  - Medications
- Clinical findings
  - Predilection for flexor surfaces of the wrists, shins, ankles of the lower extremities, sacral region, mouth, genitals
  - Fine, white lines, called *Wickham stria,* are often found on the papules and mucous membranes may be found without skin involvement
  - Pink, purple (hyperpigmented brownish red), polygonal, flat topped, papules
  - Pruritus
  - Oral ulcerations have the potential to become malignant
  - Genital involvement: annular configuration of papules is seen on the glans
  - Nail findings: nail plate thinning with longitudinal grooving and ridging, matrix can be permanently destroyed with prominent pterygium formation

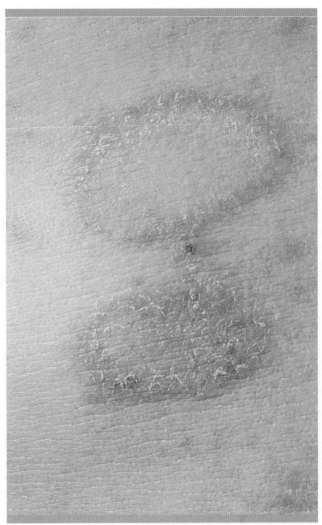

FIGURE 30-6 Pityriasis rosea. *(From Freedberg IM et al: Fitzpatrick's Dermatology in General Medicine, 6th ed. New York: McGraw-Hill, 2003, p. 446.)*

- Direct immunofluorescence: globular deposits of immunoglobulin M (IgM) and complement mixed with apoptotic keratinocytes
- Variants
  - Hypertrophic
  - Atrophic
  - Erosive
  - Follicular (lichen planopilaris)
  - Lichenoid drug eruption
    - Lichen planus-like rash caused by medications
    - Associated medications: antimalarial agents, beta-blockers, bismuth, captopril, carbamazepine, cholorpropamide, gold, hydroxyurea, meprobamate, mepacrine, methyldopa, *para*-amino-salicyclic acid, penicillamine, phenothiazine, quinine, quinidine, streptomycin, sulphonylurea, tetracycline, thiazides

- – Actinic lichenoid drug eruption is confined to sun-exposed sites; most likely drugs: quinine, thiazide diuretics
- Histology: hyperkeratosis (*without* parakeratosis), irregular acanthosis and colloid bodies in the epidermis with liquefactive degeneration and linear fibrin deposition in the basal layer, upper dermis with a bandlike infiltrate of lymphocytes and histiocytes, artificial subepidermal clefts (Max-Joseph spaces)
- Immunoflourescence: colloid bodies contain globular deposits of IgM (occasionally IgG or IgA) and complement; linear or shaggy deposits of fibrin and fibrinogen in the basement membrane zone
- Treatment: topical steroids, systemic steroids, psoralen with ultraviolet light A (PUVA), acitretin, cyclosporine, griseofulvin; immune modulating drugs that inhibit calcineurin

Benign Lichenoid Keratosis (BLK)

- Occurs on extremities and presternal area, often in sun-exposed areas
- Clinically resembles a lentigo, Bowen's disease, or a basal cell carcinoma
- Histology: solitary lesion mimicking lichen planus; parakeratosis is often present
- Immunohistochemical studies: epidermal and dermal lymphocytes are mainly CD8(+) T cells

Lichen Nitidus

- Clinical findings
  - White papules, about 3 mm
  - Usually asymptomatic
  - Age: usually children, young adults
  - Location: often trunk, upper extremities, penis
  - Köebner phenomenon
- Histology: foci of dense intrapapillary infiltrate consisting of lymphocytes and epitheloid histiocytes, forming tiny granulomas; rete ridges are bent around the infiltrate, parakeratosis
- Treatment: topical and systemic steroids, cetirizine, levamisole, etretinate, acitretin, itraconazole, cyclosporine, topical dinitrochlorobenzene, UV-B photo-therapy, and psoralen plus ultraviolet light A (PUVA)

Lichen Striatus

- Clinical findings
  - Affects children and young adults
  - Location: extremities, asymmetrical
  - Small erythematous, scaly papules in linear arrangement
  - Pruritus occasionally
  - Healing in weeks up to 1 year
- Histology: lichenoid lymphohistiocytic infiltration, exocytosis, parakeratosis, focal spongiosis, necrotic keratinocytes single or in groups within epidermis

- Treatment: topical and systemic steroids, cetirizine, levamisole, etretinate, acitretin, itraconazole, cyclosporine, topical dinitrochlorobenzene, UV-A/UV-B phototherapy, and psoralen plus ultraviolet light of A wavelength (PUVA)

Erythema Dyschromicum Perstans (Ashy Dermatosis)

- Clinical findings
  - Chronic condition
  - Asymptomatic, irregularly shaped, gray-blue hyperpigmented macules on the trunk, the arms, the face, and the neck
  - Begins as ash-colored macules, sometimes with an erythematous or elevated border
  - Slow progression
- Histology: vacuolar degeneration of the basal layer, with pigment incontinence in the upper dermis, superficial lymphocytic infiltrate; later scattered melanopages in the upper dermis
- Treatment: not many effective therapies, clofazimine, antibiotics, antihistamines, antimalarials

Transient Acantholytic Dermatosis (Grover's Disease)

- Precipitating factors: heavy exercise, heat, fever
- Clinical findings
  - Usually affects elder males
  - Trunk, sometimes the thighs
  - Brownish red, small hyperkeratotic papules, sometimes with crusts or vesicles
  - Benign course; lasts several weeks to several years
  - Usually pruritic
- Histology: several forms: spongiotic, pemphigus foliaceus-like, Darier-like, Hailey-Hailey-like, infiltration of the upper and deep corium

FIGURATE ERYTHEMAS

Erythema Annulare Centrifugum (Erythema Figuratum)

- Hypersensitivity reaction to a variety of agents, including drugs, arthropod bites, infections, and malignancy
- Clinical findings
  - Trunk, extremities
  - Urticarial erythematous annular or polycyclic lesions
  - Centrifugal spreading, regression in the center
  - Trailing scale is present on the inner aspect of the advancing edge

- Middle-aged adults
- Healing in weeks up to years
- Histology
  - Intense, superficial, and deep lymphocytic or lymphohistiocytic perivascular infiltrate in a coat-sleeve fashion in the middle and lower dermis
- Treatment: usually self-limited; treat underlying disorder; topical, systemic or injection steroid therapy

Erythema Gyratum Repens (EGR)

- Associated with malignancy in as many as 80 percent of patients; often precedes the detection of malignancy
- Clinical findings: wood-grain appearance; concentric mildly scaling bands of patches or plaques of erythema; rapid migration (up to 1 cm/day); intense pruritus
- Course of rash closely mirrors the course of the underlying illness
- Associated malignancies: lung (most common), breast, urinary bladder, uterus and/or cervix, gastrointestinal tract (stomach), and prostate
- Associated with some nonneoplastic conditions: pulmonary tuberculosis, lupus erythematosus, CREST (calcinosis, Raynaud phenomenon, esophageal motility disorder, sclerodactyly, and telangiectasia) syndrome
- Histology: spongiosis, focal parakeratosis, and a superficial perivascular lymphohistiocytic infiltrate, with eosinophils and melanophages; exocytosis of neutrophils and eosinophils
- Workup: search for common or clinically suspected malignancies
- Treatment: steroids for pruritus; symptoms disappear with resolution of underlying disease

URTICARIA

Acute Urticaria

- Mast cell stimulation results in the release of both preformed (histamine) and newly formed (prostaglandins) mediators from cytoplasmic granules
- Hypersentitive reaction to various stimuli
  - Allergic (IgE or complement-mediated: food, drugs, insects)
    - Radiocontrast media
    - Drugs: aspirin, nonsteroidal anti inflammatory drugs (NSAIDs), opiates, succinylcholine, and certain antibiotics (e.g., polymixin, ciprofloxacin, rifampin, vancomycin, some beta-lactams)
    - Contact urticaria
  - Nonallergic

- Pressure
- Vibration
- Cholinergic (triggered by heat, exercise, or emotional stress)
- Sunlight
- Water
- Cold
- Cryoglobulinemias
- Serum sickness
- Thyroid disease
- Lymphoreticular malignancies
- Clinical findings
  - White, pink, or red wheals with surrounding edema
  - Angioedema
  - Acute attacks disappear within several hours; if longer than 24 hours, consider urticarial vasculitis
  - Pruritus

Chronic Urticaria

- Urticaria that persists for longer than 6 weeks
- Dermographism can occur concomitantly with chronic idiopathic urticaria (CIU)
- Etiologies: same as acute urticaria
  - Chronic idiopathic urticaria (CIU): up to 80 percent of cases
- Laboratory tests
  - Complete blood count (CBC) with differential
  - Total eosinophil count
  - Sedimentation rate
  - Urinalysis
  - Liver function tests
- Treatment: avoidance of a trigger
  - H_1 and H_2 antihistamines
  - Glucocorticoids
  - Epinephrine (α-adrenergic effect)
  - Colchicine and dapsone for refractory urticaria
  - Monteleukast

Angioedema

- Clinical findings: well-demarcated, localized, nonpitting edema
- Acute: recurrent episodes of distensible tissues (e.g., lips, eyes, earlobes, tongue, uvula) for less than a 6-week duration
- Chronic: >6 weeks duration
- Normal or elevated complement mediated: angioedema may result from various antigen exposures—foods, drugs, parenteral exposure
- Low complement-mediated angioedema involves immune complex-mediated necrotizing cutaneous venulitis manifested as serum sickness, due to direct mast cell-releasing agents
  - Fever, angioedema, arthralgias, urticaria, and palpable purpura

- Low C1-INH
  - Hereditary angioedema (HAE): autosomal dominant, recurrent, self-limited attacks involving the skin, subcutaneous tissue, upper respiratory tract, or gastrointestinal tissue, upper respiratory tract, or gastrointestinal tract; attacks may last from several hours to 2 to 3 days
    - Type I: no protein
      - Normal inhibitor of the activated first component of the complement system (C1-INH)
    - Type II: normal or increased amount of dysfunctional C1-INH
    - Type III: normal and functional C1-INH, estrogen dependent
  - Acquired angioedema (AAE)
    - Type I: low protein; lymphoproliferative disorders
    - Type II: dysfunctional protein; anti-C1-INH antibodies
  - Laboratory studies
    - Type I HAE
      - C1-INH, C2, and C4 levels are low
      - C4 levels are low during an attack; they may be normal in between attacks
      - C1q normal
    - Type II HAE
      - Normal levels of C1-INH that is dysfunctional
      - C4 and C2 levels are low during an attack
    - Type III HAE
      - C1-INH normal
      - C4-INH normal
    - In AAE, Type I and Type II: low C1q, C2, C4, and C1-INH levels; C4 levels are low during angioedema episodes but may be normal between episodes
  - Treatment: steroids, H_1 and H_2 blockers
    - Stanazolol, danazol, for the acute phase of an attack of hereditary angioedema
    - Aminocaproic acid for maintenance replacement of C1-INH to prevent attacks
    - Treatment of the underlying disorder associated with AAE

Urticarial Vasculitis

- Form of leukocytoclastic vasculitis
- Clinical findings: generalized wheals or erythematous plaques, occasionally with central clearing, lasting for more than 24 hours in a fixed location
- Primary causes
  - Drug induced: angiotensin-converting enzyme (ACE) inhibitors, penicillin, sulfonamides, fluoxetine, and thiazides
  - Normocomplementemic: can be associated with connective tissue diseases
  - Hypocomplementemic: autoantibodies to C1q, associated with connective tissue diseases

- Serum sickness
- Type III hypersensitivity reactions
- Viral diseases: hepatitis B, hepatitis C, and infectious mononucleosis
- Idiopathic causes
- Schnitzler's syndrome
  - Urticarial vasculitis
  - Monoclonal IgM
  - Fever, lymphadenopathy, hepatosplenomegaly, bone pain with osteosclerosis, sensorimotor neuropathy
- Laboratory studies
  - CH50, C3, C4, C1q, and antibodies to C1q
  - If preceding tests are positive, evaluate renal function and urinalysis to check for the effects of vasculitis on the kidneys
- Histology: leukocytoclastic vasculitis
- Treatment: antihistamines or nonsteroidal anti-inflammatory drugs (NSAIDs), colchicine, hydroxychloroquine, dapsone, glucocorticoids, or azathioprine

Papular Urticaria

- Variation of urticaria caused by hypersensitivity to insect bites
- Lesions may last longer than 24 hours
- Type I hypersensitivity reaction
- Chronic symmetrically distributed pruritic papules and papulovesicles
- Histology: mild subepidermal edema, extravasation of erythrocytes, interstitial eosinophils, and exocytosis of lymphocytes
- Treatment: symptomatic in most cases; topical steroids

Other Figurate Erythemas (Covered in Separate Chapters)

- Bullous pemphigoid
- Erythema annulare centrifugum
- Erythema multiforme
- Glucagonoma syndrome
- Granuloma annulare
- Lupus erythematosus, subacute cutaneous
- Lyme disease
- Pityriasis rubra pilaris
- Psoriasis, plaque
- Tinea corporis

Id Reaction, or Autoeczematization

- Generalized acute cutaneous reaction to a variety of stimuli (infectious and inflammatory skin conditions)
- Symmetric, pruritic, erythematous, maculopapular, or papulovesicular eruption at a site distant from the primary infection or dermatitis
- Begins 1 to 2 weeks after primary infection or dermatitis

- Histology: superficial perivascular lymphohistiocytic infiltrate with a spongiotic epidermis and vesiculation; infectious agents not found in the specimens
- Treatment of primary eruption
  - Systemic or topical corticosteroids
  - Wet compresses
  - Systemic or topical antihistamines

Granuloma Faciale (Fig. 30-7)

- Probable immune disorder
- Clinical findings: persistent, asymptomatic, brown-red papules, nodules that affect the face (almost exclusively)
- Histology
  - Dense infiltrate of lymphocytes, histiocytes, neutrophils, and eosinophils deep in the dermis; Grenz zone; leukocytoclastic vasculitic with extravasation of erythrocytes and hemosiderin
  - Direct immunofluorescence: IgG, fibrin, (occasionally IgM) at the basement membrane and perivascularly
- Electron microscopy: Charcot-Leyden crystals, eosinophil granules, are evident within eosinophils and histiocytes
- Treatment: usually resistant to treatment; oral, topical, or intralesional corticosteroid injections; intralesional gold injections; oral bismuth; antimalarials; isoniazid; *p*-aminobenzoic acid (PABA); calciferol; topical psoralen UV-A (PUVA); radiation therapy; dapsone; surgical excision; dermabrasion; argon laser; carbon dioxide laser; electrosurgery; cryotherapy; 585-nm pulsed dye laser

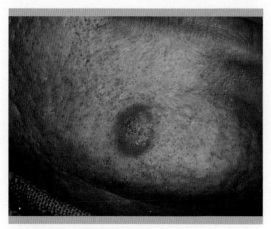

FIGURE 30-7 Granuloma faciale. *(From Freedberg IM et al: Fitzpatrick's Dermatology in General Medicine, 6th ed. New York: McGraw-Hill, 2003, p. 967.)*

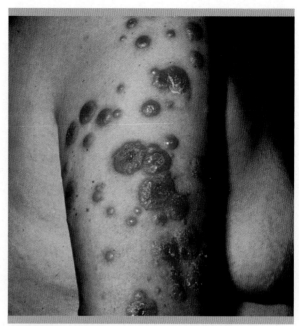

FIGURE 30-8 Sweet's syndrome. *(From Freedberg IM et al: Fitzpatrick's Dermatology in General Medicine, 6th ed. New York: McGraw-Hill, 2003, p. 951.)*

Acute Febrile Neutrophilic Dermatosis (Sweet's Syndrome) (Fig. 30-8)

- Reactive process
- Frequent association with hematologic malignancy (acute myelogendis leukemia and others), solid malignancies, Crohn's disease, and ulcerative colitis
- Drugs: granulocyte colony-stimulating factor, bactrim, all-*trans* retinoic acid, minocycline, lithium, furosemide, hydralazine, carbamazepine, and levonorgestrel/ethinyl estradiol
- Infections: upper respiratory infections (streptoccocal) and gastrointestinal tract (yersenia)
- Sjögren syndrome, Behçet disease, lupus erythematosus, rheumatoid arthritis
- Diagnostic criteria: two major and two minor clinical findings
  - Major criteria include (1) abrupt onset of tender or painful erythematous plaques or nodules, occasionally with vesicles, pustules, or bullae, and (2) histopathologic evidence of predominantly neutrophilic infiltration in the dermis without leukocytoclastic vasculitis
  - Minor criteria include (1) lesions preceded by a nonspecific respiratory or gastrointestinal tract infection or vaccination or associated with inflammatory disease, hemoproliferative disorders, solid malignant tumors, or pregnancy, (2) accompanied by periods of general malaise and fever higher than 38°C, (3) laboratory values

during onset of erythrocyte sedimentation rate greater than 20 mm/h, C-reactive protein positive, segmented nuclear neutrophils and bands greater than 70 percent in peripheral blood smear, and leukocytosis more than 8000 (three of four of these values necessary), and (4) excellent response to treatment with systemic corticosteroids or potassium iodide

- Clinical findings
  - Middle-aged adults
  - Reddish blue or violaceous papules, plaques, or nodules; edema that mainly affects upper extremities, head, neck
  - May last weeks, sometimes longer
  - Pulmonary manifestations are the most common extracutaneous finding (culture-negative pulmonary infiltrates on chest x-ray films)
  - Demonstrates pathology
- Histology: edema of papillary dermis, widespread infiltrates composed of neutrophils; malignant cells sometimes present as well
- Treatment: prednisone, dapsone, colchicine, potassium iodide

Pyoderma Gangrenosum

- Inflammatory skin disease with progressive ulceration
- Associated with other diseases (colitis ulcerosa, rheumatoid arthritis, hepatitis) in about half of patients
- Inflammatory bowel disease (ulcerative colitis or regional enteritis/Crohn's disease), polyarthritis (symmetric and may be either seronegative or seropositive); hematologic diseases/disorders, such as leukemia or preleukemic states, predominantly myelocytic in nature or monoclonal gammopathies (primarily IgA)
- Clinical findings
  - Inflammatory pustule or bulla, ulcerates with purulent discharge
  - Ulcerations with undermined, inflamed borders, sometimes with vegetations, pathergy
  - Sometimes painful
  - Intraoral form of the disease known as *pyostomatitis vegetans*
  - Heals with cribriform scar
- Histology: deep and dense infiltrate with many neutrophils, abscess, blood vessels with fibrin deposits, ulcerations
- Treatment
  - Topical therapies: local wound care and dressings, superpotent topical corticosteroids, cromolyn sodium 2% solution, nitrogen mustard, and 5-aminosalicylic acid
  - Systemic therapies: corticosteroids, cyclosporine, mycophenolate mofetil, azathioprine, dapsone, tacrolimus, cyclophosphamide, chlorambucil, thalidomide, nicotine, enteracept
  - Intravenous therapies: pulsed methylprednisolone, pulsed cyclophosphamide, immune globulin
  - Other therapy includes hyperbaric oxygen
- Surgery should be avoided because of pathergy
- Recurrences may occur, and residual scarring is common

GRANULOMATOUS PROCESSES

Granuloma Annulare (GA) (Fig. 30-9)

- Clinical findings
  - Asymptomatic red papules with elevated borders and central depression, annular arrangement
  - Often involutes following minor trauma
  - Chronic, usually self-limiting disease
  - Often in children; adults also affected
  - Predilection for the extensor surfaces of extremities and the dorsa of hands and fingers
- Clinical variants
  - Localized GA: typical distribution as above (75 percent of cases)
  - Generalized GA: few to thousands of 1- to 2-mm papules or nodules
  - Subcutaneous GA: firm, nontender, flesh-colored or pinkish nodules without overlying epidermal alteration
  - Perforating GA: one to hundreds of grouped 1- to 4-mm papules; necrobiotic material is extruded

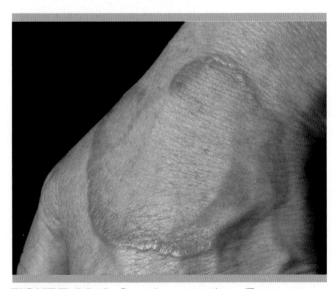

FIGURE 30-9 Granuloma annulare. *(From Freedberg IM et al: Fitzpatrick's Dermatology in General Medicine, 6th ed. New York: McGraw-Hill, 2003, p. 981.)*

through focal perforations; most often affects children; papules often coalesce to form annular plaques

- Arcuate dermal erythema: uncommon form of GA that manifests as infiltrated erythematous patches that may form large, hyperpigmented rings with central clearing
- Histology: foci of necrobiosis within the dermis, surrounded by palisading histiocytes
  - Deep forms: within the reticular dermis and can reach into the subcutaneous tissue
  - Subcutaneous granuloma annulare is situated within the subcutaenous tissue
- Treatment: intralesional corticosteroids, potent topical corticosteroids, psoralen and UV-A (PUVA), systemic steroids, dapsone, pentoxifylline, hydroxychloroquine, isotretinoin, chlorambucil, interferon-γ, cyclosporin A, potassium iodide, nicotinamide, niacinamide, salicylates, chlorpropamide, thyroxine, and dipyridamole

Actinic Granuloma (Annular Elastolytic Giant Cell Granulomas)

- Annular or serpiginous areas with raised erythematous borders
- Location on heat- or sun-damaged skin
- Present with 1 to 10 plaques
- Histology: may lack the classic palisaded arrangement observed in GA; elastosis is abundant in the middermis outside the granuloma; elastic tissue is absent from the center

Chondrodermatitis Nodularis Helices

- Unknown etiology: vascular deficiency, cold, chronic trauma
- Clinical findings
  - One or sometimes several painful nodules on helix, several milimeters in size
  - No tendency to healing spontaneously
- Histology: epidermal ulceration above a focus of cartilage degeneration, granulation tissue
- Treatment: relieve or eliminate pressure at the site; collagen injections may bring relief by providing cushioning; topical and intralesional steroids; excision; curettage; electrocauterization; carbon dioxide laser ablation; and excision of the involved skin and cartilage

Sarcoidosis

- Noncaseating epithelioid granulomas
- Delayed-type hypersensitivity, heightened helper T-cell type1 immune response
- Clinical findings
  - Lofgren's syndrome

- Presents with bilateral hilar lymphadenopathy, pulmonary infiltration, and ocular (uveitis) and skin lesions; erythema nodosum, arthritis
- Extrathoracic manifestations involving the liver, skin, heart, and/or eye are the presenting findings in 40 percent of patients
- Twenty-five percent of cases limited to skin
- Asymptomatic dark red plaques and papules are the most common variant
- Lupus pernio: red to purple or violaceous, indurated plaques and nodules on the nose; usually commonly seen with chronic uveitis and bone cysts
- Erythema nodosum (EN) is the most common nonspecific cutaneous disease
- Darier-Roussy sarcoidosis: subcutaneous nodular sarcoidosis
- Uveoparotid fever (Herendtfort's syndrome): anterior uveitis, fever, parotid enlargement, seventh cranial nerve palsy
- Neurosarcoid: lesions may occur anywhere in the CNS or peripheral nervous system
- Laboratory studies
  - Serum angiotensin converting enzyme (ACE) level is elevated, hypercalciuria, hypercalcemia
  - Chest radiography
  - Kveim test: most specific test for sarcoidosis; intradermal injection of tissue from the spleen or the lymph node of a patient with sarcoidosis; biopsy sample is obtained from the area 4 to 6 weeks after injection, and it is examined histologically for noncaseating granuloma formation
  - Pulmonary function tests
- Histology: dermal epitheloid granulomas, irregular, often mild lymphocytic infiltrate, inclusion bodies (schaumann, asteroid bodies, residual bodies)
- Treatment: oral or intralesional corticosteroids, methotrexate, azathioprine, hydroxychloroquine, chloroquine, cyclosporine, oral isotretinoin, allopurinol, and thalidomide

Foreign-Body Granulomas

- Clinical findings
  - Located in areas of trauma and surgery
  - Small, firm nodules, often surrounded by inflammation
  - Red, red-brown, or color of normal skin
  - Ulcerations and fistula
- Histology: foreign bodies (suture material, keratin, hair, traumatic foreign material); chronic inflammation with giant multinuclear histiocytes and granulocytes; some foreign bodies (silica, wood, suture material, glass) are birefringent (identify with polarized light)

INFILTRATIVE DISEASES

Papular Mucinosis (Lichen Myxedematosus, Papular Mucinosis); Scleromyxedema

- Spectrum of disease
  - Localized, less severe forms: lichen myxedematosus or papular mucinosis
  - Sclerotic, diffuse form scleromyxedema
- Lichen myxedematosus
  - Fibroblast proliferation and mucin deposition in the dermis in the absence of thyroid disease
  - Associated with plasma cell dyscrasia: monoclonal paraprotein band, usually of the IgG type
  - Slow onset of asymptomatic or mildly pruritic papules, which may be localized or generalized
  - Primary lesion is a 2- to 4-mm dome-shaped and flesh-colored or erythematous papule
  - Lesions may coalesce into grouped lichenoid papules and are found on the dorsal hands, face, or extensor surfaces of the arms and legs
- Scleromyxedema
  - Widespread progressive induration, decreased mobility
  - Cysts and urticarial lesions, leonine faces
  - Widespread erythematous, indurated skin resembling scleroderma
  - Range of motion of the face, fingers, and extremities is decreased
  - Systemic manifestations include restrictive and obstructive pulmonary dysfunction, cardiovascular abnormalities
  - Gastrointestinal symptoms (most commonly dysphagia) are related to esophageal aperistalsis
  - Severe proximal muscle weakness, polyarthritis
  - Ophthalmologic changes: ectropion and corneal opacities
- Studies
  - Serum protein immunoelectrophoresis: paraprotein (usually IgG) with lambda light chains
  - Few patients may have myeloma or Waldenström's macroglobulinemia
  - Thyroid function test results are normal
  - Histology: large depositions of mucin (hyaluronic acid) in the dermis; numerous plump stellate fibroblasts in dermis; mucin stains with periodic acid-Schiff and Alcian blue at pH 2.5 but not pH 0.4, metachromatically stains with toluidine blue at pH 3.0
- Treatment
  - Melphalan, stem cell transplant
  - Cyclosporine, prednisone, electron beam therapy, extracorporeal photopheresis

Colloid Milium

- Multiple, dome-shaped, amber- or flesh-colored papules developing on light-exposed skin
- Three variants: adult-onset type, a nodular form (nodular colloid degeneration), and a juvenile form (autosomal dominant)
- Degenerative condition linked to excessive sun exposure
- Histology: fissured eosinophilic colloid masses are seen in the dermis; solar elastosis
- Stains: periodic acid–Schiff (PAS)–positive and shows green birefringence with Congo red
- Treatment: dermabrasion, cryotherapy, and diathermy

Favre-Racouchot Syndrome (Nodular Elastosis with Cysts and Comedones)

- Multiple open and closed comedones in the presence of actinically damaged skin
- Periorbital and temporal areas
- Skin with yellowish discoloration, yellowish nodules, atrophy, wrinkles, and furrows is present
- Usually bilaterally
- Histology: comedones with significant actinic elastosis, including nodules of elastin

Erythema Elevatum Diutinum (EED) (Fig. 30-10)

- Type of leukocytoclastic vasculitis
- Deposition of immune complexes in small blood vessels
- Red, purple, brown, or yellow papules, plaques, or nodules on extensor surfaces, especially over the joints, Achilles tendons, fingers, and toes
- History of arthralgia, exacerbated by streptoccocal disease

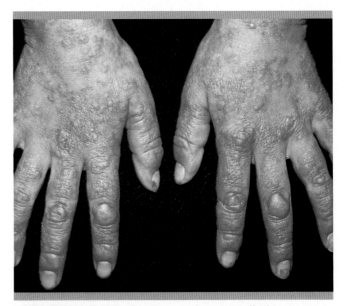

FIGURE 30-10 Erythema elevatum diutinum. *(From Freedberg IM et al: Fitzpatrick's Dermatology in General Medicine, 6th ed. New York: McGraw-Hill, 2003, p. 957.)*

- Histology: necrotizing vasculitis, older lesions with extracellular cholesterol deposits
- Direct immunofluorescence: complement and IgG, IgM, IgA, and fibrin around the damaged vessels
- Treatment: dapsone, sulfapyridine; intermittent plasma exchange, niacinamide
- Chronic disease that usually evolves over a 5- to 10-year period, at which point it may resolve

Scleredema

- Diffuse, firm, edematous induration of the skin
- Neck, upper part of the trunk and arms
- Regression after several months
- May be associated with a history of an antecedent febrile illness, diabetes mellitus, or blood dyscrasia
- Fibroblast culture: increased procollagen synthesis
- Histology: epidermis is normal; dermis is thickened with broad collagen bundles; mucin deposits; no proliferation of fibroblasts
- Treatment: systemic steroids, cyclosporine, methotrexate, psoralen with ultraviolet light A (PUVA), penicillamine, electron beam, and glycemic control with prostaglandin E1 (PGE1)

Cutaneous Myxoma

- Lesions that are myxoid and variably cellular
- Includes subungual myxomas; propensity for local recurrence
- Papular lesion
- May be seen in Carney complex (33% patients)
- Perifollicular in orientation
- Histology: localized accumulation of mucin within the reticular dermis

CALCIUM DEPOSITS

Subepidermal Calcifying Nodule

- Calcium deposits (dystrophic calcification) of unknown etiology

Calciphylaxis (Fig. 30-11)

- Necrosis of skin secondary to calcification and occlusion of small cutaneous arterioles
- Associated with: chronic renal failure, hypercalcemia, hyperphosphatemia, an elevated calcium-phosphate product, and secondary hyperparathyroidism; common in patients with end-stage renal disease (ESRD)
- Nonspecific violaceous mottling, as livedo reticularis, or as erythematous papules, plaques, or nodules
- Developed lesions have a stellate purpuric configuration with central cutaneous necrosis
- Lower extremities most common location (90 percent); proximal greater than distal, where body fat is most abundant

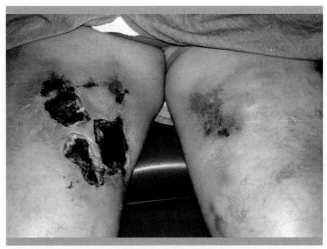

FIGURE 30-11 Calciphylaxis. *(From Freedberg IM et al: Fitzpatrick's Dermatology in General Medicine, 6th ed. New York: McGraw-Hill, 2003, p. 1493.)*

- Laboratory studies
  - Calcium-phosphate product frequently exceeds 60 to 70 mg^2/dl^2
  - Serum blood urea nitrogen and creatinine levels; calcium, phosphate, alkaline phosphatase, and albumin levels; parathyroid hormone level
  - Coagulation factors: prothrombin time (PT), activated partial thromboplastin time (aPTT), protein C, protein S, anticardiolipin, lupus anticoagulant, factor V Leiden, and homocysteine
- Histology: calcium deposits within the walls of blood vessels, mixed inflammatory infiltrate; subcutaneous calcium deposits with lobular panniculitis and fat necrosis vascular microthrombi, epidermal necrosis
- Prognosis: mortality rate of calciphylaxis is reported to be as high as 60 to 80 percent; the leading cause of death is sepsis from infected, necrotic skin lesions
- Treatment: serum calcium and phosphate concentrations must be brought to low-normal levels; aggressive wound care, parathyroid ectomy, hyperbaric oxygen

Osteoma Cutis

- Bone within the skin in the absence of a preexisting condition
- Familial occurrence of Albright's hereditary osteodystrophy (pseudohypoparathyroidism and pseudopseudohypoparathyroidism) may be present
- Face, extremities, scalp, digits, and subungual regions
- Deposits of calcium and osteomas within the dermis
- Laboratory studies: serum calcium and parathyroid hormone (PTH) levels
- Histology: mature bone is found in the dermis or extends into the subcutaneous tissue

Calcinosis Cutis

- Calcium deposits form in the skin
- Four major types
  - Dystrophic: due to trauma, inflammatory processes, tumors, infections
  - Metastatic: abnormal calcium or phosphate metabolism
  - Iatrogenic: secondary to a treatment or procedure
  - Idiopathic: no causative factor identifiable
- Insoluble compounds of calcium (hydroxyapatite crystals or amorphous calcium phosphate) are deposited within the skin
- Ectopic calcification can occur in the setting of hypercalcemia and/or hyperphosphatemia (if calcium-phosphate product exceeds 70 mg^2/dl^2)
- Multiple, firm, whitish dermal papules, plaques, nodules, or subcutaneous nodules
- Laboratory studies: serum calcium, inorganic phosphate, alkaline phosphatase, and albumin
- Histology: granules and deposits of calcium are seen in the dermis, with or without a surrounding foreign-body giant cell reaction
- Treatment: correct the underlying problem

Gout

- Increased level of uric acid in the blood
- Caused by overproduction of purines, increased catabolism of nucleic acids, decreased excretion of uric acid (idiopathic gout, about 80 percent), or decreased degradation of purines
- Chalky white deposits on intraarticular structures
- Subcutaneous deposits (tophi), sometimes discharged transcutaneously, sometimes in late stages of the disease
- Location: helix of the ear, elbow, fingers, toes
- Up to several centimeters
- Histology
  - Epidermis normal or ulcerated; large deposits of amorphous, basophilic material with parallel, needle-shaped clefts within the dermis and subcutis; lymphohistiocytic infiltrate, often with granulomatous foreign-body reaction
  - Fixation in 100% ethanol, crystals are birefingent; crystals dissolve if tissue fixed with formaldehyde; the fixation fluid can be tested for presence of urates

Hemosiderin

- Intradermal deposits of iron (hemosiderin), chemical degredation
- Associated with hemorrhage (purpura, stasis dermatitis)
- Hemoglobin
- Clinical: brown, reddish-brown macules, patches
- Histology: siderosis around foreign bodies
- Tissue stain: Perl's iron stain

PERFORATING DISORDERS

Kyrle Disease

- Large papules with central keratin plugs
- May develop in a widespread distribution pattern
- Associated with chronic renal failure
- Small papule with silvery scale, enlarges to form a red-brown papule or nodule with a central keratin plug
- Histology: parakeratotic plug, acanthosis; within the plug there often is admixed basophilic debris; necrotic cellular material and degenerated connective tissue undergo transepidermal elimination; mixed infiltrate
- Treatment: keratolytics, 5-fluorouracil, topical corticosteroids, methotrexate, mercury, chloroquine, and prednisone

Perforating Folliculitis

- Keratotic follicular papules over extensor surfaces
- Disruption of the infundibular portion of the follicular wall, with transepidermal elimination of connective tissue elements and cellular debris
- Can be associated with chronic renal failure or idiopathic
- Histology: perforation of follicular epithelium, transepithelial channel and, often, a parakeratotic luminal plug; degenerating, collagen and elastin mixed with inflammatory cells
- Treatment of underlying condition; tretinoin 0.1% cream; oral β-carotene, keratolytics, antiacne therapies, and topical corticosteroids

Elastosis Perforans Serpiginosa (EPS)

- Small papules erupt, grouped in a confined area, eventually becoming serpiginous
- Central core of each papule contains a compressed aggregate of fibrous material and cellular debris
- Sites affected most commonly: nape of the neck, upper extremities, face, lower extremities, and trunk
- Three forms
  - Idiopathic: cause unknown; genetic predisposition is possible
  - Reactive: associated with systemic, inherited, fibrous tissue abnormalities, such as Down's syndrome, Ehlers-Danlos syndrome, Marfans syndrome, osteogenesis imperfecta, scleroderma, and pseudoxanthoma elasticum
  - Drug-induced: D-penicillamine and occurs in approximately 1 percent of patients
- Histology: abnormal elastic tissue fibers, other connective tissue elements, and cellular debris are expelled from the papillary dermis through the epidermis (transepithelial elimination)
  - Acid orcein-Giemsa and aldehyde fuchsin, Verhoeff-van Gieson stains

Reactive Perforating Collagenosis (RPC)

- Focal damage to collagen followed by the elimination through epidermis
- Pin-sized lesions that grow into larger papules over a few weeks
- Linear pattern Koebner phenomenon
- Most commonly found on the extensor surfaces of the limbs and the dorsa of the hands
- Abnormal response to superficial trauma
- Inherited form presents in childhood
- Precipitated by cold or superficial blunt trauma
- Acquired form (acquired perforating dermatosis): occurs in patients with chronic renal failure, diabetes
- Histology: disrupted collagen bundles extrude through the epidermis, forming a plug with a cup-shaped epidermal depression; mild perivascular mononuclear cell infiltrate, mild acanthosis
- Treatment: topical and systemic steroids, topical and oral retinoids, methotrexate

OTHER DISORDERS

Hyperkeratosis Lenticularis Perstans (HLP, Flegel's Disease)

- Loss or decreased number of membrane-coating granules (Odland bodies)
- Red-brown papules with horny scales of irregular outline
- Measuring 1 to 5 mm in diameter and up to 1 mm in depth
- Located primarily on the dorsal feet and lower legs
- Histology
  - Discrete area of hyperkeratosis, with areas of parakeratosis, overlying a thinned stratum carneum and thinned-to-absent granular layer lymphoid infiltrate with occasional histiocytes in a bandlike pattern in the papillary dermis
- Treatment: topical 5% fluorouracil and synthetic vitamin D_3 derivative
- Oral retinoids have been successful only during continuous therapy

Degos Disease

- Progressive, small and medium-sized arterial occlusive disease, leading to tissue infarction and initially involving the skin
- Occurs both in a limited benign, cutaneous form and in a lethal multiorgan, systemic variant
- Erythematous, pink or red papules that heal to leave scars with pathognomonic, central, porcelain white, atrophic centers and peripheral telangiectatic rim
- Systemic variant: gastrointestinal tract (50 percent of cases); intestinal perforation (most severe complication and the most common cause of death); central nervous system (20 percent)

- Frequently fatal within 2 to 3 years from the onset of systemic involvement
- Ocular findings: posterior subcapsular cataracts, visual field defects, ptosis, third cranial nerve palsies, blepharoptosis, and optic atrophy
- Histology: superficial and deep perivascular, periadnexal, and perineural chronic inflammatory cell infiltrate with interstitial mucin deposition, wedge-shaped degeneration of collagen, melanin incontinence, epidermal atrophy, and a developing zone of papillary dermal sclerosis
- Treatment: No successful medical therapy is known; antiplatelet drugs may reduce the number of new lesions in some patients with only skin involvement

Anetoderma (Fig. 30-12)

- Benign condition
- Focal loss of dermal elastic tissue resulting in flaccid or herniated saclike skin (on pressure, a normal ring of surrounding skin is felt); begin as erythematous macules, plaques, nodules, or urticarial wheals that enlarge over weeks
- Upper arms, trunk, and thighs
- Primary anetoderma: idiopathic
- Secondary anetoderma: associated with multiple diseases, infections, and medications

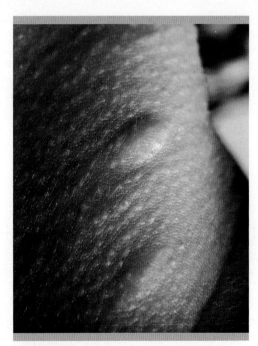

FIGURE 30-12 Anetoderma. *(From Freedberg IM et al: Fitzpatrick's Dermatology in General Medicine, 6th ed. New York: McGraw-Hill, 2003, p. 1028.)*

- Possible etiologies: defective elastin synthesis, uncontrolled release of elastase by inflammatory cells, elastophagocytosis, or an immune mechanism
- Histology: perivascular and periadnexal lymphohistiocytic infiltrate of papillary and/or upper reticular dermis, loss of elastic fibers
- Treatment: no effective treatment for anetoderma is known

Atrophoderma of Pasini and Pierini (IAPP)

- Atrophy of the skin
- Single or multiple sharply defined, slightly depressed oval areas of skin
- Lesions may be discrete or confluent
- Affected skin appears thinned and discolored and becomes depressed below the level of the surrounding skin (clifflike shelf at the borders)
- *Borrelia burgdorferi* may be involved in the pathogenesis
- Histology: decrease in the size of the dermal papillae, with flattening of the rete ridges; melanin is increased in the basal layer
- Treatment: if positive *Borrelia* antibody titer, treat with appropriate antibiotic therapy; Q-switched laser

Ainhum

- Autoamputation of a digit
- Most commonly the fifth toe; triggered by trauma
- Fibrotic band develops from a flexural groove and progressively encircles the toe until spontaneous autoamputation occurs
- Histology: shows fissuring and epidermal hyperkeratosis and parakeratosis, followed by a fibrotic reaction under the deepening fissure; as scar tissue contracts, it constricts and narrows neurovascular bundles
- Treatment: no current treatment appears to halt the progression of ainhum

Pseudoainhum

- Occurs as a secondary event resulting from certain hereditary and nonhereditary diseases leading to annular constriction of digits
- Due to a collagen band around the digit
- May be acquired or congenital
- Treatment: excision of bands, retinoids

Pseudoxanthoma Elasticum (PXE) (Fig. 30-13)

- Inherited connective tissue disorder; mutation of *ABcc6* gene, autosomal recessive
- Progressive calcification and fragmentation of elastic fibers
- Skin manifestations: small, yellow papules in a linear or reticular pattern that may coalesce to form plaques; skin takes on a "plucked chicken" appearance

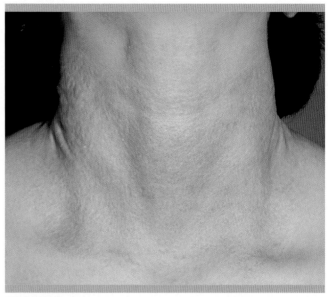

FIGURE 30-13 Pseudoxanthoma. *(From Freedberg IM et al: Fitzpatrick's Dermatology in General Medicine, 6th ed. New York: McGraw-Hill, 2003, p. 1504.)*

- Changes are first noted on the lateral part of the neck and later involve the antecubital fossae, axillae, popliteal spaces, and inguinal and periumbilical areas, as well as the oral, vaginal, and rectal mucosa
- Ocular manifestations: angioid streaks of the retina: slate gray to reddish brown curvilinear bands radiating from the optic disk
- Cardiovascular manifestations: calcification of the elastica media and intima of the blood vessels: hypertension, coronary artery disease, angina pectoris, myocardial infarction; mitral valve prolapse
- Gastrointestinal hemorrhage
- Diagnosis criteria:
  - Major: characteristic skin signs, characteristic ophthalmologic features, characteristic histological features of lesional skin
  - Minor: characteristic histological features of non-lesional skin, family history of PXE in first degree relatives
  - Category I: all major criteria
  - Category II: no skin lesions with one major and a minor or two minor criteria
- Histology: fragmented, swollen, and clumped elastic fibers are basophilic because of the calcium deposition; collagen fibers are split and are said to unwind; calcification of blood vessels
- Elastic stains: Verhoeff-Van Gieson, orcein; calcium deposit stains; Von Kossa, alizarin red
- Treatment: diet low in lipids and calcium (600 to 1200 mg/day) is recommended

Hypertrophic Osteoarthropathy (HOA)

- Digital clubbing and subperiosteal new bone formation
- Associated with polyarthritis, cutis verticis gyrata, seborrhea, and hyperhidrosis
- Divided into primary (pachydermoperiostosis) and secondary (hypertrophic pulmonary osteoarthropathies) forms
  - Pachydermoperiostosis (PDP): autosomal dominant; accounts for 5 percent of all cases
  - Hypertrophic osteoarthropathy (pulmonary hypertrophic osteoarthropathy): associated with underlying cardiopulmonary diseases and malignancies
- Treatment: nonsteroidal anti-inflammatory drugs (NSAIDs) or corticosteroids may alleviate the polyarthritis associated with PDP

Dermatofibrosis Lenticularis (Buschke-Ollendorf Syndrome)

- Autosomal dominant, connective-tissue disorder
- Cultured fibroblasts produce three to eight times more tropoelastin than fibroblasts of healthy individuals; elastin production is higher in involved than uninvolved skin
- Slightly elevated and flattened yellowish papules and nodules grouped together forming plaques in the sacrolumbar region and, symmetrically, on the extremities
- Nasolacrimal duct obstruction, amblyopia, strabismus, benign lymphoid hyperplasia, hypopigmentation, and short stature
- Osteopoikilosis in the stratum spongiosum of the epiphysis and the metaphysis of the long bones
- Histology: numerous thickened collagen fibers in the dermis; elastic fibers with various diameters; orcein stain
- Treatment: surgical excision of the dermal lesions is indicated only for cosmetic reasons

Pseudocyst of the Auricle

- Benign, noninflammatory, asymptomatic swelling on the lateral or anterior surface of the pinna, usually in the scaphoid or triangular fossa
- Swelling develops over 4 to 12 weeks
- Histologically: pseudocyst of the auricle is characterized by an intracartilaginous cavity lacking an epithelial lining, with thinned cartilage and hyalinizing degeneration along the internal border of the cystic space
- Treatment: surgical incision of the lesion with replacement of the anterior skin surface
- Without treatment, permanent deformity of the auricle may occur

ULCERATION

Pressure Sores (Ulcers)

- Clinical findings
  - Occur in immobilized patients
  - Due to chronic pressure in tissues overlying bony prominences
  - Lumbosacral region, greater trochanters, and heels are the most common areas
  - Tissue ischemia and neural damage lead to necrosis
- Varying degrees:
  - I: erythema
  - II: induration, blisters
  - III: shallow ulcers
  - IV: deep necrosis of fat and muscle
  - V: bone destruction
- Underlying a small skin defect there can be vast necrosis of deep tissues and proliferation of granulation tissue
- Histology: epidermal necrosis, subepidermal bulla, vascular proliferations, often secondary inflammation

REFERENCES

Almond SL, Curley RK, Feldberg L. Pseudoainhum in chronic psoriasis. *Br J Dermatol* 2003:149(5):1064–1066.

Arpey CJ, Patel DS, Stone MS, Qiang-Shao J, Moore KC. Treatment of atrophoderma of Pasini and Pierini-associated hyperpigmentation with the Q-switched alexandrite laser: a clinical, histologic, and ultrastructural appraisal. *Lasers Surg Med* 2000;27(3):206–212.

Freedberg IM et al. *Fitzpatrick's Dermatology in General Medicine*, 6th Ed. New York: McGraw-Hill; 2003.

Giro MG, Duvic M, Smith LT. Buschke-Ollendorff syndrome associated with elevated elastin production by affected skin fibroblasts in culture. *J Invest Dermatol* 1992;99(2):129–137.

Hoque SR, Ameen M, Holden CA. Acquired reactive perforating collagenosis: four patients with a giant variant treated with allopurinol. *Br J Dermatol* 2006;154(4):759–762.

Kim YJ, Chung BS, Choi KC. Calciphylaxis in a patient with end-stage renal disease. *J Dermatol* 2001;28(5):272–275.

Lebwohl M, Phelps RG, Yannuzzi L. Diagnosis of pseudoxanthoma elasticum by scar biopsy in patients without characteristic skin lesions. *N Engl J Med* 1987;317:347–350.

Marcoval J, Moreno A, Peyr J. Granuloma faciale: a clinicopathological study of 11 cases. *J Am Acad Dermatol* 2004; 51(2):269–273.

McKee PH. *Pathology of the Skin: With Clinical Correlations*. London: Mosby-Wolfe; 1996.

Richard G. Molecular genetics of the ichthyoses. *Am J Med Genet* 2004;131C(l):32–44.

Richie RC. Sarcoidosis: a review. *J Insur Med*. 2005;37(4): 283–294. Review.

Sangueza OP, Pilcher B, Martin Sangueza J. Erythema elevatum diutinum: a clinicopathological study of eight cases. *Am J Dermatopathol* 1997;19(3):214–222.

CHAPTER 31

DISORDERS OF FAT

ASRA ALI

NEOPLASMS OF THE SUBCUTANEOUS FAT

Lipoma

- Most common benign mesenchymal tumor
- Solitary or multiple round, lobulated, yellow masses within the subcutaneous tissue
- Histology
  - Well-circumscribed neoplasms surrounded by a thin, fibrous capsule
  - Thin strands of tissue intersect the sheets of adipocytes
- Types
  - Intramuscular lipomas: lipomas that extend into skeletal muscle
  - Fibrolipoma: thick bundles of collagen in the lipoma
  - Sclerotic lipoma: thickened collagen bundles with few persisting adipocytes
  - Myxolipomas: stromal deposits of mucopolysaccharides
  - Myelolipomas: ectopic hematopoietic bone marrow elements
  - Infarcted lipomas: necrotic fat surrounded by multinucleate histocytic giant cells, lymphocytes, and extravasated erythrocytes
- Syndromes
  - Dercum's disease/adiposis dolorosa: tender nodules, idiopathic, obese, postmenopausal women, arms, trunk, paraarticular
  - Madelung's disease/benign symmetric lipomatosis (Fig. 31-1): upper trunk, proximal (not distal) extremities, middle-aged men, alcoholics or those with liver disease; "horse collar" appearance: confluence on neck; laboratory abnormalities: hyperuricemia, decreased glucose tolerance
  - Familial lipomatosis: autosomal dominant; third decade of life; hundreds of discrete nodules, slowly asymptomatic, extremities, forearms, intraabdominally
  - Congenital lipomatosis: first few months of life; large subcutaneous masses, chest; infiltrating lipomas permeate skeletal muscle; manifests in *Proteus* syndrome (partial gigantism, autosomal recessive, hemihypertrophy, hemangiomas, lymphangiomas)
  - Bannayan-Zonana syndrome: autosomal dominant; multiple lipomas, syringomas, hemangiomas, macrocephaly, delayed motor and speech
- Other lipomas
  - Angiolipoma
    - Numerous, tender, mobile, arms, trunk, subcutaneous nodules
    - Histology: sharply circumscribed, adipocytes with prominent vascular pattern
  - Spindle-cell lipoma
    - Subcutaneous nodule, middle-aged men, back, shoulder, posterior neck; well circumscribed
    - Histology: mature adipocytes, oval to spindle-shaped cells, stroma with mucin, spindle cells, and pale cytoplasm (fibrocytes—prelipoblasts)
  - Pleomorphic lipoma
    - Clinically similar to spindle-cell lipomas; subcutaneous nodules trunk, posterior neck
    - Histology: floret cells: multinucleated bizarre giant cells with eosinophilic cytoplasm and overlapping nuclei; stroma, mucinous with foci of fibrosis; no mitoses
  - Chrondroid lipoma
    - Females > males; subcutaneous fat, muscle of hips, extremities
    - Histology: eosinophils, vacuolated cells that resemble chrondroblasts, arranged in sheets, cords, mucinous stroma (cartilage), scalloped nuclei
  - Myolipoma/lipoleiomyoma
    - Resemble large lipomas, abdomen, retroperitoneum, >15 cm, slimy, yellow-white cut surface
    - Histology: biphasic: mature adipocytes with smooth muscle cells, no atypia

403

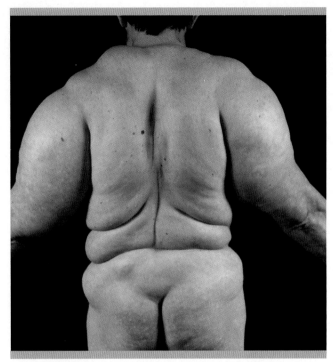

FIGURE 31-1 Symmetric lipomatosis. *(From Freedberg IM et al: Fitzpatrick's Dermatology in General Medicine, 6th ed. New York: McGraw-Hill, 2003, p. 1069.)*

- Angiomyolipoma/angiolipoleiomyoma
  - Usually in kidney; associated with tuberous sclerosis; can occur in skin (acral, elbows, ears); these are not associated with tuberous sclerosis; slow growing; asymptomatic
  - Histology: blood vessels, smooth muscle bundles, adipose tissue, vessels with thick walls
- Hibernoma
  - Red-brown, mobile, brown fat, solitary, between scapulae, lower cervical/mediastinal (most common), axillary
  - Histology: vacuolated cells, large round central nuclei with prominent nucleoli, abundant eosinophilic, granular cytoplasm secondary to mitochondria (mulberry cell)
- Lipoblastoma/lipoblastomatosis
  - Appears only in infants, first three years of life, >12 cm, solitary subcutaneous mass, trunk, limbs
  - Two variants
    ▲ Benign (circumscribed lipoblastoma): subcutaneous, well demarcated
    ▲ Diffuse (lipoblastomatosis): deep-seated infiltrates of soft tissue and skeletal muscle
  - Histology: mature adipocytes separated into small lobules by fibrovascular septa; filled with cytoplasmic fat vacuoles displacing nucleus to periphery (signet ring)
- Liposarcoma
  - Most common soft tissue malignancy; arises de novo; elderly; nonmobile; rapidly enlarging; causes pain by compression
  - Histology: well-differentiated pleomorphic adipocytes; enlarged nuclei in thickened septa; sclerosing: abundant dense and fibrillary collagen; myxoid: most common variant, mucinous stroma

LIPODYSTROPHY

- Lipodystrophy
  - Absence of subcutaneous fat with no evidence of inflammation
  - Congenital or acquired, and clinical variants include total, partial, and localized forms
  - Histology: small adipocytes and intervening hyaline or myxoid connective tissue and proliferation of small blood vessels; second type has some inflammation with lymphocytes, foamy histiocytes, and plasma cells within the small fat lobules
- Absence of subcutaneous fat
- Partial lipodystrophy (PL) (Fig. 31-2)
  - Loss of subcutaneous fat in demarcated symmetric areas of the body

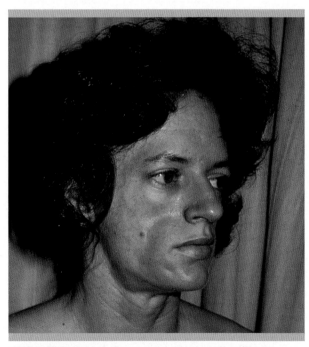

FIGURE 31-2 Partial lipodystrophy. *(From Freedberg IM et al: Fitzpatrick's Dermatology in General Medicine, 6th ed. New York: McGraw-Hill, 2003, p. 1064.)*

- Begins on the face and spreads downward, stopping at any level
- More common in females
- Occasionally correlated with onset of an acute febrile illness
- Associated with C3 nephritic factor (binds factor H) inhibitor of C3; results in uncontrolled activation of C3
- Glomerulonephritis: direct toxicity from C3 nephritic factor
- Histology: marked decrease or absence of subcutaneous fat cells
- Treatment: renal transplant for increased uremia, increased third-trimester intrauterine death
- Dunnigan-Kobblering syndrome
  - Mutations in *LMNA* gene that encodes laminins A and C
  - Subcutaneous loss of fat from limbs
  - Can be autosomal dominant
  - Metabolic problems: insulin-dependent diabetes mellitus (IDDM), acanthosis nigricans
- HIV-associated lipodystrophy
  - Associated with highly active antiretroviral therapy (HAART) therapy
  - Loss of subcutaneous fat of upper and lower extremities and from the face
  - Fat increases at the posterior neck and upper back and on the breasts
  - Laboratory findings: insulin resistance and hyperglycemia
  - Treatment: changes within or between a class of drugs, recombinant human growth hormone (rhGH), metformin, dehydroepiandrosterone, nonsteroidal anti-inflammatory drugs, liposuction of the upper back, filler substances (silicone, poly-L-lactic acid)
- Generalized lipodystrophy (GL)
  - Mutation of *seipin* gene; patients with later-onset GL do not have the mutation
  - Primary hypothalamic dysfunction with secondary adipose tissue effects
  - Patients lack both subcutaneous fat and extracutaneous adipose tissue
  - Syndromes
    - Acquired: Seip-Lawrence syndrome
    - Congenital: Berardinelli-Seip syndrome
  - Other related signs and symptoms: acanthosis nigricans, hypertrichosis, generalized hyperpigmentation, thick curly scalp hair, increased appetite, increased perspiration, heat intolerance, basal metabolic rate increased, external genitalia enlarged
  - Diagnosis: decreased glucose tolerance owing to lipoatrophic diabetes; no ketoacidosis, increased low-density lipoproteins (LDLs)

- Lipoatrophy
- Syndrome of localized lipodystrophy
- Atrophy of the subcutaneous fat
  - Loss of subcutaneous fat owing to a previous inflammatory process involving the subcutis
  - Residual process of several inflammatory conditions involving the subcutaneous fat lobules; lipoatrophy secondary to subcutaneous injections of corticosteroids
  - Histology: lipophagic granuloma surrounding a small fat lobule, with perilobular fibrosis

PANNICULITIS

- Group of heterogeneous inflammatory diseases that involve the subcutaneous fat
- Subcutaneous fat is organized into lobules of lipocytes separated by thin septa of connective tissue
- Each individual lobule is supplied by an arteriole branching from the septa to form capillaries into the lobule, and a capillary network surrounds each adipocyte

Panniculitis (Lobular)

- With vasculitis
  - Erythema nodosum leprosum
  - Lucio's phenomenon
  - Neutrophilic lobular (pustular) panniculitis associated with rheumatoid arthritis
  - Erythema induratum of Bazin
  - Crohn's disease
- No vasculitis
  - Sclerosing panniculitis
  - Calciphylaxis
  - Oxalosis
  - Cold panniculitis
  - Sclerema neonatorum
  - Lupus panniculitis (lupus erythematosus profundus)
  - Weber-Christian
  - Posttraumatic
  - Panniculitis in dermatomyositis
  - Pancreatic panniculitis
  - α_1-Antitrypsin deficiency
  - Infection
  - Factitial panniculitis
  - Subcutaneous sarcoidosis
  - Lipoatrophy
  - Subcutaneous fat necrosis of newborn
  - Poststeroid panniculitis
  - Gout panniculitis
  - Crystal-storing histiocytosis
  - Cytophagic histiocytic panniculitis
  - Postirradiation pseudosclerodermatous panniculitis

Panniculitis (Septal)

- With vasculitis (see Chap. 23)
  - Leukocytoclastic vasculitis
  - Superficial thrombophlebitis
  - Cutaneous polyarteritis nodosa
- No vasculitis
  - Scleroderma
  - Erythema nodosum
  - Necrobiosis lipoidica
  - Subcutaneous granuloma annulare
  - Rheumatoid nodule
  - Necrobiotic xanthogranuloma

Disorders Erroneously Considered as Specific Variants of Panniculitis

- Weber-Christian disease
- Rothmann-Makai disease
- Lipomembranous or membranocystic panniculitis
- Eosinophilic panniculitis

Necrobiosis Lipoidica

- Deep extension of the dermal process of palisading granulomas
- Yellow-brown, indurated plaques with an atrophic and slightly depressed center and a well-defined raised erythematous edge that radially enlarges
- Histology: palisading granulomas with histiocytes surrounding areas of degenerated collagen within widened septa; IgM and complement depositions in the walls of the blood vessel of necrobiotic areas

Scleroderma (Deep Morphea)

- Extension from the deep dermis into the septa of subcutaneous fat; process can be entirely a panniculitis
- Bound down indurated plaques or nodules, heal with atrophy
- Histology: marked fibrous thickening of the septa of subcutaneous fat

Subcutaneous Granuloma Annulare

- Subcutaneous nodules with no inflammatory appearance at the skin surface (can coexist 25 percent of the time); head, hands, buttocks, and the anterior aspect of the lower legs
- Histology: necrobiosis with peripheral palisading granulomas involving the septa of the subcutis

Rheumatoid Nodule

- Nodules in the vicinity of the joints affected by arthritis; predilection for the elbows and fingers
- Large areas of necrobiosis (homogeneous and eosinophilic) surrounded by palisaded granulomas involving the dermis and subcutaneous fat

Necrobiotic Xanthogranuloma

- Indurated plaques with yellow-violaceous coloration that are sharply demarcated and show a tendency to ulceration; predilection toward the periorbital region; chronic and progressive
- Paraproteinemia, mostly of IgG κ type
- Histology: large areas of necrobiosis (occasionally with cholesterol crystals in the center) alternating with granulomatous inflammation

Erythema Nodosum (EN) (Fig. 31-3)

- Most common type of panniculitis
- Acute
  - Sudden appearance of red, warm, tender nodules symmetric on the anterior surfaces of lower legs with fever, malaise, arthropathy (70 percent); lasts from 3 to 6 weeks
  - Erythema contusiformis: late-stage lesions with yellow or greenish appearance
- Chronic (EN migrans): several red subcutaneous nodules unilateral on the lower extremities
- Immunologic reaction triggered by several antigens: fungal, enteropathies (ulcerative colitis, Crohn's), sarcoid, drugs (oral contraceptive pills, sulfonamides, bromides), bacterial infections (tuberculosis, streptococcal infections, leprosy, tularemia, cat scratch), viral infections (paravaccinia, Epstein-Barr virus, lymphogranuloma venereum, hepatitis B), Behcet's, Sweet's

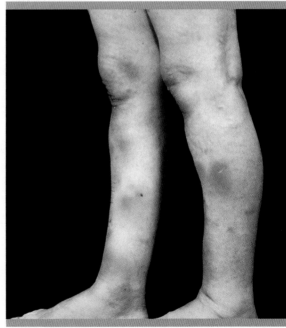

FIGURE 31-3 Erythema nodosum. *(From Freedberg IM et al: Fitzpatrick's Dermatology in General Medicine, 6th ed. New York: McGraw-Hill, 2003, p. 1056.)*

- Streptococcal infections are the most frequent etiologic factor for erythema nodosum in children, whereas drugs, sarcoidosis, and inflammatory diseases of the bowel are the most commonly associated disorders in adults
- Diagnosis: biopsy, increased erythrocyte sedimentation rate, chest x-ray, complete blood count (CBC), anti-streptolysin (ASO) titer, virologies, tuberculosis, fungal cultures
- Histology: septal panniculitis; Miescher's radial granulomas: small, well-defined nodular aggregations of small histiocytes around a central stellate or banana-shaped cleft
- Treatment: spontaneous resolution, nonsteroidal anti-inflammatory drugs (NSAIDs), oral steroids, potassium iodine

Erythema Nodosum Leprosum

- Immune complex–mediated vasculitis with painful erythematous and violaceous nodules, mostly involving the extremities of patients with lepromatous leprosy
- Histology: fibrinoid necrosis of their walls and luminal thrombi
- IgG and complement in the walls of the involved vessels

Lucio's Phenomenon

- Necrotizing vasculitis in patients with a variant of a lepromatous leprosy reaction and hemorrhagic ulcers
- Necrotizing vasculitis of the small vessels with foamy histiocytes that contain numerous acid-fast bacilli

Erythema Induratum of Bazin (Nodular Vasculitis)

- Most common form of lobular panniculitis with vasculitis
- Painless, tender, deep-seated, circumscribed subcutaneous infiltrations of both lower extremities/calves; usually in middle-aged women
- Erythema induratum of Bazin: relationship with *Mycobacterium tuberculosis;* remainder of cases are referred to as *nodular vasculitis*
- Histology: lobular panniculitis with vasculitis; ischemic necrosis of fat lobule with decreased septal involvement; tuberculoid-type granulomas

Crohn's Disease

- Abscesses, sinuses, and fistulas on the genital and perianal areas
- Histology: noncaseating granulomas composed of epithelioid histiocytes

Sclerosing Panniculitis

- Also known by a variety of names, including hypodermitis sclerodermiformis,

lipodermatosclerosis, and lipomembranous change in chronic panniculitis
- Woodlike indurated plaques with erythema, edema, telangiectasia, and hyperpigmentation involving the lower legs with a stocking distribution
- Associated with chronic venous insufficiency, arterial ischemia, and previous episodes of thrombophlebitis
- Histology: stasis dermatitis changes (proliferation of capillaries and venules in the papillary dermis, fibrosis, and abundant hemosiderin deposition), atrophy of the subcutaneous fat, areas of ischemic necrosis

Calciphylaxis (Fig. 31-4)

- Associated with chronic renal failure
- Calcification of cutaneous vessel walls resulting in necrosis and ulceration
- Abnormalities in calcium-phosphorus metabolism, with elevated serum calcium and phosphorus levels, often in the context of the secondary hyperparathyroidism associated with renal failure (normal in some patients)
- Violaceous, mottled to reticulated patches and plaques; evolve to necrotic, indurated plaques and nodules
- Symmetry, and distal parts of the extremities, thighs, and buttocks are the most frequent areas
- Histology: calcium depositions in the walls of small- to medium-diameter blood vessels
- Prognosis: mortality rate as high as 80 percent

Oxalosis

- Primary inherited oxalosis
  - Autosomal recessive
  - Type I: deficiency of 2-hydroxy-3-oxoadipate carboxylase

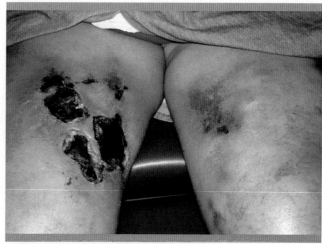

FIGURE 31-4 Calciphylaxis *(From Freedberg IM et al: Fitzpatrick's Dermatology in General Medicine, 6th ed. New York: McGraw-Hill, 2003, p. 1493.)*

- Type II: deficiency of D-glyceric dehydrogenase
- Livedo reticularis and acral gangrene
- Secondary acquired oxalosis
  - Excessive oxalate or glycolic acid ingestion, ethylene glycol poisoning, intravenous glycerol or xylitol infusion, methoxyflurane anesthesia, pyridoxine deficiency, intestinal disease, ileal resection, and in the setting of chronic renal failure, hemodialysis
  - Miliary deposits of calcium oxalate on the palmar aspects of the fingers
- Both primary and secondary oxalosis often lead to renal failure and death of the patient
- Histology: calcium deposition and oxalate crystals on the vessel walls

Sclerema Neonatorum

- Develops during first few days of life
- Affects debilitated infants, low-weight premature newborns often with severe illnesses
- Increased ratio of saturated-to-unsaturated fats
- Rapidly spreading induration of the skin; begins on buttocks to thighs, back; usually symmetric
- Histology: lobular panniculitis without fat necrosis, little inflammation, enlarged lipocytes with needle-like clefts in a radial array
- Prognosis: poor, usually death within a few days

Cold Panniculitis

- Cheeks of children sucking ice cubes, ice packs, or ice lollies (popsicles)
- Indurated erythematous plaques with ill-defined margins
- Histology: lobular panniculitis with an inflammatory infiltrate of lymphocytes and histiocytes in the fat lobules; marked edema in the papillary dermis
- Equestrian panniculitis: subtype of cold panniculitis
  - Occurs in healthy women during cold months when riding horses and wearing tight trousers
  - Painful red nodules on superior lateral thighs develop 48 to 72 hours after exposure

Lupus Panniculitis (Lupus Erythematosus Profundus)

- One to three percent of patients with cutaneous lupus erythematosus; may precede, appear simultaneously, or develop after disease has developed
- Trauma to subcutaneous fat can be a precipitating factor
- Deeply situated subcutaneous nodules or plaques on the upper arms, shoulders, face, and buttocks
- Atrophy and swelling after resolution
- Histology: fifty percent of patients with epidermal and dermal changes of discoid lupus erythematosus (atrophy of the epidermis, vacuolar change at the dermal-epidermal junction, thickened basement membrane, interstitial mucin between collagen bundles of the dermis, and superficial and deep perivascular inflammatory infiltrate of lymphocytes involving the dermis)
- Fifty percent of patients with changes confined to the subcutaneous fat; presence of lymphoid follicles with germinal centers and peripheral plasma cells
- Immunofluorescence: linear deposition of IgM and C3 along the dermal-epidermal junction

Pancreatic Panniculitis

- Association with acute and chronic pancreatitis and 2 to 3 percent of all patients with pancreatic diseases and pancreatic cancer, acinar cell
- Tender, fluctuant, erythematous subcutaneous nodules ulcerate spontaneously and exude an oily brown material (liquefaction necrosis of adipocytes)
- Pretibial area most common site, ankle arthralgias
- Fat necrosis can occur in internal organs.
- Calcium precipitation can produce hypocalcemia
- Histology: ghostlike fat cells (thick cell wall, no nuclear staining, lobular, calcification), necrotic fat cells, polymorphous fat infiltrate
- Saponification: Dystrophic calcification in ghost adipocytes (hydrolytic action of pancreatic enzymes on fat followed by calcium deposition)

α_1-Antitrypsin Deficiency (α_1-Protease Inhibitor Deficiency/Serine Protease)

- Affects homozygous patients
- Enzyme inhibits trypsin (produced in liver), also chymotrypsin, plasmin, thrombin, neutrophil-produced elastase
- Clinical findings: liver disease, hepatitis, cirrhosis, pulmonary disease, vasculitis, acquired angioedema
- Panniculitis: Lesions may occur after trauma; painful, recurrent nodules that drain a yellow fluid derived from fat breakdown
- Diagnosis: serum α_1-antitrypsin decreased
- Histology: septal and lobular inflammation, splaying of neutrophils between collagen bundles of the reticular dermis, fibrous septae, fat necrosis

Infective Panniculitis

- Bacteria or fungi may cause lobular panniculitis mainly in immunosuppressed patients
- Local cutaneous infections
  - Direct physical innoculation or from an indwelling catheter (primary)
  - Direct extension to the chest wall in pulmonary infections (secondary)
- Hematogenous dissemination

- Histology:
  - Primary cutaneous infections: epicenter of the inflammation is the superficial dermis; thrombosed vessels do not contain intravascular organisms
  - Secondary cutaneous infections: epicenter of inflammation is deeply seated; vessels are thrombosed and dilated with masses of organisms

Factitial Panniculitis

- Self-inflicted by psychiatric patients
- Histology: mostly lobular panniculitis; inflammation predominantly composed of neutrophils in early lesions and a more granulomatous infiltrate in late-stage lesions; polarization of the slide can identify the refractile foreign material

Iatrogenic Panniculitis

- Drugs injected in the subcutaneous fat, such as povidone, meperidine, pentazocine, and vitamin K_1, or substances used to correct facial wrinkles, such as paraffin, silicone, polymethyl-methacrolate (PMMA)-microspheres
- Histology: mostly lobular panniculitis; inflammation composed predominantly of neutrophils in early lesions and a more granulomatous infiltrate in late-stage lesions; polarization of the slide can identify the refractile foreign material; paraffinoma (sclerosing lipogranuloma), multiple "Swiss-cheese-like" pseudocystic spaces replacing the fat lobules, silicone multinucleated giant cells surrounding polygonal translucent angulated foreign bodies, which represent impurities in the silicone

Traumatic Panniculitis

- Accidental blunt trauma, especially frequent in women with large breasts (excessive weight affects mammary subcutaneous fat)
- Indurated nodules deeply situated on the breast tissue, surface of the skin with occassional "orange peel" appearance
- Variants:
  - Lipoatrophia semicircularis
    - Semicircular bandlike atrophy of the subcutaneous fat
    - Involves half the circumference of the anterolateral aspects of the thighs
    - Occurs in patients who repeatedly knock their thighs against a desk or chair because of their working habits
  - Mobile encapsulated lipoma (encapsulated fat necrosis)
    - Well-demarcated movable nodules in the subcutis of lower limbs, elbows, or hips after trauma

- Histology: cystic spaces of variable size and shape within fat lobules, as a consequence of confluent necrosis of the fat cells, surrounded by variable degrees of fibrosis and hemorrhage

Subcutaneous Sarcoidosis

- Subcutaneous nodules on the lower extremities without superficial cutaneous involvement
- Histology: noncaseating granulomas of the fat lobules and few lymphocytes at the periphery ("naked" granulomas); occasional calcification

Subcutaneous Fat Necrosis of the Newborn (SFNN)

- Neonatal period, benign, self-limiting
- Healthy full-term neonates
- Localized erythematous, violaceous, firm nodules and plaques; spares anterior trunk
- Greater ratio of saturated to unsaturated fatty acids than in adult fat
- Hypercalcemia of unknown significance
- Histology: granulomatous inflammation, lymphocytes, epithelioid cells, foreign-body giant cells, needle-shaped clefts (crystals of triglycerides), fat in macrophages and giant cells, calcium deposition
- Prognosis: Lesions regress spontaneously in a few days

Post-steroid Panniculitis

- Mainly in children
- High-dose systemic steroids for a short period of time with doses that were decreased quickly or steroid therapy was withdrawn suddenly
- Deep nodules appear 1 to 10 days after cessation of high-dose steroids; reinstitution of steroid therapy may help to resolve the lesions
- Histology: Lobular panniculitis with needle-shaped clefts (represent former sites of fatty acid crystals dissolved by tissue processing) within lipocytes, histiocytes

Cytophagic Histiocytic Panniculitis

- Two presentations that present with multiple inflammatory subcutaneous nodules and plaques over limbs
- Authentic panniculitis
- Histology: inflammatory infiltrate in the fat lobules composed of histiocytes and mature T-lymphocytes and with cytophagocytosis that results from macrophages that contain intact or fragmented erythrocytes, leukocytes, or lymphocytes within their cytoplasm, which produce the so-called bean-bag cells

Subcutaneous "Panniculitic" Lymphoma

- Lymphoma with appearance of panniculitis
- High-grade aggressive lymphoma, cytotoxic T cell

- Lethal hemorrhagic episodes and fever are common; adenopathy
- Histology: pleomorphic lymphocytes involving the fat lobule show marked atypia, with large and hyperchromatic nuclei, karyorrhexis, and frequent atypical mitotic figures; often atypical lymphocytes form a ring surrounding necrotic adipocytes
- Immunohistochemical: CD3, CD8, and cytotoxic granular proteins (TIA-1 and perforin); lack expression of CD4

Weber-Christian Disease

- Lobular panniculitis without vasculitis and systemic manifestations including fever and involvement of visceral fat tissue
- Term *Weber-Christian disease* should be abandoned as a diagnosis for cases of lobular panniculitis because now a more specific diagnosis may be rendered in most cases

Rothmann-Makai Disease

- Cases of relapsing nodular panniculitis without other systemic manifestations
- Obsolete term that is no longer used

Lipomembranous or Membranocystic Panniculitis

- Found in late-stage lesions of sclerosing panniculitis
- Cystic spaces in the fat lobule that result from necrosis of the adipocytes; the cystic spaces are lined with a homogeneous eosinophilic membrane with convoluted projections (stain brightly with periodic acid-Schiff and Sudan black and are resistant to diastase) into the cystic cavity

Eosinophilic Panniculitis

- Septal or lobular panniculitis in which eosinophils predominate in the inflammatory infiltrate
- Nonspecific reactive process found in many different disorders

REFERENCES

Freedberg IM et al. *Fitzpatrick's Dermatology in General Medicine,* 6th Ed. New York: McGraw-Hill; 2003.

Garg A. Lipodystrophies. *Am J Med* 2000;108(2):143–152.

Gonzalez-Garcia R, Rodriguez-Campo FJ, Sastre-Perez J, Munoz-Guerra MF. Benign symmetric lipomatosis (Madelung's disease): case reports and current management. *Aesthetic Plast Surg* 2004;28(2):108–112.

Lever WF, Elder DE. *Lever's Histopathology of the Skin.* Philadelphia: Lippincott Williams & Wilkins; 2005.

McKee PH. *Pathology of the Skin: With Clinical Correlations.* London: Mosby-Wolfe; 1996.

Misra A, Garg A. Clinical features and metabolic derangements in acquired generalized lipodystrophy: case reports and review of the literature. *Medicine (Baltimore)* 2003;82(2):129–146.

Requena L, Sanchez Yus E. Panniculitis. Part II, Mostly lobular panniculitis. *J Am Acad Dermatol* 2001;45(3):325–361; quiz 362–364. Review.

Requena L, Yus ES. Panniculitis. Part I. Mostly septal panniculitis, *J Am Acad Dermatol* 2001;45(2):163–183; quiz 184–186.

Weiss SW. Lipomatous tumors. *Monogr Pathol* 1996;38: 207–239.

CHAPTER 32

GENODERMATOSIS

MARZIAH THURBER
ADRIENNE M. FEASEL
ADELAIDE A. HEBERT

VASCULAR-RELATED DISORDERS

Von Hippel-Lindau Syndrome

- Autosomal dominant
- *VHL* gene
- Presents by fourth decade
- Clinical findings
  - Cerebellar, medullary, or spinal cord hemangioblastomas with increased intracranial pressure, spinal cord compression
  - Retinal hemangioblastomas with visual impairment
  - Renal cell carcinoma, renal and pancreatic cysts
  - Pheochromocytoma, adrenal carcinoma
  - Polycythemia secondary to increased erythropoietin

Ataxia-Telangiectasia (Louis-Bar Syndrome)

- Autosomal recessive
- Mutation in *ATM* gene; codes for protein kinase
- Defective DNA repair with increased sensitivity to ionizing radiation
- Clinical findings
  - Progressive ataxia
    - Presents at ages 2 to 3 years
    - Due to depletion of Purkinje cells in cerebellum
  - Oculocutaneous telangiectasias by ages 3 to 6 years
  - Respiratory infections owing to decreased humoral and cellular immunity
  - Malignancies: lymphoma, breast cancer
  - Hypogonadism

Osler-Weber-Rendu Syndrome (Hereditary Hemorraghic Telangiectasia)

- Autosomal dominant
- Mutation in endoglin, TGF-β receptor
- Presents in childhood to early adulthood
- Clinical findings
  - Telangiectasias in third to fourth decade: face, palms, soles, conjunctiva, oral mucosa

- Recurrent epistaxis
- Gastrointestinal telangiectasias with hemorrhage
- Pulmonary AV shunts (most serious problem)

CONNECTIVE TISSUE DISORDERS

Ehler's-Danlos Syndrome (Fig. 32-1)

- Disorders characterized by skin extensibility, tissue fragility, and joint hypermobility
- Due to defects in collagen or defective posttranslational modification of collagen
- Classical (formerly I and II)
  - Autosomal dominant
  - *COL1A1, COL1A2, COL5A1* (most common, 30 to 50 percent), *COL5A2*
  - Collagen V defect
  - *TNXB,* codes for tenascin-X
  - Clinically similar to classic Ehler's-Danlos without scarring
  - Clinical
    - Skin hyperextensibility, easy bruising
    - Wide, atrophic scars
    - Joint hypermobility with sprains, dislocations
    - May have cardiac defects
    - Molluscoid pseudotumors (calcified hematomas)
    - Spheroids (fat-containing cysts)
- Hypermobility (formerly III)
  - Autosomal dominant
  - Gene defect *TNXB;* codes for tenascin-X
  - Clinical findings
    - Joint hypermobility with recurrent dislocations, chronic pain
    - Chronic joint pain
    - Skin hyperextensibility, easy bruising
    - Mitral valve prolapse
- Vascular (type IV or arterial type)
  - Autosomal dominant
  - *COL3A1* gene mutation
  - Collagen III defect

411

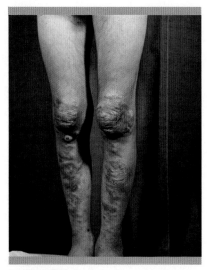

FIGURE 32-1 Classic Ehler's-Danlos syndrome. *(From Freedberg IM et al: Fitzpatrick's Dermatology in General Medicine, 6th ed. New York: McGraw-Hill, 2003, p. 1498.)*

- Clinical findings
  - Arterial rupture may cause sudden death
  - Thin, translucent skin; wound dehiscence
  - Arterial, intestinal, uterine fragility and rupture
  - Characteristic facies
- Kyphoscoliosis (formerly type VI or ocular-scoliotic type)
  - Autosomal recessive
  - Lysyl hydroxylase deficiency
  - PLOD gene

- Clinical findings
  - Generalized joint laxity with severe hypotonia
  - Progressive scoliosis; unable to ambulate by early adulthood
  - Scleral fragility; prone to global rupture
  - Arterial rupture
  - Marfanoid habitus
  - Osteopenia, osteoporosis
- Arthrochalasia (formerly VIIA and B)
  - Autosomal dominant
  - COL1A1 and COL1A2
  - Collagen I
  - Clinical findings
    - Congenital bilateral hip dislocations
    - Severe joint hypermobility with subluxations
    - Kyphoscoliosis, mild osteopenia
    - Skin hyperextensibility with bruising, atrophic scars
    - Muscle hypotonia
- Dermatosparaxis (formerly VIIC)
  - Autosomal dominant
  - Deficiency of procollagen I
  - N-terminal peptidase
  - ADAMTS2 gene
  - Clinical findings
    - Severe skin fragility
    - Redundant sagging skin (resembles cutis laxa)
    - Large hernias
    - Premature rupture of membranes at delivery
    - No impairment of wound healing

Osteogenesis Imperfecta (OI) (Table 32-1)

- Mutations in collagen I
- Mostly autosomal dominant

TABLE 32-1 Characteristics of Osteogenesis Imperfecta (OI)

OI Subtype	Characteristics
I	Thin skin, blue sclera Lax joints, kyphosis, abnormal dentition Aortic valve disease, mitral valve prolapse
II (severe)	In utero fractures, limb avulsion at delivery Perinatal death common Beaded ribs Aortic valve disease, blue sclera
III	In utero fractures Progressive scoliosis, limb bowing, crippling deformity Blue sclera
IV	Fractures at birth, abnormal teeth Improvement with age

- Four subtypes
  - Different mutations result in varying severity of disease
  - All characterized by osseous fragility
  - May develop hearing loss owing to otosclerosis

Marfan's Syndrome

- Autosomal dominant
- Mutation in fibrillin-1 (*FBN1*)
- Chromosome 15
- Clinical findings
  - Ocular, cardiovascular, and musculoskeletal defects
  - Tall stature with long extremities, arachnodactyly, high-arched palate
  - Joint hyperextensibility, hypotonia
  - Kyphoscoliosis, pectus excavatum
  - Striae distensae
  - Reactive elastosis perforans serpiginosa (EPS)
    - Transepithelial elimination of abnormal elastic tissue fibers
    - Small papules erupt and are grouped in a confined area, eventually becoming serpiginous
    - Histology: Acid orcein–Giemsa stain shows abnormal elastic fibers that are swollen and clumped in the papillary dermis (thorny appearance in penicillamine-induced EPS)
  - Ectopia lentis: upward displacement
  - Mitral valve prolapse, aortic aneurysm
- Course: premature death secondary to cardiovascular defects
- Treatment: surgery, beta-blockers

Cutis Laxa (Generalized Elastolysis)

- Autosomal recessive or acquired
- Defect in elastic fibers
- Drug-associated cases with penicillin, penicillamine
- Clinical findings
  - Loose, redundant skin lacks recoil
  - "Hound dog" facies
  - Deep voice from vocal cord laxity
  - May be confined to skin or associated with emphysema, hernias, diverticula
- Histology: Elastic fiber stains show a reduction in the number of elastic fibers throughout the dermis; fibers are clumped, granular, or fragmented

Pseudoxanthoma Elasticum (Fig. 32-2)

- Autosomal recessive
- *ABCC-6* gene
- Encodes ABC-cassette transporter MRP-6
- D-Penicillamine implicated in drug-associated cases
- Progressive fragmentation and calcification of elastic fibers in skin, blood vessels, and Bruch's membrane of the eye

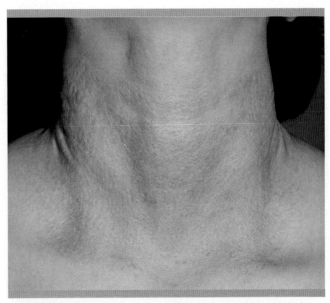

FIGURE 32-2 Pseudoxanthoma elasticum. *(From Freedberg IM et al: Fitzpatrick's Dermatology in General Medicine, 6th ed. New York: McGraw-Hill, 2003, p. 1504.)*

- Clinical findings
  - Redundant skin in intertriginous areas
  - "Plucked chicken" skin
  - Angioid streaks in eye, retinal hemorrhage
  - Claudication, hypertension, myocardial infarction (MI), cerebrovascular accident (CVA)
  - Gastrointestinal bleeds
- Histology: With hematoxylin-eosin stains, elastic fibers are basophilic because of the calcium deposition; fibers fragmented, swollen, and clumped in the middle and deep reticular dermis
- Course: decreased lifespan owing to cardiovascular disease

Tuberous Sclerosis (Bourneville's Syndrome, Epiloia)

- Autosomal dominant or spontaneous mutation
- Hamartin (*TSC1*, chromosome 9)
- Tuberin (*TSC2*, chromosome 16)
- Clinical findings
  - Triad of *epi*lepsy, *lo*w *i*ntellignce, *a*denoma sebaceum (*epiloia*)
  - Diagnosis requires the presence of two major features
    - Facial angiofibromas or forehead plaque
    - Nontraumatic ungual or periungual fibroma: Koenen's tumors (Fig. 32-3)
    - Shagreen patch (connective tissue nevus) (Fig. 32-4)
    - Multiple retinal nodular hamartomas

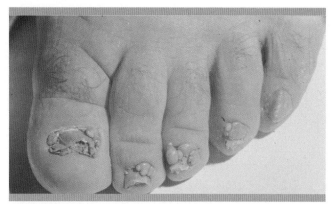

FIGURE 32-3 Koenen tumors in tuberous sclerosis complex. *(From Freedberg IM et al: Fitzpatrick's Dermatology in General Medicine, 6th ed. New York: McGraw-Hill, 2003, p. 1824.)*

  – Cortical tuber
  – Subependymal nodule
  – Subependymal giant cell astrocytoma
  – Cardiac rhabdomyoma, single or multiple
  – Lymphangiomyomatosis and/or renal angiomyolipoma
- Other findings
  - Ash-leaf macules: hypomelanotic macules (more than three) (Fig. 32-5)
  - Multiple randomly distributed pits in dental enamel
  - Hamartomatous rectal polyps
  - Bone cysts
  - Gingival fibromas

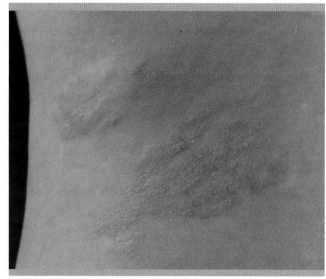

FIGURE 32-4 Shagreen patch in tuberous sclerosis. *(From Freedberg IM et al: Fitzpatrick's Dermatology in General Medicine, 6th ed. New York: McGraw-Hill, 2003, p. 1823.)*

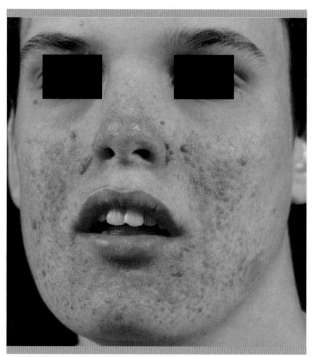

FIGURE 32-5 Ash-leaf macules. *(From Freedberg IM et al: Fitzpatrick's Dermatology in General Medicine, 6th ed. New York: McGraw-Hill, 2003, p. 1823.)*

- Nonrenal harmatoma
- Phakomas (retinal hamartomas): 50 percent of patients
- "Confetti" skin lesions
- Multiple renal cysts
- Skin tags
- Positive family history
- Focal poliosis
- Central nervous system (CNS): seizures, cortical tubers, paraventricular calcification, subependymal hamartomas, astrocytomas
- Mental retardation
- Pulmonary lymphangioleiomyomas
- Cutis verticis gyrata (CVG): folds and furrows formed from thickened skin of the scalp

Buschke-Ollendorf Syndrome (Dermatofibrosis Lenticularis)

- Autosomal dominant
- Increased elastic content in skin
- Clinical findings
  - Dermatofibrosis lenticularis disseminata
    – Yellowish papules and nodules grouped together forming plaques
    – Localized on the trunk: sacrolumbar region and symmetrically on the extremities

- Osteopoikilosis
  - Occurs in the epiphyses and the metaphyses of the long bones, especially in the fingers, the ulna, and the radius
  - No increased fracture risk
- Histology: thickened collagen fibers in the dermis; fragmented elastic fibers
- Radiologic findings: benign oval opacities on x-ray
- Normal lifespan

Focal Dermal Hypoplasia (Goltz Syndrome)

- X-linked dominant (lethal in males)
- Derives its name from the characteristic skin changes
- Clinical findings
  - Atrophic, telangiectatic streaks in Blaschko's lines
  - Fat herniations (focal dermal hypoplasia)
  - Papillomas on lips, perineum, axilla
  - Absent/dystrophic fingernails
  - Syndactyly with "lobster claw" deformity
  - Sparse, brittle hair
  - Osteopatha striata, hypodontia
  - Mild mental retardation
  - Disability owing to skeletal deformities
- Course: normal lifespan

Aplasia Cutis Congenita

- Autosomal dominant, autosomal recessive, or sporadic
- Clinical findings
  - Localized absence of epidermis, dermis, or subcutis
  - Well-demarcated erosions/ulcerations; 90 percent occur on scalp
- Treatment
  - Wound care
  - Most lesions heal with scar formation

PREMATURE AGING AND PHOTOSENSITIVE DISORDERS

Hutchinson-Gilford Syndrome (HGS, Progeria)

- Transforming growth factor β (TGF-β) upregulated
- Onset of HGS occurs at ages 6 to 12 months
- Clinical findings
  - "Elderly" appearance with atrophic, wrinkled skin
  - Birdlike facies, beaked nose
  - High-pitched voice
  - Prominent scalp veins, loss of subcutaneous fat, muscle wasting
  - Mottled hyperpigmentation
  - Sclerodermoid changes on lower extremities
  - Sparse/absent hair and dystrophic teeth
  - Large head with thin nose, micrognathia, small ears
  - Short stature

- Course: premature death in teens owing to atherosclerotic complications (angina, MI, CHF, CVA)

Werner Syndrome (Progeria Adultorum, Progeria of the Adult, Pangeria)

- Autosomal recessive
- WRN gene (RecQ helicase)
- Average age of patients at the time of diagnosis is 37 years
- Decreased growth of skin fibroblasts
- Increased urinary hyaluronic acid (abnormal glysoaminoglycan metabolism)
- Clinical findings
  - Premature aged appearance
  - Sclerodermoid changes
  - Poikiloderma
  - Loss of subcutaneous fat, muscle wasting
  - Soft tissue calcifications
  - Leg ulcers
  - Progressive alopecia
  - Short stature, osteoporosis, osteoarthritis
  - Ocular: posterior subcapsular cataracts
- Course: premature death in fourth decade owing to malignancy or atherosclerosis

Acrogeria (Grotton Syndrome, Familial Acromicria)

- Autosomal recessive
- Onset occurring up to age 6 years
- Clinical findings
  - Premature aging of extremities
  - Cutaneous atrophy and subcutaneous wasting of the face and extremities
  - Hair unaffected

Rothmund-Thomson Syndrome (Poikiloderma Congenitale)

- Autosomal recessive
- Genetic defect on chromosome 8
- RECQL4 (DNA helicase)
- Onset ages of 3 to 6 months
- Clinical findings
  - Dystrophic nails and teeth
  - Juvenile cataracts in 50 percent
  - Cataract
  - Poikilodermatous skin changes
  - Premature graying of the hair, alopecia
  - Increased photosensitivity, short stature, small skull, hypogonadism

Cockayne Syndrome

- Autosomal recessive
- CSB (ERCC6) or CSA (ERCC8)
- CKN1

- Deficiency in transcription-coupled nucleotide excision repair (TC-NER)
- Increased sister chromatid exchanges
- Cockayne syndrome I (CS-I)
  - Classic Cockayne syndrome
  - Death occurring by the second or third decade
- Cockayne syndrome II (CS-II)/Pena-Shokeir type
  - Severe Cockayne syndrome
  - Presents at birth with accelerated disease
  - Die by age 6 or 7 years
- Xeroderma pigmentosum–Cockayne syndrome complex (XP-CS)
  - No skeletal dysplasia
  - Early skin cancers
- Clinical findings
  - Erythema, bullae, scarring
  - Cachexia; large extremities
  - Sensineural deafness
  - Salt and pepper retinitis pigmentosa, cataracts
  - Mental retardation, intracranial calcifications
  - Onset during second year of life
  - Marked loss of subcutaneous fat
  - Increased photosensitivity
  - Microcephaly, progressive mental deterioration
  - Disproportionally large hands and feet
  - Protruding ears

Bloom Syndrome

- Autosomal recessive
- *BLM* gene
- *RECQL3,* DNA helicase
- Chromosomal instability
- Increased incidence in Ashkenazi Jews
- Clinical findings
  - Onset in infancy
  - Erythema, telangiectasia in butterfly distribution
  - Chelitis with high-pitched voice
  - Short stature; characteristic facies
  - Recurrent gastrointestinal and respiratory infections (low IgA, IgM)
  - Hypogonadism
- Course: increased mortality owing to neoplasm: leukemia, lymphoma, colon cancer

Seckel Syndrome

- Autosomal recessive
- Clinical findings
  - Bird head profile
  - Dwarfism
  - Trident hands
  - Skeletal defects
  - Hypodontia
  - Hypersplenism
  - Premature graying

SYNDROMES WITH MALIGNANT POTENTIAL

Dyskeratosis Congenita (Zinsser-Engman-Cole Syndrome)

- X-linked recessive or autosomal dominant
- *DKC1* (dyskeratosis congenita 1, dyskerin)
- Telomerase RNA component (TERC) defect
- Presents in first decade
- Clinical findings
  - Poikiloderma with gray-brown hyperpigmentation; "dirty"
  - Premalignant leukoplakia
  - Palmoplantar keratoderma, friction bullae
  - Hyperhidrosis
  - Dystrophic or atrophic nails; alopecia
  - Fifty percent mentally retarded
  - Pancytopenia with secondary infection, hemorrhage
  - Death in third to fourth decade owing to malignancy (usually SCC), gastrointestinal bleed, or infection

Xeroderma Pigmentosa

- Autosomal recessive
- Defective nucleotide excision repair (NER) after UV exposure (especially UV-B)
- *XPA, ERCC3* (*XPB*), *XPC, ERCC2* (*XPD*), *DDB2* (*XPE*), *ERCC4* (*XPF*), *ERCC5* (*XPG*), and *POLH* (Table 32-2)
- Clinical findings
  - Infants have sun sensitivity
  - Skin appears prematurely aged
  - Increased incidence of actinic keratosis, keratoacanthoma, squamous cell carcinoma, basal cell carcinoma, melanoma beginning in childhood
  - Photophobia, conjunctivits, corneal vascularization, and opacification (retina is spared)
  - Neurologic manifestations with progressive deterioration in 20 percent (mostly complement groups A and D)
  - DeSanctis-Cacchione syndrome: reserved for XP with severe neurologic disease with dwarfism and immature sexual development
  - Mental retardation, sensorineural deafness, spasticity, ataxia, hyporeflexia
  - Two-thirds die by third decade
- Treatment
  - Aggressive avoidance of sun exposure
  - High-dose oral isotretinoin
  - Excision of cutaneous malignancies
  - Imiquimod 5% cream, 5-fluorouracil
  - Skin screenings every 3 months
  - Ophthalmologic evaluation

TABLE 32-2 Xeroderma Pigmentosa Features and Mutations

Complementation Group	Mutation	Features
A	XPA	Neurologic abnormalities Most common in Japan
B	ERCC3	Xeroderma pigmentosum–Cockayne syndrome complex (XP/CS)
C	XPC	Most common in USA No neurologic abnormalities
D	ERCC2	DNA helicase defect XP/CS, trichothiodystrophy (XP/TTD), cerebro-ocular-facial syndrome (COFS)
E	DDB2	Mild disease, no neurologic changes
F	ERCC4	Mild disease, no neurologic changes
G	ERCC5	Neurologic symptoms only, XP/CS
Variant	XPV	No neurologic abnormalities

- Oral retinoids
- Bacterial DNA repair enzyme, denV T4 endonuclease in a topical liposome (not yet FDA approved)

Muir-Torre Syndrome (Fig. 32-6)

- Autosomal dominant
- *MSH2* gene located on chromosome 2p
- *MLH1* gene located on chromosome 3p
- DNA mismatch-repair (MMR) defect
- Presents in fifth to sixth decade
- Clinical findings
  - Numerous sebaceous tumors: adenomas, hyperplasia, epitheliomas, sebaceous carcinomas
  - Keratoacanthomas
  - Adenocarcinoma of the colon is most common cancer
  - Endometrial cancer (15 percent)
  - Other gastrointestinal, genitourinary, lung, breast, or hematologic malignancies

Cowden Syndrome

- Multiple hamartoma syndrome
- Autosomal dominant
- Chromosome 10
- *PTEN* defect (tumor suppressor gene)
  - Defect also found in Bannayan-Riley-Ruvalcaba syndrome (BRRS), Proteus syndrome (PS), and a Proteus-like syndrome

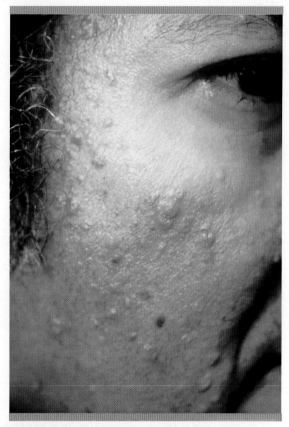

FIGURE 32-6 Muir-Torre syndrome. *(From Freedberg IM et al: Fitzpatrick's Dermatology in General Medicine, 6th ed. New York: McGraw-Hill, 2003, p. 1788.)*

- Presents in second to third decade
- Clinical findings
  - Mucocutaneous lesions: trichilemmomas, facial
  - Acral keratoses
  - Oral papillomas (cobblestoning)
  - Connective tissue nevi, epidermal nevi, and hyperostoses
  - Adenoid facies, high-arched palate, scoliosis
  - Breast adenocarcinoma
  - Most common malignancy (lifetime incidence 25 to 50 percent)
  - Thyroid cancer (follicular, rarely papillary, but never medullary)
  - Benign follicular adenomas (75 percent of patients)
  - Gastrointestinal polyps, ovarian cysts, fibrocystic breast disease

Gardner Syndrome

- Autosomal dominant
- Chromosome 5
- *APC* gene (adenomatosis polyposis coli)
- Defect also found in familial adenomatous polyposis (FAP)
- Promotes destruction β-catenin: component of a transcription factor complex

- Clinical findings
  - Polyposis of colon; most develop colon cancer
  - Osteomas of the skull and jaw, supernummerary teeth
  - Epidermoid cysts of head and neck
  - Tumors: desmoid, fibromas, hepatoblastoma
  - CHIRPE (congenital hypertrophy of the retinal pigment epithelium)
  - Predictor of colorectal polyposis
  - Skin and bony lesions in childhood
  - Gastrointestinal polyps develop by second to fourth decade
- Diagnosis: monitor with colonoscopy

Peutz-Jegher Syndrome (Periorificial Lentiginosis) (Fig. 32-7)

- Autosomal dominant or sporadic
- *STK11* gene (serine-threonine protein kinase) tumor suppressor gene
- Presents in childhood
- Clinical findings
  - Lentigines on mucosa, periorificial skin, palms, digits
  - Gastrointestinal hamartomatous polyps (more common in small intestine) may cause bleeding, pain, intussuception, obstruction; adenocarcinoma

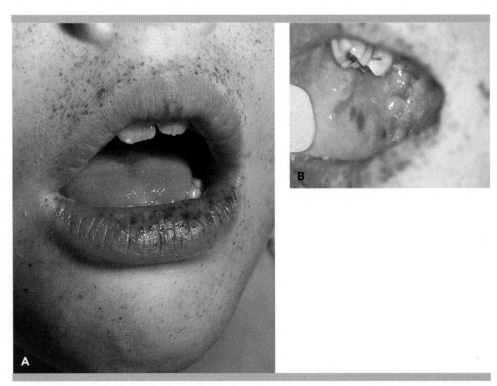

FIGURE 32-7 Peutz-Jeghers syndrome. *(From Freedberg IM et al: Fitzpatrick's Dermatology in General Medicine, 6th ed. New York: McGraw-Hill, 2003, p. 866.)*

- Ovarian cancer is most common malignancy
- Breast cancer, pancreatic cancer
- Diagnosis: monitor with colonoscopy, polypectomy
- Course: normal lifespan if malignancy detected early

Multiple Endocrine Neoplasia IIb (Multiple Neuroma Syndrome)

- Autosomal dominant
- Mutation in receptor tyrosine kinase (*RET*) protooncogene
- Chromosomal locus 10q11
- Clinical findings
  - Mucosal neuromas may result in thickened lips, eyelid eversion
  - Medullary thyroid carcinoma
  - Pheochromocytoma
  - Marfanoid habitus
  - Gastrointestinal ganglioneuromatosis with megacolon
- Course: normal lifespan with early detection and treatment of thyroid carcinoma

DISORDERS WITH CHROMOSOME ABNORMALITIES

Down's Syndrome (Trisomy 21)

- Nondisjunction at chromosome 21
- Presents at birth
- Clinical findings
  - Palmar crease
  - Nuchal skin folds
  - Syringomas
  - Elastosis perforans serpiginosa
  - Xerosis and lichenification with age
  - Alopecia areata
  - Flat nasal bridge, short broad neck, epicanthal folds, small mouth with protruding tongue
  - Mental retardation
  - Congenital heart disease
  - Duodenal atresia, acute myelogenous leukemia
- Course: increased infant mortality owing to congenital heart defects and neoplasms

Turner Syndrome

- Gonadal dysgenesis
- 45,XO monosomy
- Some cases demonstrate mosaicism
- Clinical findings
  - Short stature, webbed neck, triangular facies
  - Low-set hairline, patchy alopecia, wide-set nipples, cubitus valgus
  - Melanocytic nevi
  - Koilonychia
  - Primary amenorrhea, infertility

- Mental retardation
- Horseshoe kidneys
- Coarctation of aorta
- Treatment: estrogen replacement treatment of congenital anomalies

Noonan Syndrome

- Autosomal dominant
- Chromosome number normal (46, XX or 46, XY)
- Clinical findings
  - Resemble Turner syndrome with short stature, webbed neck, low posterior hairline, cubitus valgus
  - Cryptorchidism
  - Cardiac malformations (pulmonic stenosis)
  - Lymphedema
  - Tendency for keloid formation
- Treatment: correction of cardiac defects

Klinefelter Syndrome

- 47,XXY
- Decreased serum testosterone
- Clinical findings
  - Hypogonadism, gynecomastia
  - Tall with low hairline
  - Sparse body hair
  - Mental retardation, psychiatric problems in a third
  - Thrombophlebitis, leg ulcers
  - Risk of gonadal tumors, breast cancer
- Treatment
  - Testosterone replacement
  - Wound care

OTHER

Neurofibromatosis I (Von Recklinghausen Disease)

- Autosomal dominant
- Neurofibromin (17q)
- Clinical findings
  - Diagnosis requires two or more of the following features
    - >6 café-au-lait macules
      - ▲ >5 mm in prepubertal individuals
      - ▲ >15 mm in postpubertal individuals
    - Two or more neurofibromas or one plexiform neurofibroma (Fig. 32-8)
    - Axillary (Crowe's sign) or inguinal freckling
    - Optic glioma: tumor of optic nerves
    - Lisch nodules: hamartomas of iris; present as pigmented spots
    - Sphenoid wing dysplasia or thinning long bone cortex
    - First-degree relative with NF-1
  - Increased risk of malignancy (neurofibrosarcoma, astrocytoma, rhabdomyosarcoma, myelogenous leukemia)

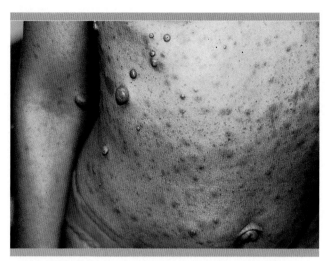

FIGURE 32-8 Neurofibromas. *(From Freedberg IM et al: Fitzpatrick's Dermatology in General Medicine, 6th ed. New York: McGraw-Hill, 2003, p. 1827.)*

- Mental retardation
- Seizures
- Kyphoscoliosis
- Endocrine disease (acromegaly, cretinism, hypothyroidism, hyperparathyroidism, precocious puberty)

Neurofibromatosis II (Bilateral Acoustic Neurofibromatosis)

- Autosomal dominant
- Schwannomin = Merlin (22q)
- Clinical: Diagnosis requires either
  - Bilateral eighth nerve masses (acoustic neuromas)
  - First-degree relative with NF-2 plus unilateral eighth nerve mass or two of neurofibroma, schwannoma, optic glioma, meningioma, juvenile posterior subcapsular opacity
- Death due to CNS tumors

REFERENCES

Disorders of Cornification

Akiyama M, Sawamura D, Shimizu H. The clinical spectrum of nonbullous congenital ichthyosiform erythroderma and lamellar ichthyosis. *Clin Exp Dermatol* 2003;28(3):235–240,

Cooper SM, Burge SM. Darier's disease: epidemiology, pathophysiology, and management. *Am J Clin Dermatol* 2003; 4(2):97–105.

Dhitavat J, Dode L, Leslie N, et al. Mutations in the sarcoplasmic/endoplasmic reticulum Ca2+ ATPase isoform cause Darier's disease. *J Invest Dermatol* 2003;121(3):486–489.

DiGiovanna JJ, Robinson-Bostom L. Ichthyosis: etiology, diagnosis, and management. *Am J Clin Dermatol* 2003;4(2):81–95.

Ikeda S, Mayuzumi N, Shigihara T, et al. Mutations in ATP2A2 in patients with Darier's disease. *J Invest Dermatol* 2003; 121(3):475–477.

Jacyk WK. What syndrome is this? X-linked dominant chondrodysplasia punctata (Happle). *Pediatr Dermatol* 2001; 18(5):442–444.

Kimyai-Asadi A, Kotcher LB, Jih MH. The molecular basis of hereditary palmoplantar keratodermas. *J Am Acad Dermatol* 2002;47:327–43.

Lam R, Armenta A, Kilic M, et al. Tyrosinemia. *Liver Transpl* 2002;8(5):500–501.

Marrakchi S, Audebert S, Bouadjar B, et al. Novel mutations in the gene encoding secreted lymphocyte antigen-6/urokinase-type plasminogen activator receptor-related protein-1 (SLURP-1) and description of five ancestral haplotypes in patients with Mal de Meleda. *J Invest Dermatol* 2003;120:351–355.

O'Driscoll J, Muston GC, McGrath JA, et al. A recurrent mutation in the loricrin gene underlies the ichthyotic variant of Vohwinkel syndrome. *Clin Exp Dermatol* 2002;27(3):243–246.

Okulicz JF, Schwartz RA, Hereditary and acquired ichthyosis vulgaris, *Int J Dermatol* 2003;42(2):95–98.

Reis A, Kuster W, Eckardt R, Sperling K. Mapping of a gene for epidermolytic palmoplantar keratoderma to the region of the acidic keratin gene cluster at 17ql2–q21. *Hum Genet* 1992;90(l–2):113–116.

Richard G, Brown N, Rouan F, et al. Genetic heterogeneity in erythrokeratodermia variabilis: novel mutations in the connexin gene GJB4 (Cx30.3) and genotype-phenotype correlations. *J Invest Dermatol* 2003;120(4):601–609.

Selvaraju V, Markandaya M, Prasad PV, et al. Mutation analysis of the cathepsin C gene in Indian families with Papillon-Lefevre syndrome. *BMC Med Genet* 2003;4(1):5.

Sprecher E, Chavanas S, DiGiovanna JJ, et al. The spectrum of pathogenic mutations in SPINK5 in 19 families with Netherton syndrome: implications for mutation detection and first case of prenatal diagnosis. *J Invest Dermatol* 2001;117(2):179–187.

Van Gysel D, Lijnen RL, Moekti SS, et al. Collodion baby: a follow-up study of 17 cases. *J Eur Acad Dermatol Venereol* 2002;16(5):472–475.

Willemsen MA, Ijlst L, Steijlen PM, et al. Clinical, biochemical and molecular genetic characteristics of 19 patients with the Sjogren–Larsson syndrome. *Brain* 2001;124(Pt 7):1426–1437.

Yotsumoto S, Hashiguchi T, Chen X, et al. Novel mutations in GJB2 encoding connexin-26 in Japanese patients with keratitis-ichthyosis-deafness syndrome. *Brit J Dermatol* 2003: 148(4): 649–653.

Disorders of Pigmentation

Barbagallo JS, Kolodzieh MS, Silverberg NB, Weinberg JM. Neurocutaneous disorders. *Dermatol Clin* 2002;20(3): 547–560, viii.

Berlin AL, Paller AS, Chan LS. Incontinentia pigmenti: a review and update on the molecular basis of pathophysiology. *J Am Acad Dermatol* 2002;47(2):169–187.

Bolger WE, Ross AT. McCune-Albright syndrome: a case report and review of the literature *Int J Pediatr Otorhinolaryngol* 2002;65(1):69–74.

Harris-Stith R, Elston DM. Tuberous sclerosis. *Cutis* 2002;69(2): 103–109.

Happle R. A fresh look at incontinentia pigmenti. *Arch Dermatol* 2003;139(9):1206–1208.

Huizing M, Boissy RE, Gahl WA. Hermansky-Pudlak syndrome: vesicle formation from yeast to man. *Pigment Cell Res* 2002;15(6):405–419.

Krishtul A, Galadari I. Waardenburg syndrome: case report. *Int J Dermatol* 2003;42(8):651–652.

Mollaaghababa R, Pavan WJ. The importance of having your SOX on: role of SOX10 in the development of neural crest-derived melanocytes and glia. *Oncogene* 2003;22(20):3024–3034.

Okulicz JF, Shah RS, Schwartz RA, Janniger, CK. Oculocutaneous albinism. *J Euro Acad Dermatol Venereol* 2003;17(3):251–256.

Reynolds RM, Browning GG, Nawroz I, Campbell IW. Von Recklinghausen's neurofibromatosis: neurofibromatosis type 1. *Lancet* 2003;361(9368):1552–1554.

Shiflett SL, Kaplan J, Ward DM. Chediak-Higashi syndrome: a rare disorder of lysosomes and lysosome related organelles. *Pigment Cell Res* 2002;15(4):251–257.

Syrris P, Heathcote K, Carrozzo R, et al. Human piebaldism: six novel mutations of the proto-oncogene KIT. *Hum Mutat* 2002;20(3):234.

Ward DM, Shiflett SL, Kaplan J. Chediak-Higashi syndrome: a clinical and molecular view of a rare lysosomal storage disorder. *Curr Mol Med* 2002;2(5):469–477.

Disorders of Vascularization

Amitai DB, Fichman S, Merlob P, et al. Cutis marmorata telangiectatica congenita: clinical findings in 85 patients. *Pediatr Dermatol* 2000;17(2),100–104.

Bedocs PM, Gould JW. Blue rubber-bleb nevus syndrome: a case report. *Cutis* 2003;71(4):315–318.

Bertucci V, Krafchik BR. What syndrome is this? Ollier disease + vascular lesions: Maffucci syndrome. *Pediatr Dermato* 1995;12(l):55–58.

Cirulli A, Liso A, D'Ovidio F, et al. Vascular endothelial growth factor serum levels are elevated in patients with hereditary hemorrhagic telangiectasia. *Acta Haematol* 2003;110(1):29–32.

Di Cataldo A, Haupt R, Fabietti P, Schiliro G. Is intensive follow-up for early detection of tumors effective in children with Beckwith-Wiedemann syndrome? *Clin Genet* 1996;50(5):372–374.

Dragieva G, Stahel HU, Meyer M, et al. Proteus syndrome. *Vasa* 2003;32(3):159–163.

Frevel T, Rabe H, Uckert F, Harms E. Giant cavernous haemangioma with Kasabach-Merritt syndrome: a case report and review. *Eur J Pediatr* 2002;161(5):243–246.

Hale EK. Klippel-Trenaunay syndrome. *Dermatol Online J* 2002;8(2):13.

Jessen RT, Thompson S, Smith EB. Cobb syndrome. *Arch Dermatol* 1977;113(11):1587–1590.

Karsdorp N, Elderson A, Wittebol-Post D, et al. Von Hippel-Lindau disease: new strategies in early detection and treatment. *Am J Med* 1994;97(2):158–168.

Kihiczak NI, Schwartz RA, Jozwiak S, et al. Sturge-Weber syndrome. *Cutis* 2000;65(3):133–1336.

Lonser RR, Glenn GM, Walther M, et al, Linehan WM, Oldfield EH. von Hippel-Lindau disease. *Lancet* 2003;361(9374):2059–2067.

Meine JG, Schwartz RA, Janniger CK. Klippel-Trenaunay-Weber syndrome. *Cutis* l997;60(3):127–I32.

Paller AS. Vascular disorders. *Dermatol Clin* 1987;5(1):239–250. Review.

Shim JH, Lee DW, Cho BK. A case of Cobb syndrome associated with lymphangioma circumscriptum. *Dermatology* 1996;193(l):45–47.

Spiller JC, Sharma V, Woods GM, et al. Diffuse neonatal hemangiomatosis treated successfully with interferon alfa-2a. *J Am Acad Dermatol* 1992;27(1):102–104.

Zvulunov A, Esterly NB. Neurocutaneous syndromes associated with pigmentary skin lesions. *J Am Acad Dermatol* 1995;32(6):915–935.

Connective Tissue Disorders

Badame AJ. Progeria. *Arch Dermatol* 1989;125(4):540–544. Review.

Beighton P, De Paepe A, Steinmann B, et al. Ehlers-Danlos syndromes: revised nosology, Villefranche, 1997. Ehlers-Danlos National Foundation (USA) and Ehlers-Danlos Support Group (UK). *Am J Med Genet* 1998;77(1):31–37.

Bergen AA, Plomp AS, Schuurman EJ, et al. Mutations in ABCC6 cause pseudoxanthoma elasticum. *Nat Genet* 2000;25(2):228–231.

Blunt K, Quan V, Carr D, Paes BA. Aplasia cutis congenita: a clinical review and associated defects. *Neonatal Netw* 1992;11(7):17–27.

Byers PH. Ehlers-Danlos syndrome: recent advances and current understanding of the clinical and genetic heterogeneity. *J Invest Dermatol* I994;103(5 Suppl):47S–52S.

Byers PH. Osteogenesis imperfecta: perspectives and opportunities. *Curr Opin Pediatr* 2000;12(6):603–609.

Chen L, Oshima J. Werner syndrome. *J Biomed Biotechnol* 2002;2(2):46–54.

De Paepe A, Devereux RB, Dietz HC, et al. Revised diagnostic criteria for the Marfan syndrome. *Am J Med Genet* 1996;62(4):4l7–426.

Duvic M, Lemak NA. Werner's syndrome. *Dermatol Clin* 1995;13(1):163–168.

Frieden IJ. Aplasia cutis congenita: a clinical review and proposal for classification. *J Am Acad Dermatol* 1986;14(4):646–660.

Goto M. Werner's syndrome: from clinics to genetics. *Clin Exp Rheumatol* 2000;18(6):760–766.

Hamada T. Lipoid proteinosis. *Clin Exp Dermatol* 2002;27(8):624–629.

Hardman CM, Garioch JJ, Eady RA, Fry L. Focal dermal hypoplasia: report of a case with cutaneous and skeletal manifestations. *Clin Exp Dermatol* 1998;23(6):281–285.

Kim GH, Dy LC, Caldemeyer KS, Mirowski GW. Buschke-Ollendorff syndrome. *J Am Acad Dermatol* 2003;48(4):600–601.

Kocher MS, Shapiro F. Osteogenesis imperfecta. *J Am Acad Orthop Surg* 1998;6(4):225–236.

Kruk-Jeromin J, Janik J, Rykala J. Aplasia cutis congenita of the scalp. Report of 16 cases. *Dermatol Surg* 1998;24(5):549–553.

Markova D, Zou Y, Ringpfeil F, et al. Genetic heterogeneity of cutis laxa: a heterozygous tandem duplication within the fibulin-5 (FBLN5) gene. *Am J Hum Genet* 2003;72(4):998–1004.

Ohtani T, Furukawa F. Pseudoxanthoma elasticum. J Dermatol 2002;29(10):615–620.

Ringpfeil F, Pulkkinen L, Uitto J. Molecular genetics of pseudoxanthoma elasticum. *Exp Dermatol* 2001;10(4):221-228.

Sule RR, Dhumawat DJ, Gharpuray MB. Focal dermal hypoplasia. *Cutis* 1994;53(6):309-312.

Thomas WO, Moses MH, Graver RD, Galen WK. Congenital cutis laxa: a case report and review of loose skin syndromes. *Am Plast Surg* 1993;30(3):252-256.

Yeowell HN, Pinnell SR. The Ehlers-Danlos syndromes. *Semin Dermatol* 1993;12(3):229-240.

Syndromes Associated with Malignancy

Braverman IM. Skin manifestations of internal malignancy. *Clin Geriatr Med* 2002;18(1):1-19.

Dokal I. Dyskeratosis congenita. *Br J Haematol* 1999;105 Suppl 1:11-15.

Drachtman RA, Alter BP. Dyskeratosis congenita. *Dermatol Clin* 1995;13(1):33-39.

Fassbender WJ, Krohn-Grimberghe B, Gortz B, et al. Multiple endocrine neoplasia (MEN)—an overview and case report—patient with sporadic bilateral pheochromocytoma, hyperparathyroidism and marfanoid habitus. *Anticancer Res* 2000;20(6C):4877-4887.

Fistarol SK, Anliker MD, Itin PH. Cowden disease or multiple hamartoma syndrome—cutaneous clue to internal malignancy. *Eur J Dermatol* 2002;12(5):411-421.

Hampel H, Peltomaki P. Hereditary colorectal cancer: risk assessment and management. *Clin Genet* 2000;58(2):89-97.

Hildenbrand C, Burgdorf WH, Lautenschlager S. Cowden syndrome-diagnostic skin signs. *Dermatology* 2001;202(4):362-366.

Kitagawa S, Townsend BL, Hebert AA. Peutz-Jeghers syndrome. *Dermatol Clin* 1995;13(1):127-133.

Lim W, Hearle N, Shah B, et al. Further observations on LKB1/STK11 status and cancer risk. *Br J Cancer* 2003;89(2):308-313.

Marrone A, Mason PJ. Dyskeratosis congenita. *Cell Mol Life Sci* 2003;60(3):507-517.

Mathiak M, Rutten A, Mangold E, et al. Loss of DNA mismatch repair proteins in skin tumors from patients with Muir-Torre syndrome and MSH2 or MLH1 germline mutations: establishment of immunohistochemical analysis as a screening test. *Am J Surg Pathol* 2002;26(3):338-343.

Mirowski GW, Liu AA, Parks ET, Caldemeyer KS. Nevoid basal cell carcinoma syndrome. *J Am Acad Dermatol* 2000;43(6):1092-1093.

Norgauer J, Idzko M, Panther E, et al. Xeroderma pigmentosum. *Eur J Dermatol* 2003; 13(1):4-9.

Parks ET, Caldemeyer KS, Mirowski GW. Gardner syndrome. *J Am Acad Dermatol* 2001;45(6):940-942.

Epidermolysis Bullosa

Bauer JW, Lanschuetzer C. Type XVII collagen gene mutations in junctional epidermolysis bullosa and prospects for gene therapy. *Clin Exp Dermatol* 2003;28(1):53-60.

Pai S, Marinkovich MP. Epidermolysis bullosa: new and emerging trends. *Am J Clin Dermatol* 2002;3(6):371-380.

Uitto J, Pulkkinen L, McLean WH. Epidermolysis bullosa: a spectrum of clinical phenotypes explained by molecular heterogeneity. *Mol Med Today* 1997;3(10):457-465.

Porphyrias

Cox TM, Alexander GJ, Sarkany RP. Protoporphyria. *Semin Liver Dis* 1998;18(l):85-93.

Elder GH. Hepatic porphyrias in children. *J Inherit Metab Dis* 1997;20(2):237-246.

Frank J, Christiano AM.Variegate porphyria: past, present and future. *Skin Pharmacol Appl Skin Physiol* 1998;11(6):3l0-320.

Frank J, Jugert FK, Kalka K, et al. Variegate porphyria: identification of a nonsense mutation in the protoporphyrinogen oxidase gene. *J Invest Dermatol* 1998;110(4):449-451.

Harada FA, Shwayder TA, Desnick RJ, Lim HW. Treatment of severe congenital erythropoietic porphyria by bone marrow transplantation. *J Am Acad Dermatol* 2001;45(2):279-282.

Lecha M, Herrero C, Ozalla D, Diagnosis and treatment of the hepatic porphyrias. *Dermatol Ther* 2003;16(l):65-72.

Moore MR. The biochemistry of heme synthesis in porphyria and in the porphyrinurias. *Clin Dermatol* 1998;16(2):203-223.

Murphy GM. The cutaneous porphyrias: a review. The British Photodermatology Group. *Br J Dermatol* 1999;140(4):573-581.

Murphy GM, Diagnosis and management of the erythropoietic porphyrias. *Dermatol Ther* 2003;16(l):57-64.

Sarkany RP. The management of porphyria cutanea tarda. *Clin Exp Dermatol* 2001;26(3):225-232.

Photosensitivity

Galadari E, Hadi S, Sabarinathan K. Hartnup disease. *Int J Dermatol* 1993;32(12):904.

Lehmann AR. The xeroderma pigmentosum group D (XPD) gene: one gene, two functions, three diseases. *Genes Dev* 2001;15(1):15-23.

Meetei AR, Sechi S, Wallisch M, et al. A multiprotein nuclear complex connects Fanconi anemia and Bloom syndrome. *Mol Cell Biol* 2003;23(10):3417-3426.

Poppe B, Van Limbergen H, Van Roy N, et al. Chromosomal aberrations in Bloom syndrome patients with myeloid malignancies. *Cancer Genet Cytogenet* 2001;128(1):39-42.

Wang LL, Levy ML, Lewis RA, et al. Clinical manifestations in a cohort of 41 Rothmund-Thomson syndrome patients. *Am J Med Genet* 2001;102(1):11-17.

Immunodeficiency

Bowen B, Hawk JJ, Sibunka S, et al. A review of the reported defects in the human Cl esterase inhibitor gene producing hereditary angioedema including four new mutations. *Clin Immunol* 2001;98(2):157-163.

Buckley RH. Advances in the understanding and treatment of human severe combined immunodeficiency. *Immunol Res* 2000;22(2-3):237-251.

Erlewyn-Lajeunesse MD. Hyperimmunoglobulin-E syndrome with recurrent infection: a review of current opinion and treatment. *Pediatr Allergy Immunol* 2000;11(3):133-141.

Farkas H, Harmat G, Fust G, et al. Clinical management of hereditary angio-oedema in children. *Pediatr Allergy Immunol* 2002;13(3):153-161.

Featherstone C. How does one gene cause Wiskott-Aldrich syndrome? *Lancet* 1996;348(9032):950.

Gennery AR, Cant AJ. Diagnosis of severe combined immunodeficiency. *J Clin Pathol* 2001;54(3):191-195.

Goldblatt D. Current treatment options for chronic granulomatous disease. *Expert Opin Pharmacother* 2002;3(7):857–863.

Koide M, Shirahama S, Tokura Y, et al. Lupus erythematosus associated with C1 inhibitor deficiency, *J Dermatol* 2002;29(8):503–507.

Shcherbina A, Candotti F, Rosen FS, Remold-O'Donnell E. High incidence of lymphomas in a subgroup of Wiskott-Aldrich syndrome patients. *Br J Haematol* 2003;121(3):529–530.

Shemer A, Weiss G, Confino Y, Trau H. The hyper-IgE syndrome. Two cases and review of the literature. *Int J Dermatol* 2001;40(10):622–628.

Thrasher AJ, Kinnon C. The Wiskott-Aldrich syndrome. *Clin Exp Immunol* 2000;120(l):2–9.

Weston WL. Cutaneous manifestations of defective host defenses. *Pediatr Clin North Am* 1977;24(2):395–407.

Metabolic Disorders

Albers SE, Brozena SJ, Glass LF, Fenske NA. Alkaptonuria and ochronosis: case report and review. *J Am Acad Dermatol* 1992;27(4):609–614.

Baumgartner ER, Suormala T. Multiple carboxylase deficiency: inherited and acquired disorders of biotin metabolism. *Int J Vitam Nutr Res* 1997;67(5):377–384.

Beck M. Variable clinical presentation in lysosomal storage disorders. *J Inherit Metab Dis* 2001;24 Suppl 2:47–51; discussion 45–46.

Brady RO, Schiffmann R. Clinical features of and recent advances in therapy for Fabry disease. *JAMA* 2000;284(21):2771–2775.

Carlesimo M, Bonaccorsi P, Tamburrano G, et al. Alkaptonuria. *Dermatology* 1999;199(1):70–71.

Cederbaum S. Phenylketonuria: an update. *Curr Opin Pediatr* 2002;14(6):702–706.

Corrent G, Rendon MI. Metabolic disease. *Dermatol Clin* 1992;10(4):717–740.

Cuthbert JA. Wilson's disease. Update of a systemic disorder with protean manifestations. *Gastroenterol Clin North Am* 1998;27(3):655–681, vi–vii.

Goskowicz M, Eichenfield LF. Cutaneous findings of nutritional deficiencies in children. *Curr Opin Pediatr* 1993;5(4):441–445.

Hill VA, Seymour CA, Mortimer PS. Pencillamine-induced elastosis perforans serpiginosa and cutis laxa in Wilson's disease. *Br J Dermatol* 2000;142(3):560–561.

Irons M, Levy HL. Metabolic syndromes with dermatologic manifestations. *Clin Rev Allergy* 1986;4(1):101–124.

Koch R, Hanley W, Levy H, et al. The Maternal Phenylketonuria International Study: 1984–2002. *Pediatrics* 2003;112(6 Pt 2):1523–1529.

Levin M, Pleskova I, Pastores GM, Gaucher disease: genetics, diagnosis and management. *Drugs Today (Barc)* 2001;37(4):257–264.

Lyon E, Frank EL. Hereditary hemochromatosis since discovery of the HFE gene. *Clin Chem* 2001;47(7):1147–1156.

Mohrenschlager M, Braun-Falco M, Ring J, Abeck D. Fabry disease: recognition and management of cutaneous manifestations. *Am J Clin Dermatol* 2003;4(3):189–196.

Muenzer J. Mucopolysaccharidoses. *Adv Pediatr* 1986;33:269–302.

Nakano A, Nakano H, Nomura K, et al. Novel SLC39A4 mutations in acrodermatitis enteropathica. *J Invest Dermatol* 2003;120(6):963–966.

Nyhan WL. Inborn errors of biotin metabolism. *Arch Dermatol* 1987;123(12):1696–1698.

Perafan-Riveros C, Franca LF, Alves AC, Sanches JA Jr. Acrodermatitis enteropathica: case report and review of the literature. *Pediatr Dermatol* 2002;19(5):426–431.

Smith WE, Kahler SG, Frush DP, et al. Hepatic storage of glycogen in Niemann-Pick disease type B. *J Pediatr* 2001;138(6):946–948.

Toussaint M, Worret WI, Drosner M, Marquardt KH. Specific skin lesions in a patient with Niemann-Pick disease. *Br J Dermatol* 1994;131(6):895–897.

Yap S, Rushe H, Howard PM, Naughten ER. The intellectual abilities of early-treated individuals with pyridoxine-nonresponsive homocystinuria due to cystathionine beta-synthase deficiency. *J Inherit Metab Dis* 2001;(4):437–447.

Chromosomal Abnormalities

Bertelloni S, Baroncelli GI, Fruzzetti F, et al. Growth and puberty in Turner's syndrome. *J Pediatr Endocrinol Metab* 2003;16 Suppl 2:307–315.

Cantani A, Gagliesi D. Rubinstein-Taybi syndrome. Review of 732 cases and analysis of the typical traits. *Eur Rev Med Pharmacol Sci* 1998;2(2):81–87.

Daoud MS, Dahl PR, Su WP. Noonan syndrome. *Semin Dermatol* 1995;14(2):140–144.

Frias JL, Davenport ML, Committee on Genetics and Section on Endocrinology. Health supervision for children with Turner syndrome. *Pediatrics* 2003;111(3):692–702.

Hayes A, Batshaw ML. Down syndrome. *Pediatr Clin North Am* 1993;40(3):523–535.

Herranz P, Borbujo J, Martinez W, et al. Rubinstein-Taybi syndrome with piebaldism. *Clin Exp Dermatol* 1994;19(2):170–172.

Patton MA. Russell-Silver syndrome. *J Med Genet* 1988;25(8):557–560.

Perkins RM, Hoang-Xuan MT. The Russell-Silver syndrome: a case report and brief review of the literature. *Pediatr Dermatol* 2002;19(6):546–549.

Roizen NJ, Patterson D. Down's syndrome. *Lancet* 2003;361(9365):1281–1289.

Russell KL, Ming JE, Patel K, et al. Dominant paternal transmission of Cornelia de Lange syndrome: a new case and review of 25 previously reported familial recurrences. *Am J Med Genet* 2001;104(4):267–276.

Slaugenhaupt SA, Gusella JF. Familial dysautonomia. *Curr Opin Genet Dev* 2002;12(3):307–311.

Visootsak J, Aylstock M, Graham JM Jr. Klinefelter syndrome and its variants: an update and review for the primary pediatrician. *Clin Pediatr (Phila)* 2001;40(12):639–651.

CHAPTER 33

CUTANEOUS TUMORS

ASRA ALI

Seborrheic Keratosis (Fig. 33-1)

- Benign lesion
- Predilection for the trunk, shoulder, face, and scalp
- Thin, sharply circumscribed, plaques with greasy crust
- Keratin-filled follicular openings
- Occurring after the age of 30 to 40 years
- Variants
  - Dermatosis papulosa nigra: lesions affect the face; small, pedunculated, and heavily pigmented
  - Stucco keratosis: gray-to-light brown, flat keratotic lesions on dorsa of the feet, the ankles, and the dorsa of the hands and forearms
  - Melanoacanthoma: deeply pigmented seborrheic keratoses in which an acanthotic proliferation of large dendritic melanocytes is identified
- Histology: papillomatous, epithelial proliferation containing horn cysts

Intraepidermal Epithelioma of Borst Jadassohn

- Considered to be clonal, seborrheic keratosis
- Histology: nests of cells and adjacent keratinocytes; within the background of a seborrheic Keratosis, eccrine peroma Bowen's disease

Nevus Sebaceous of Jadassohn

- Three clinical stages
- At birth: on scalp or face; solitary, hairless, pinkish, yellow, orange, or tan plaque with a smooth or somewhat velvety surface
- Puberty: lesion becomes verrucous and nodular
- Later in life: lesions may develop various types of appendageal tumors
  - Syringocystadenoma papilliferum
  - Tricho blastoma
  - Syringoma
  - Apocrine cystadenoma
  - Hidradenoma keratoacanthoma
  - Basal cell carcinoma, apocrine carcinoma, squamous cell carcinoma

- Neurocutaneous syndrome: mental retardation, epilepsy, neurologic deficits, skeletal deformities
- Epidermal nevus syndrome (Jadassohn nevus phakomatosis): combination of extensive sebaceous nevi with disorders of the central nervous system, bone, and eye
- Histology: papillomatous and acanthotic hyperplasia; numbers of mature sebaceous glands are increased in the dermis; ectopic apocrine glands in the deep dermis beneath sebaceous glands, reduced number of hair follicles

Nevus Comedonicus

- Found on the face, trunk, neck, and upper extremities
- Discrete, dilated follicular ostia plugged with pigmented keratinaceous material
- Nevus comedonicus syndrome: nevus comedonicus with abnormalities in the central nervous system (CNS), skeletal system, skin, and eye
- Histology: keratin-filled, epithelium-lined invaginations of the epidermis

Warty Dyskeratoma (Isolated Dyskeratosis Follicularis)

- Solitary, benign, keratotic, epidermal proliferation
- Umbilicated lesion with keratotic plug
- Usually limited to the head, neck, or face
- Histology: focal acantholysis and dyskeratosis (corps ronds), epidermal invagination, overlying parakeratotic cells (grains)

Arsenical Keratosis

- Arsenic, impairs nucleotide excision repair and enhances proliferation of human keratinocytes
  - Found in Fowler solution, which contained 1% potassium arsenite; well water
- Gray, hard, hyperkeratotic papules on palms, soles, trunk, face; can turn into squamous cell carcinoma
- Mees lines on the fingernails

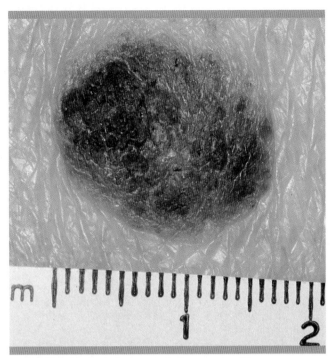

FIGURE 33-1 Seborrheic keratosis. *(From Freedberg IM et al: Fitzpatrick's Dermatology in General Medicine, 6th ed. New York: McGraw-Hill, 2003, p. 768.)*

- Histology: thick, compact hyperkeratosis and parakeratosis; may show atypia

Large Cell Acanthoma

- Solitary, slightly hyperkeratotic lesion with sharp borders, up to 1 cm; occurs on sun-exposed areas
- Histology: hyperkeratosis; keratinocytes are two times larger, lentiginous hyperpigmentation

Epidermolytic Acanthoma (EHK)

- Solitary tumor arising on the trunk of older patients
- Histology: hyperkeratosis, papillomatosis, acanthosis and variable acantholysis

Knuckle Pads

- Hyperkeratosis of the dorsal aspect of the joints of the fingers
- Histology: acanthosis, prominent hyperkeratosis

Prurigo Nodularis

- Multiple or solitary nodules, usually symmetric with excoriations present
- Extremely pruritic
- Part of the spectrum of lichen simplex
- Histology: psoriasiform hyperplasia, hyperkeratosis, hypergranulosis and focal parakeratosis, occasional spongiosis and exocytosis of mononuclear cells

Granuloma Fissuratum

- Lateral aspect of nose and retroauricular region
- Firm, flesh-colored nodule with a central groove (site of focal pressure or friction)
- Histology: acanthosis with broad rete ridges and central depressed area corresponding to the groove

Pale Cell Acanthoma (Clear Cell Acanthoma)

- Nodules and plaques, up to 2 cm, covered with a crust
- Usually solitary, located on the lower extremities
- Histology: pale, periodic acid–Schiff (PAS)–positive keratinocytes due to glycogen, acanthosis, parakeratosis, neutrophils within the epidermis, sometimes neutrophilic microabscesses, dilated capillaries

CYSTS

Steatocystoma Multiplex (Sebocystomatosis) (Fig. 33-2)

- Autosomal dominant disorder
- Abortive hair follicles at the site where sebaceous glands attach
- Flesh- to yellow-colored cysts; when punctured, oil or creamy fluid is present
- Histology: dermal, folded cyst wall composed of keratinocytes with peripheral palisading basal cells; wall embedded with flattened lobules of sebaceous glands; cyst filled with eosinophilic cuticle along corrugated keratin layer

Dermoid Cyst

- Hamartomatous lesion
- May have intracranial extension
- May have sinus tract with cheesy material
- Most commonly found on lateral third of eyebrows, nose, and scalp
- Due to sequestration of epithelium along lines of embryonic fusion
- Subcutaneous freely mobile cyst; occasionally may fix to periosteum
- Magnetic resonance imaging (MRI) is helpful in planning surgical procedures
- Histology: cyst wall lined by epidermis with mature appendages

Branchial Cleft Cyst

- Congenital epithelial cyst
- Arises on the lateral part of the neck
- Remnant of the second branchial cleft in embryonic development
- Solitary, painless mass in the neck of a child or a young adult; occurs along the lower third of the

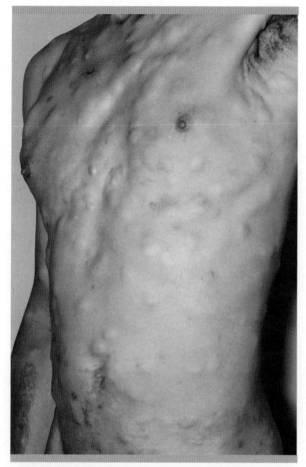

FIGURE 33-2 Steatocystoma multiplex. *(From Freedberg IM et al: Fitzpatrick's Dermatology in General Medicine, 6th ed. New York: McGraw-Hill, 2003, p. 781.)*

anteromedial border of the sternocleidomastoid muscle
- Two to three percent of cases are bilateral
- Histology: lined with stratified squamous epithelium; occasionally, cyst is lined with respiratory (ciliated columnar) epithelium; lymphoid tissue often is present outside the epithelial lining

Digital Myxoid Cyst

- Asymptomatic, elevated, dome-shaped lesion; may cause depression of the nail
- Commonly on distal interphalangeal (DIP) joints or proximal nail fold; occasionally between the proximal nail fold and the nail plate, beneath the nail matrix, or in the pulp of the digit
- Histology: variable mucin deposition, pseudocyst with a fibrous capsule, compact hyperkeratosis with a collarette of hyperplastic epidermis
- Stains: colloidal iron or Alcian blue

Thyroglossal Duct Cyst

- Congenital, vestigial remnant of the tubular thyroid gland precursor
- Midline neck, near hyoid bone
- Moves with swallowing
- Histology: lined by cuboidal, columnar, or stratified squamous epithelium; ciliated epithelium; mucous glands, thyroid follicles, lymphocytic infiltrate

Bronchogenic Cyst

- Formed from portions of foregut during development of tracheobronchial tree
- Present above suprasternal notch at birth
- Histology: intradermal, folded cyst lining, pseudostratified, cuboidal, or columnar epithelium, ciliated, with goblet cells

ADENEXAL (APPENDAGEAL) TUMORS

Appendagal Tumors with Apocrine Differentiation

APOCRINE NEVUS

- Usually present on upper chest and in axilla
- Unilateral or bilateral, soft dermal mass
- Histology: increased numbers of mature apocrine glands

APOCRINE HYDROCYSTOMA (APOCRINE TABULAR ADENOMA, CYSTADENOMA)

- Benign cystic tumor of apocrine glands
- Dome-shaped bluish nodule on face
- Histology: intradermal cystic spaces lined by a double layer of epithelium, outer layer of myoepithelial cells, inner layer of tall columnar cells

NIPPLE ADENOMA (EROSIVE ADENOMATOSIS OR FLORID PAPILLOMATOSIS)

- Unilateral nipple lesion less than 1 cm in diameter; may mimic Paget's disease
- Ductal hyperplasia of the lactiferous ducts
- Histology: mixture of intraductal papilloma and tubular glands, lined by epithelial and myoepithelial cells

SUPERNUMERARY NIPPLE (SN)

- Benign, congenital lesion
- Small pigmented or flesh-colored macule or concave or umbilicated papule
- Occurs along the embryonic milk line except for ectopic SNs (5 percent)
- Histology: identical to that of the regular nipple, pilosebaceous structure of Montgomery areolar tubercles, smooth muscle bundles

HIDRADENOMA PAPILLIFERUM

- Usually does not communicate with the surface
- Middle-aged women, small nodules in the vulva or perianal regions
- Histology: cystic tumor with two types of epithelium: tall columnar cells and underlying myoepithelial cell layer; decapitation secretion

SYRINGOCYSTADENOMA PAPILLIFERUM

- Most common on face and scalp
- Papules in a linear arrangement or a solitary plaque, in nevus sebaceous
- Increase in size at puberty
- Histology: cystic invaginations with plasma cells that communicate with the skin surface, double layer of epithelium covering papillae, columnar layer on the luminal side and a cuboidal layer on the outside, dermal tubular glands with apocrine glands

CHONDROID SYRINGOMA (MIXED TUMOR OF THE SKIN)

- Head and neck, solitary, slowly growing nodule
- Histology: located in the dermis and subcutaneous tissue, no epidermal connection, multilobulated, clusters and solid cords of tumor cells together with ductal structures set in a chondroid, myxoid, and fibrous stroma; ductal structures are lined by two layers of cuboidal cells (resembling apocrine cells), areas of ossification (pseudocartilagenous appearance)

MALIGNANT CHONDROID SYRINGOMA (MIXED CELL TUMOR)

- Typically develops de novo
- Predilection for trunk and extremities
- Solitary, occasionally painful, firm, nonulcerated nodule

EXTRAMAMMARY PAGET'S DISEASE (EMPD)

- Primary cutaneous adenocarcinoma
- Twenty-five percent associated with an underlying in situ or invasive neoplasm (eg., adnexal apocrine carcinoma)
- Nonresolving eczematous lesions in the groin, genitalia, perineum, or perianal area
- Intense pruritus
- Histology: Paget cells (large, vacuolated cells with a bluish cytoplasm) in the lower epidermis with spread along the rete ridges and adnexa (pagetoid spread); stain sialomucin with PAS and diastase, colloidal iron, and mucicarmine; Paget's cells stain with EMA and CEA
- Prognosis: recurrence 30 percent

ADENOID CYSTIC CARCINOMA

- Malignant epithelial tumor
- More common in the lesser major salivary glands (submandibular gland and sublingual gland) and the minor salivary glands
- Mass lesion; dull pain and/or paralysis of a cranial nerve (when arising from the parotid gland)
- Histology: invades nerves; irregularly shaped, dermal aggregation of basaloid cells arranged in solid and/or sievelike patterns; carcinoembryonal antigen (CEA) and S-100–positive

APOCRINE ADENOCARCINOMA

- Rare, solitary or multiple nodules and plaques measuring 2 to 8 cm in diameter in the axillae or anogenital area
- Histology: infiltrating dermal or subcutaneous nonencapsulated papillary tumor, solid or mixed pattern; apocrine secretion and cords of neoplastic cells with variable pleomorphism
- Same as chondroid syringoma with infiltrative growth pattern, epithelial nuclear and cytoplasmic pleomorphism, abnormal mitotic activity, necrosis; stains with CAM 5.2, CEA, and S–100

SIGNET CELL CARCINOMA

- Nodule or diffuse eyelid swelling; lower eyelids most commonly involved
- Can present as an expression of mammary or extramammary Paget's disease
- Histology: diffuse malignant epithelial neoplasia localized in dermis and subcutis without epidermal involvement showing variable amounts of signet ring cells (eccentric nucleus with vacuolated cytoplasm)

Appendageal Tumors with Eccrine Differentiation

CYLINDROMA (FIG. 33-3)

- Pink, firm, rubbery nodules of head, neck, and scalp in solitary and multiple patterns (turban tumors)
- Multiple tumors are not as common and are inherited in an autosomal dominant mode; *CYLD1* gene, 16q12-q13
- Malignant cylindromas may develop
- Brooke-Spiegler syndrome (BSS): autosomal dominant disease (*CYLD* gene on chromosome 9) characterized by the development of multiple trichoepitheliomas and cylindromas
- Histology: dermal tumor without attachment to the epidermis; multiple lobules of basaloid tumor cells, surrounded by a hyaline basement membrane and fit together like pieces of a jigsaw puzzle; eosinophilic hyaline sheaths and hyaline droplets are PAS-positive, composed of type IV collagen and laminin

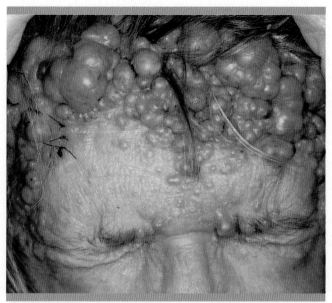

FIGURE 33-3 Cylindroma. *(From Freedberg IM et al: Fitzpatrick's Dermatology in General Medicine, 6th ed. New York: McGraw-Hill, 2003, p. 793.)*

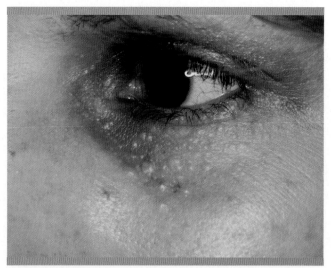

FIGURE 33-4 Syringoma. *(From Freedberg IM et al: Fitzpatrick's Dermatology in General Medicine, 6th ed. New York: McGraw-Hill, 2003, p. 795.)*

ECCRINE ACROSPIROMA (CLEAR CELL HIDRADENOMA, NODULAR HIDRADENOMA)

- Slowly growing, solitary nodule on scalp, face, or trunk
- Clear cell hidradenoma consists of pale or clear cells
- Cystic nodular hidradenoma: variant of nodular hidradenoma with prevalence of cysts (solid structures are present as well, as opposed to apocrine hidrocystoma)
- Histology: tumor well circumscribed, not connected to epidermis, two types of cells: fusiform, eosinophilic cells and polygonal, clear cells; ducts lined with hyaline cuticle

ECCRINE POROMA

- Benign neoplasm that shows differentiation toward glandular ductal cells
- Usually on side of foot, solitary; skin-colored nontender violaceous warty nodule
- Smaller than 2 cm in diameter
- Eccrine poromatosis: greater than 100 papules on palms/soles
- Histology: solid masses of cuboidal epithelial cells with ovoid nuclei, eosinophilic cytoplasm, tumor in continuity with overlying epidermis
- Variations
  - Dermal duct tumor present only in the dermis
  - Intraepidermal poroma (hidroacanthoma simplex): nests of cells with tubular differentiation; confined to the surface epidermis
  - Juxtaepidermal poroma: nests and thick cords of cells in continuity with the epidermis but also involving the superficial dermis

SYRINGOMA (FIG. 33-4)

- Adenomas of eccrine ducts
- Commonly seen in females at puberty, 18 percent of Down syndrome patients
- Small, skin-colored or yellow soft papules, lower eyelid, usually multiple
- Eruptive syringomas (Darrier and Jaquet), large crops on anterior chest, in children 4 to 10 years old
- Clear cell syringomas are associated with diabetes mellitus
- Histology: upperdermis, small ducts with elongated tails of epithelial cells (tadpole appearance) embedded in a sclerotic stroma; walls of the ducts usually lined by two rows of epithelial cells, lumen filled with PAS-positive eosinophilic, amorphous debris
- Histologic differential diagnosis: sclerosing (morphea-like) basal cell carcinoma and trichoepithelioma, microcystic adnexal carcinoma

ECCRINE SPIRADENOMA

- Solitary, tender intradermal nodule, overlying skin appears blue
- Tend to occur on the scalp, neck, and upper part of the trunk
- Histology: "big blue balls" in dermis under low-power view; no connection to epidermis; two cell types make up tumor labules: peripheral small blue cells, central large pale blue cells, connective tissue capsule

ECCRINE HAMARTOMA

- Types
  - Eccrine angiomatous hamartoma: increased number of eccrine glands with small blood vessels, nerve fibers, mucin or fat
  - Porokeratotic eccrine ostial nevus: coranoid lamellae associated with eccrine ducts
  - Acrosyringeal nevus: PAS-positive acrosyringeal keratinocytes, which extends into the dermis as anastomosing cords
  - Linear eccrine nevus with comedones: similar to nevus comedonicus together with basaloid nests in the dermis
  - Eccrine nevus: solitary, well-circumscribed area with hyperhidrosis
- Histology: dermal collection of eccrine glands and ducts, haphazardly arranged

TUBULAR ADENOMA

- Refers to a group of benign adnexal tumors
- Middle-aged adults; solitary, slowly growing, well-circumscribed nodules usually on the extremities
- Histology: numerous cystic dilated and branching tubular structures in the dermis surrounded by a compressed fibrous stroma

ECCRINE HIDROCYSTOMA (CYSTADENOMA)

- Translucent, cystic lesion 1 to 3 mm, bluish color
- Located on the head, neck, trunk, and chest
- Numbers increase in warm weather
- Secondary to retention of sweat due to malformed eccrine duct
- Histology: unilocular or multilocular intradermal cyst, lined by cuboidal cells

ECCRINE HIDRADINITIS

- Patients undergoing treatment with chemotherapy (bleomycin, cytaribine)
- Tender, erythematous macules, papules, plaques of trunk, neck, extremities; resolve after several days
- Histology: neutrophils surrounding eccrine coils, epithelial cell vacuolar degeneration and necrosis

ECCRINE CARCINOMA

- Rare carcinoma of the eccrine sweat gland
- Single, asymptomatic, nondescript cutaneous nodule or plaque
- Metastases are frequent; radiosensitive
- Histology: several subtypes (clear cell, syringoid, chondroid) classic, resembles a moderately to poorly differentiated adenocarcinoma with well differentiated tubular structures in some areas to anaplastic carcinoma in other areas

MICROCYSTIC ADNEXAL CARCINOMA

- Eccrine gland carcinoma with aggressive local invasion and indolent course
- Indurated plaques or nodules on the upper lip, chin, nasolabial fold, cheek
- Histology: desmoplastic stroma, basaloid keratinocytes, scattered horn cysts, abortive hair follicles ducts, small ducts lined by one or two layers of cuboidal cells (can have tail-like cellular extensions reminiscent of syringoma), perineural invasion
- Immunocytochemistry: epithelial membrane antigen (EMA) and CEA

POROCARCINOMA

- Verrucoid plaque or polypoid growth
- Older individuals; usually on the lower extremities
- Metastasis: about 20 percent
- Histology: large islands and small, irregularly shaped nests with infiltrative border, focal necrosis, clear cell areas, ductal structures, intracytoplasmic lumina formation, and squamous differentiation
- PAS-positive and usually diastase labile
- Immunocytochemistry: cytokeratin-, CEA-, and EMA-positive

SPIRADENOCARCINOMA

- Aggressive tumor
- Usually originates on a long-standing solitary lesion of spiradenoma on the lower extremities
- Local recurrences and metastasis
- Histology: basaloid cells and occasional ductular differentiation that invade deep dermis and extend into the subcutaneous fat; focal areas of necrosis and mononuclear reactive inflammatory cell infiltration
- Immunocytochemistry: low-molecular-weight cytokeratin, neurofilament, chromogranin, neuron-specific enolase, and EMA

Appendageal Tumors with Follicular Differentiation

EPIDERMAL INCLUSION CYST

- Implantation of epithelial elements in the dermis
- Round, mobile, flesh-colored to yellow or white subcutaneous nodules of variable size
- Central pore or punctum: when present, may tether the cyst to the overlying epidermis
- Histology: cyst is lined with stratified squamous epithelium; wall contains a granular layer and is filled with keratinous material in a laminated arrangement

PILAR CYST (TRICHILEMMAL CYST)

- Derived from the outer root sheath of the hair follicle
- Smooth, movable nodules in the scalp, usually multiple
- Histology: fibrous capsule with layers of small, cuboidal, dark-staining basal cells; solid eosinophilic-staining keratin (trichilemmal keratinization); no granular layer; cholesterol clefts in 90 percent; calcification occurs in 25 percent of the lesions

PILAR TUMOR (PROLIFERATING TRICHILEMMAL CYST)

- Arises as proliferating wall of pilar cyst with abrupt trichilemmal keratinization
- Nodule; most typical (90 percent) location is the scalp
- Usually benign
- Histology: well-circumscribed nodule with trichilemmal keratinization; horn pearls and squamous eddies

MILIA

- Benign, keratin-filled cysts
- Pearly white to yellowish, domed lesions measuring 1 to 2 mm in diameter
- Secondary lesions arise following blistering or trauma owing to disruption of the sweat duct
- Histology: identical to those of epidermoid cysts, but the cysts are much smaller

DILATED PORE OF WINER

- Comedo-like benign tumor, usually located on the face
- Histology: dilated open follicular cystic cavity filled with keratin and irregularly proliferating rete ridges

PILAR SHEATH ACANTHOMA

- Benign papule, usually on the upper lip of adults
- Histology: keratin-filled dilated follicular infundibulum; acanthosis of the follicular epithelium; cells are regular

VELLUS CYST (VELLUS HAIR CYST, ERUPTIVE VELLUS HAIR CYST)

- Congenital or acquired
- Follicular occlusion at the level of the infundibulum
- Acneiform eruption on the chest and extremities
- Histology: small cyst in dermis lined with normal epidermis with eosinophilic laminated keratinous material with small vellus hairs

FIBROFOLLICULOMA

- Small dome-shaped papules on the face, neck, and upper trunk
- Multiple fibrofolliculomas may be familial
- Birt-Hogg-Dube syndrome: autosomal dominant, fibrofolliculomas, acrochordons, trichodiscomas and pulmonary disease (spontaneous pneumothorax), renal tumors
- Histology: cystic structure with a central keratin plug and anastomosing strands of basaloid cells surrounded by a fibrous stroma

TRICHODISCOMA

- Small dome-shaped papules on the face, neck, and upper trunk
- Likely derive from the mantle of the hair follicle
- Fibrofolliculoma and trichodiscoma may represent various stages in the natural history of a single hamartoma
- Histology: proliferation of the hair mantle, small melanin granule–containing fusiform cells, thin-walled blood vessels

TRICHOADENOMA

- Rare solitary tumor located on the face, up to 15 mm in size
- Histology: groups of keratin-filled cysts connected by epithelial strands; absent granular layer

TRICHOLEMMOMA (TRICHILEMMOMA)

- Single papule or multiple, small, flesh-colored papules or warty lesions
- Cowden syndrome (multiple hamartoma syndrome; dysfunctional tyrosine kinase phosphatase enzymes secondary to a defect on 10q23): multiple facial tricholemmomas around the mouth, nose, and ear outer root sheath
- Histology: endophytic epithelial lobule with peripheral basal cell palisading; eosinophilic hyaline basement membrane zone, cells located toward the center are clear (increased glycogen)
- Desmoplastic tricholemmoma: histologic variant; lobulated tumor and cells that form narrow, irregular cords that penetrate into the dermis

TRICHOBLASTOMA

- Well-circumscribed, solitary papule
- Tumors that are poorly differentiated
- Histology: well-circumscribed dermal aggregates of epithelial (basaloid germ) and mesenchymal components increased mitotic activity

INVERTED FOLLICULAR KERATOSIS

- Verrucous lesion
- Considered to be a variant of a seborrhoic keratosis (irritated type)
- Histology: squamous eddy formation within a cytologically benign, vertically oriented, acanthotic proliferation

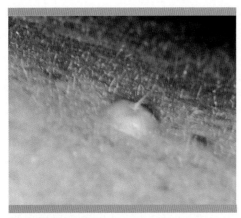

FIGURE 33-5 Trichofolliculoma.
(From Freedberg IM et al: Fitzpatrick's Dermatology in General Medicine, 6th ed. New York: McGraw-Hill, 2003, p. 804.)

TRICHOFOLLICULOMA (FIG. 33-5)

- Small, elevated papule, or flattened nodule with central depression on face
- Protruding tuft of small, short, white, or pigmented hairs
- Sebaceous trichofolliculoma: small sebaceous elements may be found within the follicular units
- Histology: cystic tumor lined by squamous epithelium, usually communicating with the surface; fully formed vellus units within cyst wall; radiating secondary follicular buds

TRICHOEPITHELIOMA (TE; BROOK'S TUMOR, EPITHELIOMA ADENOMA CYSTICUM)

- Dome-shaped papules on face, usually nasolabial folds
- Multiple lesions present as an autosomal dominant trait
- Associated syndromes: Brooke-Spiegler syndrome (cylindroma); Rombo syndrome (vermiculate atrophoderma, milia, hypertrichosis, TE, basal cell carcinoma, peripheral vasodilatation)
- Histology: palisading basaloid cells in a dense stroma; horn cysts with keratinized center; calcification; giant cell reaction; artifactual clefting is uncommon
- Desmoplastic trichoepithelioma: prominent sclerotic stroma, narrow strands of tumor cells, and keratinous cysts with calcification; pleomorphism, palisading, and peripheral clefting are not seen
- Solitary giant trichoepithelioma: deep involvement of the reticular dermis and subcutaneous tissue

PILOMATRICOMA (CALCIFYING EPITHELIOMA OF MALHERBE)

- Solitary, firm, deep-seated nodule covered by normal skin
- Superficial in skin; causing blue-red discoloration of the overlying skin

- Occurs at any age; most common in children
- Originates from hair cortex cells (shaft)
- Perforation with extrusion of contents; "tent sign" tents up skin
- Histology: irregularly shaped islands embedded in cellular stroma
- Two cell types
  - Basaloid: small, uniform, in early lesion, high mitotic activity
  - Pale, eosinophilic: areas of keratin and necrotic cells with eosinophilic cytoplasm and lost nucleus (shadow cells)
  - Transitional areas where basal cells turn into shadow cells
- Calcification and ossification present

TUMOR OF THE FOLLICULAR INFUNDIBULUM

- Solitary keratotic papule on the face
- Histology: dermal growth of epithelial cells parallel to the epidermis; peripheral palisading of the basal cells

Appendageal Tumors with Sebaceous Differentiation

SEBACEOUS HYPERPLASIA

- Whitish yellow, well-demarcated, 2- to 9-mm papules; soft, with central umbilication
- Histology: increased number of enlarged sebaceous lobules

SEBACEOUS ADENOMA

- Yellow papule or nodule, usually located on the face or scalp
- Associated with Muir-Torre syndrome
- Histology: multilobulated neoplasm with pale-staining; cells making up 50 percent of the tumor and peripheral, smaller basaloid cells

SEBACEOMA, SEBACEOUS EPITHELIOMA

- Yellowish ill-defined plaque
- Does not metastasize
- Associated with Muir-Torre syndrome
- Histology: focal sebaceous differentiation; mixed cells with >50 percent undifferentiated basophilic cells

SEBACEOUS GLAND CARCINOMA

- Presents in the sixth or seventh decade
- Firm, slowly enlarging nodule of the eyelid, often mistaken for a chalazion; can mimic keratoconjunctivitis, blepharoconjunctivitis
- Seventy-five percent arise in the periocular region: upper lid two to three times more common than lower lid tumors
- Aggressive clinical course; metastasis occurs in 14 to 25 percent of cases, first to the draining lymph nodes

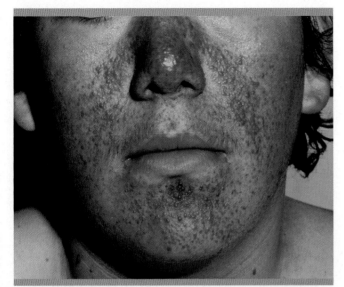

FIGURE 33-6 Angiofibroma. *(From Freedberg IM et al: Fitzpatrick's Dermatology in General Medicine, 6th ed. New York: McGraw-Hill, 2003, p. 994.)*

- Few are associated with Muir-Torre syndrome
- Histology: pagetoid spread (approximately 40 to 80 percent), many undifferentiated cells among distinct sebaceous cells in an infiltrative tumor

MESENCHYMAL TUMORS

Fibroma

- Pale brown, soft, small tumors in friction areas: neck, axillae, internal aspects of thighs
- Histology: tumors are formed by connective tissue; fibrocytes are regular and mature; mitoses are not present

Angiofibroma (Fig. 33-6)

- Small, reddish-brown papules
- Usually over sides of the nose and medial cheeks
- Associated with tuberous sclerosis
- Pearly penile papules: angiofibromas in penile coronal sulcus
- Histology: collagen with stellate fibroblasts around small vascular channels

Pearly Penile Papules

- Normal anatomic structure
- Histology: angiofibromas with dense connective tissue, rich vascular complex

Fibromatosis

INFANTILE MYOFIBROMATOSIS

- Multiple, solitary, rubbery nodules at birth

- Slow growth; may be fixed to underlying tissue
- Surface telangiectasias
- If multiple, associated with visceral involvement (35 percent)
- Histology: whorls of spindle cells; no mitosis
- Treatment: surgical excision
- Prognosis: spontaneous remission with scarring

CONGENITAL GENERALIZED FIBROMATOSIS

- Multiple: one to hundreds of nodules; bone can be involved
- Histology: whorls and fascicles of spindle cells

INFANTILE DIGITAL FIBROMATOSIS (REYE TUMOR)

- Presents at 1 month of age
- Nodules on dorsolateral digits, subcutaneous
- Histology: intracytoplasmic inclusion bodies, eosinophilic bodies (stain with Masson-Trichrome)

JUVENILE HYALINE FIBROMATOSIS

- Autosomal recessive
- Slowly growing, skin-colored spindle cell tumor, face, scalp, back
- Flexural contractures, gingival hyperplasia, papillomatosis, perianal lesions
- Histology: increased number of fibroblasts

AGGRESSIVE INFANTILE FIBROMATOSIS

- Rapidly growing nodules on the trunk; skeletal muscle involved
- Histology: immature mesenchymal cells

DUPUYTREN'S CONTRACTURE (PALMOPLANTAR FIBROMATOSIS)

- Associated with seizures, diabetes, alcoholic cirrhosis
- Nodules on tendon sheath, contracting fibrosis of palmar fascia, dimpled skin over metacarpophalangeal joint, knuckle pads, flexion deformities of fourth and fifth digits

Dermatofibroma (Histiocytoma of the Skin) (Fig. 33-7)

- Common lesion, often on the extremities
- Usually firm, solitary nodule, sometimes polypoid; pink, brown, yellowish, dimples with pressure
- Histology: mature collagen proliferation, acanthosis, increased pigmentation; foamy macrophages (and Touton cells)

Atypical Fibroxanthoma

- Locally aggressive nodule
- Located on the head, neck, dorsa of the hands of elderly people

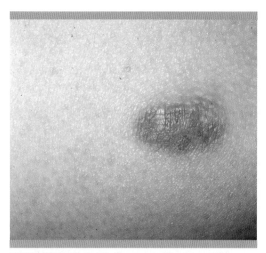

FIGURE 33-7 Dermatofibroma. *(From Freedberg IM et al: Fitzpatrick's Dermatology in General Medicine, 6th ed. New York: McGraw-Hill, 2003, p. 995.)*

- Histology: nodular tumor, spindle-shaped and pleomorphic cells, not encapsulated, mitotic activity, ulceration and necrosis, foam cells

Dermatofibrosarcoma Protuberans (DFSP) (Fig. 33-8)

- Malignant tumor, slowly growing, rare metastasis with local recurrences
- Located on the trunk, proximal parts of the extremities

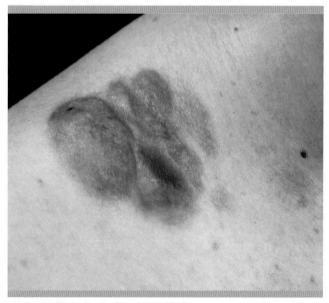

FIGURE 33-8 Dermatofibrosarcoma protuberans. *(From Freedberg IM et al: Fitzpatrick's Dermatology in General Medicine, 6th ed. New York: McGraw-Hill, 2003, p. 997.)*

- Multiple nodules
- Mainly affects younger age group
- Histology: spindle, monomorphous cells; often storiform and/or honeycomb-like arrangement; infiltration into the subcutis; myxomatous areas and polymorphous cells may be present; some mitotic activity
- Imunohistochemistry: CD34+, S-100(−)

Giant Cell Fibroblastoma

- Rare tumor, occurring in children on the chest wall, back, thighs
- Nodules, poorly circumscribed
- Histology: variable myxoid, sclerotic, dermatofibrosarcoma-like areas; multinucleated giant cells, sometimes with cleftlike, angiomatoid spaces
- Immunohistochemistry: CD34+ (regarded as a variant of DFSP)

Skin Tags

- Fibroepithelial polyp
- Polypoid tumors, small size
- Covered by the epidermis (thickened, pigmented; may resemble seborrhoic keratosis)
- Often located on the neck, axillae, inguinal areas, eyelids
- Histology: polyps covered by the epidermis; mild hyperkeratosis; stroma with fat tissue and dilated blood vessels; sometimes with groups of melanocytes present

Supernumerary Digit

- Hands, feet; usually near the fifth finger; congenital
- Skin-colored outgrowth
- Histology: fibrous stroma, many nerves, sometimes cartilage or bone, dome-shaped

Accessory Tragus

- Congenital asymptomatic papule located in preauricular area or neck
- Histology: connective tissue, fat, sometimes cartilage with many hair follicles

Acral Fibrokeratoma

- Solitary, hyperkeratotic papules on the fingers; sometimes palms, soles (but not periungual)
- Histology: fibrous stroma, prominent hyperkeratosis, often many blood vessels

Acquired Periungual Fibrokeratoma

- Periungual outgrowths with hyperkeratosis
- Accompanies tuberous sclerosis
- Histology: fibrous core, hyperkeratotic dome-shaped lesion

Vestibular Papules of the Vulva

- Vulvar papules covered with normal epidermis
- Histology: papule with fibrous stroma, covered with epidermis

Keloid

- Commonly located on sternal region, ear lobes
- Firm, nodular lesions that extend beyond trauma of skin
- Histology: thick bands of hyalinized, eosinophilic collagen within a cellular scar
- Treatment: excision, intralesional steroids or interferon, silicone gel sheets, radiation therapy

Lipoma (see also Chapter 31)

- Benign tumor of the mature fat
- Solitary or multiple elastic nodules of the subcutis
- Usually located on the arms, shoulders, back, lower extremities
- Lipomatosis: symmetric diffuse hyperplasia of the fat
- Histology: fine capsule with cells that are slightly larger than normal adipocytes

Angiolipoma (see also Chapter 31)

- Usually seen in young adults as subcutaneous lesions, sometimes painful
- Histology: lipomas with numerous vascular channels with thrombi

Liposarcoma (see also Chapter 31)

- Malignant tumor of soft tissues; rarely found in the subcutis
- Usually seen in patients over 50 years
- Four types: well differentiated (lipoma-like, sclerosing, inflammatory); myxoid; round cell; pleomorphic
- Histology: lipoblasts with cytoplasmatic lipid-laden vacuoles; causes indentations of the nucleus; variable nuclear polymorphism

TUMORS OF THE SMOOTH MUSCLE

Leiomyomas (Fig. 33-9)

- Pilar leiomyomas
  - Arise from the arrector pilorum muscle
  - Firm, pink, sometimes painful, solitary or multiple nodules
  - Histology: similar to dartotic leiomyoma
- Angioleiomyoma
  - Arise from vascular smooth muscle
  - Histology: numerous blood vessels with a thick wall, formed by smooth muscle
- Dartotic leiomyoma

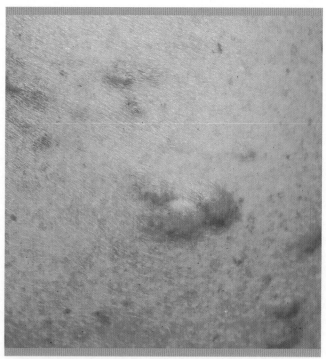

FIGURE 33-9 Leiomyomas. *(From Freedberg IM et al: Fitzpatrick's Dermatology in General Medicine, 6th ed. New York: McGraw-Hill, 2003, p. 1003.)*

- Originate in the dartos muscles of the genitalia, areola, and nipple
- Histology: fascicles of smooth muscle, blunt borders; fusiform cells with longitudinal striations, thin, cigar-shaped nuclei with blunt ends
- Malignant variant: larger lesion, cellular polymorphism, and mitotic activity
- Special stain: Verhoeff-van Gieson (yellow), trichrome (pink-red), antibodies against smooth muscle actin

Leiomyosarcoma

- Malignant tumors of smooth muscle
- Pink nodule, sometimes painful
- Often extremities but can occur elsewhere
- Capable of metastasizing
- Peak age is 50 or 60 years
- Histology: high cellularity with spindle cells cellular polymorphism, mitotic activity; occasional necrosis

Congenital Smooth Muscle Hamartoma

- Arise on trunk
- Solitary patch with or without a follicular pattern
- Diffuse skin involvement produces a "Michelin-tire baby" appearance
- Vellus hairs prominent

- Vermiculation: wormlike movements upon stroking the lesion
- Pseudo-Darier's sign: stroking induces transient induration with piloerection
- Histology: marked increase of smooth muscle fibers in the dermis; grouped fibers are in bundles arranged haphazardly and are not attached to hair follicles; basal hyperpigmentation

Adenoma Sebaceum

- Associated with tuberous sclerosis
- Multiple tiny pink or skin-colored papules on the face (chin, around the nose), periungual area, and trunk
- Histology: fibrosis, dilated blood vessels, and angiofibromas, sometimes with star-shaped fibroblasts; atrophic sebaceous glands

HISTIOCYTIC TUMORS AND PROLIFERATIONS

Giant Cell Tumor of the Tendon Sheath

- Benign neoplasm of the synovia; two forms
  - Diffuse form
  - Localized form
  - Giant cell tumor of the tendon sheath (affects especially small joints of the hand) with pain, effusion, locking of the joint; affects especially middle-aged women
- Histology: multinucleated cells, histiocytes

NEUROGENIC TUMORS

Neurofibroma

- Soft, often polypoid tumors
- Plexiform: involves an entire large nerve with its branches ("bag of worms" on palpation); can be associated with soft tissue overgrowth; pathognomonic of neurofibromatosis 1 (NF1)
- Histology: fusiform, fine, often wavy cells and fine collagenous fibers; sometimes compact, sometimes loose or even myxoid
- S-100 protein is positive

Schwannoma (Neurilemmoma)

- Benign tumors arising in any peripheral nerve
- Well-demarcated, round nodules; solitary or multiple
- Histology: well-demarcated nodule; proliferation of Schwann cells with elongated nuclei and blunted ends

- Antoni A: cells form loose fascicles with nuclei aligned in parallel arrays (Verocay bodies)
- Antoni B: less cellular areas, myxoid, edematous, S-100 protein positive

Traumatic Neuroma (Amputation Neuroma)

- Skin-colored papules, nodules at sites of trauma, scars
- Histology: irregular bundles of peripheral nerves, fibrous tissue

Neurothekeoma

- Soft, asymptomatic papules and nodules, 5 to 10 mm in adults
- Located usually face or upper extremities
- Histology: lobules of spindle and epithelioid cells in myxoid matrix
- S-100 protein, vimentin, and collagen IV positive

Granular Cell Tumor

- Asymptomatic nodules, size up to 2 cm, found in subcutaneous tissue, oral mucosa
- Usually adults; congenital form exists
- Malignant variant is very rare
- Histology: round cells with eosinophilic, granular cytoplasm pseudoepitheliomatous hyperplasia
- S-100 protein, neuron specific enolase (NSE), and protein gene product (PGP) 9.5 are usually positive

REFERENCES

Crowson AN, Magro CM, Mihm MC. Malignant adnexal neoplasms. *Mod Pathol* 2006;19 Suppl 2:S93-S126. Review.

Freedberg IM, et al. *Fitzpatrick's Dermatology in General Medicine*, 6th Ed. New York: McGraw-Hill; 2003.

McKee PH. *Pathology of the Skin: With Clinical Correlations.* London: Mosby-Wolfe; 1996.

Moor EV, Goldberg I, Westreich M. Multiple glomus tumor: a case report and review of the literature. *Ann Plast Surg* 1999;43(4):436-438.

Nakhleh RE, Swanson PE, Wick MR. Cutaneous adnexal carcinomas with divergent differentiation. *Am J Dermatopathol* 1990;12(4): 325-334.

Storm CA, Seykora JT. Cutaneous adnexal neoplasms. *Am J Clin Pathol* 2002;118 Suppl:S33-49. Review.

Wong TY, Suster S, Cheek RF, Mihm MC Jr. Benign cutaneous adnexal tumors with combined folliculosebaceous, apocrine, and eccrine differentiation. Clinicopathologic and immunohistochemical study of eight cases. *Am J Dermatopathol* 1996;18(2):124-136.

CHAPTER 34

BOARDS FODDER

BENJAMIN SOLKY
BRYAN SELKIN
JENNIFER L. JONES
CLARE PIPKIN

GENES TO KNOW

The purpose of this table is to alert dermatology residents to areas that are considered "high yield" for the mock and real boards in dermatology. This installment identifies commonly asked and highly askable factoids relating to genetic inheritance of diseases.

Disease	Pattern	Gene/Protein	Gene Function
Atrichia with Papules 'Alopecia Universalis'	AR	(HR) hairless gene	Zinc finger
Oculocutaneous albinism I	AR	TYR-tyrosinase	Melanin pathway
Oculocutaneous abinism II	AR	P gene–pink protein	Unknown
Oculocutaneous albinism III (Rufous)	AR	(TYRP1) tyrosinase-related protein 1	Stabilizes tyrosinase
Alkaptonuria	AR	(HGO) homogentisic acid oxidase	Phenylalanine and tyrosine breakdown pathway
Hereditary angioedema (Quinke's)	AD	(C1INH) C1 esterase inhibitor	Inhibits first component of complement
Ataxia-telangiectasia (Louis Bar)	AR	(ATM/ATM protein) ataxia-telangiectasia mutated	Phosphatidylinos-itol-3-kinase like domain
Baere-Stevenson syndrome		(FGFr2) FGF receptor 2	
Bannayan-Riley-Ruvalcaba	AD	(PTEN) phosphatase and tensin homolog	Tumor suppressor
Bart's syndrome	AD	(COL7A1) type VII collagen	Anchoring fibril
Gorlin syndrome (nevoid basal cell carcinoma syndrome)	AR	(PTCH) patched homolog (Drosophila)	Inhibits "smoothened" signalling; this inhibition blocked by "hedgehog"
Bloom's syndrome	AR	(BLM)	DNA helicase
			(Continued)

437

Disease	Pattern	Gene/Protein	Gene Function
Bruton's agammaglobulinemia	XLR	(*BTK* gene)	Tyrosine kinase
Bullous ichthyosiform erythroderma (epidermolytic hyperkeratosis)	AD	Keratins 1 and 10	Intermediate filament
Carney complex (LAMB [lentigenes, atrial myxoma, mucocutaneous myxomas, blue nevi], NAME [nevi, atrial myxoma, myxoid neurofibroma, ephilides])	AD	(*PRKAR1A*)	R1 regulatory subunit of protein kinase A
Chediak-Higashi syndrome	AR	LYST/*CHS1* gene/CHS protein	Lysosomal transport
CHILD syndrome (congenital hemidysplasia with ichthyosiform erythroderma and limb defects)	XLD	(*EBP* gene) emopamil binding protein/(*NSDHL* gene) 3-beta hydroxy sterol dehydrogenase	Cholesterol biosynthetic pathway
Chronic granulomatous disease of childhood	XLR (mostly)	(*CYBB* gene) cytochrome B	NADPH-oxidase complex component (respiratory burst) needed to kill catalase-positive bacteria
Citrullinemia	AR	(*ASS*) Arginosuccinate sythetase gene	Enzyme in urea cycle
Cockayne's syndrome	AR	(*CKN1*) (*ERCC6*) *XPB* DNA helicase	DNA helicase—DNA repair
Conradi-Hünermann syndrome	XLD AR	(*EBP*) (*PEX7*)	Sterol isomerase Peroxisomal gene
Cowden's syndrome (multiple hamartoma syndrome)	AD	(*PTEN*)	Tumor suppressor
Darrier-White disease (keratosis follicularis)	AD	(*SERCA2*) calcium ATPase2A2	Calcium dependent ATPase
Dyskeratosis congenita	XLR AD	(*DKC1* gene) Dyskerin (*TERC*) telomerase, RNA component	rRNA processing Telomerase RNA component
Dominant dystrophic epidermolysis bullosa (EB)	AD	(*Col7A1*) Type VII collagen	Anchoring fibril
GABEB (generalized atrophic benign EB)	AR	(BPAg2) Collagen XVII (*LAMB3*) Laminin	Structural protein
Junctional EB with pyloric atresia	AR	Integrin α6,b4/*ITGB6* gene, *ITBG4* gene	Structural
Junctional EB (EB letalis, Herlitz)	AR	Laminin 5 *LAMA3*, *LAMB3*, *LAMC2* genes	Structural

Disease	Pattern	Gene/Protein	Gene Function
EBS (epidermolysis bullosa simplex)	AD	Keratins 5 and 14	Intermediate filament
EBS with muscular dystrophy	AR	Plectin/*PLEC1* gene	Structural
Hidrotic ectodermal dysplasia (Clouston's)	AD	Connexin 30/*ED2* gene, *HED* gene	Gap junction protein
Ectodermal dysplasia with skin fragility	AD	Plakophilin 1	Structural
Ectod, dyspl., hypohidrotic (Christ-Seimens-Touraine syndrome)	XLR	Ectodysplasin	
Erythrokeratoderma variabilis (EKV)	AD	Connexin 31	Gap junction protein
Fabry's disease (angiokeratoma corporis diffusum)	XLR	Alpha-Galactosidase A	Hydrolyzes glycolipids and glycoproteins
Familial Mediterranean fever	AR	(*MEFV*) Marenstrin	PMN inhibitor
Farber's disease (lipogranulomatosis)	AR	Acid ceramidase	Deficiency leads to ceramide accumulation
Gardner's syndrome	AD	(*APC*) adenomatosis polyposis coli	Cleaves β-catenin
Gaucher's disease	AR	β-Glucocerebrosidase	
Griscelli syndrome	AR	(*MTO5a*) Myosin Va	Melanosome transport to keratinocytes
Hailey-Hailey disease	AD	(ATPase2C1)	Calcium-dependent ATPase
Herditary hemorrhagic telangiectasia	AD	Endoglin	TFG-β binding protein
(Osler-Weber-Rendu)		*ALK-1* gene activin receptor binding kinase	TGF-β receptor

VIRUSES

This is the fifth installment in an ongoing series designed to bring to light askable factoids for the dermatology boards and mock boards. This installment focuses on important (or frequently asked) disease-associated viruses. Again, by no means is the list exhaustive.

Disease	Description	Associated or Causative Virus
Boston exanthem	Mild exanthematous febrile illness with aseptic meningitis	Echovirus 16
Bowen's disease	Squamous cell carcinoma in situ	HPV (human papilloma virus) 16 and 18, mostly
		(Continued)

Disease	Description	Associated or Causative Virus
Bowenoid papulosis	Genital papules and plaques resembling Bowen's disease	HPV 16
Buschke and Löwenstein	Giant condyloma	HPV 6 and 11
Butcher's wart	Warty lesions seen in people who handle raw meat	HPV 7b
Castleman's disease	Angiolymphoid hyperplasia usually plasmacytoid in lymph nodes	HHV (human herpesvirus) -8
Condyloma acuminata	Genital warts	HPV (papovavirus-dsDNA) Low risk: Types 6 and 11 High risk: Types 16 and 18
Epidermodysplasia verruciformis	Inherited disorder of HPV infection and SCCs	HPV 5, 8, 12, and others as well as common types
Eruptive pseudoangiomatosis	As per syndrome name	Echovirus 25 and 32
Erythema infectiosum (fifth disease)	Slapped cheeks, reticular exanthem, anemia	Parvovirus B19
Gianotti-Crosti syndrome	Children with sudden onset of lichenoid papules on face, extremities, and buttocks, sparing trunk	Many viral causes, hepatitis B most common worldwide, not as much in U.S.
Hand-foot-and-mouth disease	Fever, ulcerovesicular stomatitis, acral erythematous vesicles, buttock lesions	Coxsackie virus A-16 Enterovirus 71
Heck's disease (focal epithelial hyperplasia)	Small white and pink papules in mouth	HPV 13 and 32
Herpangina	Fever, painful ulcerations in mouth	Coxsackie viruses (A-10)
Kaposi's sarcoma	Vascular tumor, various types	HHV-8
Kaposi's varicelliform eruption (eczema herpeticum)	Diffuse HSV ulcerations in eczematous dermatitis	HSV (herpes simplex virus)
Lichen planus	Purple polygonal, plateau-shaped, pruritic, papules	Hepatitis C virus
Measles (rubeola)	Viral prodrome, then enanthem (Koplick spots), then maculopapular rash spreading craniocaudally	Paramyxovirus (RNA)
Molluscum contagiosum	Umbilicated lesions common in children and HIV	Poxvirus (DNA) MCV (molluscum contagiosum virus) -1 to MCV-4 MCV-1 most common MCV-2 in HIV (human immunodeficiency virus)

Disease	Description	Associated or Causative Virus
Myrmecia	Large cup-shaped palmoplantar warts	HPV 1
Oral hairy leukoplakia	Corrugated white plaque on lateral tongue common in AIDS	EBV (Epstein-Barr virus)
Orf	Umbilicated nodule after farm animal exposure	Parapoxvirus
Papular/purpuric stocking-glove syndrome	As named	Parvovirus B19
Pityriasis rosea	Usually asymptomatic well-known exanthem	HHV-7?
Ridged wart	Wart with preserved dermatoglyphics	HPV 60
Rosai-Dorfman	Sinus histiocytosis with massive lymphadenopathy	HHV-6
Roseola infantum (exanthum subitum, sixth disease)	Infants with high fever followed by exanthem	HHV-6 and 7
Rubella	Viral prodrome, prominent lymphadenopathy, pain with superolateral eye movements, morbilliform rash, exanthem (Forschheimer's spots)	Togavirus (RNA)
Stucco keratoses	White hyperkeratotic plaques on legs	HPV 23b
STAR complex	Sore throat, arthritis, rash	Nonspecific: hep. B, parvovirus B19, rubella
Unilateral laterothoracic exanthem	Simulates zoster	EBV, HBV, echovirus 6
Variola major (smallpox)	12-day incubation, fever and malaise, then centrifugal vesiculopustular rash	Variola (poxvirus) (DNA)
Verruca plana	(Flat warts)	HPV 3
Verruca plantaris	(Plantar warts)	HPV 1 most common
Verruca vulgaris	Common warts	HPV 2 most common

HISTOLOGIC BODIES

This is the fourth installment in an ongoing series designed to bring to light askable factoids for the dermatology boards and mock boards. This installment focuses on important (or frequently asked) histologic bodies. Again, by no means is the list exhaustive.

Body	Description	Entity or Entities
Antoni A tissue	Cellular areas with Verocay bodies	Schwannoma
Antoni B tissue	Loose stromal area with relative paucity of cells	Schwannoma
Arao-Perkins bodies	Elastin bodies seen within "streamers" beneath vellus follicles	Androgenic alopecia
Asteroid bodies	Stellate collections of eosinophilic spicules and giant cells	Sarcoidosis, botryomycosis, sporotrichosis, actinomycosis, other
Banana bodies	1. Found in Schwann cells on electron microscopy 2. Crescentic banana-shaped pigmented bodies in the upper dermis	1. Farber's disease 2. Ochronosis
Birbeck granules	Racquet-shaped bodies seen on EM	Langerhans cells
Caterpiller bodies	Eosinophilic wavy collection in basal layer of epidermis, found on roof of blister	Porphyria cutanea tarda, pseudoporphyria, and erythropoetic protoporphyria
Cholesterol clefts	Needle-like crystals in fat cells	Sclerema neonatorum and subcutaneou fat necrosis of the newborn
Cigar bodies	Budding cigar-shaped PAS+ yeast (rarely seen)	Sporotrichosis
Civatte/colloid bodies	Apoptotic keratinocytes that may be found in epidermis or extruded into papillary dermis	Interface dermatitis
Comma-shaped bodies	Cytoplasmic bodies seen on EM	Benign cephalic histiocytosis
Conchoidal bodies (Schaumann bodies)	Shell-like calcium complexes within giant cells	Sarcoldosis and other granulomatous diseases
Corps grains	Dyskeratotic keratinocytes with elongated nuclei seen in the granular zone	Darier's, Grover's, warty dyskeratoma (Hailey-Hailey)
Corps ronds	Dyskeratotic keratinocytes with perinuclear halo and surrounding basophilic dyskeratotic material	Darier's, Grover's, warty dyskeratoma (Hailey-Hailey)
Cowdry type A & B inclusion bodies	Type A: intranuclear eosinophilic, amorphous bodies surrounded by a clear halo Type B: in neuronal cells	A-HSV, CMV (cytomegalovirus), and VZV (varicella zoster virus) B-polio

Body	Description	Entity or Entities
Donovan bodies	Intrahistiocyte inclusions comprised of organisms that stain positively with Warthin-Starry stain or Giemsa	Granuloma inguinale
Dutcher bodies	Intranuclear inclusions of immunoglobulins	Plasmacytoid proliferations (e.g., multiple myeloma)
Farber bodies	Curvilinear bodies seen in the cytoplasm of fibroblasts and endothelial cells on EM	Farber's disease
Flame figures	Dermal eosinophils and eosinophilic granules surrounding central masses of brightly pink amorphous collagen	Well's syndrome, arthropod bites, other
Floret cells	Multinucleated giant cells with radially arranged nuclei	Pleomorphic lipoma
Flower bodies/cells	Atypical CD4+ T cells	HTLV-1 (human T-cell lymphotrophic virus-1) and ATL (adult T-cell lymphoma/leukemia)
Giant liposomes in neutrophils	Large liposomal granules	Chediak-Higashi
Globi	Collections of AFB (acid fast bacilli) seen in foamy macrophages with Fite stain	Lepromatous leprosy
Henderson-Patterson bodies	Cytoplasmic eosinophillic inclusions in keratinocytes	Molluscum contagiosum
Kamino bodies	Eosinophilic bodies composed of BMZ (basement membrane zone) material	Spitz nevus
Lamellar/Odland bodies	Free fatty acid, ceramide, and cholesterol containing vacuoles released from the golgi in the stratum granulosum seen on EM	Normal skin, absent in harlequin fetus
Lipofuscin granules	Yellow-brown granules in macrophages	Amiodarone hyperpigmentation
Macromelanosomes	Large melanosomes	Café-au-lait macules, neurofibromatosis, Chediak-Higashi
Max-Joseph space	Artifactual separation between dermis and epidermis	Interface dermatitis, especially LP

BUGS AND THEIR VECTORS

This is the third installment in an ongoing series designed to bring to light askable factoids for the dermatology boards and mock boards. This installment focuses on important (or frequently asked) infectious disease for which there are known vectors of transmission.

Disease	Cause	Vector
Acrodermatitis chronica atrophicans	*Borrelia afzelli*	*Ixodes ricinus*
African trypanosomiasis	*Trypanosoma gambiense, Trypanosoma rhodesiernse*	Tsetse fly (*Glossina morsitans*)
Bovine farcy	*Nocardia farcinica*	Cattle
Carrion's disease	*Bartonella bacilliformis*	*Lutzomyia verrucarum* (sandfly)
Cercanial dermatitis	Cercariae of *Schistosomes* (nonhuman)	Snails
Chagas' disease (American trypanosomiasis)	*Trypanosoma cruzi*	Reduviid bug (assassin bug, kissing bug)
Chiclero ulcer	*Leishmanias mexicana*	*Lutzornyia flaviscutellata*
Cutaneous larva migrans	*Ancylostoma braziliense*	Contact with animal feces
Cystercercosis cutis	*Taenis solium*	Contaminated food
Dracunculiasis (guinea worm disease, medina worm)	*Dracunculus medinensis*	*Cyclops* water flea in drinking water
Ehrlichiosis	*Ehrlichia chaffeensis*	Tick bites
Elephantiasis tropica	*Wuchereria bancrofti, Brugia malayi, Brugia timori*	*Culex, Aedes*, and *Anopheles* mosquitos
Erysipeloid of Rosenbach	*Erysipailothrix rhusiopathiae*	Found on pigs, shellfish, and turkeys
Glanders (Farcy)	*Pseudomonas mallei*	Horses, mules, and donkeys
Leishmaniasis, new world	*L. mexicana: L. braziliensis braziliensis L. braziliensis guyanensis; L. b. panamensis*	*Lutzomyia* (sandfly)
Leishmaniasis, old world	*L. tropica; L. major; L. aethiopia; L. infantum*	*Phlebotamus perniciosus* (sandfly) Reservoir: Rodents (gerbils)
Loaiasis (Calabar, tropical and fugitive swelling)	*Loa loa*	*Chrysops* species (mango fly or deer fly)
Lyme disease	United States: *Borrelia burgdorferi* Europe: *B. garinii* and *B. afzelli*	Northeast and Midwest U.S.: *Ixodes scapularis (dammini)*, Western U.S.: *l. pacificus*; Europe: *l. ricinus*
Mediterranean fever (boutonneuse fever, S. African tick bite fever)	*Rickettsia conorii*	*Rhipicephalus sanguinous* (dog tick)

Disease	Cause	Vector
Melioidosis (Whitmore's disease)	*Burkholderia pseudomallei*	Swamp water
Myiasis	*Dermatobia hominis* (botfly) and *Cordylobia* species	Mosquito
Onchocerciasis (river blindness)	*Onchocerca volvulus*	*Simulium* species (black fly)
Plague	*Yersinia pestis*	*Xenopsylia cheopis* (rat fleas)
Rat-bite fever (Haverhill fever, Sodoku)	*Spirillium minor, Streptobacillus moniliformis*	Rat bites
Relapsing fever	*Borrelia duttonii, B. recurrentis*	*Pediculosis humanus* (louse) and *Orrithodorus tholozanii* (pick)
Rickettsialpox	*Rickettsia akari*	*Allodermanyssus sanguineus* and *Liponyssoides sanguineus* (house mouse mites) Reservoir: *Mus musculus* (house mouse)
Rocky Mountain spotted fever	*Rickettsia rickettsii*	*Ixodid* ticks, *Dermacentor andersoni, D. variabilis* and *Amblyomme americanum* (lone star tick)
Schistosomiasis	*S. mansoni, S. haematobium,* and *S. japonicum*	Snails
Scrub typhus (tsutsugamushi fever)	*Rickettsia tsutsugamushi*	*Trombiculid* red mite (chigger)
Sparganosis	*Spirometra* (dog and cat tapeworm larvae)	Application or ingestion of infected flesh from frogs or snakes
Toxoplasmosis	*Toxoplasma gondii*	Cat feces and undercooked meat
Trench fever	*Bartonella quintana*	*Pediculosis humanus* (louse)
Trichinosis	*Trichinella spiralis*	Pig, bear, and walrus meat
Tularemia (Ohara's disease, deer fly fever)	*Francisella tularensis*	Wild rabbit handling, *Dermacentor andersonii* (tick) *Amblyomma americanum* (lone star tick) *Chrysops discalis* (deer fly)
Typhus, endemic	*Rickettsia typhi*	*Xenopsylla cheopis* (rat flea)
Typhus, epidemic	*Rickettsia prowazekii*	*Pediculus humanus* (body louse) Reservoir: *Glaucomys volans* (flying squirrel)
Weil's disease	*Leptospira interrogans ictero haemorrhagiae*	Rat urine
West Nile fever	Arbovirus, RNA-virus	*Culex* (mosquito)

CONTACT ALLERGENS

This is the fifth installment in an ongoing series designed to bring to light askable factoids for the dermatology boards and mock boards. This installment focuses on important (or frequently asked) contact allergens. Again, by no means is the list exhaustive.

Allergen	Common Sources	Other Information
2-Meroaptobenzothiazole (MBT)	Rubber accelerator	
Allylisothiocyanate	Mustard, radish	
Ammonium persulfate	Bleaching agent in flour, hair bleach	
Balsam of Peru	Fragrance, adhesives	
Benzocaine	Topical amide anesthetics	
Benzoyl peroxide	Bleaching agent in flour, acne medication	
Benzalkonium chloride (Quaternium 15)	Shampoos	
Bermuda fire sponge		Contact erythema multiforme
Black rubber mix (N-Phenyl-N' Isopropyl p-phenylenediamine, N-Phenyl-N' cyclohexyl-phenylenediamine, N, N-Diphenyl-phenylenediamine)	Added to rubber products to prevent breakdown	
Calcium oxalate crystals	Dieffenbachia ("dumb cane")	
Carbamates (zinc diethyldithiocarbamate, zinc dibutyldithiocarbamate)	Rubber products	
Carene	Turpentine	
Cinnaminic aldehyde	Pastries, toothpaste, chewing gum, beverages, Bitters, lipstick	
Chromates	Leather and cement	
Colophony (rosin) (abeitic acid)	Solder, paper products, adhesives, paints, varnishes	
Diallyl disulfide	Garlic	
D-Usnic acid	Lichen	

Allergen	Common Sources	Other Information
Epoxy resin	Glues, plastics	
Ethyl cyanoacrylate	Cyanoacrylate	
Ethylenediamine	Stabilizer in Mycolog	Cross-reacts with aminophylline and hydroxyzine
Eugenol	Cloves	
Formaldehyde	Cosmetics, permanent press textile products	
Furocoumarin	Celery, dill, fig, lime, parsley, parsnip, meadow grass, St. John's wort Umbelliferae family	Phytophoto
Glutaraldehyde	Cold sterilant	
Glyceryl thioglycolate	Permanent wave solutions	
Hydrocortisone-17-butyrate	Group B and D corticosteroids	
Imidazolidinyl urea (Germall 115)	Formaldehyde releaser found in cosmetics	
Kathon CG (methylchloro-isothiazolinone)	Cosmetic preservative	Formaldehyde-like
Limonene	Orange and lemon peel, tea tree oil	
Mercapto mix (4-morpholinyl-2-benzothiazyl disulfide, N-Cyclohexyl-2-benzothiazole sulfenamide, 2,2-Benzothiazyl disulfide)	Rubber accelerators	
Methyl (chloro) isothiazolinone (Kathon CG)	Cosmetic preservative	
Methyl methacrylate	Artificial nails, dental work	
Neomycin sulfate	Topical antibiotic	
Nickel sulfate	Jewelry, clothing snaps	Eyelid dermatitis, dimethylglyoxime test (pink)
Oxybenzone	Sunscreen	Photocontact
Padimate O (PABA)	Sunscreen	

(Continued)

Allergen	Common Sources	Other Information
Paraben mix	Preservative in creams, lotions, and foods	
Paraphenylenediamine	Dark hair dye, henna tattoo additive	
Potassium dichromate	Cement, plaster, leather	
Primin	Primrose (*Primula obonica*)	

BONES, EYES, AND NAILS

This is the second installment in an ongoing series designed to bring to light askable factoids for the dermatology boards and mock boards. This installment focuses on important (or frequently asked) findings in bone, eyes, and nails. The list is by no means exhaustive.

Condition	Bone	Eyes	Nails
5-FU and AZT			Blue lunula
Acne fulminans	Osteolytic lesions		
Albright's osteodystrophy	Bradymetacarpalism		
Alkaptonuria		Pingueculae, Osler's sign	
Allezandrini syndrome		Unilateral retinitis pigmentosa	
Alopecia areata			Nail pits, red and spotted lunula
Apert's syndrome	Synostosis		One large fingernail
Argyria		Blue sclera	Slate blue lunula
Arsenic			Mee's lines
Ataxia-telangiectasia (Louis-Bar's)		Bulbar telangiectasia	
Behçet's syndrome		Retinal vasculitis, uveitis, and hypopyon	
Bushke Ollendorf syndrome	Osteopoikolosis		
CHF, connective tissue disease			Red lunula

Condition	Bone	Eyes	Nails
CHIME syndrome (colobomas of eye; heart defects, ichthyosiform dermatosis, mental retardation, ear defects)		Colobomas of retina	
Cicatricial pemphigoid		Symblepharon	
Cirrhosis			Terry's nails
Cockayne's syndrome	Dwarfism	Salt and pepper retinitis Pigmentosa with optic atrophy	
Coffin-Siris syndrome			Fifth-nail dystrophy
Congenital syphilis	Osteochondritis, saber shins, saddle nose, mulberry molars, Hutchinson's teeth	Keratitis	
Connective tissue disease and trauma			Pterygium inversum unguis
Conradi-Hünermann syndrome	Unilateral limb shortening, Chondrodysplasia punctata	Asymmetric focal cataracts	
Darier-White disease			Red and white bands, V-nicking
Ehler's-Danlos IX	Occipital horns		
Ehler's-Danlos VI		Keratoconus	
Fabry's disease		Whorl-like corneal opacities, spokelike cataracts	
Fanconi's syndrome	Absent radius or thumb	Strabismus, retinal hemorrhages	
Fe^{2+} deficiency			Koilonychia
Franceschetti-Jadassohn syndrome	Malaligned great toes		
Gardner's syndrome	Craniofacial osteomatosis	Congenital hypertrophy of retinal pigmented epithelium	

(Continued)

Condition	Bone	Eyes	Nails
Gaucher's disease		Pingueculae	
Goltz's syndrome	Osteopathia striata, Lobster claw deformity	Colobomas	
Gorlin's syndrome	Bifid rib, mandibular keratocysts, kyphoscoliosis, calcified falx cerebri, frontal bossing, etc.		
Hallerman-Streiff syndrome	Bird-like facies, natal teeth	Microopthalmia, congenital cataracts, strabismus	
Hemochromatosis			Koilonychia
High fever, surgery, and meds (chemo)			Beau's lines
Homocystinuria	Marfanoid habitus, genu valgum	Downward lens displacement	
Hyperthyroidism			Koilonychia
Hypoalbuminemia			Muehrcke's nails

INDEX

Page numbers followed by "f" indicate figures and "t" indicate tables.